PERFORMANCE MENU
JOURNAL OF HEALTH & ATHLETIC EXCELLENCE

10
YEARS

PERFORMANCE MENU
JOURNAL OF HEALTH & ATHLETIC EXCELLENCE

10
YEARS

ISBN-13 978-0-9907985-2-1

Catalyst Athletics, Inc
www.catalystathletics.com

All articles first published in the Performance Menu Journal
www.performancemenu.com

Cover by Tom Davies

CONTENTS

Introduction ix

An Interview with Art Devany 1

The Golden Ratio 9

Theories Theoretical Constructs: Max Effort Black Box 15

Power Tools 21

Yay Burpees! An Interview with Mike Burgener 24

Intermittent Fasting 28

Max Effort Black Box Revisited 34

Multidimensionality 36

An Excerpt from: The Paleo Diet for Athletes 39

Go to Bed 48

Power Bias 52

Crossfit Pregnancy 58

Alive! An Interview with Matt Thornton 64

Damn Dirty Grains: This Time It's Personal 71

Getting Stiff: A Revisionist Approach to Stretching Flexibility Part 1 78

Getting Stiff: A Revisionist Approach to Stretching Flexibility Part 2 90

Mass! A Complete Guide for Gaining Functional Muscle 103

The Big Kids' Muscle-Up 116

Intermittent Fasting: Contradictions 122

A More Civilized Approach to Bleeding: Blood Donation 125

Power Bias: Part 2 129

The Olympic Weightlifting Squat 134

Basic Principles for Strength and Conditioning for Rugby Union 138

Kettlebell Power Metrics 162

Hormesis: A Unified Theory of Performance, Health and Longevity? 165

Grappling as a Woman 172

From Glycogen to Cosmology: Nothing New Under the Sun 175

Fight! 181

Bodyweight Skill Integration 191

42 Ways to Skin the Zone 200

The Patch: Functional Training as Nature Intended 207

Joey Miller 210

Staying Fit During and After Pregnancy 214

Developing the Iron Cross 221

Kyphosis 229

Mind Freak: Part 1 233

Intermittent Fasting: No Questions Necessary! (Please) 238

Mind Freak: Part 2 243

Breathing and Breath Control for Olympic Weightlifting 247

Nightshades V: The Problem with Potatoes 249

Mass (A)gain 254

The M.E Black Box For the Family Man 262

A Closter Look at Pose Running 265

My Pre-Season Training Template For Grapplers 273

Two Roads Diverged 276

My Preparation for the CrossFit Games 283

Pulling, Pushing and Thinking 286

Lessons From Romania 291

Are You Coachable 296

There is No Evil Twin 299

Olympic Lifting in Sunnyvale 305

Plandomization 308

NorCal On-Ramp: Part 1 315

NorCal On-Ramp: Part 2 321

The Disordered Eating Chronicals 340

Bananas, Chocolate and a Big Russian Bear 345

Teaching the Olympic Lifts in a CrossFit Group Setting: Part 1 351

Teaching the Olympic Lifts in a CrossFit Group Setting: Part 2 358

Advanced Options of the Max Effort Black Box 365

Speed Training for the Non Track Athlete 368

Percentage-Based MEBB 381

Seven Days of Heaven: Planning Your Training Part 3 383

Esther Gokhale: Perfecting Posture 390

Funky lockout Blues: Fixing the Jerk 395

Get Your Hands Of My Burrito... and Other Team Building Strategies 400

So Runs My Dream, But What Am I? 405

When the Olympic Lifts Aren't Appropriate 412

Motivation 418

The Role of Strength in Weightlifting 424

The Essence of Time 428

It's Not a Race for Last 432

Reevaluating Lower Body Training 435

Pull 441

The Ritual of Competition 447

Mental Game Coaching: An Interview with Bill Cole Part 2 453

The Case for Higher Carb Paleo Diets 460

The Mental Aspects of the Handstand 465

The Mother of Invention 471

Take What Works: The Lessons of Physical Culture History 476

The Soviet System vs. The Bulgarian System of Weightlifting 481

Out with the New, In with the Old 486

Repetitive Motion Overuse Injuries in Athletes 492

The Four Phases of Weightlifting 496

Coaches Aren't That Important... Right? 502

On Losing: Seven Ways to Pick Yourself Back Up 508

Different Strokes for Different Folks: Variations in Pulling Technique 512

Optimal Strength Training for Endurance 517

GPP for the Competitive Athlete: The Lost Training Phase 521

Get Your Gump On: Hazards of Intelligence in Athletes 527

The Pull From the Floor: A Bad Time to Suck 533

Olympic Weightlifting: The Power Position 539

Upgrade Your Memory, Break Through Plateaus, and Improve Your Coaching 543

Olympic Lifting for the College Football Player 553

Locked and Loaded: A Look at Meet Week Preparation 558

Prioritizing Olympic Weightlifting Competition Training 564

Weightlifting Questions You're Afraid to Ask 572

The 10 Minute Rule 578

Immunology and Exercise 583

Creating an Annual Plan 586

Developing Independence in a Group Athletic Setting 590

How You Act... And Why It's Important 597

The Elements of a Weightlifting Teaching Progression 602

Supplemental Bodyweight Training 608

Dealing with Burnout 613

Strength Training for Football Linemen 618

Tapering for Competition 622

Training for the Tactical Athlete 626

A Great Olympic Champion... And You 631

Walking Away: Break Ups Between Coaches and Athletes 637

Programming and Progressions for Youth: Building Weightlifting's Future 642

Program Design and Recovery 647

Complexes 650

Introducing Plyometrics to the Novice Olympic Lifter 654

Strength: Easy as Pi 659

Hang Clean vs. Power Clean: Which Should Be Taught at Your Facility 665

Incorporating Olympic Lifting in Your Program to Increase Speed Development 667

Putting the Cart Before the Horse: Lifting Prerequisites 670

Does Your Athletic Experience Determine Your Coaching Ability? 673

Hey Coach, It's Not All About You. 678

Bombing Out 683

Calm Like A Bomb: Properly Applying Aggression 688

Mindfulness and Muscle 690

INTRODUCTION

I can remember the earliest meetings about the Performance Menu journal that I had with Robb Wolf and Nicki Violetti. We were living in Chico, California running our new gym, NorCal Strength & Conditioning, also known as CrossFit NorCal, the fourth CrossFit affiliate gym in the world. Ten years in the grand scheme of the universe isn't much, but in this industry, it's an eternity. The landscape of independent microgyms was just beginning to take shape, and we and a handful of other similar gyms across the country were just scraping by and struggling to build enough momentum to create sustainability.

Robb & Nicki brought the idea of a digital monthly journal focused primarily on nutrition to me sometime in 2004. At the time, like Robb and Nicki both, I was working another job in addition to the gym business and also doing website and book design on top of that to pay bills. After Nicki showed me their initial mock-up of an inaugural issue, I knew I had a moral obligation to help. More importantly, I wanted to be involved in what I knew would be something great. All successful people know the importance of being associated with and surrounded by the right people, and I knew these two were part of that for me. I was all in.

Robb in particular had a close relationship with CrossFit founder Greg Glassman, who gave us his explicit blessing on the endeavor. If you know your CrossFit history well, you know this didn't last long.

We launched the first issue February 2005. It was a pretty light issue, but we immediately got people's attention and word spread. By the end of the first year, the Performance Menu had become a significant source of information and influence in the CrossFit community and beyond.

In 2006, I moved to southern California to train full time as a weightlifter. I had effectively taken over running the Performance Menu by that point, and Robb and Nicki were obviously running the gym back in Chico, so we arranged a buyout of the Performance Menu for my one-third ownership stake in the gym. This allowed them to focus on the gym like they wanted to, and me to focus on the Performance Menu like I wanted to.

In the next few years, I changed the course of the journal considerably and put far more emphasis on training—Olympic weightlifting and strength in particular—and less on nutrition. Our readership continued to grow and eventually I brought on Yael Grauer to manage the responsibilities of recruiting contributors and collecting material for each issue. She has been instrumental in keeping the journal going this long—it would not have been possible for me to continue as the number of things I was doing continued increasing. Aimee Anaya, who would eventually marry me, helped with the layout for many issues in these earlier years when I wasn't able to fit it into my schedule.

Many of the ideas that now circulate regularly and are taken for granted as common knowledge were anything but years ago and were introduced in the Performance Menu. Things like intermittent fasting, hormesis, the intelligent programming of strength training in CrossFit got their starts in the Performance Menu journal, although this has been forgotten by many (with the help of the astonishing historical revisionism and co-opting so prevalent in the CrossFit community).

In 10 years, we have never missed an issue, and we have never put an issue out late. The Performance Menu has been a constant in my life for a long time and has spanned several major changes in my life—events like finishing college, multiple relocations across the state, getting married and opening a new gym. It's been somewhat of an anchor and a connection to a period of time of which I have very fond memories—spending time with two of the greatest people I know and launching our current careers, which I believe have surpassed in success any of our expectations from those early days.

This book is a celebration of this constant presence and this symbol of our success in this industry. The articles span the entire decade—one article from each of the 120 consecutive months—and represent both some of my favorite articles and the wide range of material and contributors we've published over the years.

Thank you for being a part of the Performance Menu and helping to allow me to experience all that I have.

— *Greg Everett*

The Performance Menu is ten years old. I've sat looking at a blank page for almost an hour, trying to come up with a pithy, meaningful condensation of emotion and experience to commemorate this event. I keep searching for how to convey all that has happened, all that we've collectively gone through with the Performance Menu and our related projects, but all I'm coming up with seems trite. Maybe a little walk down memory lane will fill in with details what I'm failing to find in meaningful writing.

I suspect some (but not all of you) know that Greg helped to co-found NorCal Strength & Conditioning (formerly CrossFit NorCal... the fourth affiliate in the world. God forgive us, we knew not what we did.) along with my wife, Nicki Violetti and me. We had little idea what we were doing. OK, we had NO idea what we were doing. The philosophy du jour on the topic of training people was "grab a broomstick and your neighbor and get training!" That approach surely got us started, but it really lacked in progression, quality control and this wacky thing (which I understand is important for a business) profits. I still see a lot of people running gyms this way. It once concerned me; now I just repeat the signature line of my good friend Eva Twardokens email: If you're gonna be dumb, you better be tough.

We learned, we changed, we grew. I was still very active on the CrossFit message board and was pinging submissions to the CF Journal on a variety of topics. Although folks really seemed to like my message board posts, most of my submissions were deemed "overly professorial" by the "editorial staff." I knew better than that. Greg and I had talked a lot (given that we spent about 14 hrs per day, 6 days per week at the gym) and we both had a lot of ideas that we felt deserved a platform besides a message board entry. We asked for permission from CrossFit founder Greg Glassman to start the Performance Menu (got it... but that's a whole interesting side story) and got cracking on topics like intermittent fasting, hormesis, dedicated strength programming and a host of other goodies. I can't say that the project "went to the Moon" but I will emphatically say that the Performance Menu has been one of the most influential sources of material in the strength and conditioning, nutrition and training realm in the past ten years. If you look at the topics we covered, from buttered coffee to intermittent fasting to a conjugate + CrossFit program (Thanks Rutman!) and what is now commonly practiced, we were really, really ahead of our time. And I'll argue, largely on-point, that feels pretty good. Figuring out how to sell several million dollars per year in buttered coffee products might have felt better, but I also think we were so early in this process that some of the ideas like that needed time to germinate and an audience to grow into. To you folks who have rode on the Performance Menu coattails: You're welcome.

If the average human lifespan is say, 80 years, we've spent more than a tenth of our lives spinning the wheels on effective nutrition, training and related topics. That's at once an eerie but powerful realization. Here is looking forward to the next ten.

— *Robb Wolf*

(R)EVOLUTIONARY FITNESS: AN INTERVIEW WITH PROFESSOR ART DEVANY
ROBB WOLF

Professor Arthur De Vany is Professor Emeritus of Economics and Mathematical Behavioral Sciences at the University of California, Irvine. He has conducted groundbreaking research in many areas of economics, but is perhaps most noted for his work concerning decentralized, non-linear systems. Professor De Vany is an accomplished athlete with an extensive background that ranges from Olympic weightlifting to professional baseball. As early as 1995, Professor De Vany had synthesized a holistic approach to health and fitness that he called Evolutionary Fitness. Many people currently involved with the CrossFit community, including me, can trace their own fitness odyssey back to Professor De Vany's Evolutionary Fitness. We are profoundly grateful to Professor De Vany for sharing with us his work and insights.

Would you please elaborate on how you came to form your ideas about Evolutionary Fitness?

I would have to say that it just happened. Like most truly complex endeavors, it is hard to identify a turning point or a key inspiration or insight. There are so many intertwined layers of science, learning, experience and so many different fields involved that I don't know at what point they came together. Nonetheless, key elements are my interests in complex systems (which was integral to my understanding of power law behavior and intermittency as components of human action) and my interest in evolution. My training as an economist was extremely helpful since it gave me the perspective required to understand how a decentralized system allocates scarce resources in the self-organized human physiology. My interests in genetics and cognition also came into play as it led me to appreciate the key role of gene expression and how diet and activity alter what the genes express.

At the Institute for Mathematical Behavioral Sciences, my true home for the last fifteen years of my career, I was surrounded by cognitive scientists, brain scientists, mathematicians, statisticians, geneticists, biologists, and information scientists. These all come into play in evolutionary fitness.

I truly began living the Evolutionary Fitness Way in about 1985 when I started cooking more at home to make our meals more healthful. My wife is a Type I diabetic and by monitoring her blood glucose we found many foods tended to promote high blood sugar. As we cut them back, we began to eat a more plant-based diet with leaner meats. I began to cook with color and texture as my guides and the results were terrific. Lots of fresh spices with their high antioxidant content, and lots of fiber and variety.

I then began to rethink my training. I began working out more in the manner of, say, a Mike Mentzer or Hitter. But, that wasn't enough; it took too much time and was tiring. I experimented, relying on Astrand's wonderful text and my understanding of power law variation to find a more natural way to balance intensity with variety. The answer was the intermittent pattern that is typical of all playful activity: wild animals exhibit power law variation in activity (proven by monitors placed on fish and wild animals), and most sports like tennis and baseball are also power law distributed activities.

Would you please describe the Evolutionary Fitness lifestyle and explain how this approach might benefit performance and longevity?

Power law variation and intermittency mean that you don't live in a narrow frequency range: you do activities that are "all over the map," with no typical or standard activity. You have intense bursts of activity and lots of languid, easy moments. Modern life is a stressor, with too much standard activity and not enough variety or true peace. Remember, our species never had more than they could carry as possessions, yet they had the whole outdoors and the gifts of nature constantly before them. Our minds are not made for the standardization of life and the quest of possessions; they can never bring true peace for that reason.

The mental peace that comes with this realization is powerful. An evolutionary perspective is truly supportive: I often laugh at myself for trying "accomplish" too much and tell myself that is just my genes talking. Remember, we are alive only because we carry the genes that got us here and they "care" only about their own reproduction. Thus, as males, we do many dangerous, demonstrative things in our youth, primarily to enhance the prospects of reproducing and sending our genes into the next generation. Women are susceptible to this as well, though it manifests itself in different ways.

As to longevity, an active lean body translates into a peaceful, playful lifeway and a powerful mind. Few people seem to realize that mind and body are one; there is no reality to Cartesian dualism. For example, children do not learn to speak if they are confined in such a way that they do not understand the force mechanics of movement, nor can they learn math unless they sense the physical relationships among things through movement. A healthy mind is the first requisite to longevity. A lean, muscular body prevents the brain from becoming resistant to the action of insulin and keeps it healthy and well-nourished. It keeps stress hormones, which are neurotoxic and cause diminished brain mass, at bay.

Body composition is one of the best predictors of longevity. Our male ancestors had about 11% body fat. Females were closer to 15%, just near the boundary where they may or may not be able to conceive. This kept population growth within bounds, along with other natural hazards. Thus, females had far fewer ovulations than a modern female and aged less rapidly because nothing ages as much as reproduction. A lean, muscular body, say 6 to 10% for a modern male and up to 17% for a female promotes low insulin levels, a key hormone in aging. I am aging at a slow rate (I think) because my insulin is so low it is outside the range for the lab. Low body fat also guarantees low blood fats, most of which come from a person's own abdominal fat rather than from their diet. But, it is body composition, not just body fat that is the issue; one must have the right balance of muscle to fat to promote the hormone drives that keep you young and your brain well balanced and nourished. Your muscle is also part of your immune system (it functions as a reservoir of protein to proliferate killer cells when needed).

Would you please explain the concept of power laws with regard to training?

First, recall that a power law is a distribution of frequencies over intensities. Such a distribution implies that the most intense activities are few, but very high in exertion. The low intensity activities are the bulk of your activities, including rest and easy walking. I do a lot of easy walking as many scientists do; Einstein and Darwin are notable examples. So did Dorian Yates when he was Mr. Olympia. For hunter-gatherers, walking is the predominate activity, by far. Modern life leaves too little of this languid, easy, "I'm not going anywhere" kind of activity.

Second, there is no typical activity with a power law so things are not compressed into a narrow frequency range: all scales of activity occur with diminishing frequency at the higher intensities.

Third, the high intensities are really very high, but their frequency is low. Again, this is far outside the Normal distribution modern life seems to encourage. If you look at hunter-gatherers again, you find that they expend about 2 to 2.5 times their basal metabolic rate in a day, most of this in a few intense bursts on the order of 10 or more metabolic equivalents. Office workers expend about 1.2 METS (equivalents of their basal metabolic rate). The hormone drives are vastly different for office worker or hunter-gatherer. The HG has higher testosterone, growth hormone, and lower stress hormone. Office Worker has many low level threats to which he/she cannot make a fight or flight response, and thus carries a stress accumulation that cannot be relieved. The HG has a higher threat threshold and does need the fight or flight response now and then. Still stressful, but the stress is periodically relieved through action with a consequent quenching of the adverse hormone profile induced by stress.

Routinized, lower intensity activities, even jogging, train the natural chaos out of the human heartbeat, making it less adaptable to stress. This pattern holds broadly for other physiological systems too.

If you want to read the research literature that investigates the ideas regarding power law training, do a search for intermittent training. You will find that it is very effective and has been studied by sophisticated scientists. This research is much harder to do than what one finds in investigations of aerobic training. That is because aerobic training is steady-state and the equations are easy to handle because they deal with equilibrium conditions. Intermittent, power law training is far-from-equilibrium training and much harder to analyze, as no steady state equations exist for intense activities that can only be sustained in brief bursts.

It is not wrong to suggest that aerobic, steady state training is often taken to be the norm for training because it is studied most. And it is studied most because that is what researchers know how to do. The far more effective intermittent training is little known because the research is harder to do. So, it is the old drunkard problem: when asked why he was looking for his lost car keys under the street lamp, the drunkard replied, "Because that is where the light is." Aerobic training is heavily studied because that is where the steady state holds. It really is nonsense. The human body is a far-from-equilibrium open energy system to which a steady state analysis simply does not hold. Such an obvious point, but it took me a long time to figure it out and see why a lot of published research has an aerobic bias to it.

Do you see a departure between the requirements in preparing for elite athleticism versus the demands faced by our Paleolithic ancestors?

Only in the way skill enters into it might there be a difference. Some sports require such a high level of skill that they require many repetitive movements. It is known that hunter-gatherers also practiced a great deal. For example, young Eskimos used to be taught to throw at an early age and even had their shoulders stretched so they could throw harpoons from a seated position with great force and accuracy. No modern person compares to the skill and endurance of ancient Eskimos in kayaking or spearing. Iroquois Indians easily out-lifted American soldiers in tests devised by a physiologist. Of course, that was in the 19th Century. Things are different now.

Few modern athletes will have the vision or bone density of our ancestors; hunter-gathers have been noted for their ability to see the moons of Jupiter by naked eye, to tolerate 50 degree temperatures naked without shivering, and to bite through iron nails. Their hearing and balance are exquisite. Remarkably, members of tribes express an almost pure type; they are similar in appearance and stature because they express their genes truly, without the alterations among modern humans that are caused by vastly different diets and lifeways. Moderns have altered gene expression greatly because we do things that vastly alter the messages our genes receive; hence, there is a very large difference among modern humans relative to the ancestral past. This would indicate that some modern humans might be better at some sports, owing to the large variation in types, but it also says that any randomly selected ancestor would be better at almost any physical task than a modern human.

One ethnologist visiting a tribe found that nearly all the males in the tribe could out sprint him even though he was a college sub-11 second sprinter. One of the games in another tribe consists of teams of men hoisting huge logs over their heads and running as far as they can go. Men of all ages participate. I have seen, on film, a New Guinea male who looks like an athletic Mike Mentzer; he had muscles on his muscles according to the speaker on the film. He "made his living" climbing great trees hunting sloth and other tree-dwelling animals. To see him go up a huge tree, fearlessly and effortlessly was mind-altering.

Your alactic and hierarchal sets are quite unique and have been found by many to be very effective. Would you please explain to our readers what they are, why you like them, and share some examples of practical implementation?

The hierarchical sets, one set of 15, one of 8 and another of 4 with increasing weight and increasing speed with no rest in between, are meant to go up the fiber hierarchy from slow to type II and I fast twitch fibers (the latter the fastest). The idea is to drop out the slower fibers with lighter weight and higher reps in the early sets, leaving the fastest, highest force type 1 fibers to carry all the load at the end. The last set also emphasizes the descending phase of the movement because eccentric movements preferentially hit the FT fibers. In addition, huge amounts of lactic acid are produced, a well-known promoter of growth hormone (GH). In addition, the genes in the muscle fibers "sense" the signal of acid or oxygen to determine whether to make fast myosin chains or slow ones. The lactic acid promotes gene expression for fast fibers. Oxygen promotes slow fiber expression. This makes sense, doesn't it, because something has to tell the muscle how to develop and it has to be a local signal, right there in that muscle fiber. This is an example of a decentralized signal that much of my economic research deals with.

It is this gene expression signaling process that hierarchical sets are designed to exploit. This process also explains how aerobic exercise promotes slow twitch muscle development and not FT development.

Alactic sets are a- or non-lactate promoting. They are done as a single rep, putting the bar down, resting 5 or 10 seconds and then doing another rep. This goes on for 2 to 8 reps. Doing a heavy weight just one rep does not produce lactic acid. But, it does use up the phosphates that fire the FT fiber. The 5 to 10 second pause between reps trains the ability of the muscle to regenerate the phosphates that fuel the FT fiber. So, you are training your recovery ability in response to intense effort. This is actually the key to endurance in many high intensity sports; it is quick recovery from intense moves, not aerobic endurance that counts in these sports. In addition, after the first rep in multiple rep sets a lot of the energy is supplied by tendon and muscle elasticity, so these reps are not as intense as the first one. It is always the first rep that is hardest in most exercises because you are starting a dead weight. So, alactic sets are extremely challenging and that is good. Finally, single reps let you handle very heavy weight without fear of failure and they stabilize the joints because of the static starting position.

In light of Evolutionary Fitness, what are your thoughts as to why brief, intense workouts elicit impressive gains in strength, power and endurance?

This is the pattern of activity to which the human genome is adapted. Through all of our evolutionary past, human physiology and metabolism adapted to a pattern of intermittency and fight or flight response. It could not have been otherwise until the advent of agricultural only 10,000 years ago. This is the pattern of activity that promotes the true expression of the human genome and produces the optimal body composition of our ancestors. To live otherwise is to cause the evolutionarily adapted genetic information to be expressed in unhealthful ways. Much has been made of the so-called "thrifty gene" as a cause of modern obesity. This is a genotype adapted to episodes of starvation that conserves energy and causes weight gain in a nutrition abundant modern world. I think this is turning evolution on its head. Humans are an active genotype, as activity was essential and obligatory to the acquisition of food. A prone-to-fat, thrifty genotype would not survive this environment and would be reproductively less successful than an active genotype. So, modern humans may fail to achieve the activity to which the active genotype encoded by evolution in their genes is adapted. The result is faulty gene expression, obesity, and ill health. When food is abundant at virtually no energy cost, the tie between activity and nutrition is broken. Activity declines and energy intake increases; that is, the real thrifty genotype and gene expression is altered adversely.

Dr. William Kraemer of Pennsylvania State University has noted an inordinate neuroendocrine response from movements such as squats, deadlifts, and the Olympic lifts, particularly when they are performed at very high intensity. From an evolutionary perspective, why might this be? How do you feel we might best capitalize on this phenomenon to obtain optimal health and elite athleticism?

It is the Growth Hormone which the movements trigger as well as the whole body coordination under maximal neural stimulation. Each type of muscle fiber has a neural threshold that must be exceeded to fire. The slow twitch fiber has the lowest thresholds, the fast twitch I (if that is the designation you use) is next, and the highest threshold fast twitch II fibers fire last. These movements go right up the fiber hierarchy and trigger all the thresholds.

Many of our readers have noted an ability to gain lean muscle mass while consuming what would appear to be a calorie-deficient diet (Paleo/Zone). You have alluded to similar phenomenon with Evolutionary

Fitness. Could you help our readers to understand some of the mechanisms possibly at play here?

Remember, caloric deficit is a steady state concept. Humans are almost never in caloric balance at a point in time, it is only through integrating moments of positive and negative balance over a longer time period that any kind of caloric balance is achieved. So, caloric balance is an averaging concept that does not apply to shorter intervals of time. It happens that when you fast and engage in intense activity of very brief duration you signal the body to conserve protein. The signal is a high level of GH, which can promote a redirection of the body's resources to retain and develop its protein pools. Remember, protein circulates through the body, in and out, and the pool goes up and down. It is possible to take in less food and still deposit protein in muscle if you lower the rate of protein wastage. This is the role of GH: it is a strong signal to conserve protein and to mobilize fat for use as an energy source. Evolutionary times would require just this mechanism. Fasting triggers a maintenance function: fat is burned for energy and protein is strictly preserved unless it is required to produce glucose (gluconeogenesis) to fuel the brain.

Would you comment on intermittent fasting and its effect on health and longevity? Do you feel that intermittent fasting is completely at odds with achieving optimum performance or can it be successfully integrated with a high-level training program?

Intermittent fasting triggers protein sparing maintenance and gene expression that underlines repair processes. Fasting also triggers brief flows of stressor hormones, which make the body more adaptable to stress. Fasting in the context of activity on an intermittent basis has all the benefits of chronic fasting without its downside.

What are your thoughts on pre- and post-workout nutrition?

Before the workout, an empty stomach to maximize GH production. After, I eat a normal meal (Paleo style) no sooner than an hour later. Usually, I hike, walk or shoot baskets after a workout. Absolutely do not drink "gainer" drinks or other high glucose supplements (they all are high in glucose). The sugar shuts down the GH response too early and we have already seen that muscle grows in a high GH environment, even in the face of brief caloric deficit. Body builders tend to have high insulin levels, even with their muscle mass soaking up the glucose. Partly, they promote this to grow and may even inject insulin to grow more. But, there is an awfully high rate of cancer among body builders and the longevity, though hard to judge since I can find no studies of it, seems rather low. Remember, things that make muscle grow, like high IGF1, 2, 3 and 4 levels also make cancer cells grow more rapidly. Cancer is just a maverick cell that doesn't obey the body's messages to cease.

Please describe "a day in the life," training, meals, play, etc?

There is no typical day. There is some pattern, but lots of variety. Since I am now retired, it is almost not fair to describe my day and hard to do as well since I do whatever I wish. Presently, I am working out three days a week in order to rehabilitate some old injuries from sports. I am also working on core stability and dynamic stability and balance. Until the injuries cease to interfere with heavy lifting, I am doing fairly light weights but at a high pace and close to failure. I am using a trainer for the first time to check my form as my injuries have caused me to lose some form and it is helpful to have another eye to watch for a loss of form. He is very good and a stickler for form. It is nice to have someone help me do negatives in safety as I thrive on them. I am a primarily fast twitch mesomorph and respond well to eccentrics.

Do you have a favorite Paleo-friendly recipe to share with our readers?

Probably my lunch salad is my favorite. A can of Trader Joe's Alaskan Salmon over a bed of lettuce, fresh spices, plenty of garlic and raw vegetables such as red cabbage, broccoli, and or cauliflower. I use olive oil and balsamic vinegar for dressing. These vegetables are not only cancer fighting, but they also block DHT (the prostate promoting metabolite of testosterone) and conserve testosterone by preventing it from being converted to estrogen. Remember, what you put in is not necessarily what you get. Inject testosterone and you get more estrogen and a shut down of testosterone production. *Finally, is there a timeline for the completion of Evolutionary Fitness?*

Well, no. I have my doubts about how it might sell. If I do finish, which this interview is encouraging me to do, it will be to put this message out there.

THE GOLDEN RATIO
ROBB WOLF

Have you heard of Phi? The Golden Ratio of mathematics? The legs of a golden triangle (an isosceles triangle with a vertex angle of 36°) are in a golden ratio to its base and, in fact, this was the method used by Pythagoras to construct phi. The ratio of the circumradius to the length of the side of a decagon is also phi, Phi is found throughout mathematics and was the basis of some quasi-religious sects finding the Devine in nature. What does this have to do with health, longevity and performance? Possibly nothing, but there does exist another Golden Ratio: namely the 40-30-30 ratio of food macronutrients espoused by the Zone, which for many holds the key to their performance goals.

Like Phi, the ratios described by the Zone have been open to broad interperatation. Unlike Phi, however, it is obvious when detractors have neither read nor followed the Zone, let alone bothered to check the numbers, when the Zone is called "low carb" or "high protein." Modern nutritional science seems to suffer simultaneously from the inability to interpret empirical findings and the lack of insight necessary to couch questions germane to health and fitness from a reasonable theoretical basis. Much of the confusion surrounding the Zone can be attributed to the developer of the Zone himself, Barry Sears, because of his omission or underplay of key information. This is unfortunate, as the Zone offers a remarkable degree of dietary precision.

I would like to set the Zone amidst a broader context and make sure people understand there are multiple facets to the Zone. I'll use myself as an example and walk through the WHOLE Zone process. I also want to look at the Zone from a Paleo perspective. To do this, I will compare it to the recommendations of Loren Cordain. I discovered a few surprising things in this process that ironically paint the Zone as a diet of extreme moderation.

The basic "How To" portion of the Zone focuses around one's protein requirements. Whether one uses the book or the handy online calculator, one must find his or her lean body mass and factor that into an activity level to discover the number of blocks needed. CrossFit founders Greg and Lauren Glassman can perform the feat of prescribing blocks based on an individual's height, weight, and visible leanness. Typically they are within one block of what the sophisticated calculators recommend, and this is based in part on the fact that most women require 10-12 blocks and most men fall in the 15-17 range.

I am 172 lbs and approximately 6-8% bodyfat. This leaves me with 158 lbs of lean body weight, and with a Physical Activity factor of .7 (158 X 0.70, Enter the Zone pg 80), this leaves me with 118. I divide the 118 by 7 (for each block there is 7g of protein) and my Zone block recommendation is 17. I have been doing 16 as per the Glassmans' recommendation, so you see this is pretty close.

The Physical Activity Factor is an important point that needs clarification. It is a surprise to most that doing the CrossFit Workout of the Day 3 on 1 off or 5 on 2 off along with martial arts training or other activity only places them in the 0.7-0.80 activity level. The WOD although very intense is not long and does not require that much energy to go through. For one to score the 1.0 level, several hours of practice in addition to a dedicated strength and conditioning program is necessary. This is an important point we will look at more later. In short, I was shocked by how "inactive" I was and pretty spooked at the prospect of dropping my calories to Zone Levels. In light of what we know from caloric restriction, intermittent fasting and the work of Art De Vany, I should not have been so nervous about the prospect of some short term caloric restriction with adequate nutrition. This was a classic example of over thinking a situation. Occasionally it pays to forget what we know in favor of what we can learn. For now, have some faith you will not wither away and starve on the appropriate block recommendations.

Remember blocks? The deal with blocks is that they are a convenient unit of measure, like the Mole in chemistry and physics or the Dozen in baking. Specifically, blocks are: protein 7g, carbohydrate 9 g, and each fat block is 1.5 g. Once one knows what a block of any given food is, constructing a two, three or four block meal is easy.

Going back to my seventeen block daily requirement, this means I need seventeen total blocks each day. That is seventeen blocks each of protein, carbohydrate and fat. Ideally these blocks are broken into five or six meals/snacks. Seventeen blocks could be split into 5 x 3 block meals with a 2 block snack. One can apportion this anyway they like, but it is better to make meals small and frequent. One need only use the May 2004 issue of the CrossFit Journal to construct meals of the proper proportions.

Let's take a moment and do a little bookkeeping with regards to caloric content and macronutrient ratios. For carbohydrates, we have 9g/block x 17 blocks; for protein it is 7g/block x 17 blocks; and for fat it is 1.5g/block x 17 blocks. This means we have 153 grams of carbohydrates, 119 grams protein (we already knew this one) and 25.5 grams of fat. Don't forget, we need to double our fat at this point, as the Zone assumes a hidden block of fat in most protein sources. That means an additional 25.5 grams of fat. My caloric breakdown (carbohydrates and protein both have 4 calories per gram and fat has 9) looks like: C-612, P-476, F-459, with total calories at 1547. If we are diligent and check our work the ratios actually come out to be: C-39.6%, P-30.8%, F-29.7%. Fairly close to 40-30-30, no?

This is one of the first places Barry Sears really loses people, and a reason why research on the Zone has gone badly awry. Sears hangs so much of his evidence regarding the Zone on the performance of elite level athletes, yet he says virtually nothing about the specifics of their process! This has made the little independent research into the Zone all but worthless. Sears asserts that this apparent caloric deficit (the ADA would put my caloric needs at around 2800 Cal vs the Zone's 1550) is fine for the rest of your life. If one is quite sedentary this may be the case, but if one is an athlete, this is not going to work forever. This is where the Athletes Zone comes in.

Barry Sears is a master of cooking and re-cooking his material in a staggering number of books but there is only one page in all of them that makes the recommendation of ramping up the mono-unsaturated fat in the diet to support activity level. In Mastering the Zone pg. 42, we get the goods, in a way. We are never told how to ratchet up the fat content, just that it can be done. I suspect the reason why Sears is virtually mute on this fact is that once one increases the fat content the original 40-30-30 is placed in a questionable light. I had never heard of the ramp up until Greg Glassman mentioned that most CrossFitters following the Zone settle at a level of 3-5 times their original fat content. In practical terms, this means that once one has leaned out on the basic Zone, they will increase fat content of each meal between 3 and 5 times. Ideally one takes a week or more at each level to get a feel for things and find their best performance with the least possible calories.

Let's see what this ramp up does both to caloric content and macronutrient ratios:

LEVEL	CALORIES	RATIOS
1X	1550	C-40 P-30 F-30
2X	1780	C-34 P-26 F-38
3X	2010	C-30 P-23 F-45
4X	2240	C-27 P-21 F-51
5X	2470	C-24 P-19 F-56

Once one has revved up to the Athletes Zone it appears one is consuming both a low carb and low protein diet! We recently had a very long debate on the CrossFit message board regarding the potential health dangers of the Zone. One of the main arguments was that the Zone is a "high protein diet." Perhaps we should only show the 5x version of this diet to the folks with this argument. Frequently, however, the Zone is called a low carbohydrate diet, which, if one is at the original 40-30-30 level, we can explain away by saying "40% of calories come from low glycemic sources, mainly vegetables and fruits." But what if we are at the 5x level? Did I just start Atkins because our carb percentage is at 24%?! Obviously the answer is no. I am still taking in around 150g of carbs per day. Low perhaps by ADA and vegetarian standards, but far above the level typically recommended by the seriously low carb crowd.

Approaching this purely from an empirical, black box perspective, we can reap all the Zone has to offer, and perhaps this is where we should leave it. But how do we know for sure the Zone is not high protein or low carb? What standards are being used here when these statements are made? When our Doctor says "high protein diets will destroy your kidneys," does this have any basis in reality, or should our health care providers have a bit more exposure to anthropology and a bit less pharmacology?

To understand what is happening here and place all of this in a meaningful context, we need to look at some studies of intermittent fasting and caloric restriction, and then some of Loren Cordain's work.

The study, "Intermittent fasting dissociates beneficial effects of dietary restriction on glucose metabolism and neuronal resistance to injury from calorie intake," looks at the effects of intermittent fasting and longevity. I want to devote a whole article to this topic in the future, but for now it can simply be used to shed some light onto our Zone understanding.

Essentially, the acts of caloric restriction and intermittent fasting increase nitrogen (protein) retention. The presence of ketone bodies from high fat intake accentuates this even further. What this means is that when one is following the low calorie 40-30-30 Zone, the mild caloric restriction combined with the by-products of body fat metabolism (ketones), greatly reduce the need for protein. Once one has leaned out it is additional dietary fat that provides sufficient calories and ketone bodies to spare protein. One question you may have is how we are getting ketosis when we are not completely glycogen depleted? In simple terms, all of our metabolic machinery is in action all the time. Under the conditions of intense exercise, intermittent fasting and increased fat intake, concentrations of circulating ketone bodies increase dramatically, even when liver glycogen has not been fully depleted. Ketones are powerful, and we will look more closely at them in the future.

The Paleo Diet

Just as a refresher, Paleo really refers to what we are eating, or perhaps more succinctly, what we are not eating. That means no grains, legumes or dairy. Unless one is a serious paleo purist, some "non-paleo" but "good" items make the cut such as olive oil and tomatoes. Now that we have established what to eat, how much of any given thing should we eat? A place many have gone to answer this question is the diets of historical and contemporary hunter gatherers (HGs). Dr. Boyd S. Eaton did this back in the early 1980's and used the Ethnographic Atlas to determine how much fish, fowl, meat, fruit, veggies, etc. our ancestors ate. From this information, he made recommendations as to what we should be eating. His paper was a powerful turning point for many researchers, including Loren Cordain.

Professor Cordain was a successful exercise physiologist teaching at Colorado State University when he found Dr. Eaton's paper. This paper was apparently a moment of enlightenment for Prof. Cordain, as he from then on approached the research of diet and exercise from the perspective of "Evolution via Natural Selection." What does this have to do with the Zone, Paleo diet, and most importantly, your performance and happiness? I'm getting there!

Prof. Cordain, being the inquisitive guy that he is, started looking at Dr. Eaton's paper and found that it was thermodynamically impossible to obtain all the calories sufficient for life on the largely plant based diet given the environment of our ancestors (pre-agriculture). What had been missed was a large amount of small game that ended up in the "Gathered Plants" section of the atlas. When Prof. Cordain made some adjustments to the previous calculations, he found that MOST HGs (over 73%) derived most of their energy (>/= 56%-65%) from animal foods. You can read the whole article at www. thepaleodiet.com/articles/AJCN%20PDF.pdf, but here are a few key points:

1. Peoples living further and further from the equator rely less and less on gathered plants and more on hunted/fished foods.
2. Regardless of location, there exist seasonal shifts in macronutrient content.
3. An "average" Paleolithic diet might look like C-23 P-38 F-39

Compared to the Zone, we have some obvious similarities but some significant points of departure. The ratios look pretty good, especially when compared to the Athletes Zone. One obvious difference is the greatly increased protein intake. Cordain's findings point toward a protein intake more than DOUBLE that of the Zone. Over 350g/day on average for me! Before the Nephrologists in all of you scream out in protest, please consider this is based upon contemporary and historical HGs. These people did not keel over from sudden onset kidney disease. There are plenty of research citation on Medline debunking the high protein = kidney disease myth.

Another apparent departure from the Zone is the total caloric content that Cordain recomends. From Cordain's perspective, I should be consuming/expending ~3900Cals. This based upon his work.

It looks like things are getting further and further apart, but if you remember we used a 0.70 Activity Factor to determine my protein/caloric needs. This was based on my activity level, which according to Cordain and these molecular geneticists: is too low. If we assume an activity level consistent with that of our ancestors and give me a 1.0 Activity Factor, my total caloric intake at a scaled up 5x Athletes Zone is 3700. The Zone is still lower in protein than Cordain's recommendations, but it is not so far off as to not make sense from a theoretical perspective, and well, the Zone just works! My main point with all of this is that if the diet we evolved on is "reasonably" safe (a remarkable number of people would argue this point) then a protein intake 50% LESS (such as we find in the Zone) is by default safe.

What can we take form all of this besides some paper to line the birdcage?

1. The Zone has a very distinctive starting phase and a ramp-up phase for athletes.

This has been seriously under-emphasized and is perhaps the primary reason the Zone has not met broader acceptance. It is interesting that a research biochemist who has lived in a world where reproducibility is everything does not adequately communicate how to reproduce his diet!

2. The Zone is perfectly compatible with what we know about human origins with regards to amounts and ratios of food. It is lower in protein but it may be that the Zone optimizes protein utilization. There is no doubt that when we increase the intake of a macronutrient we increase its utilization as an energy source. It makes sense that one would want to be fat adapted but not protein adapted. The Zone may accomplish both tasks very effectively.

3. The Zone appears to home in on a caloric and macronutrient level consistent with our energy expenditure even when the activity level is less than what may be optimum for our species. This is pretty intriguing to me. I suspect that both our performance and results would optimize when our activity reaches that 1.0 Activity Factor (or 50 Kcal/kg per day from Cordain's work) and our food is scaled to match. Art De Vany has talked at great length about living at high-energy flux. Lots of activity and lots of food. I am seeing a convergence of both clinical experience and theory.

Next Time

One troubling aspect of the Zone (I'm not the only one with this opinion) is its static nature. If we have learned anything from CrossFit and Evolutionary Fitness, it is that intermittency describes and supports optimum human performance, longevity and health. Next month I will look at a punctuated phase-shift program, The Metabolic Diet, by Mauro Di Pasquale. It is my hope that delineating the similarities between these approaches will help both in what program to choose and ultimately adherence to a healthy program for life.

THEORIES THEORETICAL CONSTRUCTS:
MAX EFFORT BLACK BOX
ROBB WOLF

Theories and theoretical constructs, we would assert, have value only to the extent that they are descriptive of reality and our past experiences and if they provide the vantage point from which further investigation may be made. In essence theories should describe where we have been and direct us where to go next. In the "What is Fitness" issue of the CrossFit Journal we are offered a Theoretical Heirarcy of Development:

> A theoretical hierarchy exists for the development of an athlete. It starts with nutrition and moves to metabolic conditioning, gymnastics, weightlifting, and finally sport. This hierarchy largely reflects foundational dependence, skill, and to some degree, time ordering of development. The logical flow is from molecular foundations, cardiovascular sufficiency, body control, external object control, and ultimately mastery and application. This model has greatest utility in analyzing athletes' shortcomings or difficulties.

Countless elite athletes have been created and indeed, our species found its way through history without overt knowledge of this theoretical template, yet it does in fact model our collective experience. With the knowledge that gymnastics (body control) and weightlifting/throwing (external object control) are natural progressions towards the end of Sport, a potential question is "what if gymnastics, and or weightlifting is your sport"? We have seen this question answered in the likes of Josh Everett and Todd Hockenburry, who have brought phenomenal strength bases to their CrossFit experiences and have excelled in truly staggering ways.

Although metabolic conditioning may be foundational to gymnastics and weightlifting according to the above template, it is the ability to generate significant power that ultimately drives higher and higher levels of metabolic conditioning. Indeed it is our strongest athletes who frequently suffer Pukies wrath the most. It appears a relatively high level of strength with a lack of metabolic conditioning, particularly in mixed modal activities, may even elicit a visit from Uncle Rhabdo. It is perhaps unfair but we find it a simple process to take a strength athlete, virtually devoid of metabolic conditioning, and turn them into a monster. We have found greater challenge turning our endurance athletes into explosive dynamos.

This month two phenomenal coaches and athletes, Michael Rutherford and Josh Everett, share with us some approaches for chasing greater strength and power within the context of a Crossfit oriented strength and conditioning program. This is NOT intended to be an exhaustive review but rather some starting points for fine tuning our own experience. In Coach Rutherford's piece we see a marriage between CF and it's cousin, the conjugate method. Usually cousins should not marry cousins, I don't think this one will end up on Jerry Springer however! UC Riverside Strength and Conditioning Coach, Josh Everett shares with us programs developed for time crunched collegiate athletes.

M.E Black Box
By Michael Rutherford, a.k.a. RUTMAN

After practicing and coaching the CrossFit methodology for over two years I am increasingly convinced the most successful athletes are those who come to the dance with the greatest strength and power. Athletes with the best strength base perform the best in this new sport called CrossFit.

Greg Amundson and Josh Everett are two perfect examples of successful, and very powerful, CrossFit athletes. Both Greg and Josh can turn "Fran" in sub 2:40 range. Greg has also been reported to 1RM a front squat/push press (a.k.a. a THRUSTER) with over 275lbs at a bodyweight of around 200lbs. I personally witnessed Josh clean & jerk 155kg while weighing in the 84kg range.

My own BLACK BOX project started last summer when I began thinking of how a template like this might go together. The final thoughts evolved during the fall when I was retained by one of the city's best high school basketball coaches. With this approach the basketball players' strength improvements continued throughout the season.

With this in mind I would like to present a permutation of the CrossFit theory. Consider this Maximum Effort CrossFit or ME CrossFit if you will. Stay with me here while we sort through this a bit.

Here are some of the components of my ME CrossFit program.

MAXIMUM EFFORT (ME): A cornerstone to the Westside Barbell training program is the Maximum Effort Day. During these sessions the athlete works with a load near his/her maximum (90% +) for that day. Repetitions range from 1-5. In this program we will be using near maximal loads for all the weightlifting movements

There are two rep ranges. The first week on a rotation, the repetitions are 5-5-5-3-3-3. Joe Kenn[1] refers to these as introductory reps. The second time through on a movement, the repetitions are 3-3-3-1-1-1. My intuition indicates that experienced athletes could stay with 3-3-3-1-1-1, or you could perform 8 x 2 or 10 x 1. The Prilepin chart may be handy in a case like this. Anything over 90%, 4-10 sets 1-2 reps with an optimal number of 7 sets.

MOVEMENT ROTATION: CrossFit athletes will recognize the following functional movements.

TOTAL BODY (T): Include Olympic Clean variations, Olympic Snatch variations, Push Presses or Jerks.

LOWER BODY (L): I like squats. I like a rotation of weighted back squats and front squats.

UPPER BODY (U): I will select standing press and weighted pull-ups for my upper body movements. You could also look at bench press and/or incline press. I find these least productive but I know they are popular and necessary in certain circles.

Again, for this discussion our movement pool includes.

TOTAL: Power Clean from the Deck (PC) and Hang Cleans (HC)

LOWER: Back Squats (BS) and Front Squats (FS)

UPPER BODY: Standing Press (SP) and Weighted Pull-ups (WP)
[Editors Note: Weighted dips and muscle ups seem fair game as well.]

What we will do with the movements is rotate them on ME days. On the first ME day we will perform a total body movement (T): power cleans from the Deck (PC); on the second ME day a lower body movement (L): back squats (BS); and finally, on the third ME Day an upper body movement (U): standing press (SP).

Crossfit Workouts

These should be familiar to everyone. One needs look no further than www.crossfit. com and the workout of the day. Whenever possible place emphasis on monostructural metabolic efforts—e.g. running, cycling, swimming—on the day following a ME workout. You could also precede ME days with more gymnastics movements. In any case, the varied if not randomized approach with CrossFit will address any weaknesses in your athletic profile and provide the GPP (General Physical Preparedness) you require to elevate your maximum strength and power.

Rest

Rest is of critical importance. I cannot improve the 3 on 1 off micro-cycling design. I think it provides excellent balance between volume, intensity and rest. Now that we have the parts, here is how it goes together.

DAY 1 - CrossFit workout (XF)
DAY 2 - ME (Total Body-PC) (introductory reps) 5-5-5-3-3-3
DAY 3 - CrossFit workout (XF)
DAY 4 - REST
DAY 5 - CrossFit workout (XF)
DAY 6 - ME (Lower Body-BS) (introductory reps) 5-5-5-3-3-3
DAY 7 - CrossFit workout (XF)
DAY 8 - REST
DAY 9 - CrossFit workout (XF)
DAY 10 - ME (Upper Body-SP) (introductory reps) 5-5-5-3-3-3
DAY 11 - CrossFit workout (XF)
DAY 12 - REST
DAY 13 - CrossFit workout (XF)
DAY 14 - ME (Total Body-PC) 3-3-3-1-1-1
DAY 15 - CrossFit workout (XF)
DAY 16 - REST
DAY 17 - CrossFit workout (XF
DAY 18 - ME (Lower Body-BS) (introductory reps) 3-3-3-1-1-1
DAY 19 - CrossFit workout (XF)
DAY 20 - REST
DAY 21 - CrossFit workout (XF)
DAY 22 - ME (Upper Body SP) (introductory reps) 3-3-3-1-1-1
DAY 23 - CrossFit workout (XF)
DAY 24 - REST

We have now rotated through the introductory reps and the foundation ME reps once. Now we rotate to the secondary foundation movement. In this case it would be hang cleans, front squats and weighted pull-ups. The athletes I have plugged into this template are continuing to improve, although they have only invested six months thus far.

Collegiate Programs

by Josh Everett

From late November to early January in the off-season, we have an eight-hour weekly training limit by NCAA rule. Two of these hours can be spent working with the athletes' sport coaches on skill practice. During winter quarter with our fall sport teams we went two days traditional lifting, one day of CrossFit, and two days of traditional running/track workouts, each session lasting an hour. So that makes for five hours of training with me, leaving two hours with their sport coaches and an extra hour for the sport coaches to do additional conditioning, film study, or team time with the sports psychiatrist.

During spring quarter our fall teams have a 4-6 week spring season. I'm currently experimenting with workouts during this time period. With volleyball, we are doing 2-3 days a week of scaled down versions of CrossFit's storms (e.g. Helen, Fran, Angie etc); with women's soccer, we are doing our traditional in-season routine; and with men's soccer, we are doing two days of traditional in-season training and one day of CrossFit. After their spring seasons, we will spend the rest of the quarter going two days of traditional lifting with women's volleyball, and two days of CrossFit and one day traditional with the soccer teams, the reason being the greater need for cardiovascular fitness of soccer as compared to volleyball, and the fact that volleyball at this point will be coming off of six weeks of just the storms. This summer I'm giving all three teams the same workout plan. I'd rather them go three days on and one off, but I feel five on and two off will be easier for them to comply with.

I set the pattern for workouts as follows:

Day 1: rounds for time (how many rounds can you do in 20minutes)

Day 2: how fast can you complete the following...(Fran, Helen, Grace type workouts)

Day 3: Focus day (squat 10x1, 10x40yd dash, etc)

My goals here are to have the athletes be the fittest they have ever been in their lives heading into season. I believe that CrossFit, while specializing in not specializing, is in fact the best program I have found to prepare athletes to specialize.

Continuing with my goals for them, I wanted to be sure to include the things that I have found that best develop & prepare athletes. I made sure to include these in the focus days so they received the proper attention and intensity. These things are the power clean, back squat, hill or bleacher sprints, sprinting full speed with full recovery, and agility work.

Lastly I have been learning much recently from our superb track coach, Irv Ray, and his system of being sure to hit each energy system each week. And while I haven't perfected it yet, I've tried to get a good balance of workouts that had an emphasis on pure anaerobic system, MVO2, lactate threshold, and endurance/aerobic. The one thing currently missing from this program is recovery workouts. I may modify the workouts to include these types of workouts, but to be honest, during the summer when it's not mandatory, I'm sure most athletes will be missing enough workouts to adequately recover. The ones who are diligent are usually smart enough and know their bodies well enough to adjust.

The rationale behind the post season soccer program is that I want to use the time right after the soccer team's season (the beginning of the off-season) to lay a good sound foundation of GPP. I find CrossFit to be perfect for this. At the same time, I wanted to prepare them for January, February and March when we do the majority of our heavy strength work. I wanted to get a gradual buildup in intensity on our two big lifts, the power clean and the back squat. Of course I'd like to go more than two days per week, but during their season they only lift two days a week. This reestablished training time fits with their class schedules, and to be honest, with just me, one part-time assistant coach, and 300+ athletes, there is only so much time in the week to train everyone. Also, I'm not too concerned, because after a long season where so much is demanded of the student athlete, the two day requirement is a good mental & physical break for them. Not to mention it gives them more free time to finish the quarter strong academically. Plus the athletes with champions' attitudes and work ethic are going to continue to train on their own anyway. I love giving them this opportunity to take ownership of their training. Unfortunately not enough of them will do this on their own; therefore the rest of the year there must have more mandatory training in order for the team to do well.

Notes
[1] The Coach's Strength Training Playbook by Joe Kenn. A must own for any coach or athlete.

POWER TOOLS
BILL FOX

Campus boards—gently over-hanging, no-feet "ladders"—became popular after Wolfgang Güllich invented one to train for Action Directe. Now Alex Huber has introduced the system wall to mainstream climbers. The latest tool in the search for greater power, the system wall overhangs more than a campus board—generally at least 30 degrees—and utilizes the feet. Huber feels this configuration provides all the benefits of a campus board, all over your body. As he says, "One's muscles extend all the way to the toes."

Despite what you may think at first glance, the system wall is not designed just to make you stronger. Strength is more efficiently built with heavy resistance training. Instead, the system wall is designed to teach and prepare your body to move with power. Many improvements gained on the system wall are neuromuscular, so the quality of your session is much more important than the quantity. A little work, done with concentration and a goal in mind, goes a long way.

To understand why the system wall works, you must first look at the relationship between power and strength. Which additional factors influence a climber's power besides his or her maximum strength?

Perhaps the single most important additional factor in the power formula is the nervous system's role in coordinating movement. In examining any complex athletic movement, we find a high level of skill. The brain, working though the nervous system, controls the actions of the muscles that produce the main forces for movement (agonists), the muscles that are involved in stabilizing and coordinating the movement (synergists), and those muscles that try to inhibit movement—the body's self-protection mechanism (antagonists).

Changes in the nervous system that optimize control over these complex movements account for a large portion of the initial increase in performance for that specific movement. This is why working a given route or boulder problem is effective. Your muscles are not getting stronger in one day; your nervous system is getting more power to the rock by teaching your body how to perform specific movements more efficiently.

A climber must also activate certain "high-threshold" motor units (groups of muscle fibers that are more difficult to access) in or der to create maximal power. Most experts agree that the ability to access these units increases with explosive training. In addition, a motor unit can "fire" at different rates. The faster the rate, the higher the force output of that unit. High-threshold units tend to have high "pulse rates," thus creating great force relative to their size. As the link is developed between these high-threshold units and the nervous system, power can increase without an increase in muscle size, a real benefit to climbers seeking an optimal strength-to-weight ratio. The system wall, through its demand for sudden bursts of power, can help train the nervous system to recruit high-threshold fibers. And, because it forces you to use your feet, the system wall prepares the whole body to perform on rock by forcing the climber to maintain tension throughout his body while training.

Just as you can develop maximum power on the wall, you can increase the speed at which you can reach it. Almost instant activation of peak power is necessary to latch onto a small hold after a dynamic movement. It is generally believed that most of the adaptations needed for this specialized movement are neuromuscular; if you drop repeatedly onto your fingers while training on a system wall, the nervous system learns how to develop power quickly, because if the power doesn't come, you fall off.

The body has many built-in mechanisms to protect itself from injury. Physical and nervous system adaptations can push back the point at which these protections kick in, thus allowing the climber to access more of his or her peak power. The golgi tendon organ, for example, is a sort of emergency brake located between the tendon and muscle. If the golgi senses too much tension developing in the tendon, usually caused by a high demand on the attached muscle, it tells the muscle to quit before it becomes injured. Theory has it that if you thicken the tendon through repeated explosive loading, it will take more and more force to cause the tendon to develop enough tension to shut down muscular contraction, thereby enabling you to access more of your muscles' power.

Another theory, but much more controversial, states that explosive or high-velocity movements cause muscle fibers to become activated out of order. Usually, a muscle activates the smaller, slow-twitch units first; it accesses the larger, fast-twitch units as needed. Some believe that the muscle can learn to violate this rule when presented with a sudden large load, preferentially firing the fast-twitch units first.

It has also been suggested that, over time, the nervous system maximizes the efficiency of all the muscles involved (agonists, synergists and antagonists) in a complex movement. By preferentially recruiting the muscles in the most efficient manner possible, including lessening the inhibiting action of the antagonists, more power can be focused in the final complex movement. The system wall may then work by slowly teaching the body to move powerfully with less intermuscular inhibition. And, by utilizing the feet, the system wall helps to strengthen the multitude of small stabilizing muscles in the torso and throughout the body, muscles that can often be the weak link in a climber's power.

Build it Yourself

You can build a simple system board in one afternoon for around $50. Use 3/4-inch plywood for the backing; a 4-foot by 8-foot piece costs about $20. Choose either 2x4s filed to round the edges, or lengths of banister wood to form the rungs. Space the rungs about six to eight inches apart from the top to the bottom of the board. You may wish to alternated larger and smaller rungs; large rungs should protrude 3/4 inch to 1 inch, and smaller ones should protrude about 1/2 inch.

Pre-drill holes for your drywall screws. Prepare the screws by dipping them into very soapy water, and back them up with liquid nails. Place the wall at a 100-to 120-degree angle. If you already have a wall at this angle in your home gym, you can skip the plywood-backing stage and place the rungs directly onto the wall.

Sample System Board Workouts

When adding the system wall to your training program, proceed with extreme caution. Any adaptation—be it in gross physiology, the thickening of a tendon, or nervous system and intermuscular coordination—that allows the body to work closer to its limits creates a serious risk of injury. This (and other training regimens) can lead to tendonitis, tendon tears, muscle tears and arthritis. Warm up gradually, and increase difficulty incrementally. Start with one session a week, and never exceed two. Always rest the day after a workout. Do your workouts fresh, and stop before you're wiped out. Listen to your body!

Now that you know what you have to gain, get to it. Watch out, Alex.

Beginner (5.11+) Match hands on middle rung, and climb as you would a ladder, using larger rungs. Repeat five times maximum.

Intermediate Keeping your feet stationary, experiment with two- or three-rung jumps, moving one hand at a time. Mix smaller and larger rungs. Do laps to build power/endurance.

Advanced Keeping your feet stationary, as above, go for maximum distance and speed with your hands—try moving both at once. Try catching with three or even two fingers.

This article appeared previously in Rock & Ice issue 72. Reprinted with the author's permission.

YAY BURPEES! AN INTERVIEW WITH MIKE BURGENER
ROBB WOLF

This month we have the honor of an interview with world-renowned Olympic Weightlifting coach, Mike Burgener. Those of you who know Coach B know that anything written by or about him should be ALL CAPS ALL THE TIME!!! This is because he is "SO FREAKING PASSIONATE ABOUT THE OLYMPIC LIFTS!!" Well, our design department nixed the ALL CAPS for the interview, but I want readers to know the boundless energy, knowledge and excitement that burns in this man. If you watch him coach, see his excitement, and do not want to become an Olympic lifter, you do not have a pulse.

If you have not checked out Coach B's site, you need to at www.mikesgym.org. Read the articles and look at the sequences he has picked out as exemplifying good pulling technique in the Olympic lifts. Once you have done that, get a broomstick, dowel or piece of PVC, and practice The Warm-up.

Read the interview, compete in the Olympic lifts, and make this man proud!

Would you give our readers some background on yourself? What are some of the athletic achievements of which you are most proud? When and how did you get involved in Olympic weightlifting?

I grew up in southern Illinois. Marion, Illinois, to be exact. My dad was a dairy man, my mom a beautician. I have two sisters who still reside in the Midwest. I played football at Notre Dame and was a defensive back under Ara Parseghian, who brought Notre Dame back to prominence in 1964. My strength coach, Fr. BHB Lange, was an Olympic lifting coach who taught me the lifts, and I competed in the off season.

When you begin coaching a newbie in the Olympic lifts, how important are overall conditioning and athleticism?

Overall conditioning and athleticism are very important to be a high-caliber Olympic weightlifter. Having said that, everyone can have loads of fun training the lifts and participating in contests at the local and even national levels.

How do you gauge the attributes you find desirable for success in the Olympic lifts and what are some ways you address possible weaknesses in these areas?

Flexibility is the number one attribute that I look at when identifying a potential athlete. I also look at size: long levers and shorts limbs are ideal to be successful at a high school level. However, I have seen many motivated men and women who have big hearts and lots of motivation that do not have those attributes but have been successful. There really is not much that I can do about somotyping, but we can address weaknesses of individuals with certain exercises to enhance the strength in various positions.

Coach, you teach the Russian style of pulling in the O-lifts; tell our readers a little about this style and why you like it.

I like the Russian style of the pull because of its vertical position. I have found that when we are pulling in the straight up and down position, we can put more momentum on the bar. Also, the Russian pull is what most kids in the USA identify with, i.e. the vertical jump. I have found it easier to teach us ing this system because of our youth knowing how to vertical jump. When I can get them to jump with a barbell in their hands, putting momentum and elevation on that barbell, then learning to pull their bodies under the barbell, the light goes on and they become addicted to the sport.

What are some other styles that are effective on the international level?

The Bulgarian style is more of a horizontal thrust if you will… a big arc or a C-pull. Many Olympic champions, the pocket Hercules, use this style and have been very successful.

Do you see any benefits or short-comings of these styles relative to the Russian style?

I choose to teach the lifts with the Russian style because of the ease with which the kids learn them.

You have included things like The Patch and kettlebells in the training of your athletes for some time. This seems to fly in the face of "conventional" wisdom. What do you feel these tools bring to your athletes?

Functional strength, core strength, core stabilization. It is amazing to see the athletes become much more functionally strong when doing the patch, kettlebells and CrossFit. What I am after is better Olympic weightlifters, and using these modalities has made my lifters stronger and more powerful.

When did you first hear about CrossFit?

In February 2004.

Did you expect it to take such a prominent role in your coaching?

I was not sure. I started reading about what Greg and Lauren were doing and the fact that the military and special forces and secret service were using it. I was intrigued to say the least. Let's just say I am a good learner, so I was open to the CrossFit family and how it could make me a better coach.

Would you share with us some of your successes using this combined approach?

I use CrossFit daily in my teaching of physical education. Josh Everett, a CrossFit mad man, uses CrossFit and the Olympic lifts to better his lifting. My son Cody and my daughter Sage are both athletes and lifters who use CrossFit to aid their performance.

You are the Strength and Conditioning Coach at Rancho Buena Vista High School. Could you tell us about your experiences with CrossFit and the Olympic lifts at the high school level?

My final exam is the snatch, clean & jerk, back squat, front squat, and ten kettlebell exercises. Now I am adding a CrossFit workout to that final. The students will be allowed to choose between Angie, Grace, Helen or Fran for their finals. We will have a minimum standard for the students to perform to pass.

Please fill us in on your desire to bring CrossFit to high schools everywhere.

It's a no-brainer: CrossFit brings us back to the hardcore, physically fit lifestyle that we used to have—back in the day. It does not take much money, it's easy to administer, and the kids will love it. Believe it or not, kids want to be worked hard. Kids want to be in shape. They may not know it initially, but I have found that the harder I work the kids, the better they like it. Putting the ladies' names on the board and the kids' names on the board that accomplish the workout has done amazing things within my weight room. Braggin' rights are abundant!

Do you modify how the O-lifts are performed if you are training people for sports besides the Olympic lifts?

Not really. I may not use a full clean or a full snatch if I see a potential problem with flexibility, but I will always work toward getting that full range of motion.

Coach, the Olympic lifts are not popular in the US. What can we do to change that?

Get them into the schools: high school, middle school, and elementary school. Getting back to the fitness age, i.e. getting our kids fit again and introducing them to all kinds of activities… other than football, basketball, baseball and track. There are many sports and fitness activities that everyone can perform. That is why I like CrossFit: it is written across the board and everyone can do the workouts… scaled down, sure, but everyone can do them!

INTERMITTENT FASTING
ROBB WOLF

I wrote a paper on Intermittent Fasting almost two years ago but I have sat on it because… well, I am not entirely sure why, but I think some of it had to do with the unknown. Not like the meaning of life, what happens when you die, or something heavy like that… just, What is going to happen if I release this thing and it does not work? I have ruminated for a while on how best to implement this thing (sorry… I am slow), but I realized a few weeks ago that it does not matter. I say this because every other nutritional plan from the Zone to NHE is only a starting point. The Zone has all the trappings of high science and sophistication, but the base Zone is simply a point to deviate from. This is obvious when you consider the marked difference between the basic Zone and Athlete's version. In Issue 2 we looked at this topic and there is simply no comparison between 40-30-30 and 20-17-63! Beyond this there seem to be as many exceptions to the Zone as consistencies. I know smallish hard-gainers who should be on 16 blocks that make little or no progress. These people get bumped up to 19-20 blocks and take off like monsters. Why? It just seems to work and clinical implementation has shown this result. No theory, no proof, just inputs and outputs. The Zone is a good starting point, and if one is meticulous it can be adapted to get a good air/fuel ratio. But it is an art, not a science.

Similarly, Intermittent Fasting (IF), as presented herein, is a starting point. It is not meant to be an exhaustive final word on the topic, but rather an introduction that will enable you to tailor it to YOUR goals. I love the Straight Blast Gym philosophy of avoiding the Cult mindset, remaining grounded, and using one's own experiences to evaluate the efficacy of this or that approach… but always with an eye on self improvement within the framework of one's OWN goals. This may equate to elite performance in a relative sense, but then again it may not; that is up to you.

In chemistry and physics there is something called a triple point that describes a set of conditions under which a substance, like water, transitions between solid, liquid, and gas. A graphical representation of this triple point shows pressure on one axis, temperature on another and a phase line. Altering the temperature or pressure can shift the relative position of the phase diagram to some degree and thus emphasize one phase over another. Thinking about the triple point is what inspired me to write this paper: I see Performance, Health and Longevity as similar to the phases of the triple point and I suspect that IF may bring about an optimization of these parameters.

Consider this example: If your one and only purpose is to live as long as possible, there will be implications from the IF information that will make for some compelling arguments. Optimizing lifespan (in the IF scheme this seems to be feast one day, fast one day) will likely by extension bring Health (an acute measure of longevity) near optimization, but Performance may suffer. Eating one day and fasting one day may not yield elite athleticism. One may be able to be quite good, but perhaps not elite and this is the similarity of altering the pressure/temperature conditions to shift the triple point to a different emphasis of solid, liquid or gas. I think it is obvious that some may desire to optimize performance and the pursuit of performance may necessitate levels of activity (wrestler Dan Gable does not get around so well on his very worn knees) and food consumption that are not conducive to longevity. Some degree of IF should still aid performance, but it may be different in duration and frequency than the person looking for maximum longevity.

Please just keep in mind that we try to present material that is germane to as broad an audience as possible and in such a way that people can make decisions about how best to implement a given technology to their betterment. It is not for me or anyone else to put forth dictates as to how (or why) to live or what the goals of the individual should be.

As Governor AHHHnuuuld might say: Enough Talk.

Program Optimization: Intermittent Fasting

For some time there appeared to be only one way to extend the average and total lifespan of organisms (anything from yeast to fruit flies to mice to monkeys): caloric restriction with adequate nutrition (CRAN). This involved feeding organisms about 60% of what they would normally eat. The results included: increased lifespan and ability to learn throughout life, significantly reduced body weight, reduced body temperature, modulated immune function, decreased blood glucose and insulin levels and an acute adrenal cortical response (short duration of elevated cortisol levels). It appears that the caloric restriction reduces non-enzymatic glycosolation of proteins (sugar sticking to proteins) and increases the organism's ability to withstand stress via an increase in heat shock proteins and other cellular stress mechanisms. This is great stuff, but CRAN guaranteed that one was to be skinny—really skinny. Recently a protocol has emerged which appears to do everything desirable from CRAN, only better and seemingly without the downsides.

Intermittency represents life and natural processes far better than any type of steady state model. This considered, it should not be surprising that a protocol of intermittent fasting (IF) bestows maximum Longevity, Health and perhaps, if properly tinkered, Performance. Recent research has shown that animals on an IF protocol in which they fast one day and eat all they want the following day receive all of the benefits of CRAN with noted improvements.

Many of the metabolic alterations found in CRAN are encountered in IF, but there are some notable differences. In both protocols there is a marked increase in beta-hydroxy butyrate (BHB), which is a ketone derivative of fat metabolism. The BHB appears to have a plethora of functions that are only now being explored4., but it appears ketosis is not the monster it has been portrayed as.5. Ketosis has been shown to prevent muscle wasting even in hypocaloric conditions and appears to be a preferred state for muscle accretion as well. In a specific study, IF conferred a greater neuroprotective effect than CRAN against a chemical irritant which mimics the oxidative stressors thought to induce Alzheimer's and Parkinson's. The IF protocol produced markedly higher levels of BHB that in other studies has proven to be a powerful agent in preventing lesions under toxic stressors.6.

It is important to note that these protocols induce markedly increased levels of ketone bodies despite the fact the experimental animals are fed a very low quality, high carbohydrate diet. According to most nutritionists, this is impossible, much like gaining muscle while on a hypocaloric diet. Those familiar with CrossFit, Evolutionary Fitness and the Zone know the latter to be untrue if the conditions are correct. This is the case with CRAN and IF in which ketosis is achieved despite adequate liver glycogen levels. The why behind this has to do with the redundant systems devoted to fat accretion and sparing glucose for the brain. Sorry if that is vague, but that is a whole other paper. It is also interesting to note that one of the main indicators of a heightened level of conditioning is the utilization of fat as a preferred fuel source. The acts of CRAN and IF dramatically increase the utilization of fat and so in effect increase one's level of fitness independent of any other factors. This is what Arthur DeVany refers to as Metabolic Fitness.

The next action of IF I want to look at is particularly interesting in light of the action of growth factors and the well fed vs. fasted states. In this study several parameters were measured including blood levels of various biomarkers such as growth hormone (hGH) and insulin like growth factor (IGF). IGF and hGH are crucial in actions such as tissue repair, hypertrophy, DNA repair, lypolysis, and, to some degree, strength. It is important to note that in recent years IGF has been linked to various forms of cancer due to its mitogenic (cell growth) effects.7. This appears to be due to excessive caloric and or carbohydrate consumption.

A brief digression into reproductive biology may be helpful here… especially for those of you who suffer from insomnia. All organisms express different characteristics under varying conditions. During times of relative plenty (lots of food), resources are directed to reproduction. This state is typified by high androgen levels and mitogens like insulin, IGF, epidermal growth factors, endothelial growth factors… it's like spring for your body: everything is in bloom. During times of scarcity, resources are directed towards survival, and this state is typified by an adrenal cortical response (cortisol, epinephrine) and low androgen levels. This stress response increases cellular protection mechanisms such as heat shock proteins and apoptosis.

These 2 states have obvious survival implications and in normal circumstances there is a seasonal balance and interplay between them. It is interesting to note that in general these two states are highly distinctive and show no metabolic overlap... except for one situation: Intermittent Fasting. In the IF state we have elements of both the well fed state and the acute stress state. As we will see below this is in stark contrast to CRAN.

It was found that the CRAN animals showed decreased levels of IGF. They also showed decreased rates of all cancers, as well as cardiovascular disease and neuro-degeneration. The IF animals showed even greater reductions in disease states but with an increase in IGF. It appears that IF and CRAN act via different mechanisms. Professor Art DeVany made the point recently that there are a surprising number of redundant systems in place for fat accretion. This metabolically costly venture shows how important fat gain was to our ancestors and allows for quite a number of mechanisms to be underway with interventions such as CRAN and IF.

It is worth mentioning a few other important results found in the CRAN/IF protocols.

Both reduce blood glucose levels and insulin levels.6. An inevitable consequence of blood glucose is Advanced Glycation End products (AGE). This is a non-enzymatic addition of glucose to various body proteins. The faster this process is, the faster you are aging. This is why diabetics age faster than other people. For its part, insulin acts as a growth agent and is a factor in accelerated aging. Both protocols dramatically drop insulin and glucose levels, but IF is actually much more effective on both counts.

We are getting close to the practical application of all this information, but there are a few more theoretical items I want to consider. I mentioned previously that my goal is to find an optimized nutritional protocol for Performance, Health and Longevity. A key feature of both optimum performance and "effective" aging is a reserve of muscle mass. The IF protocol, as mentioned previously, does not leave the organism in an emaciated state. Simple energy balance seems to account for most of this, as the IF animals consume on average the same amount as the ad-libitum controls and consequently do not lose weight. Add to this the finding that IF improves body composition and that IF with a low carbohydrate diet improves it even further. We also have an increase in IGF and neuroendocrine response to exercise.8. All of this bodes well for muscle mass and performance.

Implementation

Lots of theory thus far, but how does one do this? Whatever one's approach, it is important to on average eat as much as one would have done with regular day-to-day feedings. This is an important distinction between CRAN, which usually peels off up to 40% of the individual's body weight, and IF, which maintains bodyweight, muscle mass and overall body composition. With that in mind, here are a few ideas.

Feast/Fast

Eat one day, don't eat the next day… repeat. If one is following the Zone and eating say 16 blocks per day, this may mean a 32-block day. That is a lot of food! I suspect one's protein needs are diminished due to the elevated hGH levels that induce improved nitrogen retention, so you may be able to swap out some protein for increased fat intake. One may also need to increase fruit intake in place of some of the vegetables. This will mean both larger and more frequent meals on your "eat" days. Have fun with that, Zoners!

If you are "just eating," then I guess just eat! Keep protein in most meals; make sure to add fat in the form of nuts, avocados and olive oil (remember, IF combined with high fat intake produces the best results). If you are feeling flat and not recovering from training, you may need to increase your fruit intake. For those seeking long life this may be the way to go. There may be other approaches, but the data has shown this to be effective.

15 Hour-ish Plan

This is what I do most days and it seems pretty easy. Eat your last meal at 5 P.M. and fast until the following day. The duration is up to you, but if you can fit in some training while on an empty stomach, that is preferable. Once you break the fast it is time to get down and eat! Zoners, fit in all those blocks some way. Eaters… well, eat! Are you going to win the Arnold Classic doing this? Likely not, but if your results are similar to mine, you will be lean, feel very good and, depending upon your total caloric intake, possibly add some muscle mass. I am unsure if this abbreviated fast still produces high levels of BHB and IGF/hGH. If this is in fact the case, this may be the best way to optimize performance assuming one can take in adequate nutrition to support activity level. In essence this plan may increase anabolic hormone status, improve fat utilization, improve insulin sensitivity, produce an acute adrenal cortical response, allow for adequate nutrition and perhaps even offer the life extension benefits of the feast/fast plan.

An additional tweak could be to combine the two approaches and this is essentially what Art DeVany suggested on the July 11 post at his site. Scott Hagnas of CrossFit Portland has a good account of a mixed approach here.

This is all the information you need to get started, but IF may not be the best way to go for you. I love it and I have been getting a lot of positive feedback. Tinker with it if you like, ask questions, and keep track of the results. Send us your experiences, good and bad, and we will follow up on this in a few months.

Notes

1. Cordain L. The nutritional characteristics of a contemporary diet based upon Paleolithic food groups. J Am Nutraceut Assoc 2002; 5:15-24.

2. Evolutionary health promotion. Prev Med 2002; 34:109-118. Eaton SB, Strassman BI, Nesse RM, Neel JV, Ewald PW, Williams GC, Weder AB, Eaton SB 3rd, Lindeberg S, Konner MJ, Mysterud I, Cordain L.

3. The human metabolic response to chronic ketosis without caloric restriction: preservation of sub maximal exercise capability with reduced carbohydrate oxidation. Metabolism. 1983 Aug;32(8):769-76 Phinney SD, Bistrian BR, Evans WJ, Gervino E, Blackburn GL.

4. Prostaglandins Leukot Essent Fatty Acids. 2004 Mar; 70(3):309-19

5. Trans Am Clin Climatol Assoc. 2003; 114:149-61; discussion 162-3

6. Intermittent fasting dissociates beneficial effects of dietary restriction on glucose metabolism and neuronal resistance to injury from calorie intake. Proc Nat'l Acad Sci U S A. 2003 May 13;100(10):6216-20. Epub 2003 Apr 30

7. Glycemic index, glycemic load and risk of gastric cancer. Ann Oncol. 2004 Apr; 15(4):581-4

8. Wan, R., S. Camandola, and M.P. Mattson. 2003. Intermittent food deprivation improves cardiovascular and neuroendocrine responses to stress in rats. Journal of Nutrition 133(June):1921-1929.

9. Exercise and insulin sensitivity: a review. Int J Sports Med. 2000 Jan;21(1):1-12

MAX EFFORT BLACK BOX REVISITED
MICHAEL RUTHERFORD

In April, Coach Michael Rutherford unveiled an elegant template that draws from the success of Joe Kenn's Tier System and of course, CrossFit. We have received numerous comments as to the efficacy of the program and we are hoping to post before and after stats as they come in. Smart manipulation of training helps not only to maintain the crushing metabolic conditioning of CrossFit but also builds elite levels of strength and power.

Profile

This athlete is eighteen years old. He will be entering his freshman year in college this fall and plans on playing linebacker in college. He was highly successful as a high school athlete. In football, he recorded the highest number of tackles totaled over two seasons and is the single season record holder for his school. This record stood for over sixteen years. His senior season, he placed third in the Kansas State Wrestling Championships with only one defeat all season. His high school weight room accomplishments include all time school best in the Power Clean, Jerk and the third best back squat in school history.

This background is important because it shows that the subject was trained but also highly motivated.

Practice

For the last eight weeks, he performed the ME BLACK BOX template (see The Performance Menu April 2005). He missed one week practicing for the Metro All Star football game. The athlete rotated the following exercises during the time frame:

- T= Hang Cleans / Squat Cleans
- L= Back Squats (Olympic) / Front Squats
- U= Bench Press / Incline Press

Reps

- 1st Rotation= 5x3
- 2nd Rotation 5x1

In addition to these changes the athlete modified his dietary practice, reducing additional servings on what was already a solid dietary practice for an 18-year-old male.

The results have been rather significant considering the initial level of fitness for this athlete. Below are some measurable results.

Pre:

- Height: 71"
- Weight: 211 lbs
- Clean & Jerk: 301.4 lbs
- Thruster: 245 lbs
- Back Squat: 380 lbs x 6

Post:

- Height: 71"
- Weight: 202 lbs
- Clean & Jerk: 313.5 lbs
- Thruster: 275 lbs
- Back Squat: 405 lbs x 6

Real World Vertical Jump (Two-Hand Basketball Dunk)

- Pre: Close, but no cigar
- Post: Clean two

CrossFit Diagnostics (post)

- Grace 2:29
- Fractured Fran 3:39
- Karen 7:05

MULTIDIMENSIONALITY
ROBB WOLF

Functional training has become quite a buzz-term of late, almost to the point that op-ed pieces on the topic are themselves a trendy item (this contribution excluded of course). The flow of these pieces has been lamentably predictable... THIS is functional training... THAT is not. This tactic is occasionally helpful in that terms like BOSU and Pilates are set in the proper context: limited functionality. People who Olympic lift, practice gymnastics, MMA, highland games, and track and field, to name a few, "get" the fact that what passes for functionality for many has no basis in reality when performance really matters. Previous issues of the CrossFit Journal have delineated what functionality is to an amazingly sophisticated degree: Core to extremity, universal motor recruitment patterns, and neuro-endocrine response are concepts and or results of functional training. This is a profound insight and an area that is ripe for further investigation, but I would like to put forward a simple theoretical construct for evaluating the functionality of various activities. Let's call it "Multidimensionality."

In the book Contact (or this may only happen in the movie... it has been ages since I read the book, so my apologies if I missed this), it appears some scientists on earth have received millions of images that contain information from an alien civilization. These images appear to fit together in some way but no one can quite figure out how the system works. One aged and dying billionaire engineer makes the observation that a superior intelligence would not be constrained to sending information in the two dimensions typical of writing, but would instead take advantage of three dimensions to increase the information density of their communications (the images fit together like a puzzle and were then decipherable). Thus I would assert that functionality has a high degree of multidimensionality.

For an example of multidimensionality, let's consider permutations of the pull-up. If you have been anywhere near the CF message board at any time in its history, the often heated debate of the kipped vs. dead-hang pull up can be seen. People from the gymnastics and CrossFit community regard the kipped pull-up as more functional (multidimensional) for a variety of reasons: increased power output, ballistic load ing of the shoulder girdle, full body coordinated movement initiated by an explosive hip flexion/extension, improved proprioception due to moving ones body through space... The list is long and can have many iterations. The Dead Hang crowd has complained that the kipped pull-up generates inadequate strength in an absolute sense. I argue against that assertion, but let's assume for a moment that a dead hang pull up has merit for the sake of increasing absolute strength or simply for another training stimulus... is the standard dead hang pull up the best? For relative experts on the DHPU, I would look to the climbing community and/or Pavel Tsatsouline. One of Pavel's best contributions has been a concept of full body tension or hyper-irradiation. Not only does this technique improve strength, but also it protects joints and prevents injury.

So... the dead hang pull up practitioner (DHPP) would fasten a weight about their waist, grasp the bar, tighten every muscle in his or her body (hopefully) and grind away at pull-ups. Effective strength training to be sure, but what about a multidimensional move like the L-sit pull-up? In the L-sit, the task of a full body contraction is requisite to the activity. One CAN do DHPU's without full body tension but L-sits, front and back levers necessitate contraction of every muscular element, and there is no middle ground. An additional feature of the L-sit PU is the rotational moment at the hips, which must be overcome by increased (relative to DHPU) grip force. This increased grip force increases the "hyperirradiation" of the exercise. Those concerned with progressive overload need only borrow a trick from Coach Sommer and take a 2-3' piece of Theraband and tie it into a loop. Thread the Theraband through the opening of a 1 1/4 lb weight and then slide the feet through the loops of Theraband. The weighted L-sit PU, because of the lever arm of the legs, is amazingly challenging. All of the benefits mentioned above are greatly increased with what appears to be minute loading. The core is trained in a highly effective way, something that becomes very obvious to the L-sit PU practitioner. If the L-sit PU seems unchallenging to the DHPU crowd, perhaps the front lever PU could be of interest.

This whole idea of multidimensionality occurred to me after the discussions found here. Somewhere deep in that discussion I make the point that it is the very complexity of gymnastics and the Olympic lifts that makes them desirable for athletic training and are in fact the only route to elite fitness as defined by CrossFit. This statement was made to a person who claimed a Westside Barbell approach to training would yield superior fitness, that swings, deadlifts and keg tosses are superior to the Olympic lifts for athletic preparation. This seems an easily tested claim, particularly in the case of simplistic one-dimensional training trumping complexity. Swings and keg tosses are not superior modalities to the snatch. This is fairly easily proven by the fact that an individual proficient in the snatch can perform swings and keg tosses with the best of that crowd, but the reverse is not true. Push-ups, pull-ups and sit-ups are gateways to levers, press to handstands and basic tumbling. Sledgehammer work will never be a hammer throw. These basic movements are subsets of a greater whole that encompasses multiple training stimuli and therefore elicit a more integrated and impressive training effect.

When one chases the multidimensional training effects to be found in gymnastics, throwing events, the Olympic lifts and martial arts, progress will be obtained in all the parameters of fitness while avoiding the dead-end of fringe athleticism and sub-par fitness.

AN EXCERPT FROM THE PALEO DIET FOR ATHLETES
LOREN CORDAIN, PH.D.

The following is excerpted from *The Paleo Diet for Athletes: A Nutritional Formula for Peak Athletic Performance* by Loren Cordain, Ph.D, and Joe Friel, M.S.

Chapter 9: The 21st-Century Paleo Diet: Special Dietary Needs of Modern Athletes

As a serious athlete, you have a lifestyle and activity level that are far different from that of the average American. Chances are your training patterns also vary significantly from the daily activity patterns of our Paleolithic ancestors. They were unlikely to ever run 26.2 miles as fast as they could, nonstop. Nor would they work and run at high-intensity levels day after day, week after week. The only reason for doing so would be under extreme conditions in which their lives were continually at risk, and the only way to survive would be to run far and fast every day. Such situations would be rare. As you will see in the next chapter, the more typical manner of "exercise" for the Paleolithic athlete would have involved long, steady hunts and foraging expeditions conducted at a moderate pace until the kill was imminent or the gathered foods were hauled back to camp. At these times their effort would increase, but they would no doubt rest at every opportunity. Ceremonial dance would also provide nearly continuous "exercise," but the intensity would be relatively low.

What all of this means for you is that your diet must be modified slightly to accommodate your "unusual" high-level training patterns that are a requisite for peak performance during competition. These modifications, as you are now well aware, involve exactly when and what you eat before, during, and immediately following exercise. These critical dietary nuances were discussed extensively in Chapters 2, 3, and 4.

Now let's get down to the crux of this chapter: What should you eat for the remainder of your day, from the time short-term recovery ends until just before the next workout begins? During this period, you should be eating in a manner similar to that of your Paleolithic ancestors. You'll quickly discover that your day-to-day recovery is greatly enhanced and, as a result, your performance will improve.

21st-Century Dietary Tweaks

Let's make it clear from the start: It would be nearly impossible for any athlete or fitness enthusiast living in a typical modern setting to exactly replicate a Paleolithic hunter-gatherer diet. Many of those foods are unavailable commercially, no longer exist, or are totally disgusting to modern tastes and cultural traditions. Do brains, marrow, tongue, and liver sound appealing to you? Probably not, but to hunter-gatherers, these organs were mouthwatering treats that were gobbled up every time an animal was killed. For hunter-gatherers, the least appetizing part of the carcass was the muscle tissue, which is about the only meat most of us ever eat

Most of the familiar fruits and veggies that we find in the produce section of our supermarkets bear little resemblance to their wild counterparts. Large, succulent, orange carrots of today were nothing more than tiny, purple or yellow, fibrous roots 1,000 years ago. The numerous varieties of juicy, sweet apples that we enjoy would have resembled tiny, bitter crabapples a few thousand years ago. Thanks to thousands of years of selective breeding, irrigation, and, later, fertilizers and pesticides, we now eat domesticated fruits and veggies that are larger and sweeter, and have less fiber and more carbohydrate, than their wild versions. Does this mean that you need to go out and forage for wild plants and animals to stock your pantry for our lifetime nutritional plan? Absolutely not! Nearly all of the performance rewards and health benefits of the Paleo Diet for Athletes can easily be achieved from modern-day foods and food groups that had a counterpart in Stone Age diets.

The fundamental dietary principle for the Paleo Diet for Athletes is simplicity itself: unrestricted consumption of lean meats, poultry, seafood, fruits, and vegetables. Foods that are not part of the modern-day Paleolithic fare include cereal grains, dairy products, high glycemic fruits and vegetables, legumes, alcohol, salty foods, high fat meats, refined sugars, and nearly all processed foods.

The exceptions to these basic rules were fully outlined in Chapters 2, 3, and 4. For instance, immediately before, during, and after a workout or competition, certain non-optimal foods may be eaten to encourage a quick recovery. During all other times, meals that closely follow the 21st-century Paleolithic diet described here will promote comprehensive long-term recovery and allow you to come within reach of your maximum performance potential.

Animal and Plant Food Balance

A crucial aspect of the 21st-century Paleolithic diet is the proper balance of plant and animal foods. How much plant food and how much animal food were normally consumed in the diets of Stone Age hunter-gatherers? There is little doubt that whenever and wherever it was ecologically possible, hunter-gatherers preferred animal food over plant food. In our recent study of 229 hunter-gatherer societies, published in the American Journal of Clinical Nutrition, my research team showed that 73 percent of these cultures obtained between 56 and 65 percent of their daily subsistence from animal foods. In a follow-up study published in the European Journal of Clinical Nutrition, involving 13 additional hunter-gatherer groups whose diets were more closely analyzed, we found almost identical results. Our colleague, Mike Richards, PhD, of the University of Bradford in the United King dom, has taken a slightly different approach in determining the plant-to-animal balance in Stone Age diets. He has measured chemicals called stable isotopes in skeletons of hunter-gatherers that lived during the Paleolithic Era. His results dovetailed nicely with ours and confirmed that hunter-gatherers living 12,000 to 28,000 years ago were no different from contemporary hunter-gatherers—the majority of their daily calories also came from animal sources.

Based upon the best available evidence, you should try to eat a little more than half (50 to 55 percent) of your daily calories from lean meats, fish, and seafood. Avoid fatty meats, but fatty fish such as salmon, mackerel, and herring are perfectly acceptable because of their high concentrations of healthful omega-3 fatty acids and cholesterol-lowering monounsaturated fats. Table 9.1 lists some of the animal foods you should include in your diet as well as those you should avoid.

How About Fatty Meats?

Some people who have adopted what they think are "Paleolithic diets" have embraced fatty meats such as bacon, T-bone steaks, and ribs as staples. Even some of the diet doctors with high-fat, low-carbohydrate weight-loss schemes have tried to jump on the Paleolithic bandwagon by suggesting that fatty meats would have been normal fare for Stone Agers. Let's take a look at the real story.

Because animals had yet to be domesticated, Stone Age hunters could eat only wild animals whose body fat naturally waxes and wanes with the seasons. In contrast, virtually all of the meat in the typical US diet comes from grain-fattened animals, slaughtered at peak body-fat percentage regardless of the time of year. For instance, modern feedlot operations typically produce an obese (30 percent body fat or greater) 1,200-pound steer ready for slaughter in about 14 months. These animals are produced like clockwork, 12 months a year, no matter whether it is spring, summer, fall, or winter.

That's quite the opposite of wild animals such as caribou, whose body fat changes with the seasons, as shown in Figure 9.1. Note that for 7 months out of the year, total body-fat averages less than 5 percent. Only in the fall and early winter are significant body fat stores present, but these values are one-half to two-thirds less than the obese feedlot-produced steer!

Even more telling is how the types of fat change seasonally in the carcasses of wild animals. Remember, hunter-gatherers relished all edible body parts—they ate everything except bones, hooves, hide, and horns. By analyzing the total amount of fat and the kinds of fat in muscle, storage fat, and all of the edible organs, our research team was able to show how the animal's total body content of saturated fat varied with the seasons. Take a look at Figure 9.2 on page 168; you can see that for 7 months out of the year, the saturated fat from the edible carcass averages only 11.1 percent of its total available calories—meaning that hunter-gatherers simply did not have a high, year-round dietary source of saturated fat. To lower our blood cholesterol levels and reduce the risk of heart disease, the American Heart Association recommends that our dietary saturated fat intake be 10 percent of our total daily calories—remarkably close to what hunter-gatherers could have obtained from eating wild animals on a year-round basis! For this reason, we recommend that you always eat the leanest cuts of meat.

There is absolutely no doubt that hunter-gatherers favored the fattiest parts of animals. There is incredible fossil evidence from Africa, dating back to 2.5 million years ago, showing this scenario to be true. Stone-tool cut marks on the inner jawbone of antelope reveal that our ancient ancestors removed the tongue and almost certainly ate it. Other fossils show that Stone Age hunter-gatherers smashed open long bones and skulls of their prey and ate the contents. Not surprisingly, these organs are all relatively high in fat, but, more important, analyses from our laboratories showed the types of fat in the tongue, brain, and marrow are healthful, unlike the high concentrations of saturated fats found in fatty domestic meats. Brain is extremely high in polyunsaturated fats, including the health-promoting omega-3 fatty acids, whereas the dominant fats in tongue and marrow are the cholesterol-lowering monounsaturated fats.

Most of us would not savor the thought of eating brains, marrow, tongue, liver, or any other organ meat on a regular basis; therefore, a few 21st-century modifications of the original Paleolithic diet are necessary to get the fatty acid balance "right." First, we suggest you limit your choice of meats to very lean cuts, but don't worry about fatty fish--they're good for you, just like the organ meats our ancestors preferred. Second, we recommend that you add healthful vegetable oils to your diet. By following these simple steps, together with the other nuts and bolts of this plan, the fatty acid balance in your diet will approximate what our Stone Age ancestors got.

From our analyses of 229 hunter-gatherer diets and the nutrient content of wild plants and animals, our research team has demonstrated that the most representative fat intake would have varied from 28 to 57 percent of total calories. To reduce risk of heart disease, the American Heart Association recommends limiting total fat to 30 percent or less of daily calories. On the surface, it would appear that, except for the extreme lower range, there would be too much fat in the typical hunter-gatherer diet--at least according to what we (the American public) have heard for decades: Get the fat out of your diet! The Food Pyramid cautions us to cut out as much fat as possible and replace it with grains and carbohydrate. Not only is this message misguided, it is flat-out wrong. Scientists have known for more than 50 years that it is not the total amount of fat in the diet that promotes heart disease but, rather, the kind of fat. Plain and simple, it is a qualitative issue, not a quantitative one! Polyunsaturated fats are good for us, particularly when we correctly balance the omega-3 and omega-6 fatty acids. Monounsaturated fats are heart-healthy, and even some saturated fats such as stearic acid (found in animal fat) do not promote heart disease. Deadly fats are three specific saturated fats (palmitic acid, lauric acid, and myristic acid) and the trans fats found in margarine, shortening, and hydrogenated vegetable oils, as well as processed foods made with these products.

Now let's get back to the fat content of our ancestral hunter-gatherer diet. They frequently ate more fat than we do, but it was almost invariably healthy fats. Using computerized dietary analyses of the wild plant and animal foods, our research team has shown that the usual fat breakdown in hunter-gatherer diets was 55 to 65 percent monounsaturated fat, 20 to 25 percent polyunsaturated fat (with an omega-6-to-omega-3 ratio of 2:1), and 10 to 15 percent saturated fat (about half being the neutral stearic acid). This balance of fats is exactly what you will get when you follow our dietary recommendations.

Foods Not on the Paleolithic Menu

Let's get down to the specifics of the diet. Table 9.2 on page 172 includes an inventory of modern foods that should be avoided. These recommendations might at first seem like a huge laundry list, with seemingly needless elimination of entire food groups. Most dyed-in-the-wool nutritionists wouldn't object to our advice to cut down or eliminate sugars and highly refined, processed foods. They would have no problem with our suggestions to reduce saturated and trans fats and salt, and they would be ecstatic about our recommendations to boost fresh fruit and vegetable consumption. But they would, guaranteed, react violently to the mere thought of eliminating "sacred" whole grains from your diet. If they heard we also advocate reducing or eliminating dairy products, they almost certainly would brand this diet unhealthful, if not outright dangerous. You may wonder why, just because hunter-gatherers did not regularly eat grains or dairy products, you should follow suit. After all, aren't whole grains healthful, and isn't milk good for everybody? How can you get calcium without dairy? And won't eating a lot of meat increase blood cholesterol levels?

In science, decisions should be made based upon what the data tell us, and not upon human bias and prejudice. With these ground rules in mind, let's take a look at the reasons for and potential benefits of eliminating or severely restricting entire food groups with the Paleo Diet for Athletes. One of the major goals of any diet, for both athletes and non-athletes alike, is to supply you, the consumer, with a diet rich in nutrients (vitamins, minerals, and phytochemicals) that promote good health, which in turn promotes good performance. Table 9.3 on page 174 shows the nutrient density of seven foods groups.

From top to bottom, here's the ranking of the most nutritious food groups: fresh vegetables, seafood, lean meats, fresh fruits, whole grains and milk (tied for second to last), and nuts and seeds. Why in the world would the USDA place grains at the Pyramid's base if the goal is an adequate intake of vitamins and minerals? This strategy makes no sense for the average American, much less athletes like you. Had we included refined grains in the list, they would have ended up dead last because the refining process strips this nutrient-poor food group even further of vitamins and minerals. Unfortunately, in the United States, 85 percent of the grains we eat are highly refined, and grains typically make up 24 percent of our daily calories.

Not only are grains and dairy foods poor sources of vitamins and minerals, they also retain nutritional characteristics that clearly are not in your best interest, whether you're an athlete or not. From Chapter 5, you now know all about the glycemic index and acid/base balance in foods, along with how they impact your performance. Virtually all refined grains and grain products yield high glycemic loads. Further, all grains, whether whole or refined, are net acid producing. Dairy products are one of the greatest sources of artery-clogging saturated fats in the American diet, and cheeses produce the highest acidic loads of any foods. If that's not bad enough, a recent study found that dairy products, despite having low glycemic indices, spike blood insulin levels similar to white bread. Do yourself a favor—get the grains and dairy out of your diet and replace them with more healthful fruits, veggies, lean meats, and seafood.

If you, like most Americans, have been swayed by those milk mustache ads, you probably are part of the mass hysteria, largely generated by the dairy industry, suggesting there is a nationwide calcium shortage that underlies osteoporosis. Not true! Calcium intake from dairy, or any other food, is only part of the story behind bone mineral health. More important is calcium balance, the difference between how much calcium goes into your body from diet and how much leaves in urine. You will be out of balance if more calcium leaves than what comes in, no matter how much milk you drink. What we really need to pay attention to is the other side of the equation—the calcium leaving our bodies. Dietary acid/base balance is the single most important factor influencing calcium loss in the urine. Net acid-producing diets overloaded with grains, cheeses, and salty processed foods increase urinary calcium losses, whereas the Paleo Diet for Athletes is rich in alkaline-yielding fruit and vegetables that bring us back into calcium balance and promote bone mineral health.

Dietary Staples: Lean Meats

With the Paleo Diet for Athletes, you'll be eating lean meat and seafood, and lots of it, at almost every meal. Should you be worried about your blood cholesterol levels rising? Absolutely not, and here's why. In the 1950s, when scientists began to realize that saturated fats promote heart disease, a nationwide campaign was initiated to reduce dietary fats, and meat became a primary target. As this strategy gained momentum in the late '60s and early '70s, meat, and red meat in particular, became vilified. In the eyes of overzealous vegetarians, nutritionists, and physicians, meat consumption was the scapegoat underlying the epidemic of heart disease and cancer in the United States. But the problem was oversimplified—they threw out the baby with the bathwater. It was not meat, per se, that was the problem; rather, it was the fatty meats such as hamburger, T-bone steaks, bologna, and hot dogs that had become the norm in the US diet.

This fact was strikingly demonstrated by my colleague, Andy Sinclair, PhD, from the Royal Melbourne Institute of Technology, with a clever dietary intervention in which people were fed a diet either of lean beef trimmed of visible fat or with the trimmed fat added back in. When lean beef was consumed, LDL (bad) cholesterol in the blood declined, but (not surprisingly) it increased when the fat was added back in. These results have been duplicated numerous times in independent labs. In fact, experiments by Bernard Wolfe, MD, at the University of Western Ontario have decisively shown that when low-fat animal protein replaces dietary saturated fat, it is more effective in lowering blood cholesterol and improving blood chemistry than are low-fat carbohydrates. In nutritional interventions such as Dr. Wolfe's, the key to scientific credibility is replication—replication, replication, replication! It is absolutely essential that other scientists get similar results from comparable experiments. To the surprise of some party-line nutritionists, a series of four recent (2003) papers from independent researchers around the world confirmed Dr. Wolfe's earlier work.

Is there a limit to a good thing? You now know that lean animal protein lowers your blood LDL (bad) cholesterol levels, increases HDL (good), and provides muscle-building branched-chain amino acids. How much protein should—or can—you eat?

There is a limit to the amount of protein you can physiologically tolerate. Nineteenth- and 20th-century explorers, frontiersmen, and trappers who were forced to eat nothing but the fat-drained flesh of wild game in late winter or early spring developed nausea, diarrhea, and lethargy, and eventually died. Studies conducted in the laboratory of Daniel Rudman, MD, at Emory University have examined the causal mechanisms underlying the protein ceiling and found that toxicity occurs when the liver can't eliminate nitrogen from the ingested protein fast enough. Nitrogen is normally excreted as urea in the urine and feces, but with protein toxicity, ammonia and excessive amino acids from protein degradation build up in the bloodstream and produce adverse symptoms. For most people, the maximum dietary protein limit is between 200 and 300 grams per day, or about 30 to 40 percent of the normal daily caloric intake. On the Paleo Diet for Athletes, you will never have to worry about protein toxicity, as you will eat unlimited amounts of carbohydrates in the form of fruits and vegetables. Further, in the post-exercise window, as fully explained in Chapters 2, 3, and 4, you will be encouraged to consume high glycemic, alkaline-yielding carbohydrates to fully replenish your glycogen stores.

From our analyses of hunter-gatherer diets and the nutrient content of wild plants and animals, our research team has shown that the protein intake in the average hunter-gatherer diet would have ranged from 19 to 35 percent of daily calories. Since the protein intake in the normal US diet is about 15 percent of daily energy, we recommend that for peak performance during Stage V of re covery (the period following short-term recovery, lasting until your next pre-exercise feeding), you boost your protein intake to between 25 and 30 percent of daily calories. At values higher than 30 percent of energy, some people may begin to experience symptoms indicative of the physiologic protein ceiling.

Macronutrient Balance

We've already mentioned that the fat content in Paleolithic diets (28 to 57 percent total calories) was quite a bit higher than values (30 percent or less) recommended by the American Heart Association. We suggest consuming between 30 and 40 percent of your Stage V energy as fat. But remember, you will be eating the bulk of your fats as healthful monounsaturated and polyunsaturated fats (particularly the omega-3s). How about carbohydrates? In hunter-gatherer diets, carbohydrate normally ranged from 22 to 40 percent of total daily energy. Because of your special need as an athlete to restore muscle glycogen on a daily basis, you should boost these values a bit higher. We suggest that Stage V carbohydrate intake should typically range from 35 to 45 percent of calories. As you personalize the Paleo Diet for Athletes to your specific training schedule and body needs, you will be able to fine-tune your daily intake of carbohydrate, fat, and protein.

Nutritional Adequacy

Regardless of your final ratio of protein to fat to carbohydrate, you will be eating an enormously enriched and nutrient-dense diet, compared with what you were probably eating before. We've partially addressed this concept in Chapter 1, where we compared the Paleo Diet for Athletes with the recommended USDA food pyramid diet, and also in Table 9.3 on page 174. An even better way to appreciate how much more nutritious your diet will become when you adopt the Paleo Diet for Athletes is by looking at what the average American eats. Figure 9.3 shows the breakdown by food group in the typical US diet. Notice that grains are the highest contributor to total calories (23.9 percent), followed by refined sugars (18.6 percent) and refined vegetable oils (17.8 percent). When you add in dairy products (10.6 percent of total energy) to grains, refined sugars, and refined oils, the total is 70.9 percent of daily calories. None of these foods would have been on the menu for our Paleolithic ancestors, as fully discussed in Chapter 8.

Refined sugars are devoid of any vitamins or minerals, and except for vitamins E and K, refined vegetable oils are in the same boat. Think of it: More than a third of your daily calories come from foods that lack virtually any vitamins and minerals. When you add in the nutrient lightweights we call cereals and dairy products (check out Table 9.3 on page 174), you can see just how bad the modern diet really is. The staple foods (grains, dairy, refined sugars, and oils) introduced during the agricultural and industrial revolutions have displaced more healthful and nutrient-dense lean meats, seafood, and fresh fruits and vegetables. Once you begin to get these delicious foods back into your diet, not only will your vitamin, mineral, and phytochemical intake improve, but so will your performance.

MEATS & SEAFOOD TO EAT	% PROTEIN	% FAT
BEEF		
VEAL STEAK	68	32
SIRLOIN STEAK	65	35
LEAN FLANK STEAK	62	38
POULTRY		
SKINLESS TURKEY BREASTS	94	5
SKINLESS CHICKEN BREASTS	63	37
PORK		
LEAN TENDERLOIN	72	26
LEAN CHOPS	62	38
ORGAN MEATS		
BEEF HEART	69	30
CHICKEN LIVERS	65	32
BEEF LIVER	63	28
SEAFOOD		
BOILED SHRIMP	90	10
ORANGE ROUGHY	90	10
POLLOCK FISH	90	10
BROILED LOBSTER	89	5
RED SNAPPER	87	13
DUNGENESS CRAB	86	10
BROILED HALIBUT	80	20
STEAMED CLAMS	73	12
BROILED TUNA	68	32
BROILED SALMON	62	38
GAME MEATS		
BUFFALO ROAST	84	16
ROAST VENISON	81	19

MEATS TO AVIOD	% PROTEIN	% FAT
BEEF		
T-BONE STEAK	36	64
GROUND BEEF (15% FAT)	35	63
BEEF RIBS	26	27
POULTRY		
CHICKEN WINGS	38	59
CHICKEN THIGHS/LEG	36	63
PORK		
RIBS	27	73
SHOULDER ROAST	45	55
LAMB		
SHOULDER ROAST	32	68
CHOPS	25	75
PROCESSED MEATS		
HAM LUNCH MEAT	39	54
DRY SALAMI	23	75
LINK PORK SAUSAGE	22	77
BACON	21	78
LIVERWURST SAUSAGE	18	79
BOLOGNA	15	81
HOT DOG	14	83

GO TO BED
ROBB WOLF

Go to bed. Well, maybe not right this minute, but sooner rather than later. It is fall, heading in to winter, and the days are getting short, the nights are cool and some of you may be feeling a bit squirrelly with the changes. Especially if you are up late, lacking sleep or some horrid combination of the two. If you have hung around the CrossFit message board for a while, you will know that I make a yearly call for people to read Lights Out: Sleep, Sugar and Survival.

This is that call and a synopsis of the key points for the book. Dan John reads this book every fall. I do too. So should you.

The Big Idea

Lights out is written by T.S. Wiley and Bent Formby, the dynamic duo who between them have PhDs in Medical Anthropology, Biophysics and Biochemistry. They are bright people who do a pretty amazing job of wedding evolutionary biology, modern medicine and even some aspects of alternative medicine such as acupuncture into a coherent message: Eat, Sleep and Live with nature, not against it. How does one do that?

Mangia!

Eat meat vegetables and seasonal fruits. Avoid sugar and processed foods like the plague. Enter ketosis for a period of the year, just like our ancestors did. Specifically they recommend that between June and September one can consume all the naturally occurring carbohydrates one likes. From October through May, however, a lower carbohydrate, ketogenic diet is the recommendation. This is an interesting point that is perhaps worth a moment of digression. Most people following a CrossFit style training regime will not be able to recover or sustain the level of intensity AND frequency they are accustomed to with this relatively limited carb intake. Training will need to shift towards heavy low rep training with ample rest and slower walks and hikes. Metabolic conditioning can still happen but the workouts themselves will likely have to be shorter than some of the longer CF-style death marches and, as mentioned previously, less frequent. This sounds like an interesting way to allow food intake to dictate periodization. Stated another way: Olympic lifting and gymnastics in the fall and winter; metabolic conditioning and generally running wild in the spring and summer.

Another approach is Intermittent Fasting. Let's back up for a moment before we dig into that. Wiley and Formby make the point that one must have a period of "fasting" or "starvation" to avoid the scourge of metabolic disease. Their approach, as mentioned above, is to undertake a ketogenic diet for several months of the year. This creates an environment of low insulin levels and ketone bodies, both of which have far reaching effects on the expression of genes central to aging and degenerative disease. Intermittent fasting also reduces insulin levels AND creates ketosis even when carbohydrate is NOT a limiting factor. This punctuated stressor appears to enhance DNA repair, apoptosis (programmed cell death, typically in cells which may be heading down the road towards cancer) and nitrogen retention to name a few benefits. Intermittent Fasting can provide all this and will accommodate any activity level.

To recap, Lights Out recommends that we have a period of "fasting" in which we eat a ketogenic diet. If one follows this recommendation some modifications may be necessary with regards to training to accommodate lower muscle glycogen levels. Another approach is Intermittent Fasting, which meets the recommendations of Wiley and Formby while allowing a high activity level.

Sorry, one more digression. What about people eating a standard Zone or Athletes Zone? Well... I'm not sure. The AZ is quite high in fat at the 3-5X levels and may create a state of Ketosis similar to that seen in IF. It is, however, static. This may matter a little, a lot, or not at all. What we have planned to answer this question is a small study looking at some people on the Zone and some people doing IF. We will look at amounts and ratios of food consumed, sleep, activity levels, etc. We will then look at fasting levels of insulin, blood glucose, glycated Hemoglobin (A1c), triglycerides, aploprotien A, C-reactive protein and beta hydroxy butyrate. This will give us some direct comparisons between these two nutritional plans and what types of effects they have on these complex but very interesting mechanisms.

ZZZZZ...

So we have a very good idea of what Wiley and Formby had in mind when they were talking about eating. I may in fact have beat that horse so badly that the recommendation to sleep might be a little late as most readers drifted into a coma several paragraphs earlier. If you are an insomniac, a nerd or my mom, you are possibly still reading this, so let's talk about sleep. The Lights Out perspective on sleep focuses on two key points: One, get a bunch; two, do it in the dark.

Let the Excuses Begin

How much is a bunch? About 9.5 hours. Yes…9.5 HOURS. How do you fit that into work, school, kids, training and watching "Lost"? I have no idea; you just need to do it. We need about 6 hours of dark before we release prolactin which has effects on melatonin and a whole slew of other goodies. The 9.5 hours allows for melatonin production and complete restoration of our immune system and neurotransmitters.

This brings us to the second point about sleep. Absolute, complete total—no light peeking through—dark. Think it's a crock? Black out your bedroom completely, such that you cannot see your hand in front of your eyes anywhere. Cover the alarm clocks and fire alarm LEDs. Do this for a week and tell me you are not sleeping better, are better recovered and generally more sane and happy. Just to completely belabor this point, I will use an analogy. Roger Harrell, when coaching gymnastics, frequently says, "Straight is straight. A little bent is NOT straight." Similarly, dark is dark. A little light is NOT dark. If the preceding has become annoying I am just starting to make some progress. If you need convincing, find Dan John's experiment of sleeping 10 hrs per day and the results he obtained. So our sleep recap is short and sweet. 9-10 hours per night of blissful sleep in a completely dark room. Easy-Peezy.

La Vida Loca

The final portion of the Lights Out prescription involves exercise and a few supplements. I am assuming our readers participate in CrossFit, Olympic lifting, gymnastics, strongman or something along these lines. If so, you need not worry about exercise: you are indeed PERFECT. The Lights Out supplement list is mercifully short. We may do a more in depth supplement review at some point; if we do, these will top the list again.

Fish Oil

Unless you have been hiding in a cave for many years, you are likely already using some fish oil. I love the Costco Kirkland brand, as it is inexpensive and good quality. If you are sick, have insulin/blood sugar issues, depression or some other serious ailment, you likely need 10-20 grams of fish oil per day. That is a lot of capsules and it may be easier to go for the more expensive but very convenient liquid fish oil. Keep all fish oil in the freezer.

Alpha Lipoic Acid

This is a common constituent in grass-fed meat but it is completely missing in grain-fed meat. It acts as both a fat- and water-soluble antioxidant and improves insulin sensitivity. 500-1000 mg per day should do it. Jarrow formulas (http://www.jarrow.com/) has a very good quality product that is inexpensive.

Acidophilus

Our guts are inhabited with symbiotic microorganisms. Lots of them. They play an amazing role in a surprising number of processes far removed from digestion. They act as our first immune system protecting us from pathogenic gut organisms and even influence neurotransmitter status in the brain. Cool, huh? Jarrow has a good product but most health food stores have decent options. Make sure you buy something that is refrigerated and is far from its expiration date.

That's it! This is your primer for navigating the change of seasons more gracefully. Please do make it a priority to read all of Lights Out. For some the tabloid type writing style and frequent conspiracy theories make for tough reading, but from my experience it is one of the most amazing books written; I'm just not sure people are ready for the implications
of its message.

POWER BIAS
ROBB WOLF

I have a major bias: I love explosiveness in athletics. Yes, I understand Iron Man is demanding both physically and mentally, but it just does not inspire much passion for me. I have always been more intrigued by sports like weightlifting, boxing and sprinting than I have by marathons, triathlons or the The Tour.

Like I said, I'm biased. This bias has carried me along not only in my own training but also in my intellectual pursuits surrounding athletics. This is what brought me ultimately to CrossFit.

When I first found CrossFit, my training bias allowed me to perform some fairly impressive tricks. I could jump on top of objects that were chin high, and at the Sequoia-like height of 5'9" (175cm), I could dunk a tennis ball from a standing jump. What my bias did not allow me was the ability to survive the CrossFit met-cons. They crushed me and I initially thought the WODs to be beyond human capacity. I was wrong about the human capacity part: the WOD is very hard but certainly doable. But for me it came at a price: my two footed jumps now bring me only a few inches up the basketball net and jumping on top of something navel high is a fairly challenging affair. I am undoubtedly fitter by any measure, but I must admit some lamentation about the loss of top-end power.

Perhaps this explains my interest in concepts like the Max Effort Black Box template offered by Coach Michael Rutherford and the work of Jay Schroeder, who most of you will recall turned Adam Archuleta into a monster. In the case of Archuleta, it appears his training involved a combination of conventional strength moves performed as quickly as possible, throwing and catching weights (as in the bench press), smart use of functional isometrics, and finally, plyometrics. The intention according to Coach Schroeder is to make the athlete as quick as possible and to teach the athlete how to absorb and transmit force. Watching Archuleta's Freak of Training DVD got me thinking about my power bias and how we might tweak traditional CrossFit programming to improve our maximum power output. Greater emphasis on Olympic lifting, as it trains one to maximally accelerate an outside object and to absorb ballistic loading, might be one way to approach this. Perhaps less obvious would be gymnastics elements such as round-offs, handsprings, blocking, and work on the parallel bars, rings and high-bar. A third area that may offer opportunity in both maximum power output and metabolic conditioning are ballistic/plyometric derivatives of traditional callisthenic movements such as pull-ups, push-ups, sit-ups and squats.

Before we look at these derivatives, let's consider the attributes of some of the CrossFit mainstays:

Angie

- 100 Pull-ups
- 100 Push-ups
- 100 Sit-ups
- 100 Squats
- For time

Barbara

- 20 Pull-ups
- 30 Push-ups
- 40 Sit-ups
- 50 Squats
- 5 rounds for time

Chelsea

- 5 Pull-ups
- 10 Push-ups
- 15 Squats
- Every minute on the minute for 30 minutes

These WODs offer a fairly high volume of work that develop strength, localized lactate tolerance and overall metabolic conditioning. These workouts also remind me vaguely of distance running with the relative volume and lack of higher strength and power demands. I tend to opt for Mary (5 HSPU, 10 One Legged Squats, 15 Pull-ups - rounds in 20 minutes) and have come within 5 Pull-ups of 17 rounds. So, toss out push-ups, squats and sit-ups? No, of course not, but I think we can modify these movements by making them ballistic/plyometric, thus increasing their training stimulus and value. This can be accomplished by using clap variations of the push-up and pull-up, medicine ball throws for the sit-ups and jump squats for a revved-up version of our old standby. Let's look at each of these movements in more detail and then we can talk about how to incorporate them into our training.

The clapping Pull-up is initiated like a standard kipped variety, but the body is launched violently upwards such that the hands leave the bar to complete a clap and then re-grab the bar (hopefully) on the way down. One may do these as singles but they lend themselves very well to multiple repetitions. Of the basic callisthenic movements, the clapping pull-up may offer the least benefit if one has been performing kipped Pull-ups with excellent form, as the standard kipped pull-ups already offer a potent plyometric loading of the shoulder girdle. The Big Fat Pull-Up is an extreme example of this, but I think it illustrates perfectly the points of power and plyometric loading. As one gains confidence in the clap variety it is possible to get first the chin and eventually the shoulders above the bar at the apex of the kip.

Everyone has likely seen the clapping push-up. One stays in a tight, standard pushup position and violently explodes upwards. The hands leave the floor and clap before returning. Gymnasts do a variation of this movement in which the arms are kept completely straight and the movement is completely a product of scapular protraction and retraction. Our variant is a full range of movement that maximizes work output.

For our ballistic sit-up, we will add a medicine ball throw and anchor our feet to allow for rapid cycle time and maximum velocity on the ball. At CrossFit NorCal, we set a crash pad against a wall, slip the feet under the pad and then get hucking! We use a 6-pound Dynamax ball for our stronger athletes, so do not be afraid to go as light as 2 pounds, especially in the beginning. If you use a Dynamax ball, it is crucial that you throw to a padded surface lest you destroy both the ball and contact surface. Technique involves holding the arms high over head with a fully engaged shoulder (shoulders in the ears). Pull the abs in, creating pressure and stability in the midsection. The sit-up can be performed through a full range of movement, but also through partial range of movement that minimally flexes the spine and takes advantage of the abdominals' primary role in midline stability. In either case, the medicine ball is released with as much speed as possible, and with a little practice, one's accuracy and precision will improve to the point that the ball hits the same point every throw and bounces right back to the hands, allowing for rapid cycling of the movement.

The jump squat is perhaps the most intuitive of the movements, as virtually all of us have jumped at some point in our lives. The movement is executed with standard Olympic-style-squat positioning and range. With your feet shoulder-width apart, torso erect and eyes toward the horizon, pull yourself down violently with the hip flexors. As quickly as possible, reverse this downward movement and explode upward, your feet leaving the ground. You should be in the classic triple extension (ankle, knee, hip) while airborne. This may be a news flash to some, but you will reach a maximum height and then return to the ground (nothing to see here folks... standard Newtonian physics). The landing occurs in the exact reverse order of the take off, with toes landing first, followed immediately by a roll to the heels that initiates the flexion of both knee and hip. Over time, you will learn to use the energy from one jump to transition to the next.

Now that we have some familiarity with these ballistic varieties of our standard callisthenic movements, I want to make a strong case for why we should incorporate these into our training. I want to look at power/work output and some considerations related to muscle fiber type and super-compensation.

First, let's look at the components of power and work to critically evaluate our movement choices:

Work = F * d
F = force and d = distance moved (displacement)
Power = Work / Time

I think most of you, based on the fact that you are reading this publication, have a good understanding of these concepts and are on the lookout for ways to increase the amount of both work and power you can generate. The ballistic movements by their very nature involve greater travel (increased work) and greater power (the work is performed faster) than their less springy relatives... per repetition. One may make the case that over the course of a workout like Angie, one's average power will decrease due to the greater segmentation of sets, but this will only be true until one has adapted to the greater demands of the ballistic movements.

In our limited pool of participants, we have noted rapid progress with the ballistic derivatives that transfers quite well to the non-ballistic parent movements. As we have noted in previous PM issues, this implies multi-dimensionality of the ballistic movements AND the necessity for a path dependant approach to training. In essence, the ballistic movements offer more opportunity for growth regardless of the testing parameter. Not to beat this to death, but there is an interesting finding that training non-explosively might make you, well, non-explosive. Do check out a great article by Kenny Croxdale and Tom Morris here. Here is a small excerpt from that article:

Another obstacle when training for an explosive bench press (even at lower percentages of 1 RM) is the deceleration of the bar during the lift. "Research has shown as much as 75% of a movement can be devoted to slowing the bar down." (Flannagan, 2001). Elliot et al. (1989) revealed that during 1-RM bench presses, the bar decelerates for the final 24% of the range of motion. At 81% of 1-RM, the bar deceleration occurs during the final 52% of the range of motion. The accompanying deceleration phases result in significantly decreased motor unit recruitment, velocity of movement, power production and compromises the effectiveness of the exercise. (Berry et. al., 2001)

What I take form this is that high-volume non- explosive calisthenics can make one slower in an absolute sense. No, I am not saying the non-ballistic movements have no place in training. I am suggesting a re-evaluation of some movements used in general programming.

It is also interesting to note that throwing athletes (shot, discus, hammer) frequently have elite level careers that extend into their late 40s. These athletes are concerned with one thing: Moving objects as fast as possible. This training seems to forstall much of the age related decline in power production.

I want to look at some aspects of muscle fiber type to complete my sell for these ballistic movements. For our purposes we will keep things very general and lump fibers into fast and slow twitch categories. The slow twitch fibers are generally termed type 1 fibers and are small, produce relatively little power, have high mitochondrial density, are highly vascularized and are therefore perfect for long-duration aerobic activities as they fatigue slowly. Fast twitch fibers are divided into type 2A and 2B fibers. The type 2A fibers are much larger than the type 1 fibers and therefore produce much more force. They have an impressive mix of both power and endurance as they are fairly well vascularized and contain large amounts of Glycolytic enzymes in addition to a fair mitochondrial density. The type 2b fibers are very large, have virtually no oxidative potential and are the elements responsible for maximum power output.

It is perhaps not surprising that different training stimuli affect the various fiber types differently. When one must recruit maximally and or quickly, the type 2b fibers are the prime movers. Moderate intensity longer durations activities involve the type 2a fibers while low intensity efforts rely upon the type 1 fibers.

Here are some other interesting tid-bits. High power output training that is followed by long stretches of relative low intensity activity tends to improve large motor-unit recruitment, which innervates the type 2b fibers. Two situations, however, cause a conversion of type 2b fibers to type 2a. Endurance training, whether it is anaerobic threshold training or classic long distance cardio cause a 2b-to-2a shift with aerobic training possibly even converting type 2a to 1 fibers. Any way you cut it, this represents a significant decrease in the ability to produce maximum power. High-volume high-intensity training actually causes a conversion of some 2b elements to 2a. This happens after a high volume block of work that lasts several weeks to a few months. If one now dramatically decreases volume, there tends to be a rebound of fiber type to even higher levels of type 2b. It appears some of the 2a fibers can switch type. This represents the standard tapering period seen for most sprint athletes.

The implication is that smart use of ballistic calisthenics movements will allow not only for crushing metabolic training but also for maximum power output, even for single repetition efforts. Additionally, we might be able to structure blocks of training in which volume is cycled to take advantage of these neurological and morphological changes.

Implementation

Sorry for the long-winded lead in, because implementation is simple: Start slow! Cindy is a good place to start: 5 Pull-ups, 10 Push-ups, 15 squats-rounds in 5 minutes. Then 10 minutes etc. we have also been doing 1/10th or 1/5th of Angie as a warm up (10 or 20 of each movement instead of the standard 100). These efforts have been amazingly taxing but produce some impressive results. Try adding these movements into your programming for a month and then go back and check your performance on the conventional workouts. Let us know what your results are.

CROSSFIT PREGNANCY
ROBB WOLF

This month we have a case study of one woman, Casee Sumter, her pregnancy, the birthing process and concurrent CrossFit training. The mystery and awe of pregnancy are enough to make this an interesting and fun endeavor for all concerned, but we had the added bonus of helping an already healthy mom get healthier, thus facilitating the birth of an amazing new baby boy. What more could one possibly ask for?

Before we get to the story, however, let's look at something that has been talked about a bit, but for which no quantifiable numbers have been run. CrossFit seems to get people pregnant. Brian Mulvaney astutely commented on this observation and offered a fantastic free market solution to the infertility crises that seems to strike well-to-do mid-30s couples. Seemingly healthy, these couples find it near-impossible to conceive a child, and find themselves in one of the highest mark-up businesses in the world. The problem? Insulin. Elevated insulin levels in one's youth lead to a state of hyperfertility caused by decreased production of Sex Hormone Binding Protein. A decrease in SHBP results in more free estrogen and testosterone. This means increased youth fertility, acne, PMS and a slew of other problems. This is the very situation that caused the massive population explosion our species encountered when we switched to starchy foodstuffs as the basis of our diet. Neither the crushing levels of activity inherent in early agriculture nor even breastfeeding could stop this process that normally matched our population exactly to our food supply. Hyperfertility is the short term result of elevated insulin. The long-term result is premature sterility due to an ever more deranged metabolism that becomes deaf to its signal of high sex hormones and insulin.

In a normal menstrual cycle, estrogen and progesterone play a game of tag. Estrogen climbs to a peak in response to the maturation and release of an egg within the ovaries with progesterone following quickly behind. At a crucial point, progesterone passes estrogen in concentration and estrogen levels then drop to a low baseline for 10-14 days, during which estrogen begins climbing in concentration again in a continuous cyclical manner. If a fertilized egg is in the proper location, progesterone encourages implantation of the egg and growth. If no egg is present the uterine lining is shed.

If one is insulin resistant, this scenario can shift from the hyperfertility of youth to a form of sterility amid remarkably high estrogen levels. With high insulin comes a higher fat mass. This fat mass plays a role in aromatizing testosterone to estrogen. This feeds into even higher levels of estrogen due to decreased SHBP which eventually leads to estrogen receptor burnout. This means ever higher levels of estrogen and an eventual inability of progesterone to surpass estrogen and facilitate either egg implantation or shedding of the uterine lining. This is the hormonal environment in which we find uterine fibroids, polycystic ovarian syndrome, polycystic breast disease and endometriosis to name but a few conditions.

These mechanisms are quite well known and hyperinsulinism is obviously understood to be a player in these events as insulin lowering drugs are the first intervention for infertility. Call me cynical, but it appears we have a situation of extreme laziness on the parts of both medical professionals and our populace—we appear incapable of adopting the recommendation of nutrition and exercise that is consistent with health. Metformin (an insulin lowering drug with the brand name Glucophage) will reduce insulin levels for a time, but it is not a long term solution to problems that go far beyond infertility.

In very simple terms, the adoption of sound nutritional practices and a short duration, high intensity exercise program will set right the condition of hyperinsulinemia and make the numbers a bit more favorable for not only conception but lifelong health.

If you have a female in your life whose health and well being you value (you know… wife, daughter, mother… yourself), buy the book Sex Lies and Menopause. Read it and strongly consider its message. Be warned! If you have strong political leaning to either the right or left you will likely be enraged by some aspects of the book. If you are middle of the road, you may simply shake your head in disbelief at some of the implications raised by the book.

OK, enough of the intro on pregnancy! Here is the story of one mom and her experience doing CrossFit while pregnant. Casee had been training with us for approximately one month prior to becoming pregnant. We have had three women become pregnant within the first month of training with us in the past year.

First Trimester

During the first trimester, I was really tired, so the toughest part about working out was dragging my butt out of bed at 5:45 am to get to CrossFit. Sometimes I had great energy during my workouts and during others I could feel a lag, but all in all I think I held my own with all of the workouts.

Second Trimester

Fourteen Weeks

Although I had only gained about six pounds, immediately into the second trimester I found out the hard way that I needed to curb the weight I was lifting. I think it was a workout that contained three rounds of deadlifts at 35 pounds. That wreaked havoc with my back. I was out of commission for about a week. After that, I resolved to keep the lifting under 20 pounds. Robb and Nicki were great and they worked with me to adjust the routines in a way that wouldn't take me out. They showed me stretches for my lower back and I started spending more time cooling down and stretching after workouts. [As one gains weight during pregnancy, the abdominal wall distends forward, which can both weaken the abdominal wall and tends to put the low back into a state of hyperlordosis. This condition can lead to back pain and certainly destabilizes the core and can make lifting dangerous. Stretching the hip flexors and hamstrings with generous helpings of "sit-to-stands" keeps this problem at a minimum.]

Eighteen Weeks

No more back issues. Yeah! My morning energy is rockin' and I'm loving the workouts. I feel really strong at squats right now. [We only perform sit-to-stands with our expectant moms as it would obviously be madness to have them squat] My upper body is becoming stronger and running and rowing seem to be agreeing with me too.

With the growth of the baby, my stomach is starting to pull and stretch. All of a sudden hanging from the rings to do knee ups doesn't feel so great. No worries—doing knee ups on the parallel bars is the solution.

Twenty Weeks

The workouts are becoming more challenging. My times are longer, but I'm able to complete the workouts, and my recovery is slower. My running is slow and steady. Just need to breathe and take it easy.

Twenty-two Weeks

I have gained about 14 pounds and am feeling it in my pelvis and left hip and leg. Lifts involving squats are tougher than they were a few weeks ago, but I will keep persevering because these will help with labor and delivery.

Robb and Nicki say my negative pull-ups are getting strong enough to start kipping. I'm game! [Casee was VERY close to a pull-up at this point. Her weight outstripped her performance, however, and we will have to wait for the first one.]

Twenty-six Weeks

Over the last two weeks I've experienced Braxton-Hicks contractions with regularity, so I'm stepping the intensity down yet another notch. This week, no running, rowing, jumping rope or weight. I will monitor how I feel and adjust as I go. I still get a pretty darn good workout from the things I can still do. Yesterday I did five rounds of wall ball (20 reps with a 6-lb ball) with OHS (15 reps with PVC pipe only). Kicked my butt!

Twenty-Seven Weeks

Instead of the 200 meter run, Robb and Nicki had me do a 200 meter farmer's walk. This felt a lot more comfortable and was a great workout for me. [Tthe farmers walk can be a great alternative for anyone who can not run. However, in the case of an expectant mom, keep the loading very moderate and make sure they do not have to death grip the weight. Extreme contraction of the hands can dramatically increase the mom's blood pressure.]

Third Trimester

Twenty-eight Weeks

I've gained 20 pounds. Only got to CrossFit twice this week. Had a good upper body workout doing three rounds of a 200 meter run, 10 dips and one rope climb. [Casee climbed approx five feet up our fifteen-foot rope three times to count for a full ascent. She is a VERY good rope climber, but this seemed a prudent modification. Two layers of crash mats were also provided "just in case".]

Twenty-nine Weeks

I felt pretty strong today. Did Fran with rowing (800 m, 400 m, 200 m) instead of thrusters. My negative pull-ups were OK but took some time because my belly tends to tighten up. I also practiced kipping.

Looks like I'm back to being able to do the runs—they're more of a powerwalk-run combo, though. Kickboxing Friday with Robb got my cardio going pretty well, and then I practiced kipping. [Casee has a wicked right cross. Upper body is feeling stronger each week.]

Thirty-two Weeks

Due to family schedule changes, I am only able to go to CrossFit one day a week. I can already feel a difference in my body. I am so bummed!

Did the "Carry." Nicki and Greg had us carry a variety of weighted whatevers to the back fence and back. I did the Farmer's Walk, Waiter's Walk, Suitcase Walk, pulled the sled, negative pull-ups and some kipping. [Dan John would have been proud.]

Thirty-Three Weeks

The baby is in an uncomfortable position that makes it painful to even walk at times. I have decided to begin my temporary leave of absence from CrossFit. I look forward to resuming in two months!

Thirty-six to Forty Weeks

(10 days past due date) Thankfully my temporary leave of absence was short-lived. The baby shifted and I am on maternity leave so I look forward to my mornings at CrossFit. I basically come in to waddle around, stretch out and talk to everyone about how big I'm getting and when is that baby due?! All in all I really do still feel great and am keeping on top of my nutrition as well. Robb has been a great source of information for my nutrition and physiology questions. My pregnancy could not possibly be going any better.

Labor and Delivery

I couldn't imagine getting through the weekend marathon labor I had without my CrossFit training. The true meaning of the word "labor" really hit me. I had almost no sleep during my 36 hours of contractions, dilated to seven centimeters at home, and pushed my 9-lb 3-oz baby boy out CrossFit style in 20 minutes! I had complete confidence in my body's strength and ability to do what Mother Nature intended us goddesses to do. Incidentally, this was a natural (drug-free) VBAC (vaginal birth after cesarean) and I felt like I had conquered the world! [Casee had to do quite a bit of work to convince her doc to allow a VBAC. Read up on it. Interesting topic.]

Recovery

My recovery has been amazing. I went back to CrossFit one month after delivery, and two months after the birth I was back to my pre-baby weight. The workouts are bringing my strength and body shape back in an unbelievably short period of time. The nurses at my OB's office couldn't believe how quickly my body recovered, and I actually feel like I am in better shape now than I was before I got pregnant!

A Few Words More

I try not to give unsolicited advice, but I would tell anyone who is trying to get pregnant or is pregnant that CrossFit training is the only way to go. The combination of the extraordinary knowledge of Robb, Nicki and Greg and the satisfaction of completing the unique conditioning classes gave me an inner and outer strength that totally complemented my "holistic" aspirations for my pregnancy. If you are ready to take control of your body and health, then CrossFit NorCal is where you need to be.

ALIVE: AN INTERVIEW WITH MATT THORNTON
ROBB WOLF

I had the good fortune of spending some time with Kelly and Juliet Starrett, founders of San Francisco CrossFit this past weekend. They are some of my favorite people in the world and Kelly is a GENIUS of physical therapy and rehab. If you get hurt, you want it to happen near this guy. Kelly told me a story of one of his colleagues getting very upset at Kelly's statement that the Swiss Ball has limited rehab value. Kelly made come cogent arguments regarding basic functionality, motor-unit recruitment, common sense and experience. This exchange did not start well and it devolved to the point that Kelly's colleague, when feeling boxed in, I assume, made a statement to the effect "Show me your research. If you do not have research supporting this it CAN NOT be true."

I imagine this scenario plays itself out in many arenas, but I have seen it particularly in medicine, strength & conditioning and martial arts. Medicine has played party to the lie that fat is the causative agent in diseases ranging from type II diabetes to cancer to Alzheimer's. The Soft Science of Dietary Fat broke the seal on the medical establishment's denial of the role dietary carbohydrates play in modern disease. Things seemed to improve for a time, but the old dogmas have crept back in. The newest study is touted as being the most comprehensive to date… and shows NO benefit to eating a low fat diet for either body composition or health and longevity. No benefit. So the interesting thing is even in the face of insurmountable evidence, it appears to be fairly easy to spin or ignore the data to maintain the dominant paradigm. I guess that is human nature and to be expected. It is interesting that the market seems to sort this out fairly effectively as the Zone empire grows slowly but surely. This growth occurs because people try the Zone and it works. Personal experience wins out occasionally!

The martial arts have witnessed a similar avoidance of reality to that seen in the medical establishment. Pressure points, Kata and hierarchy have received greater value than conditioning, delivery system and progression. It took nearly twenty years for the Gracie phenomenon to convince most that a ground game was integral to effective combat. We see a decided advantage to those who embrace critical thinking and personal experience over those clinging to dogma and tradition.

This month we are proud to present an interview with Straight Blast Gym

International founder Matt Thornton. Matt is a true pioneer in Mixed Martial Arts and has been somewhat of a controversial figure, particularly in the Jeet Kune Do world, because of his insistence upon authentic, alive training. Matt has a keen mind and his constant analysis of curriculum and teaching methods have created an environment where fighters competing at the highest levels of MMA are trained with the same methodology as children and grandparents. SBG modifies intensity and volume; they do not change workouts. Sound familiar?

Tell our readers about yourself including athletic, educational and martial arts background.

I started martial arts with boxing as a kid, and discovered JKD when I left the military, about fourteen years ago. I liked it because they used boxing hands. Then I had the privilege, of meeting Rickson Gracie, a year or so before the first UFC, and that got me hooked on BJJ. Our curriculum evolved over the decade to what we have today.

Matt, you talk at length about "Aliveness" on your website, in your seminars and other interviews… so much in fact that I feel guilty asking about it again! But here goes: What is "Aliveness", who trains this way and how can our readers who may not be familiar with martial arts discern a school or group who trains this way?

Personally I think Aliveness is the most important concept within all martial arts. Without that concept as a core basis, everything else kind of just falls apart. So Aliveness needs to come first. It keeps everything authentic, functional, and above all else, healthy.

We put up a huge Aliveness Q & A at our website, www.straightblastgym.com, which anyone can access. It deals with nearly all the questions that come up regarding Alive training. But in short Aliveness means timing, energy, and motion, the three key ingredients to functional training. And when Aliveness is maintained, then everything else seems to come right in the end; it will fall into place if it's going to.

From your writings it seems you had some trepidation about switching your curriculum to alive training because your friends and instructors felt you could not make this type of training commercially viable. What was that process like? How does it feel now that SBG has grown so much?

I wouldn't so much say trepidation, but more that I had resigned myself to the fact I would always have to keep a second job, in order to feed my family. And I believed that because at the time absolutely everyone told me that nobody wanted to train this way. That people loved dead patterns, and nobody would want to sweat. That was more or less where the JKD as a majority was at that time, and that was pretty much where traditional martial arts are in the country. So I just accepted it. I was actually amazed at the really positive influx of new students that kept arriving weekly when I first opened my tiny little gym. We were way ahead of the curve of MMA at the time, and I was, and am, happy to prove my old critics wrong. People do want to train this way, and yes, you can make a comfortable living if you work hard and are good at what you do. You don't need any of those old dead patterns or methods. There is a better, healthier way.

Why do you feel that training Alive as an athlete helps in character development?

Great question! I think the key word is probably authenticity. It's authentic, in the sense that when you roll in BJJ, or box, or wrestle, the matches are not choreographed. It is not based on one and two step sparring patterns. It is real in that sense. It contains that combination of timing, energy, and motion. So as time goes by the athlete develops a real sense of self confidence, based on what they know their body can, and cannot do. And that can't be faked. And I think that process can be an incredible form of Yoga. In the sense of self actualization that Yoga can imply.

I don't think it is a given that training Alive will make people nicer human beings. I think that Alive training has to go hand in hand with a healthy environment, mature role models, and a caring community. The combination of the two can be really powerful in terms of the positive aspects it can have on people's lives. People of all ages, by the way. And although I don't think Alive training is enough alone, it is certainly is required within martial arts. Because if what you are doing is based on a lie, that is, it is not authentic, then I don't think it will be useful as a tool for happiness.

That is why I am a big believer that the Alive training should go hand in hand with a really intense introspective process. And that is a very personal subject, so I speak about it in general terms, but I think it is crucial. It is an uncomfortable topic for many people. But I think it is so vital. All forms of Yoga contain both parts. A physical part, which has to be honored. And an introspective part, which also has to be honored. I think that when our intentions regarding the activity we are engaging in are clear, honest, and open, then that 'thing' (activity-event) becomes incredibly healthy. It becomes a kind of Yoga. But for that to occur we must be clear within ourselves about our own personal intentions. And although most people believe they already are, I think its pretty clear we usually are not. So that ruthless bent towards introspection also has to be there, I think. Again, it is all about authenticity.

The respect, humility, and honor of martial arts is actually, when we tell the truth, only ever found in Alive training. It's just imitated in the other kind of training. It's about being authentic. In other words, I can pretend to be humble, I can bow to you and all that, or I can actually be humble. But obviously, I can't be both at the same time. Aliveness takes us there.

People who accuse Alive training of not having that actually have things completely upside down. Alive training has all of that, and recognition of it is what helps create that healthy culture we share together.

You have had success with the Zone in the past. How did you hear about the Zone and what were your performance changes while implementing it?

I was never really a jock. Boxing was the first sport which ever interested me. And at that time I did plenty of cardio, but not much else. And once I stopped going to the boxing gym, conditioning kind of took a backseat for me. It wasn't until maybe the second year after opening my own gym that I decided I was going to get serious about my own personal level of fitness. I needed to in order to push my BJJ skills as far as I wanted to at that time. So I did tons of research on diet, exercise, etc. This was around 98 or 99. The zone made the most sense to me, so I stuck with that religiously for a couple Years. I may have taken in a few less carbs then normally prescribed within that diet, but all in all I stuck with it. I didn't drink at all, and I was lifting heavy and doing anaerobic HIT cardio routines 2 – 3 times a week. I went from about 260 lbs, with a body fat in the high teens, to about 255, and 5-6% body fat, when I hit my peak period of emphasis on conditioning. My body, and its capabilities, completely changed.

How do you balance learning basic motor skills and aliveness? For example, when learning boxing and Thai boxing, how much emphasis is placed on basic combinations (jab, cross, right round kick)? Can you give an example of the progressions a beginner might see as they work their way through the SBG curriculum?

We don't have a beginner, intermediate, advanced curriculum, in terms of technique. I am a big believer that there are only fundamentals, and those fundamentals when done really well, at just the right time, are advanced technique. So the progression then becomes one more of intensity, and levels of resistance, and not so much of technical movement. That said, a beginner will work out in much the same way and with the same skill sets and techniques. The only difference is how hard the practice is, and how loose or tight the drill parameters may be.

In terms of passing on a basic technique, any technique, be it from boxing, wrestling, BJJ or whatever, then the method typically used is what I call the "I" method. The "I" method is a three phase process. The first step is introduction, and that is where we work the basic mechanics of the movement without resistance. This usually takes anywhere from 5 to 15 minutes. This is followed with a drill phase, this is the isolation stage. Progressive resistance is used in various ways so that the feel and timing of the movement is acquired. We finish with integration, where we put that skill, technique, or tool, back into the complete game that they are training for. The really important part is that the isolation stage, which follows the introduction stage, is never skipped. I never teach a class that is just introduction stage. Even on day one, people train Alive when they are training with me.

The "I" method is the primary method in the beginning, but as the athletes progress we move into different types of curriculums, the progression I usually follow is as follows:

'I' method, which develops skillsets. Then a more conceptual method, which helps develop a well rouded game, and various types of pressures. The progression for that is usually objectives, concepts / pressures, and games… with emphasis being on creating a fun training environment that allows more freedom for the athlete then is always found in an "I" method type course.

The last method I use is the Inquiry method, and again this is a pretty simple three-phase process: objective (or challenge), questions define the games, and students discover & articulate concepts/pressures. This is a type of class that requires participation in the direction of what is being taught by every student present. So usually the athletes we coach using this method already posses a game.

Your writing alludes to a sense of obligation to be honest and seek the truth with regards to martial arts training and in fact all areas of life. What are your thoughts on this topic regarding strength and conditioning? What do you feel works when preparing for fighting or life?

That is potentially a huge topic, so let me answer as practically as I can. I think looking at the latest studies and ideas that are related to athletic conditioning is a solid thing to do. Especially for a coach, but I also believe that most of what we need to know, we already know. How to lift for strength, how to develop a large gas tank, and how to eat clean and healthy. Again I think it comes down to fundamentals, done well, and done regularly. That said, I still like to see what new ideas and innovations come around when it comes to conditioning athletes.

Matt, you said, "Fundamentals done really well… those are advanced techniques." This is eerily similar to what some have noticed in athletic training. Fundamentals like the Olympic lifts, sprints, jumps, tumbling, rope climbs seem to deliver a level of athleticism impossible to obtain using the parts and pieces bodybuilding approach. Does this resonate with you? Share any thoughts you might have on this.

Exactly… that is absolutely my opinion. There are a few individuals that can get by with sloppy technical skill in any sport, by making up for it with superior attributes, drugs, or genetic gifts. But even these people would be better served by working on good, technical, core fundamentals, or whatever skill set they are trying to learn. So my focus as a coach is always on those with fundamentals, with all the athletes I work with.

Please take our readers through your "I" method. This seems deceptively simple yet it is rare in the teaching of martial arts. How did you come to it?

Most everything that I have come up with regarding the gym has been a description of what already was, and not something I created or invented. So I was teaching using an "I" method progression for years, and then when I started to receive attention, and promote the Aliveness concept, people would always ask me, "Well how do you teach someone the basics Alive if they don't know anything yet?" etc., so I began describing what I was doing, and that description was given a name for sake of easier explanation. The same is true for Aliveness, adaptability, delivery systems, non-attribute-based training, and all the other terms which have been identified with SBG. It is a process of evolution in terms of language, for ease in communication and the sharing of knowledge and skills. Like everything else I suppose.

We have noted that the conditioning needs of military and law enforcement personnel are not met by conventional segmented training (bodybuilding M-W-F, long slow run T-Th) but rather by constantly varied mixed modal training. Do you see parallels here with regards to martial arts training in these populations? How has your ISR matrix addressed this issue?

ISR is the brainchild of SBGi VP Luis Gutierrez, and he put a tremendous amount of thought, effort, and experience into that program. I think it is light years ahead of everything else I have seen that is usually taught within those professions. The reasons are not just the techniques taught, though all of them are simple, powerful, and functional fighting fundamentals; the reason is the training method. Again, Luis brings back Aliveness into that training, along with cutting edge delivery system technology, so the classes, while staying safe, actually do teach these people how to control their suspects and stay safe.

In linguistics, the term "pidgin" refers to the overlap of two different languages and the initial incomplete integration of these languages. Creole refers to a much more sophisticated integration of the two languages, typically performed by the children of the pidgin speakers. The Creole is more advanced in both grammar and content and takes on the characteristics of a fully formed stand-alone language. Where do you see SBG with this regard if we use boxing, Muay Thai, BJJ and Greco-based clinch as the parent languages? Does this analogy work? If so, where do you see this process going in the next 5-10 years?

That's an interesting analogy. I think, however, that the opposite is often true. I say often because there are always exceptions. But in general terms I think pure BJJ, or sport submission grappling, is more complex then MMA. The amount of technique variables actually increase. I think MMA, although it involves stand up skill, wrestling skills, and clinch skills, as well as BJJ or ground skills, is actually a simpler sport in that one specific sense. And by simpler I don't mean less refined, or less technical. I mean simpler in terms of the volume of techniques and fundamentals that are needed in that arena. I actually think that sport BJJ, with the gi, is probably the most complicated combat sport that exists in terms of volume of technique required. Again I am generalizing, and there will people in all of the above that are exceptions. But speaking for just the delivery systems, I believe the above stated is absolutely true.

But that does not mean that BJJ is any more of an art then MMA is. Art can be defined in so many ways. As an example, just the mental preparation that goes along with training for an MMA bout can be an art in and of itself. And I am not talking about pop psychology or any particular technique even. But just the trials these athletes go through in terms of nerves, uncontrolled thoughts, anxiety, anticipation, and all of that. So in terms of art, I don't think any one craft is inherently more artistic. Even the simplest tasks can become fantastic forms, or movements of art.

In closing, is there anything you would like to say?

I'd just say that loving whatever you are doing has always been the key for the moments of happiness I have had. So if you love MMA, or BJJ, then just relax and enjoy it for what it is in that very moment. And forget any destinations, goals, desires, or fears you have at the moment. Just be with that activity one hundred percent. Just try giving it that space. I have come to believe that this is truly honoring the process, and I believe that is a good thing. And I would encourage everyone to test that theory for themselves. To go into it themselves. And I would echo what the late great Tim Leary always encouraged: question authority and think for yourself.

DAMN DIRTY GRAINS: THIS TIME IT'S PERSONAL
ROBB WOLF

Do you ever feel like you have something completely dialed? You know the issue inside and out, can argue it from every angle and… discover you were at best wrong, but more accurately, you were delusional. Such was my foray into vegetarianism. I mean EVERYBODY knew fat was bad, meat was full of toxins and the enlightened humane thing to do was to not eat critters. So my fare revolved around beans, rice and whole grains. I'm handy in the kitchen. I made it work. The fruits of my labors included high blood pressure, horrible blood lipids and gastrointestinal problems that were eventually diagnosed as gastritis. I was a pudgy bloated mess who was dying from doing what I thought was right.

Concurrent to and actually preceding my downward spiral into vegetarianism, my mother had been battling a slew of health problems. Fatigue, lethargy, diffuse but intense bouts of pain. My mom had not been doing well for a very long time. Eventually a diagnosis of Rheumatoid Arthritis and Lupus were issued from a specialist. Immune suppressing drugs were prescribed in an attempt to cool the over active immune response that seemed bent on dispatching my mom. Along with the Lupus and RA diagnoses, an afterthought of a condition was also discovered: Celiac Sprue. In technical parlance, Anti-glidan enteropathy. My mom was experiencing a profound reaction to wheat, dairy and a long list of other problematic substances.

The autoimmune diseases I had heard of, but this Celiac Sprue was news to me. When I started researching the topic I got the feeling that the CS was THE problem and likely the causative factor in the other interrelated autoimmune conditions. What became clear was that humans were not designed to eat cereal grains. That obviously was a position that not many people were talking about and it seemed to be outright heresy at the time. I think that was late 1998 or early 1999. Suffice to say I was stumped. I knew the Standard American Diet had some serious problems but now it appeared all the rice, beans and whole wheat bread I'd been eating might actually be killing me. If vegetarianism was not going to work, what would? I thought about science, evolution… evolutionary biology… hunter-gatherers… I remembered hearing someone mention of the term "Paleolithic Diet" once. I put that term in a search engine (before Google…

crappy returns) and found www.paleodiet.com. From there I found Art Devany's site and things really started to make some sense.

If my meandering down memory lane was a bore, I apologize, but I do have a point and it does pertain to performance, health and longevity. Most of you folks who read this publication also likely participate in some form of high-level physical activity like CrossFit or Olympic Lifting. I think it is safe to say that the people who are drawn to CrossFit and its affiliated specialists are people who are looking for the BEST. The best training, the best performance, the best health possible. That being the case, the question of nutrition inevitably arises and it is hoped that the best nutritional recommendations are made. For many communities, even beyond CrossFit, that nutritional answer of answers is the Zone. The Zone is the genius of Barry Sears and it is waiting with open, warm, non-judgmental arms, ready to bring you in regardless of your food preferences, so long as you partition your slop into the Golden Ratios of 40-30-30. It has been put forward that cottage cheese and a snickers bar can fit the bill for Zoners. Now obviously the Zone recommends "good" carbs like veggies and fruit, but if we are about Elite Fitness and the health that should be associated with that fitness, is an anything-goes Zone really the answer? Is that the best we can do?

Let me use an analogy here and let's assume for a moment we are looking at fitness through the eyes of CrossFit and the four-part definition of fitness as described in the CrossFit Journal. Some of the key points of that definition are to create as broad an adaptation as possible and that segmented training produces segmented results. These concepts fit together in that if you are training in a segmented fashion you will be lacking in some breadth of adaptation. A bit chicken-and-egg, but stay with me. Now we can make the argument that from a "fitness" perspective, things like Olympic weightlifting, sprinting and gymnastics yield enormous benefit, especially when compared to marathons, Pilates and Jazzercise. No arguments there, and I think no one would argue that an individual who O-lifted one day, did sprint work the following day and some gymnastics the day after that in some fashion that allowed for recovery… well, this person would be pretty "fit".

According to the CrossFit definition of fitness, however, this individual would be segmented and it would not be hard to cook up a workout that would expose that segmented training. Interestingly, the exploration of that segmentation (CrossFit style, multi-modal training) would likely improve the game of this person in all of their activities as that very segmentation is likely limiting performance. Make sense? So this is why, from the broad, highly-refined definition of fitness that CrossFit offers we need to do both specialized skill work in the areas of O-lifting, sprinting and gymnastics, but also multi-modal work.

Back to food. Taken that this all-encompassing definition of fitness requires non segmented training and performance, we can infer that we indeed want a complete "fitness", and since nutrition—the molecular basis of health—is the FOUNDATION of an optimized fitness regime, we should want the very best nutritional strategy we can find, especially if our definition of fitness includes ALL parameters of health. If that is indeed the case, then before we start slicing and dicing our food into exacting proportions we need to have the right stuff on the plate. Grains are not among those things. We can be apologists and try to be all things to all people, but much like the argument that too much power lifting or long distance running will hamper your overall fitness, so too will consumption of foods that are at odds with health. This is a long introduction to what is destined to be a longer paper on grains: what they are and what they do to us when we eat them, especially if they take a prominent role in our diets.

Anatomy of the Grain

You have likely heard terms like Bran, Kernel and Germ as they relate to grains, but I want to take a moment to cover what exactly these structures are and what they contain.

Bran: The tough outer coating that contains proteins, vitamins and minerals. That's the standard ADA position. (Eatright.org... what a damn farce. Keep your eyes open for that topic and others at our new blog... Sorry, back to bashing grains.) So the bran appears to be a bountiful harvest of nutrition. We will take that fallacy apart in greater detail later. For now just know that bran is also home to most of the antinutrients and gut-irritating protein constituents.

Kernel: This is where most of the nutritional action is, at least with regard to caloric content. This is where we find most of the carbohydrate in grains. If you have seen white rice you have seen the kernel.

Germ: This is actually the plant embryo and it contains a fairly dense source of fatty acids, mostly n-6, some protein and assorted vitamins and minerals.

This is your average grain, and it is representative of grains ranging from wheat to rice to popcorn. A detailed understanding of grain taxonomy and structure is not my intent here, but it is important that you understand the components grains, as we will be talking about processing methods that may remove certain problematic fractions but inevitably leave others.

The Real Problems

Most of the problems related to grain consumption can be lumped into one of two categories: those related to hyperinsulinemia and those related to irritant/toxicant properties inherent to the grains. It is interesting to note that these properties of irritation and inflammation via hyperinsulinemia may be multiplicative with regards to deleterious health effects, i.e. one makes the other worse.

Did the food pyramid make all the Dieticians Chubby or did the Chubby Dieticians make the food pyramid?

Possibly the longest introduction for a paragraph you have ever seen but it is at the crux of the first problem with grains. Grains are mostly starchy carbohydrate, and starchy carbohydrate, when consumed in any amount, causes the release of a significant dose of insulin. The starch in grains can be subdivided into two basic forms, amylose and amylopectin.

Amylose is a long chain of glucose molecules and amylopectin is a highly branched, interwoven structure also comprised of glucose molecules. Think of amylose as a rope and amylopectin as a dust bunny. Grains are made up of differing amounts of amylose and amylopectin, and this variation accounts for differences in the glycemic index of various grains.

Starches are digested by the enzymes salivary amylase and pancreatic amylase. Amylase acts on the last glucose molecule in the polymer, whether it is amylose (rope) or amylopectin (dust bunny). I think it's pretty clear that the rope has far fewer locations for the amylase to attack in the digestion process than the dust bunny does. The more locations for the enzyme to attack, the faster the digestion, the quicker the rise in blood glucose levels, and typically the larger the insulin release. Any type of processing (cooking, milling) breaks up both the varieties of starch molecules, thus facilitating digestion. Easier digestion means a greater insulin response. The making of pizza crust fractures the starch grains in such a way that the body produces more insulin in response to pizza crust than raw glucose! No one knows why, but the processing inherent in most grain products can increase the insulin response far above what would otherwise be expected.

So grains can have a fairly wide-ranging glycemic index and thus insulin response and various forms of processing can greatly increase both those numbers and consequently their impact on our health. One of the fallacies that is still spewed forth by the likes of the ADA is that slow-releasing carbs (beans, whole grains) causes a flat insulin response and consequently do not pose a problem. This is true only if one is consuming grains as condiments, as in a tablespoon here and there. Eat them a cup at a time, and not only does blood glucose level rise dramatically, but it stays elevated for a long time. Research is pretty conclusive that the insulin spike is more detrimental than the lower level chronically elevated insulin, but the end results are the same: Syndrome X, AKA the Metabolic Syndrome (You always need multiple names for things in science and medicine to ensure that as few people as possible have an idea of what is going on). Grains, both processed and unprocessed, are a major player in metabolic derangement in that they are almost entirely carbohydrate and they are typically consumed in large quantities.

Now that we understand the relationship of grain consumption and the inevitable and deleterious rise in insulin levels, let's look more closely at what Syndrome X is. The word Syndrome is defined as "A collection or group of signs and symptoms that occur together and characterize a particular disease or abnormality." The signs and symptoms of Syndrome X include high triglycerides, low HDL cholesterol, high blood pressure, high risk of stroke and heart attack… and a bunch of other stuff. Professor Loren Cordain wrote a paper that sheds some light on some of that "other stuff" Called "Syndrome X: Just the Tip of the Hyperinsulinemia Iceburg" That other stuff runs the gamut from cancer to myopia, but many diseases that have been associated with Syndrome X and hyperinsulinemia are slowly being put under the umbrella of Chronic Inflammation. We know that we are onto something hot when Barry Sears has a new topic that allows him to re-hash his Zone offerings. The Anti-Inflammation Zone is his most recent contribution to the Zone book club.

[Just a small digression here, but I think we are going to adopt Barry Sears's approach to rehashing material and combine that with the consistent subject lines of my Spam and we will start re-releasing the P-Menu with catchy titles like "The Anti-Penile Dysfunction P-menu" or the "Better than Cialis P-Menu". No new content… just a new topic to hang the material from.]

Anyway, inflammation has many factors, including antioxidant and essential fatty acid status, but one of the key contributors to the condition we call inflammation is insulin level. Here is a detailed Look at what happens with elevated insulin levels (Scroll down to insulin dysregulation).

The insulin and inflammation topic is absolutely huge and far beyond the scope of this article or publication for that matter. The main point is grains pack a potent impact with regards to insulin response and that can lead to a variety of problems.

Irritant/Toxicant

The next broad category I want to look at falls under the irritant/toxicant label. Let's look first at antinutrients. Grains are essentially a reproductive structure and contain not only a dense energy source for the developing embryo, but also a number of control mechanisms that prevent both predation and abnormal germination. Sequestering away key nutrients like calcium, zinc and magnesium prevents abnormal germination. One of the main antinutrients is a chemical called Phytic acid of which there are several varieties, all going by the general term "phytates".

Now the phytates are powerful chelators; that is they bind to metal ions very tightly. This is postulated to be the main reason why cultures that consume large portions of their diets as grains and/or legumes tend to be shorter than their westernized transplants. The Okinawan vs. Japanese story is clearly illustrative of this. Okinawans have historically been significantly taller than their Japanese counterparts. The diets of the two groups differed in that the Okinawans consumed more protein and most of their carbohydrates in the form of highly nutritious tubers and only a modicum of rice. Japanese Americans show a markedly different phenotypic expression than their rice and tofu-eating ancestors. Just look at Jeff Oji.

It is interesting to note that phytates are used in some alternative medicine circles as an anti cancer agent. Apparently phytates exert some influence on the growth of tissues by removing metal ions such as calcium, magnesium and zinc that are important for growth. This seems like a nice closed system: feed people grains, let them get cancer from the elevated insulin levels then use grain extracts (phytates) to try to treat their condition.

This antinutrient concept is found in all eggs including those of birds and reptiles. Avidin binds to biotin, which is an important growth factor for bacteria. Hide away the biotin and it's hard for the egg to spoil. These antinutrients are so powerful that avidin has even been genteically engineered into some grains… to extend their storage. Avidin is destroyed with cooking but phytates are not. Bon appetite!

Another sub category of irritants/toxicants includes items such as gluten. Gluten is a protein found in wheat and other grains. It is also categorized under a huge family of molecules called lectins. Many of these lectins actually damage or destroy the gastrointestinal tract. In the small intestine we have structures called microvilli that interact with the food in our intestines. Microvilli are covered with enzymes that help to digest and transport food particles into the blood stream or lymph. Certain proteins such as gluten found in wheat, rye and barley cause a severe autoimmune reaction in some individuals, which is called Celiac Sprue. Celiac is a full-blown autoimmune reaction in which the microvilli of the intestines are destroyed. This condition makes it nearly impossible to absorb fats, minerals and many vitamins.

Not everyone shows a full blown celiac response; however, irritation is present with virtually all grain consumption. This lower level irritation has been broadly labeled as "leaky gut syndrome" and is emerging as a primary player in all autoimmune disorders. The theory is that once the gut lining is damaged, large food particles are able to make their way into the blood stream. Once there, the immune system mounts an attack against the foreign, undigested food particles. These particles may have elements that are similar in structure to body proteins and thus antibodies are produced that have affinity for one's own tissues. The seed of autoimmunity has then been sown (nice grain cliché, no?). This is something that has been kicked around for many, many years, but some other very interesting disease processes have been uncovered, like schizophrenia and congestive heart failure, which appear to owe their existence, at least in part, to leaky gut. Nay Sayers (read also: The Ignorant) frequently make the point that not everyone gets celiac. That is true, but across all species tested, grains cause gut irritation. Check PubMed. This knowledge has even allowed the design of experiments looking at gut permeability and autoimmunity.

It is worth mentioning that dairy is a potent cross reactor for celiacs. It is fairly easy to assay dairy and get high concentrations of grain lectins. It has also been noted that grass-fed dairy shows little or no cross reactivity in celiacs. I'm going to look at some of the other deleterious effects of grain consumption for animals later, but this is obviously a source of grains that most people would not have considered.

Just to completely beat this into the ground, let's look at Quinoa. Quinoa is similar to a grain in its carbohydrate content and layout as a reproductive structure, but Quinoa is botanically a fruit, and if you remember your botany, is a dicotyledon, whereas wheat, obviously a grain, is a monocotyledon. Relevance? They differ phylogenetically at the class level. To put that in perspective, mammals are a class, as are fish, as are reptiles. This is a huge difference and denotes ages since a common ancestor. Despite that fact, Quinoa still has a protein fraction that can cause problems with celiacs. What I take from this is nature found a similar answer to reproductive strategies with quinoa and grains, and not surprisingly, quinoa presents similar potential problems.

I want to mention just a few more things here. Grains also have a highly addictive nature beyond the carbohydrate content. They contain opiate-like substances that can be very problematic. Not surprisingly, these opioid constituents can be concentrated in dairy. Makes one look at pizza in a new and frightening way.

Grains are not just bad for humans; they give livestock some serious problems as well, ranging from creating heat and acid resistant forms of E. Coli to completely altering the fatty acid and nutrient content of meat. Grass-fed meat should contain significant amounts of n-3 fatty acids, alpha lipoic acid, CLA, Vitamin E and loads of carotenoids. Grain fed meat is the protein version of cardboard.

You Have It!

So, there you have it! Likely more than you EVER wanted to know about grains. But considering that our mission with the Performance Menu is to provide the best possible information on how to feed, water and exercise your person to optimize performance, health and longevity, avoiding such thoroughness with the topic would be a dereliction of our responsibilities. We advocate a Paleo/Zone approach to nutrition and jazz that up with some Intermittent Fasting. We feel strongly that both anecdotal and scientific research supports these positions. Grains obviously play a major dietary role for many people, but I hope this exploration helps to clarify why they may not be a wise choice for optimized health.

GETTING STIFF: A REVISIONIST APPROACH TO STRETCHING AND FLEXIBILITY PART 1
GREG EVERETT

The reigning notion of flexibility and stretching is that its relationships to both athletic performance and injury protection are positive and linear; that is, as stretching and flexibility increase, so do athletic performance and injury protection. With this in mind, advice from nearly everyone for nearly everyone is to stretch as much as possible.

The actual research and experience of coaches and athletes, however, have failed to convincingly demonstrate this or any other relationship. The research hasn't done much of anything beyond making the subject even more confusing by producing a continual stream of contradictory conclusions, and it's easy to find coaches and athletes willing to supply emphatic anecdotal support for any conclusion you'd like.

Research in the arenas of fitness and nutrition are inherently difficult simply because of the enormous number of variables involved and the impossibility of true control subjects. Studies of stretching and flexibility are no exception. In fact, they offer a number of unique problems in addition to those more universal. Studies of stretching's effects on injury prevention and athletic performance have extremely limited application and are not exceptionally reliable. Anecdotal evidence simply contributes another layer of corroboration and contradiction.

Ultimately both coaches and athletes need a reliable flexibility and stretching prescription regardless of how difficult its development may be. In this issue, we'll discuss the research, some biomechanics and other fundamentals related to stretching and flexibility to build a solid foundation on which we'll develop the appropriate prescription in the next issue.

Definitions

The first step through the sludge of stretching and flexibility is to clearly understand the terminology involved. Often the definitions of flexibility and related terms are remarkably flexible. Unfortunately, the degree of flexibility of a term's meaning is proportional to the term's usefulness: The less precise the definition, the less useful the term. To avoid confusion, we're going to clearly define a few terms for the purposes of this discussion

Flexibility: The degree to which a muscle can be extended beyond its resting length, which will have a positive relationship with the range of motion of the associated joint(s).

Range of Motion: The degree to which the body can move about a given joint.

Stretching: The set of several methods of increasing flexibility

Hypermobility: More often called Joint Hypermobility. Decreased joint integrity and excessive possible joint movement as a result of congenitally defective connective tissue development.

Acquired Hypermobility: Non-congenital joint hypermobility arising from injury or joint abuse.

Minimal Flexibility: The minimal degree of flexibility required to properly achieve and maintain specified positions and ranges of motion.

Optimal Flexibility: The degree of flexibility for a particular pursuit that allows the greatest performance and provides the greatest injury protection possible.

Hypoflexibility: Flexibility to a degree short of minimal flexibility.

Hyperflexibility: Flexibility to a degree beyond optimal flexibility.

The terms stretching and flexibility are often used interchangeably in reference to research. For reasons that will become clearer as we progress, this is a serious mistake: they are not the same thing. The terms hypermobility and hyperflexibility are also often used synonymously, but they are not the same condition, and the distinction between the two is only somewhat less crucial than between stretching and flexibility. Hyperflexibility refers exclusively to muscle characteristics: more specifically, a muscle's capacity to be lengthened beyond what has been determined to be its ideal maximum length. Hypermobility, whether congenital or acquired, refers to the joint structure and the excessive possible motion and diminished integrity thereof. The reasons for my insistence on clearly distinguishing the two will become more apparent later.

The Research

Relatively little research on the effects of stretching and flexibility on injury prevention and athletic performance exists. That which does exist provides conclusive evidence of virtually nothing. Particularly in the realm of injury prevention, the research demonstrates little other than that it's nearly impossible to conduct useful, reliable and broadly applicable research of this nature.

Studies can be categorized according to their focus on the contributions of either stretching or flexibility to either injury prevention or athletic performance. It's important here to reiterate the distinction between stretching and flexibility: stretching is an activity typically employed as a means to increase flexibility; flexibility is the actual capacity for a muscle to extend beyond its resting length, which is associated with the range of motion of the body about the corresponding joint or joints. They are absolutely not the same thing.

The structure of studies and the wording of their conclusions are critical. For example, we cannot misinterpret a study that compared the injury rates of two groups, one who stretched and one who didn't, that concluded that stretching was associated with decreased rate of injury to mean that increased flexibility reduces the risk of injury. Nor can we misinterpret a study concluding that increased flexibility improved a certain aspect of performance in a certain group of athletes to mean that stretching improves athletic performance. And we cannot misinterpret a study that determined stretching was associated with any effects on injury prevention or performance to mean that all types of stretching will produce the same effects. We must be extremely careful to use the data and conclusions of studies for exactly what they are and nothing more, provided of course that we deem the studies reliable at all.

Let's consider a varied sample of the available research

A two-year cohort study of over 100 high-level soccer players, Gaelic football players and hurlers determined that "flexibility scores were not found to be significant predictors of injury." An RCT study with about 1500 army recruits for 12 weeks had the test group perform pre-exercise static stretching, while the control performed no stretching. Both groups performed a warm-up prior to stretching and/or exercise. The researchers concluded that "a typical muscle stretching protocol performed during pre-exercise warm-ups does not produce clinically meaningful reductions in risk of exercise-related injury in army recruits."

A study similar to the last of about 300 military trainees, in which the test group performed three hamstring stretching sessions in addition to the normal PT program through which both they and the control group went, concluded that "the number of lower extremity overuse injuries was significantly lower in infantry basic trainees with increased hamstring flexibility." A cohort study of Belgian soccer players during a single season determined that "players with an increased tightness of the hamstring or quadriceps muscles have a statistically higher risk for a subsequent musculoskeletal lesion" A study of a Division III collegiate football team comparing the injury rates of players during two successive seasons, during the second of which the players added static stretching prior to training, found that there was an "association between the incorporation of a static stretching program and a decreased incidence of musculotendinous strains."

An epidemiological study of military personnel data cited both low and high degrees of flexibility as factors for injury risk

It has been demonstrated that passive stretching may temporarily disrupt nerve function, resulting in diminished force production capacity and delayed reaction to proprioceptive input. This means the possibility of slightly less strength and power and greater injury risk if passive stretching is performed prior to activity. A study using college sprinters similarly found that sprinting speeds following passive stretching were reduced. Another study found that vertical jump height diminished immediately following passive stretching. Research regarding flexibility and running economy—cardiovascular efficiency—hasn't generated consistent conclusions. A study of sixteen powerlifters concluded that increased flexibility improved bench press performance over time.

The Bottom Line

These are just a few of maybe a hundred studies. While not an exhaustive sampling, it is accurately representative of the existing research and should help make clear its overall inconclusiveness.

Studies regarding flexibility and injury risk have almost invariably attempted to demonstrate infinitely linear relationships. In other words, they have sought to show that increasing flexibility or the practice of stretching either increases, decreases or doesn't affect the risk of injury, and that this relationship is the same regardless of the degree of flexibility. But what if the relationship—if there even is a relationship—isn't linear? What if there are static points along the plot of increasing flexibility at which the relative relationship suddenly shifts in terms of its rate of change or even direction?

There is also a great deal of variation among existing studies in terms of purpose, subjects of measurement and evaluation, the methods of measurement and evaluation, the subjects, the types of activities, the frequency and intensity of the activities, the duration of the study, and, possibly most important, there is enormous variation in the actual stretching protocols prescribed to the test subjects or studied retrospectively. Some studies focus merely on the presence or absence of any type of stretching in an athlete's training, some focus on the incorporation of a defined stretching protocol—which may or may not align with what we deem appropriate—and others focus exclusively on the degree of flexibility possessed by the athletes regardless of the methods employed to obtain it. These are all very different things and the associated data communicate very different messages.

On average, studies undertaken in an effort to determine the effects of flexibility and stretching on athletic performance are more useful than their injury counterpart studies: these studies more often focus on the given intervention's effects on specific physiological characteristics, such as those cited above regarding the effects of pre-activity static stretching on strength and power production.

Ultimately, there has been one unequivocal conclusion generated by the existing research: Pre-activity static stretching has the potential to negatively affect factors of athletic performance such as strength and proprioception. This conclusion is transferable to the realm of injury prevention because a reduction of normal strength and proprioception obviously both subject an athlete to a greater risk of injury.

In short, it can be asserted that static stretching generally has no place in pre-training activity, but all other relationships remain less certain according to research results.

Some Biomechanics

Let's briefly indulge in some biomechanics to illustrate some of the most important aspects of optimal flexibility.

The spine is a vertical stack of bone segments that articulate on cartilaginous disks. In its normal, stable position, it curves through lordosis in the lumbar region and kyphosis in the thoracic region. In this naturally curved position, compressive forces are balanced over the surfaces of the vertebrae and intervertebral disks. Maintenance of these curves provides the greatest possible structural integrity, while shifting of them transfers increased pressure either ventrally or dorsally to smaller areas of the vertebrae and disks, reducing structural integrity and increasing the risk of damage. Additionally, the spinal erectors' mechanical disadvantage is exaggerated when the lower back loses its lordotic curve—back strength is greatest with the spine in its normal curvature.

In its natural posture, the spine is curved through kyphosis in the thoracic region and lordosis in the lumbar region. Maintenance of these natural curves provides the greatest possible structural integrity and mechanical advantage, while shifting of them transfers increased pressure either ventrally or dorsally to smaller areas of the vertebrae and disks, reducing structure integrity, exaggerating mechanical disadvantage, and increasing the risk of damage.

The vast majority of back injuries involve the vertebrae L4 to S1—the point at which the spine and pelvis join. The primary reason is pervasive hip extensor and flexor inflexibility, which prevents proper spinal curvature in anything but an upright position and results in hypermobility of the lumbar spine, which must compensate for the lack of pelvic rotation during body flexion.

Flexion and extension can occur at both the hips and the lower spine. Differentiating between the two movements is remarkably difficult for many people. When I ask my clients to point to their hips, their fingers nearly invariably land on the iliac crests of their pelvises—our sense of anatomy has been distorted by idiomatic English. The hip is the joint of the femur and the pelvis, well below the bony ridges we mistakenly refer to as our hips. Were I to draw a line around the circumference of their bodies at this point, it would be right around the L4 – S1 vertebrae—the joint of the spine to the pelvis. (Figure 3)

Public education regarding lifting technique centers on the trite, oversimplified instructions to lift with the legs. But employing the legs in a lifting motion does not necessarily place the back in a biomechanically sound position as the technique ostensibly intends. The ineffectiveness of this advice is related to the misunderstanding of the involved joints as described above.

The lack of distinction between the back and hips becomes problematic during any movement involving bending at the waist ("waist" for our purposes referring to the area comprised of the lumbar spine and hip joints). When the torso changes position relative to the legs, as it does when we squat or lean over to pick something up, little or no control is exercised by the average person regarding at which joint this flexion occurs. This results in the bulk of the work being performed by the joint offering the least resistance—in most cases, the lumbar spine.

This is the primary source of the acquired lumbar hypermobility mentioned earlier. If the pelvis is not allowed to rotate adequately by tight hip extensors, the lower back must hyperflex, reversing the natural lordotic arch. It should be easy to see how the frequent repetition of this movement over many years can result in serious laxity in the lumbar spine, all while enabling the hamstrings—unusually resistant to stretching as it is—to grow even tighter.

No matter how strong your spinal erectors are, their activation across a hypermobile spine simply cannot overcome the far greater strength and relative mechanical advantage of the hamstrings. This means that strengthening of the spinal erectors, while absolutely integral to resolving this problem, cannot be considered a solitary solution—it must be accompanied by increased hamstring flexibility. Nor is the problem resolvable simply by "fighting" the stubbornly static pelvis position while performing the motions during which the problem arises. Direct hamstring stretching is an absolute requirement.

The best illustration of this—partly because it's the most common situation in which this "fighting" is posited as an independent solution—is the squat. As the depth of the hips increases during a squat, the angle of the back relative to the upper legs decreases, demanding lengthening of the hamstrings. If the hamstrings are not adequately flexible, they will pull the pelvis with them, leaving the lumbar spine to absorb the remaining necessary flexion. No amount of fighting with the strength of the mechanically disadvantaged spinal erectors over a hypermobile spine will defeat the strength and relative mechanical advantage of short hamstrings.

The idea that improper squat positioning due to inflexibility can be fixed by nothing more than doing squats to only the greatest depth at which lordosis can be maintained and then attempting to incrementally increase that depth over time while maintaining lordosis is not sound. While squatting will increase strength in both the spinal erectors and hamstrings, this ratio of strength and mechanical advantage will remain constant, resulting in no net improvement of the spinal erectors' ability to fight the hamstrings. Compounding the problem is the limited range of motion, which will encourage further shortening of the hamstrings.

And now another joint gets involved: the knee. When performing a proper, full range of motion squat, the knees are not subjected to any excessive degree or unusual type of force. The squat is an entirely natural movement and position for the human body, and, performed properly, will fortify the structures and abilities of the body, not harm them. That doesn't mean, however, that all variations of the squat are equally beneficial or without risk. If a squat is stopped short of full depth, undue stress is placed on the knees.

In a properly-positioned full-depth squat (hips below the knees), tension in the hamstrings balances the forces on the knee joint by opposing the force of the quadriceps. If the depth of the squat is not sufficient to generate this hamstring tension, the tension of the quadriceps on the knee is disproportionately great, resulting in potentially damaging shear force.

In short, as a method of attaining adequate flexibility for proper movement and position in the squat, the protocol of squatting only to the depth at which lordosis can be maintained and attempting to incrementally increase that depth over time is ineffective at best and potentially harmful at worst. The protocol must include additional stretching.

While hypoflexibility can create serious problems as described above, hyperflexibility may not necessarily be a substantially better condition.

The most obvious potential problem is related to the above discussion of the undue stress to the knees in the partial squat. As described there, hamstring tension at the bottom of the squat provides knee stability by balancing the forces on the joint. With hypoflexible hamstrings, if a full-depth squat is performed, this hamstring tension is not developed because of pelvic rotation shortening the distance between the muscles' origins and insertions, whereas if a partial depth squat is performed to maintain lordosis, the hamstrings are also not lengthened sufficiently to generate the necessary tension.

On the other hand, hyperflexible hamstrings may also fail to develop adequate tension on the tibia in this bottom position, thereby contributing to similar shear force on the knee. However, while the potential for this shear force is similar with hypoflexible and hyperflexible hamstrings, hyperflexibility is far less of a concern: with conscious effort, the hamstrings can be activated sufficiently throughout the squat to create the necessary tension, and, in fact, this activation of the hamstrings is requisite to a proper squat.

Some Finer Points

My explanation to many of my clients that they have hypoflexible hamstrings, hyperflexible spinal erectors, and hypermobile lumbar spines is often countered by complaints of lower back tightness, and insistence that their spinal erectors must therefore be stretched and their abdominals strengthened. But the naming of tight spinal erectors as the cause of lumber spine tightness is commonly erroneous. More often than not, the actual source of their discomfort is a combination of tight psoas, hamstrings or a combination of the two

The psoas is a hip flexor that inserts with the iliacus on the femur, originating on the inferior thoracic and lumbar vertebrae. Tension in the muscle pulls these vertebrae toward the leg, resulting in an exaggeration of the lumbar curve called hyperlordosis—or Hairdresser Back—and the associated feeling of a tight lower back.

The psoas originates along the inferior thoracic and lumbar vertebrae and insert on the femur to serve as a hip flexor. Tight psoas exaggerates the lordotic arch, creating compression in the lower back. This is often mistaken for tight spinal erectors.

Responding as is typical to this condition by stretching the lower back and performing more abdominal—or worse, hip flexion—work compounds the problem by reducing the stabilizing pull of the spinal erectors, strengthening the psoas, and increasing the mobility of the likely already hypermobile lumbar spine, exacerbating existing hyperlordosis and the feeling of back compression.

If the hamstrings are also tight, the summation of their tension on the pelvis and the tension of the psoas on the lumbar vertebrae further exaggerates the compression of the lumbar spine. In this case, posture may actually appear correct in terms of pelvic rotation and spinal curvature because of the balance of anterior and posterior tension. But while the position is normal, the amount of compressive force on the spine is not.

It's critical to be aware of what is and isn't actually tight, and to stretch and strengthen accordingly. Assessments and programming will be discussed and demonstrated in the next issue.

Flexibility and Stretching: The Revised Version

It's my contention that the relationship of flexibility to both injury and performance describes a modified bell curve; that is, both hypoflexibility and hyperflexibility increase the risk of injury and may limit performance. However, in close proximity to the apex representing optimal flexibility—the degree of flexibility associated with the least risk of injury and the greatest performance—hypoflexibility is associated with greater injury risk and greater performance inhibition than is hyperflexibility.

The relationship of injury protection and performance to flexibility describes a modified bell curve. The apex represents optimal flexibility—the degree of flexibility that allows the greatest performance and provides the greatest protection from injury. Note that the curve is steeper on the hypoflexibility side of the apex—in proximity to optimal flexibility, a given degree of hypoflexibility impedes performance and increases the risk of injury to a greater extent than that same degree of hyperflexibility.

Evidence that has shown stretching to be associated with increased injury rates can be explained by improper flexibility programming and implementation. In short, the increased rates of injuries were due to joint instability or muscle damage caused by improper stretching or from the negative effects of pre-activity static stretching—not a state of hyperflexibility. The vast majority of studies testing whether or not stretching reduces the risk of injury have involved pre-activity static stretching, which, as mentioned earlier, increases injury risk regardless of a subject's flexibility. Additionally, stretching is an activity that very few people do correctly, exposing their connective tissue to potentially damaging stress, as we'll discuss in greater detail in the next issue.

Another part of my resistance to believing hyperflexibility to be the cause of increased injury rates in these studies is the simple fact that I have yet to meet a single human being, athlete or otherwise, who could be considered hyperflexible. I've seen photographs of Thomas Kurz doing the splits in between two folding chairs, but that position is anything but common. In my experience, the vast majority of people—including long-time, competitive athletes—are actually surprisingly inflexible, and, more importantly, possess unbalanced degrees of flexibility among joints. They are unable to properly achieve positions and ranges of motion demanded by their sports, and are therefore accurately described as hypoflexible, not hyperflexible as careless interpretations of stretching studies may suggest.

Some research, like the powerlifter study cited previously, has demonstrated improved performance over time with increased flexibility of the athletes. But these results are very specific to conditions in the study: they don't demonstrate a reliable linear relationship between flexibility and strength, for example. More likely, the athletes in question were hypoflexible to the point of impeded performance, and the flexibility training they performed as test subjects simply reduced that impediment. There is no evidence that further increasing their flexibility would have continued improving their performance.

It's important to understand the difference between reducing or eliminating a performance-limiting factor and actually improving performance. It's also important to visualize this trend on the bell curve described previously and note that past the apex, the increasing flexibility that initially improved performance may begin to harm it instead. In terms of athletic performance, optimal flexibility will not improve in any dramatic manner strength, power, speed or any other physiological capacity. It will simple eliminate hypoflexibility-related performance limitations. If those limitations in a particular athlete are extraordinarily great, however, the improvement in performance gained from increased flexibility may be dramatic.

Requirements

One of the key parameters necessary to developing a proper stretching prescription is an athlete's flexibility demands. There are two categories of flexibility requirements— universal and sport-specific. That is, there is a defined set of positions and ranges of motion that are requisite to functional, healthy human life, and these obviously apply to everyone of human genetic construction. And then there is a set of positions and ranges of motions that are defined by the demands of your chosen athletic pursuits. The degree to which your sport-specific requirements differ from the universal requirements is dependent on the unique demands of your sport.

All athletic activity involves movement and the attainment and sometimes maintenance of certain positions (e.g. static holds in gymnastics). Some sports demand those things in the presence of significant loading or forces far exceeding bodyweight. Sport-specific positions may be functional, reflective to varying degrees of some of our universal positions and movements, while others may be wholly non-functional in this sense.

For example, a flare in gymnastics is a movement demanding of a high degree of flexibility, but it is not functional in the fundamental sense of the word—it's not a movement the human body would ever need to perform in the course of practical existence. A squat, on the other hand, is found in numerous variations in many sports, but also epitomizes functionality.

The reason this idea is important is that when determining your flexibility requirements, you need to first recognize and understand the demands of your existence and their demands of flexibility. In most cases, your sport-specific flexibility requirements will involve a greater degree of flexibility than the universal requirements, but this is not a rule without exception. If you do nothing more than run, for example, you have relatively little demand for athletic flexibility; your sport requires a very limited range of motion of all joints. On the other end of the spectrum are sports like gymnastics and Olympic weightlifting, which demand movement and the control of great resistance through ranges of motion beyond those found in the universal requirements.

The manner in which optimal flexibility improves athletic performance also varies greatly depending on your sport, but more importantly, on its relation to your previous flexibility status. As I suggested earlier in reference to the powerlifters whose bench press performance improved with the incorporation of stretching into their training, optimal flexibility is not technically a performance enhancer, but an impediment reducer. This is important to keep in mind when considering the flexibility-injury-performance curve: increasing flexibility will increase performance and decrease risk of injury if you are presently hypoflexible. But that trend will not continue indefinitely. Beyond the apex of the curve representing optimal flexibility, the trend prior will invert, and it's likely that increasing flexibility will increase the risk of injury and decrease performance.

My focus within the context of injury protection is connective tissue injury. That said, I don't disregard strains entirely. A severe enough strain can cause long term or permanent deformity and compromise function. But I would argue that strains of that severity are rarer and more difficult to incur than connective tissue injuries. My primary concern is actually not severe, acute injuries, but long term or even permanent damage to ligaments and joint structures. More specifically, my focus within the context of joint structure injury is cumulative connective tissue damage, which, in my opinion, is far more insidious than even fairly severe acute injury.

For example, if you rupture your ACL, you will most likely notice. The condition is relatively easy to diagnose reliably, and surgery to repair the rupture and subsequent rehabilitation seem to fairly successful. On the other hand (or leg), consider gradual loosening of knee ligaments due to some unspecified activity repeated regularly over a long period of time. No acute injury and its associated sudden pain, noise or unnatural joint movement exists to alert you of a problem that you can then address; the minutely incremental lengthening of the ligaments is completely unnoticeable day to day, and it therefore continues unnoticed until an acute injury, facilitated by this condition, occurs and suddenly draws your attention to your unusual joint laxity.

By this point, the ligaments are probably going to stay stretched. Reattaching a ligament is one thing—making a ligament shorten is another. Thermal capsulorrhaphy— surgical application of heat to the joint capsule to cause microscopic restructuring and subsequent tightening of the joint might work. Of course it also poses the risks of motor nerve damage, over-tightening, and burns to a degree beyond reconstruction. The only practical solution to joint laxity is preventing it.

The Y-Word

I would be derelict in my duties if I failed to discuss at least briefly the Y-word. Yoga has somehow developed a reputation of being a legitimate method of developing flexibility, at least among people with no exposure to real stretching. The truth is that it's surprisingly ineffective. More importantly, its positions frequently violate what I consider the single most crucial rule of flexibility training: stretching shall never place undue stress on connective tissue or joints. I won't argue that yoga may be a wonderful way to relax and relieve stress. I have no intention of denying anyone stress reduction; as the Cortisol Kid,

I encourage it emphatically. But there are many methods of stress reduction that do not concurrently damage the body. I assure you that experiencing a joint injury precipitated by lax connective tissue will not reduce your stress levels.

The Bottom Line

In short, a flexibility prescription is concerned with two areas: injury prevention and performance impediment elimination. In terms of injury prevention, the goal is to reduce the likelihood of musculotendinous, ligamental or other injuries, with its primary focus being the reduction of potentially damaging stress to connective tissue and the maintenance of joint integrity. In terms of performance, the goal is to eliminate any impediments arising from either hypo- or hyperflexibility.

In order to achieve these goals, the prescription must be predicated on determined flexibility requirements, of which there are two types: universal and specific. Universal requirements are those that apply to everyone; specific requirements are unique to each sport or activity and must be determined individually for each athlete. The protocol must employ proper stretching methods that achieve the desired goals but do not at all threaten joint integrity or performance.

Until Next Time

That's it for this installment. In the next issue we'll finish the process with a revised flexibility training prescription based on the information presented in this article, including flexibility assessments and how and when to perform what stretches. Until then, lay off the pre-activity static stretching and drop out of your yoga class.

GETTING STIFF: A REVISIONIST APPROACH TO STRETCHING AND FLEXIBILITY PART 2
GREG EVERETT

There is no universal stretching program. There are guidelines to which everyone must adhere to be successful, but success also requires understanding of individual requirements. As discussed in the last issue, every individual has two sets of flexibility needs: universal and specific. The universal requirements are those that apply to all human beings regardless of the physical activities in which they choose to engage as recreation or profession. The specific requirements are dependent on the nature of the demands involved in those physical activities.

The protocol for developing individual flexibility training programming includes a few steps. First and foremost, we must define and understand the program's goal, which we did in the last issue: achieving optimal flexibility to reduce performance impediments and the risk of injury as much as possible. Next, we must determine the requirements to define the individual's optimal flexibility. Once we know our requirements, we can develop the actual training methods to satisfy them. Of course we then must actually implement our program consistently. And finally, we must continue re-evaluating our flexibility status and adjusting our training accordingly.

Universal Requirements

The universal flexibility requirements are simple and few, but not necessarily easy to achieve. The first and second requirements are the abilities to maintain proper spinal curvature through the entire range of motion of two movements: a full-depth squat and hip flexion to a minimum of 90 degrees relative to the legs. The third requirement is the ability to achieve a proper overhead position.

In the last issue, we discussed the various problems arising from hypoflexible hip extensors and hypermobile lower backs. Inflexible shoulder girdles are another commonly overlooked cause of lower back injuries and pain. If the shoulders are unable to open fully (extend the arms vertically), the overhead position is not actually overhead. Therefore, when attempting to lift the arms overhead, the lumbar spine tends to hyperextend, rotating the torso backward to allow the arms attached to the partially opened shoulders to extend vertically. The ability to fully open the shoulder, then, is integral to long-term functionality and injury prevention.

Specific Requirements

In addition to the universal requirements, each athlete will have sport-specific requirements. The degree to which sport-specific requirements differ from the universal requirements is dependent on the nature of the sport. It's possible that your sport-specific requirements are less than the universal requirements; in the case of running, for example, the sport-specific requirements are far less than the universal.

The Compromises of Multi-Sport Athletes

For a single-sport athlete, determining optimal flexibility is simple. But for the multi-sport athlete, the process becomes more complicated. As we discovered previously, sport-specific optimal flexibility will vary dependent on the demands of the sport. Multiple sports mean multiple sets of demands, not all of which will necessarily be identical or even remotely similar. If an athlete's sports are long-distance running and cycling, the variation in sport-specific optimal flexibility is minimal. If, however, an athlete is a gymnast and weightlifter, contradictory flexibility requirements arise: the greater degree of flexibility required for gymnastics may increase the risk of injury during weightlifting.

Unfortunately, multi-sport athletes must compromise. That is, they must decide what their priorities are: a balance of performance and safety in all their sports, or an imbalance that provides greater potential performance and injury protection for a particular sport at the cost of a degree of those things for the other sports.

This decision may best be made based on the respective injury risks of each sport as the athlete intends to engage in it. That is, our multi-sport athlete may decide that the risk of injury during weightlifting is greater than during gymnastics both because of the sports' individual natures and because he is a competitive weightlifter but only a recreational gymnast, and he would therefore benefit more overall from optimal flexibility that favors weightlifting and may reduce somewhat his performance capacity and injury protection for gymnastics.

In short, it must be accepted that participation in multiple sports may increase on average an athlete's risk of injury, and may negatively affect performance in one or even all sports.

Determining Specific Requirements

Your specific flexibility requirements are simply a product of the positions and ranges of motion of your sport or sports. If you're uncertain what those things are, give up now.

Assessment

Now that we have the universal and specific guidelines described, we need to determine our present flexibility's relation to them. The closer an athlete is to optimal flexibility, the more difficult assessment becomes. For instance, if a new weightlifter cannot in a squat lower his hips below his knees, it's obvious he falls short of the universal squat requirement and a crucial sport-specific requirement. On the other hand, if a long-time weightlifter can squat to full-depth and has been doing so with great loads for a considerable amount of time, but experiences a slight loss of lordosis near the bottom of the squat, it most likely goes unnoticed or ignored. These are the athletes for whom optimal flexibility offers the most protection—they are engaging nearest their bodies' biomechanical limits at the greatest intensities.

Active and Passive Flexibility

Passive flexibility is the static flexibility limit attainable with external assistance, e.g. you or someone else pulling a limb as far as it will travel with no muscular assistance from that limb. Active flexibility is the static flexibility limit of agonist muscles attainable with only the power of antagonist muscles, i.e. how far a limb will travel being pulled by only the muscles that control it.

There are existing arguments that the gap between your active and passive ranges of motion should be reduced as much as possible, predicated on the idea that if your passive ROM is greater than your active ROM, you essentially have a realm of movement through which you have inadequate muscular support. The possibility of problems arising from this and those potential problems' severity is both equivocal and variable dependent on activity: there may not be any risk at all associated with large differences in passive and active ranges of motion. However, there are certainly no problems with having no difference between the two, provided of course the shared ROM meets the athlete's flexibility requirements.

The disparity between passive and active ranges of motion is a function of inadequate strength, not hyperflexibility. Unless an athlete is currently hyperflexible, the solution is not related to stretching, but to strength training; that is, that athlete needs to improve the strength of the antagonist muscles, particularly in their inside ranges of motion, not reduce the flexibility of the muscles being stretched. In the case of a hyperflexible athlete, the excessive flexibility should obviously be eliminated, but some degree of strengthening will likely remain necessary.

Universal Requirements

The assessment process here is quick and easy: if you can't perform a full-depth squat with proper lordosis, bend at the hip 90 degrees with proper lordosis, and achieve a genuine overhead position, you have work to do. That work is a flexibility training program comprised of the stretches you determine to be necessary based on your assessment.

Specific Requirements

With specific requirements, you're pretty much on your own. Identify any potentially challenging positions or ranges of motion and evaluate your ability to achieve them. If all of your require positions and ROMs are attainable, continue with business as usual. Otherwise, determine the appropriate collection of stretches and associated parameters to remedy existing hypoflexibility.

Getting Stiff

As touched on above, while uncommon, there are athletes who may determine that they're hyperflexible. In these cases, static stretching of the hyperflexible muscles should be discontinued. Dynamic stretching during pre-training activity and active stretching following training should continue. When optimal flexibility has been achieved with the reduction of hyperflexibility, static stretching may need to be reintroduced at an appropriate dose to maintain it.

Training

The flexibility training protocol will depend primarily on your sport or sports and the gap between your present flexibility and optimal flexibility. If your assessments have placed you at or near optimal flexibility, your training will be minimal and serve more as a means to preserve rather than develop flexibility. If you're instead nowhere near your requirements, your training may be more aggressive and frequent.

Warming Up

Warming up adequately is the most important pre-training activity. Increased body temperature produces positive effects such as improved blood flow in muscles, improved sensory nerve sensitivity and accelerated nerve impulses. Even dynamic stretching alone is not a sufficient warm-up, particularly in cold conditions. Were it not ignored so commonly and completely, it would seem absurd to clarify the obvious, but warming up literally means raising your body temperature. Failure to do this is not warming up.

As you already know, static stretching should never be performed prior to training or athletic activity, and is therefore not a part of appropriate pre-training activity. Dynamic Range of Motion (DROM) stretching can and should be, although it should be performed only following an adequate warm-up.

Warm-ups should generally begin with some type of low-intensity monostructural activity such as rowing. Particularly in cold weather, rowing is a much better option than running or even jumping rope, at least initially, because of the impact involved in the latter two—that impact is better saved until after the body is already somewhat warm. Following this general warm-up, DROM stretching and more training-specific warming up can take place before and during training.

Judgment

A certain degree of judgment will need to be exercised by the coach or athlete in terms of whether or not certain movements in the athlete's training should be modified based on inadequate flexibility. For example, if it's determined that the athlete is incapable of achieving a full depth squat with perfect lordosis, it must be decided whether or not it's necessary to restrict and how to restrict the performance of the squat by that athlete: Should the athlete perform only bodyweight squats until adequate flexibility is attained, or should the athlete be permitted to perform weighted squats even with his compromised bottom position?

Obviously the most prudent decision in terms of injury prevention is to not allow an athlete to perform loaded squats if his squat technique is not sufficiently developed. However, there are numerous instances in which the athlete is a high level performer and needs the stimulus of a loaded squat—and may have been performing loaded squats for years already. In these cases, it may be decided that the benefits of loaded squatting, even with somewhat compromised form, may outweigh the risk of injury. It's then necessary to decide how the movement will be modified; with the squat, for example, the athlete can either squat to less than full depth with proper back positioning or squat to full depth with a compromised back position. Again, neither is ideal; these decisions need to be made with the understanding that there are legitimate risks involved with improper movement mechanics and positions.

Putting it Together

A basic training sequence would be a general warm-up, DROM stretching, specific warm-up, training, static stretching. Depending on your present flexibility status, post-training static stretching may be very limited, or fairly extensive.

In the case of significant hypoflexibility, stretching may need to be performed even on non-training days, although without the aid of training's warming effect, non-training day static stretching should be less aggressive than that performed following training. In the absence of training, stretch when as warm as possible, such as following a hot shower or hot tub. Accept the fact that you simply may not be as flexible at these times and don't be spastic.

When presently in possession of optimal flexibility, static stretching can be greatly reduced in both frequency and intensity. Some experimentation and evaluation may be necessary, but essentially the goal is to reduce the volume of stretching as much as possible. If you're able to maintain optimal flexibility stretching two minutes—or not at all—after each training session, don't do more. But if you notice a reduction in flexibility over time with a given protocol, it obviously needs appropriate adjustment, whether in terms of volume, intensity or selection of stretches.

If you're currently hyperflexible in any area, eliminate static stretching of the area in question. Continue training through full, normal ranges of motion, continue including DROM stretching prior to training, but do not continue statically stretching muscles that are already too flexible. When you have returned to optimal flexibility, employ the minimal amount of stretching necessary to maintain it without returning to hyperflexibility.

DROM stretching upon rising in the morning can help improve flexibility throughout the day. The morning is not the time to go for extensive ranges of motion—this should be gentle, incrementally increasing movement nowhere near the ranges of motion you're able to achieve later in the day when warm. DROM stretching is also a good way to break up long hours of sitting at a desk.

Stretching Mistakes

The most pervasive problem with stretching in my experience is the failure of hamstring stretches to stretch the hamstrings and their success in stretching the spinal erectors instead. Consider the stretch of touching the floor with straight legs, the equivalent to the bench press in terms of the movements' use for measuring success within their respective disciplines. The ability to achieve this position is almost universally believed to signal flexible hamstrings. But if you watch the performance of this movement by nearly anyone, you'll notice little pelvic rotation and a great deal of lumbar spine rounding:

they're performing back flexion, not hip flexion, hyperflexing the spine and leaving the hamstrings nearly unaffected. This mistake is present in all hip-extensor-related stretches you can think of, from long-sitting to the butterfly to the straddle—the pelvis is not rotated forward, and therefore the hamstrings are not stretched. Worse, the back is stretched even more, contributing to the lumbar spine's existing hypermobility.

The Moves

The most important rule governing all stretches is that they should never place excessive stress on connective tissue. That means never introducing unusual torque on uniaxial or biaxial joints in a direction through which they are not intended to rotate, and never stretching to an extent at which pain is felt in any joint.

Following are descriptions and demonstrations of several stretches that can be incorporated into your training. If you're unsure what a movement stretches, try it—it's the muscles that get tight. This is by no means an exhaustive list, but for most people, this will be an adequately thorough collection. If you're hypoflexible in some particular way that isn't addressed by these stretches, get creative and find an appropriate stretch, keeping in mind the rules regarding stretches we've discussed.

Dynamic Stretches

As mentioned earlier, DROM stretches can be an effective pre-training activity provided an adequate warm-up has already been undertaken. DROM stretches use movement to achieve the desired range of motion; however, this does not mean limbs are carelessly forced into extreme ranges of motion. The ranges of motion of all DROM stretches are increased incrementally from conservative starting points. In the case of leg stretches, an external brake is applied to arrest movement. This convinces the nervous system that the involved muscles are not in danger and will gradually allow greater ranges of motion to be attained. DROM stretching should never be painful or even uncomfortable.

Arm Circles

Begin by circling a single arm slowly. Shrug as the arm passes overhead. Gradually increase the speed and range as you feel the shoulder loosen. After both arms have been done independently, circle them together, starting again with less speed and range and gradually increasing both. 10-20 reps of each arm in each direction, 10-20 of both arms together in each direction.

Torso Rotation

Begin with torso rotations in an upright position. Allow the foot on the side from which you're turning away to pivot to avoid placing excessive torsion on the knee. Turn your head with the rotations. 10-20 reps.

Next, bend the knees and flex at the hip to an angle as great as parallel with the floor. It's important to flex at the hip, not the back, to maintain proper spinal curvature in this position. Once in position, perform rotations as you did while standing upright. 10-20 reps.

Leg Kicks

In the leg stretches, use your hand to stop the motion of your leg. That means actually kicking your hand. Every time. Holding your hand in the air above your kicking leg without the two ever meeting just makes you look stupid. Don't. And notice I didn't say drop your hand to your leg. Start with your hand at a level you know you can reach. Kick to it and let your hand lift slightly in preparation for the next kick. Continue elevating your hand and increasing the ROM of the kicks. Do not avulse your hamstrings from the bone.

It's critical here to again distinguish back and hip flexion. This is a hamstring stretch—maintain normal spinal curvature throughout the movement, not allowing your pelvis to rotate up with the kicking leg. This will likely reduce your ROM greatly, but this is not Jazzercise and higher kicks due to lumbar spine flexion do not impress women.

Perform kicks to the front, followed by kicks to the side. 5-15 reps each direction and each leg. Don't do so many reps that you fatigue.

Butt Kickers

The most important point of this movement is that the name refers to your own butt. Someone else's may be remarkably gratifying, but it doesn't in this case achieve our goal of stretching the quads, in particular the rectus femoris, and the psoas. In order to hit these effectively, make sure you're striving to open the hip as fully as possible, not just flexing the leg.

Shoulder Dislocates

Despite the name, this movement should not dislocate your shoulders. Nor should it cause any pain; never force yourself through the ROM. Start with a generously wide grip with which you can easily pass through the full ROM with straight arms. Remain at this width for at least a few passes to warm-up to the movement. Then narrow your grip incrementally as your flexibility allows, always shrugging your shoulders as your arms pass overhead. If using this following training, you may want to pause at the tightest point in the ROM and hold as a static stretch. 10-20 reps.

Kip Swings

If you're not sure what a kip is, check out Eva T's instruction (http://www.crossfit.com/cf-video/eva-on-kipping.wmv) Like the other dynamic stretches, ease into it and gradually increase the range of motion. 10-20 reps.

Active Stretches

Active static stretches use antagonist muscle contraction to stretch the agonist muscle. Because of this, the actual stretch produced is minimal if even existent: with the exception of strength imbalances around a joint, it's difficult to produce enough force in this manner to achieve a stretch of any significant degree. That being said, active stretching is not without utility; it's an excellent method of developing static strength at end ranges of motion and for postural purposes. If you decide to incorporate active stretches into your training, perform them like passive static stretches following activity.

Get a Leg Up

Like the DROM leg kick, maintain your spine position while raising your leg in front of you as high as you can and hold. Next, raise it to the side and hold. Finally, raise it behind yourself and hold. If you want to get jiggy and work on some balance, perform all three positions without replacing your foot on the floor. Hold each position for 10-20 seconds.

Overhead Squat

Using a length of PVC or dowel, drop into an overhead squat, maintaining proper spinal curvature and active shoulders (shrug), and hang out. You can also add shoulder dislocates and presses from the bottom position.

If you're beyond the point at which the standard overhead squat offers much of a stretch, narrow your grip and stance incrementally until your feet and hands are touching. Holding your arms overhead without an implement also makes all overhead squat variations more difficult.

Static Stretches

Passive static stretching should never be performed prior to training or athletic activity. Stretched positions should be achieved slowly and gently, and then held for 20-60 seconds. The stretched position should not be painful. Overly aggressive static stretching is counterproductive. Most importantly, no unusual strain should be placed on joint structures.

Lunge

Keep your hips in line with your shoulders, facing forward, and drop them as low as possible while keeping your torso upright—this is more of a hip flexor than extensor stretch, so don't lean forward.

The Death Stretch

From the lunge position, you can flex your leg and stretch the quads, but I don't like the pressure on the patella in that position. Instead, I prefer hanging the foot from a box and achieving a similar position. Again, keep your torso upright. This is not only a quad stretch, but a potent hip flexor stretch, primarily for the rectus femoris.

If you are hypoflexible enough that this position is not practical, instead use a standing quad stretch, holding the leg with the opposite hand, keeping your hips square and open.

Butterfly

It never has been the most intense-sounding stretch, but it's a good one anyway. The key is maintaining proper spinal curvature—you're wasting your time without it. If you're fairly hypoflexible, that means you may not even be able to sit perfectly upright—hold your ankles and drive your pelvis forward to get your back in line.

Piriformis

This is basically a butterfly on one side with the other leg behind you, knee pointing to the floor. The stretch is commonly performed in a way that places too much torque on the knees. Keep the leg being stretched in contact with the floor entirely from the hip to the knee to the outside of the ankle. Allowing your hip to rise rotates the femur at the knee joint in a way it's not supposed to rotate. Don't. This may prevent you from rotating your hips all the way over—that's fine.

Lying Hamstring

There's nothing worse than a hamstring that won't tell you the truth. But really. Use something, like an AbMat (http://www.abmat.com/), to maintain lordosis when lying on your back (if you don't have anything, try to hold it yourself—but if you're at all hypoflexible, this will be difficult).

First, bring your knee to your chest and hang out for a bit. Do not let your pelvis move at all—remember, this is a hamstring stretch, not a lower back stretch. Without letting your pelvis or knee position change, attempt to straighten your leg. With your knee at your chest, you may be far from straight—that's fine. Keep your knee where it is. Pulling a straight leg to your face doesn't mean much if your pelvis is coming with it. This is a good stretch in which to use a little PNF love (see Getting Jiggy below).

A good alternative is elevating one foot on a box around knee level while standing. With a slight bend in the knee, flex at the hips—with proper spinal curvature, of course. After holding the position for a while, you can also try turning your hips into the elevated leg—this will shift the emphasis of the stretch to the lateral hamstrings, which are often tighter than expected.

Straddle

Like in the butterfly, proper spinal curvature is critical in this stretch. If you can't achieve anything that resembles a straddle with proper spinal curvature, lose this stretch until your hamstrings loosen up enough.

The Growler

This is a direct method of improving deep squat positioning. Drop into the bottom of a squat and grab your knees. Using your own legs as anchors, rotate your pelvis into position to achieve proper lordosis. Do this while no one is watching.

Getting Jiggy

PNF (proprioceptive neuromuscular facilitation) stretching is a reliable method of improving the effectiveness of static stretches. It's generally far more easily accomplished with assistance, although some stretches can be performed alone such as the lying hamstring described above.

There are a number of PNF methods, but we're going to stick with simple and effective. First, achieve the static stretch position in question and hold it for 15-30 seconds. Then contract the agonist muscle isometrically against the resistance, whether from a training partner or yourself, for 5-6 seconds. Each time you relax after a contraction, try gently increasing the static stretch in preparation for the next contraction. Repeat 2-5 times.

PNF stretching is taxing on muscles. Don't be overly aggressive. Keep the volume in each session and the frequency of sessions low: 2-5 sets of the above described protocol 2-3 times each week at the most.

Don't Slouch!

Stretching when, where and how appropriate will unquestionably provide results. But keep in mind how much time in a day you're not moving through your body's full ranges of motion—this is when habits and postures are created. Combat the products of your daily life by remaining vigilant about your posture and positions. If it's good to maintain proper spinal curvature during a back squat, it's good to do so while sitting at a desk.

There's no need to stretch all day long—but try to move as much as possible. If you're stuck at a desk for long hours each day, try setting a timer to force yourself to get up and move around regularly, whether that involves simply walking, going through a series of DROM stretches, or doing a few bodyweight exercises like squats and push-ups.

So here's to injury prevention, performance enhancement, and the end of an article that's far longer than it ever should have been.

Notes
[1] Shellock FG, Prentice WE. Warming-up and stretching for improved physical performance and prevention of sports-related injuries. Sports Med. 1985 Jul-Aug;2(4):267-78. http://www.ncbi.nlm.nih.gov/entrez/query.fcg i?db=PubMed&cmd=Retrieve&list_uids=3849057&dopt=Citation

MASS! A COMPLETE GUIDE FOR GAINING FUNCTIONAL MUSCLE
ROBB WOLF AND GREG EVERETT

Hang around any fitness site long enough and the question of weight gain, or more specifically, muscle gain, will be raised. If you frequent the bodybuilding sites, the question, "How do I gain muscle?" will put you in the company of everyone from the pre-pubescent to the peri-andropausal; in other words, everyone. Make the desire to gain muscle known around a fitness-oriented site and you may be met with equal parts disdain and confusion: disdain because it's obscene to want to gain muscle (most equate this desire with purely aesthetic motives) and confusion because few people have a solid understanding of how to gain functional muscle mass.

The question of how to gain muscle mass, whether for aesthetic or performance reasons, is one of the most common in sporting and athletic circles. The only close runner-ups I can think of are, "How do I get lean?" and, "What's the proper form for a reverse curl?" The answer to the lean question can be complex and is beyond the scope of this article, but the reverse curl answer is simple: perform the movement in the middle of a busy street so you will be removed form the gene-pool and neither sire nor bear demon spawn who also desire to "curl". Where was I? Oh! Gaining muscle. The simple answer to the mass gain conundrum: perform some resistance exercise, eat prodigious amounts of food, and rest adequately. Trips to Tijuana can be an effective solution to this universal problem, but that can also leave one with "huevos como pasas" or as the guest at a federally sponsored sleep-over program called "Da Big-House". What's a poor skinny dude/dudette to do if your last name is not Fragoso, Twardokens or Savage? Well, you need to get smart and use the best of what's available.

Le Programme
Or for non-French Speakers, The Program

As I mentioned above, the key elements of gaining muscle include resistance training (notice I did not specifically say weight lifting—various gymnastics movements can be quite effective in adding size and strength), nutrition and lifestyle. We have put together a training template using Olympic lifts and O-lift derivatives with a few gymnastics moves. Nutritionally we are offering several approaches, starting with the Zone and Cyclic low carb, and incorporating elements of intermittent fasting to optimize hormonal response. Finally, we will crawl up your lifestyle hoo-ha (metaphorically, of course) to ensure you are doing everything possible to optimize recovery and growth.

Let's take a close look at the training first, work our way through the nutrition, and wrap it all up with lifestyle.

Train, Train, Train… Train of Fools

I want to make a point here, and some of my own training experience makes that point pretty well. For several years when I was powerlifting, I had floundered with my training as I took every workout, virtually every set of every workout, to huevo-busting levels of intensity. I screamed, yelled, shook… and made very little progress. I had very poor sleep, a racing pulse and constant irritability. Yes, I was going through puberty, but my already dicey mental state was made far worse by my lame program and chronic overtraining.

Two guys who were former world champion powerlifters, either out of kindness or a desire to have peace in the gym, decided to apprentice me in the sport of powerlifting. My training was simple: move heavy weights and use looooong rest periods between sets. It was normal to rest 3-5 minutes between sets when we were in a peaking phase.

Although most people would consider the training archaic, we used a simple linear periodization model of higher reps and lower weight cycling down to low rep, high weight work. Monday was squat day. Most of the year I squatted using an Olympic-style high-bar, narrow stance, ass-to-ankles squat. This type of squatting was very demanding and made the competition powerlifting squat seem like cheating! On Monday I also did some accessory movements for the bench press, abs and basic bodybuilding stuff. I benched on Wednesday and did pull-ups, rowing, shrugs and tripe like that. On Friday I deadlifted, but early in the cycle, I performed lots of power cleans to work speed off the floor. I used the same linear periodization on the bench and deadlift. The only other nifty stuff I can think of was using the power rack to target sticking points with isometric work.

The results? At 19 years of age, 5' 9" and 181 lbs, I had a 565 lb squat and deadlift and 345 lb bench. The only supportive gear I wore was an Inzer lever belt for squats and deadlifts. No hydraulic bench shirts or poly-metallic alloy exoskeleton. Now, I was not FIT by any stretch of the imagination. Walking up a flight of stairs put my heart near redline, but I was pretty strong and could dunk a tennis ball standing flat footed under a basketball hoop. My nutrition was abysmal… high carb and low fat, and that put my body fat at about 15%. With what I know now, both with regards to nutrition and general physical preparedness, I could have been the same bodyweight with almost 20 lbs more muscle!

This trip down memory lane does have a point. The time in my life that I was the strongest and heaviest was when I had a VERY conservative training program that focused on putting more weight on the bar from workout to workout. I was also absolutely sure I had adequate recovery form one session to the other. If you are at all a hard-gainer and/ or have difficulty with recovery, a stripped-down program is critical to success.

If one has a goal of gaining muscle mass, a key point needs to be kept in mind: Stimulate, don't annihilate. In practical terms, we want to send ENOUGH of a stimulus to ensure a favorable adaptation. A workout that sidelines us for 3-5 days is in the annihilation category.

The stimulus should ideally have two features. The first is a mild-moderate amount of protein degradation caused by training volume. The second is to try to add resistance to each movement in a consistent manner. This ensures development of the neurological aspects of strength and it encourages growth of muscular contractile elements, not satellite cells and edema due to excessive volume. These factors considered, our training plan includes alternating mesocycles of moderate weight, moderate volume hypertrophy-specific training and moderate-high volume, heavy strength work. We are including a dash of metabolic conditioning and active recovery not only to enhance performance, but to also make those long climbs up two flights of stairs a little easier.

The Little Things

The training program is fairly straightforward. It's based on 1-week microcycles, each of which belongs to either a hypertrophy or strength mesocycle, each of which ends in an unloading microcycle. A single 7-week macrocycle consists of 3 hypertrophy microcycles, 1 unloading hypertrophy microcycle, 2 strength microcycles, and 1 unloading strength microcycle. 1RM testing is built into the schedule for both the measurement of progress and calculations of training loads.

Let's address some details:

Set/Rep Notation

The sets and reps when following a weight or percentage are in the order of reps x sets, e.g. 90% x 2 x 10 means 10 sets of 2 reps of 90% of the 1RM load. If a load prescription is absent, the format is the conventional sets x reps, e.g. 3 x 10 means 3 sets of 10 reps.

Prescribed Loading

Training loads are prescribed by percentage of 1RM. Most are based on the 1RM of that movement itself, but some are based on the 1RM of an associated movement—this is noted where applicable. Not a single rep in this entire training program should be taken to failure—don't do it. During the first hypertrophy microcycle, in fact, the loads should feel almost too light.

The template calls for the addition of 2%/week to the loads. What increases are actually possible is dependent on a number of variables, so it will range greatly both among individuals and movements. This will be something that requires some flexibility and experimentation by each individual. Some may find that greater increases are possible, and others may find 2% far too large of a jump. In the case of the latter, bump up the weight as little as your equipment will allow and/or perform less than all prescribed sets with this increased load, then drop down to the last microcycle's load for the remaining sets.

The loading percentages listed in the descriptions of microcycles are the percentages for the first microcycle. For example, the hypertrophy microcycle description lists 60% x 6 x 6. This is for week 1. Week 2 would be 62% x 6 x 6, and week three 64% x 6 x 6. If you find the initial percentage too heavy for a particular movement, drop it. Remember, if you're approaching failure in the first sets during the first microcycle, you're going to struggle to make it through. Start lower and make sure you're increasing the load each week.

Interset Rest

During the hypertrophy phase, rest between sets should be 1 minute, except when performing circuits, in which case rest should be limited to only that which is necessary. During the strength phase, longer interset rest is appropriate, from 1-3 minutes. You should feel well-recovered before jumping into the next set.

Abs-Back Circuit

In both the hypertrophy and strength phases, the prescription calls for "Abs-Back Circuit". During the hypertrophy phase, this should be higher volume work, such as a circuit of an ab movement, such as GHD sit-ups, hanging leg raises, knee-to-elbows, etc., and a back movement, such as GHD back extensions, reverse extensions, etc. During the strength phase, this work should drop in volume but increase in intensity—that is, where applicable add weight to the movements and perform fewer reps. Or this can mean using a movement like the hanging leg raise, of which you may be capable of only doing 5-6 reps unweighted. During the unloading microcycles, this circuit should follow the same format, but with about 50% of the volume used during the rest of the mesocycle.

Push-Pull Circuit

On Fridays of the hypertrophy microcycles, you'll see "Push-Pull Circuit." Like the abs-back circuit described above, this is a circuit of one pushing movement with one pulling movement performed in moderate to high volume. An example would be alternating between 10 kipping pull-ups and 10 clapping push ups as many times as you can in 10 minutes. Change this circuit each week for variety and try increasing the volume each week.

Strength Cycle Max Days

The strength cycle is based on Coach Mike Burgener's training template. Saturdays are contest days; that is, you'll work up to your heaviest snatch, clean & jerk and front squat. Remember, these are your maxes for the day; you may not always get a new record.

Unloading

Unloading microcycles appear at the end of both the hypertrophy and strength mesocycles—these lower volume and lower intensity weeks will allow you some periodic recovery while preventing detraining.

Rest Days

Rest days should include some active recovery efforts such as light sled pulling, wheel barrow walking, boxing technique work, o-lifting technique work with PVC. This work should be non-taxing—no lactic acid production, vomiting, tunnel vision or anything related—keep in mind, this is rest. Follow it if you can with a cold plunge.

Testing Days

Testing days are scheduled at the end of unloading microcycles. This is when you'll determine your 1RMs to calculate your training loads for the following cycle. Remember, you're testing 1RMs for the movements you'll be using in the NEXT cycle—not the one you're finishing.

Record Keeping

Record keeping will be a critical component of success with this plan. Because it's predicated on consistent load increases, knowing the loads you've used from cycle to cycle will be important. Unless you're Rain Man, don't make the mistake of thinking you'll remember all the numbers. Pens are neither expensive nor difficult to find (Speak to your local pharmaceutical rep for complimentary writing implements).

Good Eats!

If you want to grow you will need to eat… an amazing amount. That may be an enjoyable scenario if pizza and donuts are your main food groups, but we actually care about body composition and health a little, so expect to get the preponderance of your foods from meat, fruit, nuts, oils and yams. If you are in a serious hurry, you can use the Ido Portal method that we will look at later. I have some trepidation with this approach as it involves some serious insulin spiking… but it does appear to work very well. Before we get to that, let's look at how to use the Zone and cyclic low carb to best effect. Put on your feed-bag!

The Zone

The advantage of the Zone is that you know EXACTLY how much food you are eating and thus can assess your situation critically and subsequently make informed decisions. You can dial up or down protein, carbs or fat to run as lean or hot as you like. This regimentation virtually guarantees success, as you will be able to alter you nutrition to continue to move towards your goals. For an in-depth how-to for the Zone, you can check out issue two (http://www.performancemenu.com/backissues/index.php?show=issue&issueNum=2) of the Performance Menu or you can get help with the calculations directly from Barry "I Don't Follow My Own Diet" Sears (http://www.enterthezonediet.com/learn/zone-diet-calculator.html).

As an example, I weigh 173 lbs and am about 8% body fat. That means I have 159 lbs of lean body mass. My activity level is about a 0.8 considering I O-lift, kickbox a little, and do about 2-4 WODs per week. That 0.8 multiplier leaves me with a unit-less number of 127, which I divide by 7 to get my block allotment of 18 blocks. So that is:

173 lbs x 0.08 BF = 13.8 lbs fat
173lbs - 13.8 = 159 lbs LBM
159 x 0.8 = 127
127 / 7 = 18 blocks

If that process doesn't make sense, check out the Issue 2 Performance Menu and/or the link to the Zone website for a more patient and thorough discussion.

So my base Zone is 18 blocks, but to support my activity level, I have ratcheted up the fat content by a multiple of 5. Since our goal is mass gain, an appreciation of how many calories we are taking in might be helpful. Each Zone block has approximately 90 calories (trust me), so that puts my base level caloric intake at 1640 calories. Pretty skinny, and that's why people on the base Zone drop fat like crazy. That's also why I need to ratchet up my fat content so my energy intake approximately matches my output. When I have ratcheted up my fat blocks to 5X, I am taking in 2610cals per day. That is some pretty serious eating, but again, that is a maintenance level. If you want to add muscle, you will need to eat more! The easiest way to do that is to add another block… or two. If you are at 5X for your fat multiplier, add 1 block every 2 weeks. That represents approximately a 200 calorie increase. Even if your fat multiplier is 2-3, it might be a good idea to just step things up one block every 2 weeks. This will allow your digestion to adapt to the increased food intake and it provides you an opportunity to monitor your progress.

This brings up two digressions. The first digression relates to the ability to digest fat. Some people have reported they do not handle the ramped up fat content very effectively. These hearty souls have mentioned digestive problems and the condition "steatorhea" (http://www.diagnose-me.com/cond/C634635.html). If you actually read that link you likely understand that if fat absorption is an issue, a high-fat diet can be, shall we say, unpleasant. One can investigate what the issue is, such as potential parasitic infection or lack of adequate bile salts from the gall bladder, or just eat less fat! If you find the ramped up fat level to be too much, simply find the fat level you are comfortable with, typically baseline to 2X, and then add 2 blocks every 2 weeks instead of 1 block every 2 weeks for the 3-5X fat crowd. Ok, that's digression number one.

Digression number two has to do with fat gain. I have in the past endorsed the plan to get as lean as possible before trying to gain muscle. The argument for this is that with a low body fat level, one will tend to partition excess calories to muscle instead of fat. If one is at a lower body weight, the amount of testosterone that is aromatized to estrogen tends to be minimized. Sounds like good stuff, and for certain I am not advocating the classic powerlifter approach to mass gain: 1 gallon of chocolate milk and 3 peanut butter and jelly sandwiches IMMEDIATELY before bed! The reality, however, is that when one is gaining muscle, it is fairly normal to gain some fat in the bargain. Your abs may soften up for a while, but there is a reality that a higher body fat level CAN be a highly anabolic environment due to elevated IGF levels. My main point is that if you REALLY want to gain a significant amount of muscle, you may need to temporarily take a small hit with regards to body composition. A common obstacle for people trying to gain mass is the inevitable meltdown they experience at the realization that their body fat level has increased (although usually nowhere near as much as they believe), and their consequent cessation of increased eating—this results in a lot of time wasted in a 1-step-forward, 1-step-backward routine. The way we are structuring our programming, you should be able to keep fat gain to a minimum, and the smart use of intermittent fasting may help to keep insulin sensitivity rocking. More on that later.

Something you are likely wondering is how much do you increase your food intake? That is difficult to say. For some people muscle gain may come in a fairly linear fashion. Add 2 blocks, and a month down the road they will have gained 1-2 lbs of lean body mass. Other people will add 3-4 blocks at 5X fat (600-800 calories) and still not see change in the scale, performance or measuring tape. A good standard is to increase your intake approximately 5 blocks (1, 000 cals) and stay at that point for at least a month. See how your body reacts to this, and if you need to add more weight to reach your goal, you can start this process again. If you are gaining too much body fat, you might try dropping 25% of the carb blocks and replace each carb block with 3 blocks of fat. Don't multiply that fat by 5!! Just add in another 3 blocks of fat for every carb block you delete.

Ok, let's shift gears and look and another approach to this whole process!

CLC: The Revenge

If the Zone is not to your liking, you can use a cyclic low carb approach. The strength of the Zone is that you know exactly how much food you are taking in, but there is no reason we cannot have that precision with other approaches. Let's look at my situation again as an example. If you recall, my maintenance level Zone is 18 blocks at 5X fat. That means I am taking in 18 blocks (126 grams) of protein, 18 blocks (162 grams) of carbs and 90 blocks (135 grams) of fat in a given day. Most cyclic low carb programs recommend somewhere between 20-60 grams of carbs per day. The Metabolic Diet recommends that you ratchet your carbs up to match your recovery needs, plus occasional high carb days. That seems like a good approach, and it looks a bunch like following the Zone, but it does appear that a caloric excess more from fat than from carbs will likely result in less fat gain. Sounds good to me, so let's run with this.

Since a block of carbs is 9 grams, you can dial in your carb level pretty easily. And for every block of carbs you delete, just add 3 fat blocks to your day's total. So let's say that I am doing a fairly liberal carb level and am taking in 7 blocks of carbs. Keep in mind all of your carbs should come from multi-colored, low-glycemic-load vegetable matter. That leaves 18 blocks of protein since we have not altered that, and since I have deleted 11 blocks of carbs, I need to add 33 blocks of fat to my daily total, which puts me up to 123 blocks of fat. Let's see what that looks like with regards to both calories and grams.

18 blocks protein = 126 grams protein = 504 calories
7 blocks carbs = 63 grams = 252 calories
123 blocks fat = 184 grams + 27 grams in protein = 1899 calories
Total = 2655 calories

This is almost identical to my ramped-up Zone calorie level. Another way to do it if you are deleting 11 blocks of carbs is to add 5 blocks of protein and 18 blocks of fat (11 − 5 = 6; 6 x 3 = 18 blocks fat). A nice way to step up the calories is to add 2 blocks of protein and 11 blocks of fat every 2 weeks. One additional carb block every month would likely be fine as well.

Since we are discussing cyclic low carb, we need to look at the carb load phase, which can be approached a few different ways. The first way is to have a full day of high carb intake with a total of 300-500 grams of carbs every 3-5 days. Alternatively, you can simply do 1-2 meals every third or fifth day and again take in 300-500 grams of carbs. Choose sources like yams, sweet potatoes, turnips, berries, melons and grapes. These sources are all either starchy or have a high glucose:fructose ratio and thus will preferentially fill muscle glycogen. You can also drop protein intake on your carb load day to very low levels: this will allow more room to accommodate your carbs and it makes your system a bit more thrifty with regards to protein usage. Make sure to keep fat intake low (base Zone block levels) on your carb load day or at least for high carb meals.

Low Carb by the Seat of Your Pants

The previous was a very detailed plan and perhaps a bit stifling for some. Here is a seat of the pants approach for the free spirits: 4-7 meals per day, each meal containing 20-50 grams of protein, loads of fibrous, nutrient-dense vegetable matter, and as much fat as you can stand. Every third to fifth day, implement a carb load as per the recommendations above. Pretty damn simple, no? This is the method I have typically gravitated towards. It does not provide one the level of detailed information to follow progress, but it works remarkably well. This is the first time I have mentioned meal frequency but I need to look at that topic separately... so let's get to it!

Fast and Grow Big

Sorry about that heading. It either sounds like very bad grammar or some kind of oxymoronic-hippy, but the smart implementation of intermittent fasting may be a key to success in your Mass Plan. If you are interested in a detailed account of intermittent fasting (IF), you can check out Issue 6 and Issue 16. If you are not interested in the details of IF, shame on you, and here is a minimalist explanation: Brief fasts appear to enhance insulin sensitivity, decrease inflammation, enhance performance, improve anabolic status, favorably alter nutrient partitioning... and possibly increase lifespan. There are two main methods that have been employed: alternation of fasting and eating days—fast day 1; eat like crazy day 2; repeat—or compression of daily eating into a 5-9-hour window (eat all your meals in this time frame and fast the remainder of the day).

Intermittent fasting is in stark contrast to the standard bodybuilding dogma that advocates 6-8 small meals per day and even waking up in the middle of the night for one extra slug of nutrients. That method undoubtedly works, but at what price, and is it really optimal? If one can get that same number of calories in during a six-hour feeding time, are there benefits? We think so. Several people have reported gaining a significant amount of muscle mass on this approach. These same people have had limited success on the "eat all day" plan. You might consider a hybrid approach in which you intermittent fast every second or third day. The benefits of improved insulin sensitivity are remarkable. Give some consideration to this technology.

The Last Straw

This final approach is a recommendation from our good friend, Ido Portal. Ido is an amazing strength coach and a hell of an athlete: he boasts a low 3 minute Fran, 3X BW deadlift, 5% BF level, planche push ups and does workouts like 130 standing back flips for time—he knows what he is doing. Ido's plan involves using the seat-of-your-pants low-carb approach: protein, fat and greens at every meal, carb load every 3-5 days. Protein at a level of 2-3 g/lb of body weight/day... that's a lot! And one small tweak: Ido recommends a post-workout shake that includes 150ml of grape juice, 40g of branched chain amino acids, and 40g of protein powder, preferably whey protein isolate. It's not paleo, and it may spike insulin to amazing levels, but he guarantees its efficacy. Ido is NOT a fan of IF, so he recommends many meals throughout the day. I think IF could improve this situation due to its effects on insulin sensitivity, but Ido is frankly aghast at the idea. The bottom line is that plan is effective—but it requires participants recognize and accept potential consequences of regular, enormous insulin spiking. It's not the healthiest approach, but as a temporarily means to an end, it will likely not kill you before you reach your weight goal.

Lifestyle

Recovery is something that is generally dismissed as inconsequential, but I find that those who ignore this topic are either gifted themselves or focus their efforts on those who have extraordinary natural recovery. What about the genetically average? I saw this in the Capoeira group I was formerly a part of. Super long classes, late hours, after practice parties… Lots of fun to be sure, but what this selected for was the young and the strong. If you were a little older or of average recovery, you were burnt to a crisp by this schedule.

Stay tuned for a thorough accounting of recovery in a future issue, but for now here are a few things to keep in mind:

Sleep: Get 8-10 hours per day if you can. If it gets you fired or divorced, go for less, but try to awake sans alarm.

Fish Oil: Take 3-10 grams per day with meals. Keep capsules frozen to prevent oxidation.

Cryotherapy: Fancy term for sitting in a cold body of water. Eva Twardokens got clever and bought us a watering trough used for livestock. Fill it with cold water. Jump in. If you want it to be very effective, dump a bag of ice in with yourself. Jump in as soon as you can post workout and stay in as long as you can stand. Do not pass out. Do not drown.

Stress: Don't do it. It'll kill ya.

Wrap It

All right, folks, there you have it. A training plan and four different nutritional approaches. Even some help with your rambunctious lifestyle. Remember that this is a long term commitment to make significant progress, and that you may need to temporarily sacrifice some aspects of your fitness like extreme metabolic conditioning to save energy for growth and repair. Once this process is over, however, and you find yourself heavier and much stronger, you can shift gears and see what you can do with that bigger engine.

HYPERTROPHY MESOCYCLE

The hypertrophy mesocycle is a series of 3 hypertrophy microcycles and 1 unloading microcycle (4weeks total). Clean pull % based on clean 1RM.

Hypertrophy Microcycle

Monday
Back Squat: 70% x 6 x 6
Press: 70% x 6 x 6
Weighted Chins: 60% x 6 x 6
Abs-Back Circuit

Tuesday
Rest

Wednesday
Push Press: 70% x 6 x 6
L-pull-up: 60% x 6 x 6
Abs-Back Circuit

Thursday
Rest

Friday
Clean Pull: 80% x 6 x 6
Push-Pull Circuit
Abs-Back Circuit

Saturday
Rest

Sunday
Rest

Hypertrophy Unloading Cycle

Monday
Back Squat: 70% x 3 x 6
Press: 70% x 3 x 6
Weighted Chins: 60% x 3 x 6
Abs-Back Circuit

Tuesday
Rest

Wednesday
Clean Pull: 80% x 3 x 6
Push Press: 70% x 3 x 6
L-pull-up: 60% x 3 x 6
Abs-Back Circuit

Thursday
Rest

Friday
Testing Day: Find 1 RM for movements to be used in the next strength mesocycle

Saturday
Rest

Sunday
Rest

STRENGTH MESOCYCLE

The strength mesocycle is comprised ot 2 strength microcycles and 1 unloading microcycle (3 weeks total).Pull % based on associated lift 1RM; Snatch balance % based on 1RM snatch; Rope Climb % basedon Weighted Pull-up 1RM.

Strength Microcycle

Monday
Back Squat: 80% x 2 x 10
Snatch Pull: 100% x 3, 105% x 3, 110% x 3
Snatch Balance: 5 x 1 (work up to heaviest singlefor the day)

Tuesday
3 Position Cleans: 65% x 3 x 5
1-arm Sotts Press: 30% x 2 x 10
Weighted Pull-ups: 70% x 2 x 10
Abs/Back Circuit

Wednesday
Front Squat: 75% x 2 x 10
Clean Pull: 95% x 3, 100% x 3, 105% x 3
Rack Jerk: Max for day; 80% of that x 1 x 3

Thursday
3 Position Snatch: 65% x 3 x 5
Push-Press: 80% x 2 x 10
Weighted Rope Climb: 10% x 2 x 10
Abs/Back Circuit

Friday
Rest

Saturday
Work up to 1RM Snatch
Work up to 1RM Clean & Jerk
Work up to 1RM Back Squat
Abs/Back Circuit

Sunday
Rest

Strength Unloading Microcycle

Monday
Front Squat: 80% x 1 x 5
Snatch: (60% x 1, 70% x 1, 80% x 1) x 3

Tuesday
Rack Jerk: 80% x 1 x 5
Snatch: 60% x 1 x 10

Wednesday
Back Squat: 75% x 1 x 5
Clean & Jerk: (60% x 1, 70% x 1, 80% x 1) x 3

Thursday
Snatch Balance: 70% x 2 x 4
Clean & Jerk: 60 % x 1 x 10

Friday
Rest

Saturday
Testing Day: find 1RM for movements in next hypertrophy mesocycle

Sunday
Rest

THE BIG KIDS' MUSCLE UP
GREG EVERETT

The muscle-up has become a standard measure of an individual's development in the realm of real fitness (in contrast to the more common measure of the loading of a supinating dumbbell concentration curl). There is a large, bold line separating the haves and have-nots, and those have-nots invest a great deal of time and energy into the pursuit of their monumental first muscle-ups. A very generous definition of the movement—simply getting your center of mass from under to over a pair of rings—seems to have become an acceptable standard. This is unquestionably an accomplishment of which to be proud, but continuing progress demands the development of a strict—or strict—muscle-up.

The rudimentary variation of the muscle-up excludes full extension at both the beginning and end of the movement—the two most difficult points in terms of strength. In addition, epic kips are employed. To clarify, the kip itself is not necessarily problematic—it's an excellent tool for helping develop the pull-up, for example, and has numerous benefits of its own. But in the case of the muscle-up, the kip is used to effectively bypass the transition from under to over—the most technically difficult aspect, and the development of which is necessary for a strict muscle-up. That being the case, continued performance of rudimentary muscle-ups without additional specific work prevents the development of the strict muscle-up.

Power Grab with a False Grip

The idea of optimizing power generation is a popular one—that is, performing a maximal amount of work in minimal time. In this context, the rudimentary muscle-up has found a welcoming home. The elimination of two inches each at the initial and end stages of the movement results in a relatively small reduction in total work because of the movement's unusually great range of motion—more than double that of a squat or pull-up. A reduction of 4 total inches of travel will reduce the work of a pull-up by over 17%, but will only reduce the work of a muscle-up by 9%.

More importantly, because time has a greater influence on power than the distance of travel, the reduced time for completion for the kipped muscle-up results in an enormous increase in power despite the reduction in work resulting from the reduced travel. A muscle-up with a range of motion shortened by 4 inches and performed in 2 second results in greater than 50% more power in comparison to a full range of motion muscle-up completed in 4 seconds.

What this means is fairly simple: depending on your individual objectives, the rudimentary muscle-up may have a place in your training. If your goal is achieving the highest power output possible—for example, for metabolic conditioning—clearly the rudimentary muscle-up is the better choice: it has the potential to deliver far more power than the strict muscle-up because of its high speed of execution.

So What's the Problem?

It's mathematically demonstrable that a muscle-up performed with greater speed, even with a reduced range of motion, results in far greater power output than a strict, full range of motion muscle-up, which by its nature requires more time to execute. So does it make sense to spend time and effort developing a strict muscle-up? That depends on your individual goals (which I assume confidently that you have clearly defined). If your only goals don't extend any further than repeatedly and indefinitely getting your metabolic rocks off, the rudimentary muscle-up will suffice. If, however, you have greater athletic aspirations, the inherent limitations of the rudimentary muscle-up will be an important consideration in your programming.

Once you've achieved a rudimentary muscle-up, performing the movement regularly will undoubtedly result in the ability to perform more and more of the same movement. Eventually, however, the stimulus will not be adequate for continued strength gains (unless you're continuously gaining bodyweight). Imagine deadlifting the same load for ten years—day one, that load may allow you to perform only a single rep. Eventually you'll likely be able to perform several successive reps—some day, you may be able to 100. But the ability to perform 100 reps of a given movement with given a load does not translate into the ability to lift a significantly greater load with that same movement (think Jazzercise practitioners—they can move a two-pound dumbbell about a million times). Beyond a certain threshold, strength development is replaced by local muscular endurance development. To continue developing strength, the resistance must be increased incrementally. This is the most basic concept of resistance training—progressive overload.

This idea results in a fitness progression resembling graphically a stair-step: that is, time must be spent developing a foundation of strength, then building on that strength base a greater degree of metabolic conditioning and stamina. Failure to develop the strength base unavoidably results in eventual stagnation.

The Point, Finally

All of that is simply to say that in order to continue to progress, the development of a strict muscle-up is a necessity—and the repeated performance of the rudimentary muscle-up will never produce this result. Just like you wouldn't (I hope) progress your deadlift though a spastic, limited range of motion, nor should you do so with your muscle-up; a requisite foundation for continued strength development in the movement is the development of the movement in its most precise form.

My personal recommendation is that people make learning the strict muscle-up a priority over achieving the rudimentary muscle-up—that is, they patiently develop both the requisite strength and technique for the strict movement instead of grasping for anything that even vaguely resembles it simply to have one more movement to throw into the metCon pool. The reasons are based on both motor learning and path-dependent transferability. It's very difficult to learn a new movement pattern that is very similar to an existing one: the transition movements of the two muscle-up variations are similar enough to cause neurological learning difficultly, but different enough that the movement pattern of the rudimentary muscle-up will not translate effectively to the strict muscle-up. And in terms of transferability, if you're capable of performing a strict muscle-up, you're without question also capable of performing a rudimentary muscle-up; the inverse, however, is clearly not true.

Developing the Big Kids' Muscle-up

Whether you have several rudimentary muscle-ups already or none at all, the progression to developing the Big Kids' Muscle-up is the same.

False Grip

Just about anyone will tell you the false grip is key number one for a muscle-up. If you're not yet familiar with the term, a false grip is the deep placement of the hand on the rings. A common mistake is gripping the ring on its side—this will result in an awkward support for the pressing portion of the movement. Be sure to place the false grip at the bottom of the ring—remember that this position should be the same you would use during a dip because that's exactly what you'll be transitioning into. Also, the use of chalk to keep the hands dry, particularly when performing multiple successive reps, will help immensely in maintaining the false grip.

Development: Perform static hangs with a perfect false grip. If you're unable to hang with your entire weight, support yourself with your feet initially and incrementally reduce the amount of support over time until it's no longer necessary.

Beginning Extension

As discussed above, the rudimentary muscle-up avoids full arm extension and shoulder opening at the beginning of the movement, and for good reasons—this position is both the most difficult in which to maintain a false grip and from which to initiate a pull-up. Full extension requires the hands be pronated (palms facing forward)—this is necessary to fully open the shoulders.

Development: Practicing the beginning extension can be accomplished in the same way described for the false grip—they are of course conveniently linked.

Transition

The transition of a strict muscle-up often seems far more complicated to many people than it actually is. Typically those who have the most difficulty learning it are those who are already capable of performing kipped muscle-ups, both because of the motor learning obstacles mentioned previously and the frustration that tends to develop when they abruptly go from being able to relatively easily get above the rings to repeatedly stalling below them.

The mechanics are simple—the elbows need to move from under to over the shoulders in order to transition from a pulling position to a pushing position. A common mistake is a staggered transition of the arms—"putting on a sweater." This allows the individual to partially unload one side in order to more easily move the corresponding elbow into position, which then allows them to support themselves at a higher elevation, making the transition of the second elbow shorter and easier. Not only does this look stupid, but it places the individual in a risky position from which it's easy to over rotate forward and do some potentially serious damage to a shoulder. Unlearning this habit is very difficult—the solution is to never develop it.

Learning the transition with barely adequate strength is difficult—this typically encourages a kip—sometimes subtle, more often not—to power through the sticking point. This is a mistake—as mentioned above, overpowering through the transition alters the mechanics enough to make the development of strict mechanics far more difficult. A much better option is to reduce the load to allow perfect technique practice.

Development: Lower your rings to a level at which you can comfortably grasp them with a false grip while seated on the floor, legs extended in front of you. In this case, don't worry about full extension—you're not working on developing that ability here and that extra effort will only take away from the practice of the movement on which we're focusing—but make sure to use the false grip.

From this position, pull the rings to below your armpits—keep them and your elbows as close to your body as possible—rotating them 90 degrees from the initially pronated hand position to a neutral one. At the peak of this pull, quickly flip your elbows back and up to a position above your shoulders. From here, press out, again keeping the rings as close to your body as possible and your elbows pointing backward.

If you struggle to press out after the transition, make sure you really know where your elbows are—they may be lower than it feels like. Get them as high as you can. Pushing the chest forward as if you're attempting to break a sheet of glass with your face (not recommended) will both elevate your elbows and increase the involvement of the chest musculature. Ideally and eventually, the strict muscle-up should be performed with as little forward lean as possible—this requires both greater strength and flexibility.

Pressing Initiation

For many who seemingly have the strength and technique for a strict muscle-up, the sticking point is the initiation of the press out of the bottom immediately following the transition. Most individuals perform bar and ring dips with a comparatively shallow range of motion and suddenly find themselves in a position from which they've never had to initiate a dip and are therefore unable to—don't underestimate the increased difficulty associated with what may appear to be only a minor extension of the range of motion.

Development: Consistently perform your dips through a full range of motion—this should go without saying, but absolute full ROM dips are humblingly difficult even for those appearing strong in the movement and therefore widely avoided. Practice preferentially on rings and with the torso as upright as possible.

Finishing Extension

The rudimentary muscle-up forgoes full extension at the top as well as the bottom. Full extension requires complete elbow extension, active shoulders (in this position, depression of the scapulae—the opposite of a shrug), and partial external rotation of the arms (rotating the rings outward about 45 degrees). It's remarkably common even for individuals who can perform high numbers of successive ring dips for this final extension to be nearly unachievable initially.

Development: Perform static holds on the rings with active shoulders and tight, complete arm extension with the rings turned out. Like with the beginning extension position, partially support your weight with your feet as needed initially. Once static holds in this position have become reasonably easy, practice performing the last inch or two of a ring dip, finishing each rep with a strong, full extension and static hold. Eventually, this should become part of every ring dip you perform.

Other Considerations

The muscle-up is no joke. Obviously it demands a certain level of strength and stability—depending on your current abilities, the requisite degrees of each may be distant, but they're ultimately within reach. Continue developing your pulling and pressing strength—remember, this requires progressive overloading, not just the execution of a continually greater number of reps. Prior to developing the strength for a single bodyweight dip or pull-up, this can be achieved through negatives and/or partially leg-supported reps; following development of higher numbers of bodyweight dips and pull-ups, external weight can be added to the waist or held between the feet. Specificity of movements is important also—that is, false grip pull-ups and dips, both on rings and through absolutely full ranges of motion, will transfer better than any alternative movements.

Shoulder hypoflexibility is a limiting factor for some who would otherwise likely have the strength to perform a strict muscle-up. The combination of practicing the transition as described above and increasing the range of motion of your dips will likely be adequate for developing the requisite degree of flexibility. If you're impatient or want to be even more pro-active, include some specific shoulder stretching to your regular routine.

The Wrap

You now know far more about the muscle-up than you ever imagined necessary. Don't misinterpret this as belittlement of the rudimentary muscle-up—its achievement is cause for its very own celebration and pride. But don't make the mistake of considering it a final accomplishment—it should be a milestone along the path to ultimate studliness.

INTERMITTENT FASTING: CONTRAINDICATIONS
ROBB WOLF

We have received much positive feedback regarding intermittent fasting over the past few months. People have taken the basic premise of a high quality paleo/Zone diet and either compressed their feeding schedule or, in a few cases, adopted an alternate day fast with good success. What type of success? People have reported fat loss, muscle gain, improvements on CrossFit diagnostic WODs and increases in 1 rep max strength efforts. Keep in mind that the people reporting these results are not new trainees but rather athletes at or near the top of their game. That's all pretty nifty, but no matter how good something is there is usually a population that is ill-suited for a given protocol. Could that be the case with intermittent fasting? Well, I think there are a few situations that certainly warrant some caution when implementing IF.

Clinically Obese

Ironically the population that might benefit the most from IF is a group that really needs to be cautious with implementation. Overweight individuals are by definition insulin resistant. This peridiabetic condition lends itself to severe blood sugar crashes when feedings are not consistent. Thus these individuals must eat every 2-3 hours or face severe mood swings, lethargy and for some the difficult to remedy condition of DEATH. Why? Severe insulin resistance can prevent the facilitated diffusion of ketones through membranes such as the blood-brain barrier. This can lead the condition ketoacidosis which is often characterized by both high blood glucose and high blood ketone concentrations. This can lead to a low blood pH… and that can be very bad. What to do? Reestablish euglycemia by implementing a paleo/Zone or cyclic low carb diet. As insulin sensitivity is reestablished brief fasts should be both safe and therapeutic. Keep in mind that insulin resistance has two major contributors. The first is chronically high insulin levels which tend to down regulate the number of insulin receptors. The second factor involves damage to the insulin receptors themselves via non-enzyme mediated glycation due to chronically high blood glucose levels. Individuals with hyperinsulinism not only have fewer insulin receptors but the few they have are in effect broken. That considered, a therapeutic fast could be one of the most effective means of re-establishing insulin sensitivity; however, if the pathology is of sufficient magnitude, ketoacidosis and The Big Nap could occur.

Clinically Busy

With regards to life extension and disease amelioration, caloric restriction and intermittent fasting appear to work via mechanisms in which acute stressors increase the expression of heat shock protein genes (HSPs) and modulate immune function favorably. Sounds good so far, but the key term in the previous sentence is "Acute Stressors". What happens when an otherwise favorable stressor becomes chronic and overwhelms our adaptive ability? The short answer is "Bad Things". Let's look at IF like it's a drug. Drugs have physiologic effects, characteristic dose/response curves and therapeutic ranges. Dose response curves represent what level of physiologic response can be expected for a given dose. For example, how much pain relief one garners from a given dose of aspirin. The therapeutic range is the approximate amount of drug that may be administered and, in general, deliver a beneficial effect. Below the range one experiences little or no effect, and above the range we have too much collateral damage—also called Side Effects. In ideal situations a drug provides benefit at fairly low doses and negative side effects are not experienced until much higher doses. The reality is that most drugs have a fairly narrow window and interestingly things like age, sleep, general health and stress can greatly affect this therapeutic window. As with drugs, so too with intermittent fasting. Some can go a long way. If you are really sick you may need a lot more (remember last month when Dr Seyfried talked about ketogenic diets, fasting and cancer? One might elect to take a much larger IF dose if one is dealing with cancer than if one is simply looking to improve performance). If you are chronically besieged by other stressors, ANY dose of drug (or IF) may be too much. How are you to know? We should have an expectation of intermittent fasting improving body composition and performance. These are immediate, measurable effects. Assuming one starts IF and things go favorably initially but then say one gains a layer of fat about the midsection, sleep is disturbed or performance slumps it may be prudent to alter your dose in some way. That may mean a smaller dose (12 hour fasts instead of 18), fewer doses (every 3 days instead of every 2) or maybe you need the anti-stress effects of a very consistent Zone diet. If your life is VERY complicated and stressful it may be too much to add any type of IF to the mix. Always keep in mind that a surefire way to ruin your health and athleticism is to not eat sufficiently during an intermittent fasting protocol. Don't do it. You won't like it.

Medicated

In addition to the situations I described above remember that Dr. Seyfried mentioned extended fasts can alter liver metabolism and thus alter clearance rates of drugs. If you are heavily medicated (I wish I were right now), seek medical advice before jumping into this.

A MORE CIVILIZED APPROACH TO BLEEDING: BLOOD DONATION
GREG EVERETT

The promotion of blood donation is invariably approached from the angle of altruism. Promotional strategies emphasize the need for 38,000 pints of blood every day in the US—a pint almost every 2 seconds—for the regular and emergency treatment of a range of individuals, from cancer patients to burn victims to premature infants (who are in all probability thoroughly adorable).

But hat if you're cruel, selfish and uncaring by nature? It turns out there might be some good reasons for you to donate too.

The most common reasons to be found in the research are predicated on excess iron storage. Iron is requisite to human and most non-human life on the planet. In the body, iron's primary function is aiding the transport of oxygen by red blood cells as hemoglobin, but it also plays a number of other roles, including assisting in the synthesis of DNA, collagen, and other protein structures. At the same time, iron poses serious risks to life as a potent pro-oxidant. Because of this, the treatment of iron by the body is remarkably careful: the absorption, distribution and storage of iron is reliant on a well integrated system of protein structures that prevent iron's direct exposure to the rest of the body.

Iron Absorption & Storage

There are two types of dietary iron: heme and non-heme. Heme iron is the form found in meat and is the more efficiently absorbed type (15% - 35%). Non-heme is found in plant foods and is less easily absorbed (2% - 20%), although its absorption rate is more greatly influenced by accompanying dietary factors. Meat, vitamin C and fructose all enhance the absorption of non-heme iron, while soy, calcium, phytates (nutrient-binding protein found in grains) and tannins and polyphenols (both found in tea) reduce its absorption.

When dietary iron enters the guts, it is taken up into enterocytes, epithelial cells lining the walls of the intestine. If systemic iron levels are low enough to require uptake, the iron is encased by the transferrin molecule and distributed through the body as appropriate. Otherwise the iron remains in the enterocytes, which regularly die and pass from the body, bringing the unabsorbed iron along. Average daily iron loss though mechanisms such as sweating, urination, and the regular sloughing of integumentary components is around 0.9 mg (pre-menopausal women may lose an additional 15-20 mg per month through menstruation). These losses are easily covered by anything that remotely resembles a decent diet.

So in theory, this combination of controlled absorption and regular dietary replenishment should maintain ideal iron levels in the body. Unfortunately it's not a flawless system, particularly when challenged by unnatural modern factors.

Nearly all grain foods in the US are fortified with easily absorbable iron. Many people take daily multivitamin/mineral supplements with sometimes enormous amounts of iron. High-fructose corn syrup is used to sweeten nearly every packaged food in addition to soda. In short, there is an epic assortment of variables that can potentially override the body's controlled absorption system and leave us with more iron in storage than we need.

The body has no internal mechanism for excreting excess iron. It simply contains it in protective protein molecules and stores it in tissues, preferentially glandular tissue such as that of the liver and pancreas. In the past, humans did have a way of dropping excess iron—we were full of parasites, creating continuous minor gastrointestinal bleeding—iron contained in the hemoglobin was in this fashion dumped from the body. This constant blood loss was likely the reason we evolved with mechanisms to protect iron and none to eliminate it.

Those of us living in developed areas of the world are now free of the parasitic bleeding that reduces iron stores, but also subject to unnatural foods that are either fortified with iron, enhance the absorption of iron, or both. Over years, this can result in dangerously high levels of iron in the body.

So What's the Problem?

The primary problem with iron is its pro-oxidant characteristics: it's very good at helping create free radicals—molecules with unpaired electrons with consequently low stability and high reactivity—such as the hydroxyl radical.

In heart attacks and strokes, the bulk of the tissue damage is actually not due to oxygen deprivation, but instead to the re-introduction of oxygen. When an artery is occluded, tissues beyond the blood's reach are deprived of the accompanying oxygen and begin dying. Necrotic cell death is not orderly—pieces essentially fall apart freely—and this allows the free exposure of formerly safely stored iron. When the vessel occlusion is repaired, whether medically or naturally, a huge influx of blood bathes these broken tissues and the exposed iron, which reacts with the new oxygen. This violent reaction can result in severe tissue damage.

Excessive iron storage may also be a factor in the development of certain cancers such as of the liver, atherosclerosis, reduced insulin production and insulin resistance. The research on which these ideas are founded is—like almost all research in similar areas—not conclusive, but does appear relatively convincing.

Regular flushing and replacement of iron also means the body will have fresh material for hemoglobin and other iron-dependent structures instead of relying on continual recycling. The benefit of this is entirely speculative, but no potential drawbacks seem to exist.

Testing Your Iron Level

If you're interested in having your stored iron level tested, don't let your doctor test your hemoglobin level—this is common but inaccurate method. Instead, ask for a serum ferritin test, which measures the amount of ferritin in the blood. This number is 10 times lower than your iron level; that is, if your serum ferritin number is 70, you have 700 mg of stored iron. Certain individuals may show inaccurately high ferritin levels, including alcoholics and those with infections, severe inflammation, and cancer.

A healthy amount of stored iron is around 500 mg. 1000 mg may be problematic. 150 mg is a safe low-end threshold. Less than 100 mg is indicative of iron-deficiency anemia.

Donating Blood

Getting rid of blood is not hard—there are a lot of people out there more than happy to relieve you of some. They won't even charge you for it.

My own blood donations have been consistently positive experiences. Aside from enjoying scintillating conversation with the lovely phlebotomists and volunteer post-drainage babysitters who like to remind me I was born in 1980 while making continual subtle advances toward my defiant position with the donut tray, I've noticed a significant improvement in energy in the days following the donations. I've also been perfectly able to train at adequate intensity and volume within several hours of donation, despite my repeated and convincing assurances to my concerned caretakers that I would never dream of engaging in such reckless behavior—but of course my longstanding habit of lying to women is not relevant to this particular discussion. Performance in high-metabolic-demand training such as CrossFit will be below average with a pint less blood in your system, but generally donation frequency is limited to eight weeks—a regular blood donation schedule that coincides with a week of limited training volume and intensity could be a simple method of ensuring periodic active recovery in your long-term training strategy.

The bottom line is actually very simple: while the potential health benefits of regularly donating blood have yet to be demonstrated conclusively, with proper nutrition and lifestyle, and with consideration of known contraindications, blood donation poses little if any risk. That being the case, the prudent course of action is to make regular blood donation a habit. The worst case scenario is that your blood helps save the life of some cute little baby and your metabolic conditioning is compromised for a week every two months.

American Red Cross
www.givelife.org

POWER BIAS: PART 2
ROBB WOLF

Waaay back in issue 11 I introduced some material I called the Power Bias. In that issue we looked at some strategies for pushing power output of CrossFit WODs further towards max power. To do this I encouraged the use of ballistic/plyometric type movements such as clapping pull-ups and push-ups, jump squats and medicine ball throw sit-ups. This month I want to look at a few ways to squeeze more juice out of your programming by examining intervals in the context of mixed modal training. Some might call it intervals within intervals. These people are myopic, sarcopenic and generally do not get out much, but that is the gist of this piece. What I am proposing straddles a no-mans land between metabolic conditioning and peak power production. I'm a greedy, biased bastard (at lest where power is concerned) and I want it all.

First I want to sell you on why this is a good approach, and to do so we need to look at some key elements such as peak and average power as well as a few other goodies.

First There Was Matter And Energy...

I'm sure you folks remember that Work is defined as Force X Distance (w=fd) and Power is work per unit time (P=w/t). Contrary to propaganda from the Young Physicists Association of America, spouting these equations willy-nilly will not help your dating life. They do however help to conceptualize relative work and power outputs. Work is typically associated with some measure of power, as any activity requires some amount of time to complete. Thus, whenever we measure or think about work, we should consider power as well. OK, if you are still awake I do not think there are any arguments about the Wee-Ones physics lesson. So here is my main point: If power output is synonymous with intensity (this works for Pavel-esque definition of percentage of 1 rep max, but I am thinking more along the CrossFit/HIT puke in your shoes scenario) what is our best approach to optimizing power output and the associated adaptations? Also, what is most important, average power or absolute power?

Let me use the CrossFit classic Helen (3 rounds for time of a 400 m run, 21 1.5 Pd. KB swings, 12 pull-ups) as an example. The world Record (to my knowledge) is 7:35 by Greg Amundsun. That is flat out moving, but let's look at where time is allocated in this workout. Three rounds of 21 KB swings and 12 pull-ups means 63 kb swings and 36 pull-ups (we will look at the 1,200m of running broken into 3 pieces in a moment). From video analysis, KB swings and pull-ups require 1.25-1.5 seconds per cycle. For this analysis we will assume a bit slower cycle time on these movements. The reason for this is that a multi round workout of this type necessitates a moderate (relative) approach if one is to survive and turn in the best AVERAGE time. Although this is a grueling workout, I'm not sure it is where maximum adaptations lie… but I'm getting ahead of myself.

Back to accounting: we are looking at 99 total movements performed at an average rate of 1.5 sec/cycle with a total time spent on pull-ups and swings of 148 seconds. This is an estimate, but again, from video analysis this is quite close. Now, Greg completes this workout in 7:35 which is 455 seconds. If we subtract the Pull-up/swing time from the total, we will have the time to complete all three 400m runs (455-148=307 seconds). Dividing 307 by 3 gives us an average 400m time of about 102 seconds. Like I said previously, that is really moving, and that time represents a remarkable degree of power output, ON AVERAGE. But what if this scenario was altered a little? What if Greg performed the same amount of work divided like this:

400m SPRINT- 2 Minutes rest
21 KB swings AS FAST AS POSSIBLE (1.25s/cycle)-2 min rest
12 pull-ups AS FAST AS POSSIBLE,-2 Minutes rest
Repeat the circuit 2 more times.

This alteration brings 400m times down to the 60-70 sec range, and cuts 0.25 second off each swing and pull-up repetition. In essence, peak power is greatly increased.

Lucy, You Got Some 'Splainin

Now I need to back up a little and make the point that mixed mode (classic CrossFit) training is both hard and efficacious. Taxing one energy system/movement pattern and then shifting to another to increase systemic demand is good stuff, but the power output and potential adaptations of the 7:35 Helen vs the Interval Helen are similar to the differences between the mile and 200-400m sprints. Bold statement? Not really, just a Power Bias. "We" (coaches, scientists, smarty pants PMenu readers) have known for a very long time that interval training is beneficial for building endurance at both high and low power outputs. More recently, a study in the Journal of Applied Physiology showed that bouts of 30-second sprint intervals produced marked improvements in aerobic capacity. You may be wondering what the hell happened? Weren't we talking power? Now "aerobic capacity" is tossed around? Well, yes. It's a dirty word (or concept), but I'm interested in how we can have the best of both worlds. How can we be strong, explosive AND have crushing levels of cardiovascular capacity. There are limits to this scenario, and I will touch on that later, but see if this all makes sense, then go out and try it and see what happens. For now, look at what Stephen Seiler has to say about intervals

So back to the interval Helen. Why might this approach be efficacious for improving power output? Why might one want to allocate some training time to this interval-interval format? One answer comes from an editorial in the same issue of the Journal of Applied Physiology as the above study and is actually in response to those findings. Loads of good information can be found in this editorial but the money shot is most assuredly this paragraph:

"It is likely that the potency of all-out sprint interval training is derived in large part from the high level of motor unit activation. All-out sprint training especially stresses recruitment and adaptation of type II (i.e., fast twitch) muscle fibers that are remarkably and equally responsive as type I (i.e., slow twitch) muscle fibers in their ability to increase mitochondrial enzyme activity to high absolute levels (4, 5, 7). In fact, the low-intensity aerobic exercise that is typically prescribed for endurance training or health is not very effective at increasing aerobic enzyme activity in type II muscle fibers, which comprise approximately one-half of the fibers within the thigh (vastus) and calf (gastrocnemius) muscle in most people (6). Thus low-intensity aerobic training is not a very effective or efficient method for maximizing aerobic adaptations in skeletal muscle because it generally does not recruit type II muscle fibers".

One finds maximum adaptations ONLY when one achieves maximum recruitment of the fast twitch fibers and this can only happen for limited periods of time (intervals) otherwise power output (fiber recruitment) drops below what is likely an optimum level. If we segment mixed mode workouts like Helen, we can reach near maximum power output many, many times on a variety of movements. That's the theory. Our clinical experience has been interesting for both our top-end and raw beginners, and it reflects self-similarity. Our top-end athletes find the interval Helen to be brutal. They report peaks of discomfort not achievable with the standard Helen in which one endeavors to clock the best average time. That said, the small break between elements allows for some relief and the thought, "Just a little more, then I can rest." Most importantly, most have found an improvement in the non-interval Helen after a few exposures to this variant. For our beginners, comments are along the lines of, "The workout seems less overwhelming." Our beginners clock greater peak intensity both in magnitude and duration with this method. As I think all of you know, intensity is where we find the adaptations which we are interested.

A great question is why is this format not used more frequently? This format does not lend itself well to large groups. Timing every interval becomes impossible unless a large wall clock (or wrist watch for each client) is used and the clients track their own rest intervals. The second problem with this method is it does not create a "top dog". If the focus is "who is elite among this group" the interval method is decidedly unsatisfying. Noting beats a pack of people starting on a foot race and encountering obstacles in the form of pull-ups and KB swings! People will even watch marathons on television! At the end a definitive winner is established, as are the also-rans. This format can be a powerful motivator but if one has shifted coaching to one-on-one training, the interval method can bring about this competitive edge by pitting the client against SELF. Each round is an opportunity to best previous efforts and it affords the coach greater opportunity to provide performance crucial cues. We use 1-2 large group, classic CF style WODs each month as a "Game Day" workout… but that is another article.

Outer Limits

When the term "Elite Fitness" or "Elite Athletics" is tossed around, it is important to define the testing parameters. For example if you hear the phrase, "We have the fittest athletes in the world…" I think it quite important to ask the question "Fit for WHAT?" I think the CrossFit definition of fitness (http://www.crossfit.com/cf-download/CFJ-trial.pdf) is the most all encompassing I've ever seen. Arthur Devany offers a similar definition and I think both border on genius. That's nifty, but what if we are talking the elite levels of Olympic lifting, 100-200m sprinting, high jumping, javelin, shot-put and a host of other activities? Being "Fit" for these activities means having a mountain of type IIb (fast, non-oxidative, easily fatigued) fibers. If one is born with a bunch of these highly coveted fibers and one engages in loads of sprint intervals, Fran's, Helen's… essentially bathe the muscle in lactate, this person will now be fit for MMA, boxing, and being a cop, but they are most assuredly NOT fit for elite power sports. Does this type of mixed modal training have application with these athletes? Sure, off season, changing things up, addressing body composition issues and improving connective tissue integrity, but drop a few of these WODs into the lineup a few weeks out from competition for a power athlete and watch a contender become an also-ran.

Some have mentioned success with powerlifting and the use of mixed modal activities, but the powerlifter simply needs to complete the movements under any time frame, frequently up to 5 seconds for max efforts. When type IIb fibers are taxed, they convert to more fatigue resistant type IIa fibers that are slower (lower power) but are capable of the same maximum force. This works for powerlifters as evidenced by WestsideBarbell (http://www.westside-barbell.com/) and their successful inclusion of copious GPP and lactate tolerance work. Power athletes of the types I've mentioned, however, cannot tolerate this fiber conversion if they are to be "elite". Some have also made the point it is important to be a craftsman and not a tool peddler. Too true. This must be said of mixed modal training. It is a tool that is enormously beneficial when used appropriately. It is not, however, the cure for all ills athletic.

Wrap

In simple terms "we" will never have the power capabilities of true power athletes using mixed mode activities. That said, the only way to push the envelope and have as much of both worlds as possible is to strive to be stronger at fundamental movements. This can be achieved by an integrated approach such as the ME Black Box or blocks of training alternating between max strength development and strength-endurance (metCon) work. Ultimately the movements used within metCon activities must shift towards those activities that allow for peak power production if we are to become truly Power Biased.

THE OLYMPIC WEIGHTLIFTING SQUAT
GREG EVERETT

The squat is foundational to the Olympic lifts as a position, a movement and a strength exercise. Without a well-developed and consistent squat, neither pulling technique nor pulling power will produce entirely successful Olympic weightlifting. The great natural physical variation among athletes dictates that there will never be a universally perfect prescription for body positioning, but irrespective of this variation, the fundamental principles remain consistent. Continued reliance on them will ensure that modifications from the strict prescription are rational and sound instead of haphazard and likely improper.

Because the squat, more so than any other element of the lifts, will be affected by temporary impediments such as limited flexibility, a greater deal of modification will be necessary and allowable during an athlete's advancement. However, even in the cases of lifters for whom the strictest positioning prescription is initially impossible, this prescription will remain the ultimate goal, and continued efforts toward that end should be made.

Be cautious of defying the underlying principles with the excuse of individual variation—often this is inappropriately cited when the actual cause of an athlete's inability to adhere to these prescriptions is entirely correctable over time, such as flexibility-related limitations or simply stubborn habits. It's necessary to critically evaluate each athlete individually to make accurate determinations—avoid allowing an athlete to continue poor habits due simply to laziness or frustration with slow progress and, more importantly, increase the risk of injury.

Depth

The depth of an Olympic squat should not even be a topic of discussion, but because there has been and continues to be discussion among coaches and athletes in sports outside of weightlifting, it warrants at least clarification: proper depth is full depth; full depth means full depth. That is, full depth is not parallel, nor is it breaking parallel—it is squatting to the lowest position possible without surgical alteration of body parts while maintaining correct posture. To simplify, we want to close the knee joint maximally while maintaining a correctly arched back.

Depth is measured by the position of the hips, and the depth of the hips is governed by the position of the knees, the degree of dorsiflexion of the ankles, the absolute and relative lengths of the upper and lower leg, the horizontal position of the hips relative to the feet, the width and degree of external rotation of the feet, and the mass of the upper and lower legs. These factors are largely interdependent, and a change in one will typically effect change in others.

If the knees are prevented from moving forward over the feet, as is taught by many coaches and trainers, the hips must travel farther back behind the feet. With the hips behind the athlete's base, the torso must be inclined forward to a greater degree in order for the athlete's center of mass to remain balanced over the feet. If the hips are lowered from this position, flexibility will restrict the spine's ability to remain correctly arched, forcing the athlete to curl forward, again to remain balanced. For what should be fairly obvious reasons, neither of these positions will allow the safe and effective support of a barbell in the positions it must be received in the snatch and clean. (Note that very short-legged athletes will be able to achieve a proper squat depth and position without the knees passing significantly forward of the toes.) Moving the knees in front of the toes is not a goal itself, but something that must be allowed to happen in order to achieve the depth and trunk orientation we need.

Inadequate ankle flexibility can also result in the knees remaining too far back— if the ankles are unable to dorsiflex to a great enough degree, the lower leg cannot reach an angle sufficient to bring the knees into a position that allows the hips to reach their intended placement. This is the reason for the lifted heel of weightlifting shoes—elevation of the heel effectively increases the ankles' range of motion.

Femur length will affect the depth of each athlete's squat simply by dictating how far away from the knees the hips will be. Athletes with great flexibility and long femurs will display extraordinarily deep squat positions, while their shorter-femured counterparts will appear higher even when at their maximal depth. For some athletes, femur length will exceed what can be compensated for through ankle flexibility in the basic squat position, and adjustments will need to be made to allow a better bottom position.

For individuals with largely muscled legs and who are capable of very upright torso positions in the bottom of the squat, the hips may not be particularly low relative to the knees even when the knees are closed completely.

The Basic Squat Position

As the base from which all movement and positioning originates, the placement of the feet will dramatically influence the squat. The width of the stance and degree of external rotation will affect the movement and position of the hips and back, and will often be the deciding factor in whether a squat is successful or failed, mechanically sound or injurious. Individual variation notwithstanding, the feet must be positioned in a manner that allows and encourages proper biomechanics of the legs, hips and back, while allowing the greatest possible range of motion and supporting the unique positional and movement characteristics of the Olympic lifts.

Anthropometrics—in particular relative leg segment lengths—and hip anatomy will dictate appropriate width and rotation of the feet. Flexibility limitations and similar impediments may prevent an athlete from immediately achieving this ultimately proper positioning, but again, these are temporary obstacles that should be corrected.

The starting foot placement will be slightly outside hip-width at the heels with the toes turned out comfortably—generally between approximately 20-35 degrees from center. With the athlete sitting at the bottom of the squat in this basic position, adjustments can be quickly made according to leg segment and trunk lengths, hip anatomy, and ankle and knee alignment to place him or her in the proper position.

From here, there are two basic criteria with which we're concerned: When viewed from directly above, the foot and thigh are approximately parallel with each other; when viewed from the front of the toe, the foot is approximately underneath the knee. The hips should sit in between the heels somewhat; in other words, the heel will not be directly under the thigh, but slightly outside of its centerline. This positioning will keep the knees and ankles aligned well, but will also allow for slightly improved depth, and, more importantly, a more absorptive bottom position—that is, the final position will be structurally sound without having an abrupt and jarring stop.

With these relationships established—assuming the hips are at full possible depth—the remaining positional relationships will be unavoidably correct. This allows for a wide range of potential external rotation—athletes will in general naturally find what is most comfortable for them. That said, some athletes will need to be told explicitly to spread the knees farther than they wish; occasionally athletes will prefer a stance that prevents the hips from reaching adequate depth between the thighs due to the structures of the upper thighs being pushed into the forward edges of the pelvis. If the athlete is unable to achieve adequate depth and back extension, particularly if he or she is also feeling pressure near the front of the hips, a more externally rotated stance is more than likely needed.

What this positioning achieves is simple but important—biomechanically sound alignment of the involved joints, optimizing performance and reducing the risk of injury.

These relationships of the feet and leg segments should be maintained for the duration of the movement—in other words, the knees should follow the line described by the angle of the feet as the athlete descends and recovers. For many athletes, this will, at least initially, require they consciously make an effort to push the knees out to the sides as the tendency will be for the knees to collapse inward.

From this basic position, there will be a degree of adjustment possible without considerable violation of these relationships. That is, once in this starting position, the athlete will find he or she can move the feet in and out and turn the toes in and out slightly and continue to meet the criteria fairly well. This small range will allow some latitude for personal preference, and the lifter is encouraged to experiment within this range until the most comfortable position is found.

The effect of hip width on foot placement should be self-explanatory—this is the origin of the legs and consequently the starting point for the stance. Relative leg segment length affects how far back the foot travels relative to the thigh as the knee flexes. The longer the lower leg is relative to the upper leg, the farther toward the hip the foot will be when the knee is closed—this means that the longer the lower leg is relative to the upper leg, the closer the feet will be in a sound squat position. In other words, the overall length of the legs is not enough to determine squat stance—how that length is created is what matters.

The foot position should be identical for all squat variations—back squat, front squat, overhead squat—and all receiving positions except the split in the jerk—snatch, clean, power snatch, power clean, power jerk, squat jerk. Many athletes will assume different foot positions for each type of squat—this is an indicator that the athlete has not learned and developed a correct squat position, and is likely in need of improved flexibility.

BASIC PRINCIPLES OF STRENGTH AND CONDITIONING FOR RUGBY UNION
JAMES EVANS

"I think it is fair to say that as a nation we are more concerned and interested in the playing of an organized game than with the tedious but necessary business of getting fit and mastering the basic skills. Most players, at all levels, prefer to play less well with less training and coaching rather than work really hard to become better performers."
--Gerwyn Williams, Modern Rugby, 1964

Despite the fact, or perhaps in spite of the fact, that Rugby Union at the highest level became a professional sport nearly 12 years ago, I think that Gerwyn Williams's words still ring true. Regardless of the huge increases in size and strength seen amongst the game's top players, rugby remains mostly a sport played by admittedly pretty physical men, and women, with a generally amateur and social ethos. This has always been one of the wonderful things about the sport as a whole: a game for people of all shapes and sizes who smash seven bells out of each other for 80 minutes before enjoying a beer—or many beers—together in the clubhouse afterwards. In many circles, training has been positively frowned upon.

Sadly, while this may be one of the great things about rugby, it is completely counterproductive to bringing off decent performances on the pitch. If you want to participate in a sport where you put nothing in away from the field of competition, go and play golf. I have played rugby when I've been off the pace and I've hated it. And I've played rugby when my team mates have been off the pace and I've hated them. I enjoy tackling, but I do not enjoy tripling my tackle count because I'm the only one doing it. I'm not challenging the great spirit of the game; I'm commenting that playing a very physical contact sport with little preparation seems to me to be mindless.

Every rugby player can get stronger and faster and for longer. On paper the ways and means are really not rocket science.

The (Very) Basics of Rugby

I've quite often seen posts on sites like Crossfit.com requesting advice regarding rugby training and noticed that they usually do not get answered or if they do, get answered badly. Indeed it was a question on the Performance Menu forum that led me to finally give some answers myself. The silly thing is that the internet has brought a wealth of information to anyone able to post on a message board should they bother to look. In comparison to the in-depth discussion on the correct way to perform Moldavian Fanny Hammers (barbell or cable stack?), it's quite poor. But the stuff is there. Even in the UK the source material with regards to actual books on the subject is limited so I realise the USA will be at a considerable disadvantage. One problem is often the people searching for answers are really not that familiar with the game. So let's have a look at it.

Rugby is a sport played at high intensity by two teams of 15 players over a period of 80 minutes. Players require stamina, strength, power, speed and flexibility. You could take the attitude that the dominant attributes of a middle distance runner, an Olympic weightlifter, an NFL lineman, a 100 metre sprinter and a gymnast all blended together would make the Frankenstein's perfect rugby player. Complicating this is the makeup of the 15 players in a team, all require these attributes but in varying degrees. Each position has differing fitness and, very importantly, skill requirements. Backs are characterised by their speed and mobility (and usually their ability to handle the ball) running for lengths varying between 10–60 metres. Forwards are typically of much bigger builds and are required to do much more work in a game, typically tackling, mauling, hitting the ball up in 5–15 metre bursts alongside the set piece work of the scrum and lineout. Strength and stamina are at a premium for forwards.

Let's break down the positions further:

15. Fullback Speed is a big requirement for the modern fullback because that makes him very dangerous in the counterattack and as an extra player in the attacking line. Speed is also necessary for the cover tackling and other defensive work required of the fullback. The player is the last line of defence and the ability to knock an opponent down in a one on one tackle, often head on, require good strength alongside technique

14/11 Wings The fastest players on the field, wings are there to score tries. There is no substitute for pace on the rugby field. Rugby is not necessarily about linear speed and the ability to change direction is vital to all backs, but out and out pace is what we are talking about here. It is not uncommon for wings to display the greatest relative strength amongst their team mates.

13/12 Centres The pairing of 12 and 13 can display different attributes (a playmaker alongside a basher) or be identical in make up. Here is not the place to debate this but the centre should have good speed, exceptional acceleration and power to both break and make tackles. Centres are likely to have much heavier forwards running at them and the strength to deal with this is vital. The outside centre tends to have the furthest to run when the back line realigns in both defence and attack and this can hit the stamina reserves.

10 Fly Half Fly halves are the generals of a side, the closest to a quarterback. Like centres, acceleration is a must alongside good speed generally. They are often slighter in build than the other backs and alongside regularly being the most talented player on the field can go the mantle of being a show boating puss. Tackling is not optional for any player, especially fly halves and opposition back row forwards are always going to run hard down the 10's channel. Dan Carter of New Zealand is the world's best fly half if not best player full stop. He knocks people backwards in the tackle as did Jonny Wilkinson of England before his body broke down. Fly halves need to lift weights and bring a level of physicality to their game.

9 Scrum Half The 9 is often the smallest player on the field (an exception would be the 6' 3" Mike Griffiths of Wales). Excellent endurance is required to follow the forwards through play and make the ball available to the fly half. The scrum half is the link between the backs and the forwards. Speed off the mark allows for breaks from the scrum and the ruck. Good strength levels the playing field for a position that finds you often tangling with forwards enjoying a 56 lb advantage over you.

6/7/8 Back Row (Flankers and No. 8) The back row are ball winners, tacklers and ball carriers. Their endurance levels must be up there with the scrum half. They need the strength to make tackles and rip the ball from their opponent. Power from the base of the scrum allows them to make hard yards. They are the transition between the requirements of being a back and being a forward. A decent vertical jump gives their side added line out options.

4/5 Second Row Usually the tallest players in a side (at international level anything between 6'4" and 6'10") the second row must provide ball from the lineout and provide the drive from the engine in the scrum. Since lifting was permitted in the lineout, pure jumping ability has not been as necessary because the second row will be lifted by a prop who is built like an ox. Second rows in the modern game should be able to make repeated bursts with the ball in hand, driving into the opposition forwards. Upper body strength is necessary for tackling and mauling for the ball.

1/3 Props The players with the highest levels of absolute strength. Strength is a must across legs, back, arms, and traps. They need to scrummage strongly and lift their jumpers in the lineout. Props are the players who look closest to powerlifters and strongman competitors. Modern rugby has put a lot of emphasis on the increased mobility of props. In the past they just walked from scrum to scrum and existed purely to practice the black arts of the front row. They are now expected to run around the park, carrying the ball forward and making tackles. Some, and we are talking about 250-lb-plus guys here, will have startling 40 metre times. This is a good thing but nonetheless if you're a prop and you cannot scrummage then you are as useful as a chocolate fireguard to your side.

2 Hooker This player should combine the attributes of the prop with that of the back row. A dynamic, powerful hooker is an asset to the team. Unfortunately many hookers haven't got over the fact that they haven't been picked in the back row and don't spend enough time practising their key skills: throwing the ball in at the lineout and hooking for the ball in the scrum.

That was a pretty simplistic look at the positions; now let's think about the game as a whole. Consider the following:

1. A study originated within the New Zealand camp in the early 1990s suggested that the ball was actually in play during an international game for 25 out of the full 80 minutes. That's just over a quarter of the match. For 25 minutes you are running, tackling, pushing, jumping, being smashed to the ground. The remainder of the game you are standing around with your hands on your hips listening to the self-important interjections of the referee, waiting for a player to receive medical treatment (the clock stops for this in the top level games), or watching someone climb over a fence to retrieve the sole match ball that has been kicked from the field of play. In the highest echelons of the professional game the number of minutes will often be higher, although not always. Yet it won't really have changed much at the amateur level particularly as skill levels will be lower leading to more technical infringements and therefore stoppage of play. To train for rugby you need to be preparing for 30 minutes of actual power based bursts of activity interspersed with jogging/walking/standing breaks. A forward will move more for most of the game. A wing can stand alone for 70 minutes and then suddenly be given the opportunity to win the match with a run to the try line from 45 metres out. I've stood on the wing for a full 80 minutes and the ball hasn't come near me and nor has anything else. That's a tedious way to spend an afternoon.

2. The following is derived from The Rugby League Coaching Manual by Phil Larder. It applies equally to both codes of Rugby. A rugby pitch is 100 metres long, goal to goal, maximum. Imagine a fullback or a wing counterattacks from his own try line. He covers 100 metres of the pitch (assuming he just breaks the defensive line and heads straight up field, more allowing for dummying/swerving/sidestepping/changes of angle). Just before scoring a stunning try he is tackled and stripped of the ball, his opponent immediately launching an attack in the opposite direction. Grimly our man gets to his feet and tracks back in defence at top speed. In total he covers 200 metres. This is very rarely going to happen, certainly never going to happen for a front five forward. Even a 100 metre all out sprint is going to be unusual. The ability to run 5, 10, 20, 30 metre sprints though, often involving a collision, is going to be necessary.

Theories of Rugby fitness

In the UK we tend to view the USA as a land of overweight burger-stuffers. Please don't take this too personally—I have a point to make here. This denies our own sad state of the nation. Britain suffers from rising obesity, chronic heart disease, binge drinking, etc. Sport has been systematically eradicated from the nation's state funded schools. Recreation fields are being built upon to meet the demand for affordable housing. I run to a park where I believe there to be pull up and dip bars and the dip bars have been vandalized and the pull up bars built for elves. Our understanding of nutrition is chronically deficient. The rise of a multi-million pound fitness industry where people go to Fitness First once a month to walk for ten minutes on a treadmill, complete a set of lat pull downs and dream of Brad's abs does not make this better. When I read about the things the likes of Dan John and Mike Burgener get their kids to do at school I'm astounded. An American can walk into Wal-Mart and buy a kettlebell; I live in London and I have to get a blacksmith in Yorkshire to make me one and fly it to London.

I'm simplifying matters, I know, but bear with me.

What I'm getting at here is that although we have a long tradition of sport in this country, we don't have the physical culture of the US. Many rugby players are big guys because, well, they happen to be big guys. They have started the game at early age, discovered an aptitude for the sport, often because of their physiques, and stuck with it. The idea of a game for people of all shapes and sizes is very misleading. Yes, props are traditionally seen as hulking potbellied brutes and scrum halves as little whippets, but many people have tried and abandoned the game because they don't suit it. A man of 6'7" is going to have an easier career than a man of 5'7" who lacks speed.

Another defining factor of the past concerns social background. The private school methods seen in the UK have of course seen a lot of players graduate to the senior game. I went to a public school that took rugby very seriously; in fact the fixture between Cheltenham and Rugby School (after which the game is named) is the oldest fixture in the sport. We were in extremely good shape at school, but we could have been much better. A constant diet of push ups, interval sprints, burpees if we were lucky, and a bitch of a three-mile run if we were really very lucky, half of which was up an increasingly steep hill, certainly had its benefits. I also think that a lot of rugby skills and drills if performed properly do condition you and we did lots of them. On the other hand, though, weight training for example was almost unheard of. I learned about lifting through rowing; in fact I learned about most intelligent training through rowing, not rugby. What I did get from rugby was a high volume of actually playing rugby. I've heard many times that you cannot actually get fit from playing a sport. I totally disagree within certain conditions, mostly dependent on position. I played in the back row until I was 17 when I moved out to the backs and there I felt my conditioning levels drop off because I didn't have to do as much in a game anymore. I think this applies to all positions outside the forwards and the scrum half.

What made us good at any sport at school was that we trained five days a week and ate and slept properly. My week could look like this:

Monday: Circuit training; weights with the Rowing Club.

Tuesday: Rugby practice for around 1 1/2 hours (this normally followed by a 20-minute knock around game with my friends)

Wednesday: Some sort of physical activity: a long run, knock around game of rugby, game of soccer, etc.

Thursday: Rugby practice as per Tuesday followed by circuit training and weights with the Rowing club.

Friday: Around 70 minutes of rugby practice working on moves, set plays, etc. for the competitive match on Saturday.

Saturday: Match day

Sunday: Couple of hours out with my dogs working on my kicking and sprinting. Other than after the odd benching session in the gym, I didn't know what muscle soreness was as a teenager

This was interspersed with the general fooling around with friends, pull up and press up challenges, quick games of soccer, etc. that teenage boys cram into their lives.

And this all seemed to work, but it ignored the fact that we had a well equipped gym, we had a running track and we had a swimming pool. If I had been a prop, for instance, I might have left school with a fairly high level of technique, but I don't believe that I would have been physically prepared for stepping up a level.

Rugby is often seen as a very middle class sport, but that is unfair. In the past many players came from physically demanding jobs or jobs that demanded these players to be physically capable. So alongside the privately educated individual who carried on their rugby (and often the other sports that they were equally talented in) at university and beyond to their working careers, rugby players included farmers, miners, construction workers, policemen, firemen, soldiers. These guys got their conditioning from their jobs and fit in alongside the doctors, lawyers and bankers.

This is not to be underestimated. The relative decline of Welsh rugby from the 1970s onward has often been linked to the closure of mines and steelworks. Rugby in New Zealand and Wales has been intrinsically linked with farming. Colin Meads of New Zealand, a player who trained as well as farmed used to do hill sprints with logs on his back while he was working and handled his sheep like he was on the rugby pitch. Indeed the very heritage of many former colonial countries, such as New Zealand, Australia, South Africa, Canada and Argentina, has left them ideally prepared for contact sports. In the case of New Zealand and Australia, add in the genetically gifted Pacific Islanders to the mix and you have a pretty potent formula for success.

There is of course no reason why this couldn't be applied to the USA.

But problem arise when you professionalise a sport—you cannot have some players lifting kegs, some players running with rucksacks full of rocks, some guys sprinting on the track and the rest doing their altitude training on a barstool while reverse curling Guinness for reps. Rugby in the late 1980s and early 1990s had its weights work and its shuttle runs on the pitch. England had started to stretch out, very noticeably in its use of the Concept 2, a model being loaned to every squad member. I remember being impressed by an England player doing handstand push ups in the changing room as a warm up before a game (and partly, I suspect, as a gesture to the television cameras). English players were bigger and stronger than the Celtic nations of Ireland, Scotland and Wales and the conditioning provided by methods like the Concept 2 combined with Anglo-Saxon discipline saw them match France's combination of Gallic flair and brutal forward play. A lot of the French didn't even lift weights. It was against their mentality. Laurent Cabannes, a brilliant flanker who played for France in the 1990s, is a good example. Later in his career he came to play for the London club Harlequins. After a couple of poor performances by Cabannes, the Harlequins coach Dick Best approached him and asked what was up. Cabannes replied that he had never lifted weights in his life and the heavy schedule at Harlequins was leaving him absolutely crushed. This was a guy who had his body wrecked by a car crash in his early 20s and had rebuilt himself after 9 months in a wheelchair to be one of the best players in his position in world rugby. He is one of those athletes that stand out for having amazing natural talent, like his fellow Frenchman Serge Blanco who smoked forty a day and ran like the wind. I remember another Frenchman who did lift weights, Philippe Sella, being described as a bodybuilder. I don't know if he spent a lot of time split training or whether that reflects the ignorant perspectives of the past. Who lifts weights? Arnold. Therefore all people who train with weights are like Arnold.

So you had this mixture of different types of players doing different things. These guys were training but in comparison to the NFL or even the original professional code of rugby, Rugby League, standards were not that high or indeed homogenised across the board. Intelligently, rugby started to look at other sports and adopt many of the principles that they saw there. NFL, Rugby League, NBA, soccer, rowing, and very recently Judo (I would have had a look at that ten years ago myself) have all been plundered for ideas. And, less intelligently, bodybuilding. Oh dear. If anything winds me up it is a man who cannot pass a rack of dumbbells without picking one up to bang out a curl. Curls were actually a strength test at Harlequins for the Under 21 side when I was a student. Trivia connected to that is that the then captain was the US international Jason Keyter (who has incidentally just been banned for taking cocaine, a sad end to his career). I've seen sets and rep ranges that have been 2 x 15 with machines (and you could tell by the way the team played) and routines that took around 80 minutes at a time with only minimal rest time (you didn't want to go into the gym for month after that because it was so bloody boring). You cannot just adopt the phenomenal training demands of NFL and apply them to a sport that is played to a very different tune. Nor can you adapt the philosophy of training method used for aesthetics and expect your athletes to be dynamic as a result.

But, as you're reading this in the first place, I think you already know that. And I really want this to be conveyed to you as a reader—you already pretty much know what to do.

Doing Things Properly

- Master your own body weight. Press ups and pull ups are underestimated outside the armed forces and Crossfit type circles. Burpees eat you up. Mike Boyle is one of many coaches who observes that often people bench press when they aren't able to do that many press ups. Greg Glassman has pointed out that it seems pointless to squat with weight when you have a poor body weight squat.
- Learn to squat and deadlift—properly.
- Learn the Olympic lifts.
- Sprint.
- Learn how to stretch and stretch regularly.
- Sprint some more.
- Realise that professionals in any sport are looking for an edge. Do you need to use rotational work on the cable stack when you cannot squat your own bodyweight? Do you need to buy a parachute for sprint work when you only sprint once a month? Kettlebells are very useful but they don't own you. Powerbags are a very cool tool but you could make do with a home made sandbag.
- Sprint up some hills.
- Row.
- Surf to www.rossboxing.com and www.rosstraining.com. The routines Ross Enamait employs are excellent and have fantastic carryover to sports other than martial arts.
- Don't waste your time. Go back to the idea of the player sprinting the length of the pitch and back, some 200 metres. Why spend hours training for a marathon? If that's what you enjoy then you are better off running a marathon. I love distance running and I don't think it's as evil as many make it out to be, but there is a time and place for it.

Something we cannot escape from as amateur sportsmen is time. We do not have the luxury of fixed and structured training blocks, adequate rest time (although some would argue neither do professional rugby players), top notch nutritional support, etc. Unless we are unemployed or still studying, we have the tricky matter of having to work for a living alongside balancing family commitments and other domestic matters. You can learn from the professionals but if you try to train like them you'll fail. Part of the genius of Crossfit is the intensity of its workouts across a number of disciplines in a relatively short space of time. I think you could experiment with training for rugby by doing CrossFit, but I would advocate taking certain elements and using those alongside methods more commonly used in the sport. Despite CrossFit's emphasis on learning new sports and skills, I think a lot of time is devoted to getting better at CrossFit. You need to work on your rugby skills, not your planche. Using the Coach Rut format would be a viable approach with its Monday/Wednesday/Friday workouts.

I've set out a fairly strict strength routine below. I would be more flexible with elements like plyometrics. You can become weighed down with different facets of physical training. Try to do a little well rather than everything poorly. Strip little bits and pieces from the methods of others and give them a go.

Of course a lot depends on what is expected of you from your club, or rather what your club provides you. Most amateur clubs train 1-2 nights per week in this country, focusing on team skills. Some fitness benefit can be gained from this, but not much. Get together with some team mates and plan out a program that you can stick to

Structure of the Year

I don't want to cover this in too much detail, and I think there are better places to read about microcycles and periodisation, but we break up the year as follows:

Off season: Following the last game and covering a period of 4 weeks. Players need to recover from the demands of the season (up to 2 weeks of rest) whilst minimising a loss of fitness through a variety of non-specific work. Do something you enjoy.

Pre-season: This is the preparation phase. High volumes of work are performed over a period of 12 weeks to improve conditioning

In season: The period of competition lasting approximately 36 weeks. Many sports have relative short competitive seasons—NFL for instance—and simply look to maintain fitness in season. Pre-season is too short in the case of elite players to have a large impact on fitness and they play too many games in season. Amateurs are at an advantage because they don't play so many games, but fitness levels will drop off if only a maintenance program is followed. A balance of periods of fitness development, maintenance and recovery must be employed in season.

This is of course a guideline; your season will probably be shorter, but that gives you more time to prepare in the pre season period. You should use that wisely.

Strength

We can all be stronger. Below is a table of fitness standards and strength training prescription for aspiring professionals from the Welsh Rugby Union. This is a player's 1RM:

POSITION	BENCH PRESS (KG)	BENCH PULL (KG)	SQUAT (KG)
FULLBACK	132	107	171
WING	127	105	186
CENTRE	139	110	179
HALFBACK	131	102	176
BACK ROW	139	114	194
SECOND ROW	137	113	185
HOOKER	144	114	203
PROP	155	121	223

A chin up test should have been included in this table, but for some reason it is missing. Mike Boyle gives some numbers in Functional Training for Sports and elite males come out at 30 chins, with a NFL skill position pushing 15-20 and a lineman at 320 lbs shooting for 7+. I know that Neil Back (217 lbs or so), the former Leicester and England player consistently topped his club's testing of this with around 35. These would be dead hangs, not kipping.

We will work on the basis of a twelve week pre-season. This would be a standard template for strength gains. The twelve weeks are split into 3 phases.

Weeks 1 – 4

Exercises

MONDAY	WEDNESDAY	FRIDAY
SQUAT	CLEAN PULL	SQUAT
BENCH PRESS	RDL	BENCH PRESS
BENT OVER ROW	UPRIGHT ROW	BENT OVER ROW
MILITARY PRESS	HAMSTRING CURLS	MILITARY PRESS

Sets & reps

WEEK	SETS	REPS
1	4	12
2	4	10
3	4	10
4	3	12

Intensities of all exercises as a percentage of best lift

WEEK	MONDAY	WEDNESDAY	FRIDAY
1	65%	65%	65%
2	70%	70%	65%
3	75%	75%	70%
4	70%	70%	65%

All recoveries should be around 90 seconds and strictly adhered to. This period aims to maximise hypertrophy.

Weeks 5 – 8

Exercises

MONDAY	WEDNESDAY	FRIDAY
POWER CLEAN	CLEAN PULL	POWER CLEAN
SQUAT	RDL	SQUAT
BENCH PRESS	PUSH PRESS	BENCH PRESS
BENT ROW	HAMSTRING CURLS	BENT ROW

Sets & reps

WEEK	SETS	REPS
5	4	5
6	4	5
7	4	5
8	4	5

Intensities of all exercises as a percentage of best lift for last 4 weeks

WEEK	MONDAY	WEDNESDAY	FRIDAY
5	80%	80%	75%
6	82.5%	82.5%	77.5%
7	85%	85%	80%
8	82.5%	82.5%	77.5%

Recoveries in this phase should be around 3 minutes.

Weeks 9 – 12

Exercises

MONDAY	WEDNESDAY	FRIDAY
POWER CLEAN	CLEAN PULL	POWER CLEAN
SQUAT	RDL	SQUAT
BENCH PRESS	PUSH PRESS	BENCH PRESS
BENT ROW	HAMSTRING CURLS	BENT ROW

Sets & reps

WEEK	SETS	REPS
9	4	3
10	3	3
11	3	2
12	1	1

Intensities of all exercises as a percentage of best lift for the last 4 weeks

WEEK	MONDAY	WEDNESDAY	FRIDAY
9	87.5%	87.5%	82.5%
10	90%	90%	85%
11	92.5%	92.5%	87.5%
12	NEW MAX	NEW MAX	NEW MAX

Recoveries should be around 3 to 5 minutes

Note again that this is for the pre-season; you are not going to be making strength gains while you are playing. Rugby Football Union (England) studies have shown that players' strength and body mass drops off dramatically through the season.

I am by no means advocating this as the only way to train strength; this is an actual recommendation for players by the Welsh Rugby Union. You could of course adapt other methods depending on your knowledge and experience, but I like the concept. It employs some key lifts (hamstring curl excluded), uses intelligent set & rep ranges, measures progress and won't keep you in the gym all day. Nor will it leave you crushed. Both these points are important because you have some other things to do.

Power Training

I don't think I need to explain what power is. We are amongst other things aiming to move heavy weights (90% 1RM) as dynamically as possible for 2-3 reps with very high rest periods to allow the nervous system to recovery. Work up into the Olympic lifts from the power clean and power snatch at the end of your strength phase.

To enhance this we shall add in some ballistic and plyometric exercises. I suggest we keep these simple and avoid hammering our bodies. I'm not going to lay down all the arguments about a player being able to lift this weight before he can attempt to do that jump as I'm not qualified to express this view. Think sensibly though as to whether you really need to be doing depth jumps.

Here is a table of plyometric exercises illustrating intensity:

LOW INTENSITY	MODERATE INTENSITY	HIGH INTENSITY	VERY HIGH INTENSITY
TUCK JUMPS	TWO LEG BOUND	DROP JUMP	DROP JUMP TO SINGLE LEG BOUND
BOX JUMPS	ALTERNATE LEG BOUND	STANDING TRIPLE JUMP	
SQUAT JUMPS	TWO LEG LATERAL HOP	SINGLE LEG HOPS	PLYOMETRIC TO SPRINT ACTIVITY
WHEEL BAR-ROW WALK	MED BALL BACK TOSS	UPHILL BOUNDS	
STANDING LONG JUMP	LUNGE JUMPS	DROP CLAP PRESS UP	

As we are trying to keep things as simple as possible I'm going to suggest you work the following movements:

- Box jumps
- Ball slams
- Tuck jumps
- Single leg hops
- Squat jumps

Complete your strength training program and then introduce these plyometrics. Start with around 50 reps (be it a throw, a jump or a step) divided up into sets within a session. One session a week will be ample and adequate recovery between sets is necessary. 100%

effort on every repetition is the key.

Complex Training

Complex training is defined as weight training combined with sport specific methods in pairs. Here are a couple examples:

- Bench press @ 85% for 4 reps followed by med ball chest passes for 5 reps
- Power cleans @ 85% for 4 reps followed by hurdle jumps for 5 reps

These pairs would be repeated with adequate rest between sets. From a certain point of view, CrossFit can be perceived as involving complex training and I would like to expand the concept to a slightly wider range of methods. I think as well as great power benefits, you can gain a considerable conditioning-related bang for your buck.

I like Dan John's idea of Litvi sprints. Get outside with a weight like a dumbbell, a kettlebell or a sandbag. Perform reps of an exercise (say swings with the kettlebell or cleans with the sandbag) and then dump the weight and immediately sprint 10,15,20 metres. Vary the directions of your sprint. Place a ball in your path that you have to dive on and then return to your feet before progressing.

Alternatively you could try something like a variation of Ross Enamait's Quantity over Quality:

- Perform 12 Burpees
- Immediately sprint 30 metres (I've reduced the distance)
- Perform 10 clap press ups
- Jog back and repeat 6-10 times

Or his Sequential Fatigue Challenge:

- 10 Burpees
- Sprint
- 10 Clap press ups
- Jog back
- 10 Diamond press ups
- Sprint
- 10 Tuck jumps
- Jog back and repeat 5 times

Now we are starting to move away from pure power work and into the realms of the endurance requirements that a rugby player needs to develop, but I think that this combination of power movements, strength and sprinting is very important. And I think CrossFit can be very useful here. These are what I consider to be the most appropriate named CrossFit workouts:

- Fran – Thruster s @ 95 lb, Pull ups, 21-15-9 reps for time
- Grace – Clean & Jerk @ 135 lbs, 30 reps for time
- Helen – 400 metre run, 1.5 pood kettlebell swings x 21 reps, 12 pull ups, 3 rounds for time
- Linda – Deadlift 1.5X bodyweight, Bench bodyweight, Clean .75X bodyweight, 10-9-8-7-6-5-4-3-2-1 reps for time

Work on your own variations. Mix up lifting with sprinting and vary the distances and directions. Try to do a couple of sessions per week with adequate recovery between sessions. This should really come in after the strength base has been developed and will work well in season—but avoid thrashing yourself close to a game.

Endurance

Rugby players need to develop both aerobic and anaerobic energy production. Like power, I don't think I need to go into too much detail on the nature of these two energy producing pathways.

Aerobic training

Aerobic training serves as a base for players to develop from and on which to build other components of fitness. I could, and perhaps should, have started this discussion on training methods with an explanation of aerobic training, but I wanted to move away from the idea of long, continuous steady state runs. Aerobic endurance accelerates the rate of recovery in rest periods during a game and after both intensive training and matches. By delaying the onset of a player's fatigue, they will be helped to maintain concentration, focus and decision making capabilities. Players who have this solid endurance base will be able to utilise greater quantities of energy from fat stores prior to using muscle glycogen.

Rugby is of course a game played at speed over short distances so continuous steady state exercise is counter-beneficial to a player. Long distance runs at a constant pace have a role to play in off season, very early pre-season and rehab, but should be generally avoided. Intervals are far more efficient, particularly from a time perspective. I would avoid Fartlek, however, as I think it is too unstructured. Fartlek is very easy to cheat at.

I prefer variations of interval like this: 1 minute running, 1 minute walking for 30 minutes, 2 minutes running, 1 minute walking for 30 minutes 7 minutes running, 3 minutes walking for 30 minutes. Run as hard as you can for the duration of each interval with the aim of always completing every interval. Don't go so fast that you step into anaerobic training.

The killer that I employ is the 1 minute on, 1 minute off, 2 minute on, 1 minute off up to 7 minutes running with a minutes rest back down to one minute again. Seven minutes has never felt so long (other than when playing seven a side rugby) and one minute so short when you're gasping for air.

Mix in with these the odd 5 km or 3 km run which you perform at 70-85% of your max heart rate.

Perform a session twice a week, and as pre-season continues, start to reduce the distances you are running in an interval but also the recovery period. By the end of this period of training this would be something like 3 sets of 6 100 metre pieces, jog recovery between reps and 3 minute rests between sets.

Alternative to running is our friend the Concept 2. Here are a couple of aerobic sessions created by Wayne Proctor, conditioner of Llanelli Scarlets in Wales:

Session 1

3 x 1000m
Target pace:
Rep 1 sub 3 mins 15, Rep 2 sub 3 mins 20, Rep 3 sub 3 mins 30

3 x 500m
Target pace:
All sub 1 min 40-42

Session 2

3 x 2000m (3 mins recovery between reps)

Anaerobic Training

Rugby's requirements for frequent high intensity periods of activity interspersed with periods of recovery makes anaerobic capability a cornerstone of a player's potential. Add to this that rugby is chaotic; neither intensities nor the duration of the activity or the recovery can be predicted, so therefore training must at times be chaotic.

Anaerobic training should again be based around intervals but performed at a higher intensity than the aerobic work. Here are some examples:

- 300 metre runs: 2 sets of 4 reps aiming for 50 seconds per rep. 3 minutes walk between reps, 10 minute active movement between sets.
- 150 metre runs: 3 sets of 4 reps at 22 second target. 2 minutes walk between reps, 5 minutes active movement between sets.
- Hill runs: 3 sets of 1 minute up and down a short steady slope. 100% up the slope, jog back down. One minute rest between reps, 5 minute rest between sets.

Game specific work is the most efficient way to improve anaerobic fitness, so shuttle runs and relays are particularly good, but it does not mean that other methods such as rowing, cycling and well designed circuits should not be employed. If you are a big forward, don't flog your joints into the ground just for the sake of it. I would recommend that you Google 'Concept 2' & 'rugby training'. Goldmine of information there.

Do not forget that muscular, aerobic and anaerobic endurance are extremely important. Rugby is not like the short, sharp bursts of power interspersed with long recoveries seen in NFL. A forward can find themselves in a mauling situation similar to a round on the wrestling mat, and when the ball passes through multiple phases of play without stoppage, you will feel your lungs start to burn. Many games see the points rack up in the later stages of the second half as one team starts to tire.

Speed

Finally we come to what is arguably the most important component (accepting that a balance of all the elements of fitness are vital to performance). Top players will obviously display different levels of speed, but all will be working to improve those levels. As I have said above, there really is no substitute for pace on the rugby field.

Speed will be improved as you become stronger and more powerful with the various training methods outlined above, and this is why running-focused work is of an advantage. But you should incorporate specific drills as well. Speed and agility training improve the ability to accelerate, increase top speed and teach the ability of an athlete to manage their own body weight when changing direction at pace.

Speed is about frequency of stride and stride length. Good running form is a prerequisite.

Although I think it is unnecessary to explain a power clean, I should probably talk about sprinting technique:

Leg cycle

- Legs individually go through a three phase cycle per stride:
- 1. Support phase: the purpose of the leg is to support the weight of the body;
- 2. Drive phase: as the body passes over the foot, the ankle, knee and hips are extended, driving the body upwards and forwards;
- 3. Recovery phase: the leg finishes the drive phase, the ankle is tucked up behind the hamstring and the knee is brought forward and upward. As the knee comes to the end of its motion, the lower leg is extended, ready to move into the support phase again.
- The height at which the knee is raised and the closeness of the ankles to the hamstring depends upon the velocity achieved.
- During acceleration, the knee raise and foot tuck are not as great as when running at full velocity.
- When accelerating you are taking fast, short strides rather than the longer cyclic movements required for top end speed.

Arm action

- Arms should remain locked at 90° with the shoulders relaxed to allow a fluid motion.
- Arm action opposes that of the legs: as one leg moves forward, so does the opposite arm.
- The extremes of motion of the arms are best measured using the fists, which should be relaxed, neither clenched or fully splayed (imagine pinching a potato chip between the thumb and first finger).
- The most forward position is when the fist is level with the jaw.
- The rear drive of the arm assists the forward leg drive of the opposite leg and is the most important part of the arm action. If you have done much sprint training you will know how sore the arms can be afterwards. Sprinters don't just have big guns for vanity reason.
- In the rear drive, the fist should move backwards until it is at least level with the hips.
- Elbow bend should remain at 90° for the entire cycle.

There are many drills to assist with running form and you may have seen some of these if you have ever watched track athletes training. These would include skips, butt kicks, arm swings. Colin Jackson, the British hurdler, used to practice arm swings with light dumbbells.

A drill I have a lot of time for is 40 x 10m sprints. Really drive your arms and legs for each rep and then walk back and repeat. This is particularly good for forwards.

If you can, go down to a track and get a little coaching. It will be extremely worth your while.

Sport loading

This is sprinting while being resisted by some means. Sleds, weight vests, parachutes etc. I would actually avoid training like this as an amateur. Resistance can often impair technique and you want to focus on your running form. An amateur's time is precious and you don't need to introduce too many methods. However, hill sprints remain extremely useful and I would include those. For speed work, keep the distances short, 5 - 30 metres, reps low, 4 - 8, and recovery from 1 - 3 minutes. I recently did a set of 9x20m hill sprints off a 5 burpee start and 2 minute recovery. And I really knew about it.

Over-speed

This is preparing your muscles to make them move faster, a neurological adaptation to training. It can involve being dragged along by a harness so that the body becomes used to moving at speeds greater than previously experienced or running down gentle slopes. I would opt for running down a slope. You will notice how your stride turnover increases.

Once again, focus on correct form and posture.

Both methods should be executed by the athlete while free of fatigue and high recovery periods should be used. Do this while fresh and focus on what you are doing.

Speed endurance

After developing a solid speed base it is important to work up to maintaining high speeds for longer. Work on speed endurance at the end of a session or in a separate session entirely. Pure speed sessions usually will not involve sprints further than 40-50m (and this has specificity to rugby as a game); speed endurance sessions on the other hand will cover distances of over 100-200m. Start with high quality work even if it means shorter distances and longer recoveries. Extend the distances and reduce the recoveries as you improve.

Gear Work

Rugby is not played at a flat out pace for 80 minutes. Nor is every break by a player executed at top speed. Often a player will slow down while looking for support and then accelerate again as they spot a gap in the defence. Many very dangerous players will seemingly be running at full throttle only to be able to step on the gas yet again to pull away from a defender.

Practice running lengths of the field slowly increasing your speed. Start off jogging, finish with a balls-to-the-wall sprint.

Agility

You must be able to move over short distances quickly, change direction efficiently and manage your own body weight while doing so. Deceleration is as an important part of agility as acceleration.

Drills using hurdles, speed ladders, cones and so forth are used to imitate movements that would occur on the pitch.

You should work on an element of reactive training, responding to a training partner dropping a ball for instance or dodging tennis balls being thrown at you by team mates.

Once again, concentrate on form and posture.

Comments on the Above

I've set all these ideas out to give you an overview of the training methods utilised by top level players. I have not written a concise 12 month plan and I have not touched on periodisation. All the methods above need to supported by a dedicated flexibility program, intelligent work to secure core stability and a balanced approach to nutrition. Despite emphasis on strength and speed, these last three areas are the glue that hold everything together.

I'm not suggesting you do all of this, but be intelligent, assess your strengths and weaknesses and work where work is needed and work hard. Yes, you are an amateur, so be practical in how you apply your time and be selective in what you do. Swimming is a great activity and excellent recovery for rugby, but don't spend your life swimming when you need to work on your sprint. Likewise, don't do a massive deadlift session the day before a match. I read a hilarious article once by a guy who had trained for marathon purely by using kettlebells. Needless to say, he didn't do that well. OK, it was an experiment, but what a doughnut.

Just for the sake of completeness, here is a table that will help you when thinking about planning your training. It is based around a European season running roughly from September to April. Once more, I thank the Welsh Rugby Union for this.

Generalised Macrocycle for Rugby Union

MNTH	M	J	J	A	S	O	N	D	J	F	M
PERIOD	OFF SEASON				IN-SEASON OR COMPETITION PERIOD						
AEROBIC WORK	DEVELOP		MAINTAIN								
ANAROBIC WORK	NON SPE-CIFIC	DEVELOP			MAINTAIN - ATTEMPT TO DEVELOP IF PERIODS OF INACTIVITY ARE PRESENT						
STRENGTH	NON SPE-CIFIC	STRENGTH ENDUR-ANCE	MAX STRENGTH	RATE OF FORCE DEVELOP-MENT	MAX POWER	SPEED STRENGTH	MAX STRENGTH	MAX POWER	RATE OF FORCE DEVEL-OPMENT	SPEED STRENGTH	MAIN-TAIN
SPEED	NON SPE-CIFIC	EMPHASIS ON TECHNIQUE		Top end speed	ACCEL-ERATION	AGILITY	GAME SPECIFIC				
VOLUME	LOW	TREND HIGH. START LOWERING TOWARDS SEASON			VOLUME TO REMAIN HIGH. WILL DECREASE IF VOLUME INCREASES.						
INTENSITY	MEDIUM	TREND MEDIUM, INCREASING TOWARDS SEASON									

The Rise of the Freaks and Some Final Thoughts (and Words of Caution)

In the Rugby World Cup in 1995, a certain Jonah Lomu took to the fields of South Africa and took the game by storm. In the build up to the semi-final between New Zealand and England, the rather typically snooty English press dismissed Lomu's athletic abilities. Surely he was more likely to be around 6'2" - 6'3" and 210lbs? No, he really was 6'5", over 260lbs and able to cover 100m in under 10.9 seconds. He scored 4 tries as England were mauled 45-29 by the All Blacks. So began the start of a legend and of a legacy.

Jonah was huge; therefore everyone had to get bigger. This coincided with the start of professionalism and indeed to this day, everyone playing professional rugby has become considerably bigger. Yet a point was missed. Jonah Lomu was big because he was born that way. When Will Carling, the England captain described him as a freak, he was inadvertently correct. But rugby has ploughed on, looked at other sports, fallen in love with the players of Rugby League, and missed a vital point.

It has worked for a while. The England team that won the 2003 World Cup were the best prepared rugby team of all time, possibly one of the best prepared teams in any sport. They had probably played their finest rugby at a peak some six months prior to the tournament, but they had reached a point where they were so well conditioned physically and mentally that they just didn't lose games even when playing badly. They possessed a very talented pool of players at their disposal, and of course this was a massive advantage.

Since then England have declined abysmally and I think the rot was there before the World Cup. The English Club competition is confrontational and attritional. Most crucial to the decline is the drop in skill levels. It doesn't matter how big or fast you are in rugby if you do not have mastery of the basic skills. Union looked at League and saw these wonderful athletes with very developed skill levels and thought, "We want some of that." But League is a less complex game and there is less specificity between positional requirements. Rugby League players have more time to train hard and work on the basic skills, particularly handling the ball. They don't have competitive scrums, lineouts, ruck and maul situations to contend with.

The English situation is being hotly contended at present, but the English are not alone, and after a series of Autumn international matches, only New Zealand and Ireland seemed to be on track for the sixth World Cup in France next year. Come that tournament, sure, other nations will be competitive, but the game as a whole needs to look at itself. Former England international Austin Healey recently hit out at the young players who were becoming 'gym monkeys' to the detriment of their games:

"The strongest athletes are gymnasts who never go in a gym in their lives. It should all be own bodyweight stuff. A lot of players are too big for their frames."

I take most things that Austin Healey says with a pinch of salt and I know that he certainly didn't build his physique without the use of weights, but he's spitting in the right direction. You have to work on your skills. I'll say it again: You have to work on your skills.

Basic requirement for all players:

- To pass the ball off both hands when both stationary and on the move
- To catch the ball from a pass
- To catch a high ball from a kick
- To tackle

Basic requirement for backs:

- To kick strongly and competently off at least one foot

Work on these as much as you work your bench or your vertical leap. Likewise, if you are 5'10" and the coach tells you that you are too small to play back row, work your arse off to prove him wrong. Master the skills of the position and do your time in the gym and train smart. If you can't kick, you're never going to be a fly half, just as if you can't run quickly, you're not suited for the wing. Buy your own rugby ball and get used to handling it when you're watching TV or walking round the house. Get out with the guys you play with at your club and kick and pass the ball around. If the training program at your club is poor or non-existent, hook up with the guys who want something more and train together.

While preparing for this article, I have been watching New Zealand's unbeaten tour around Europe and it has changed a few of the ideas I was going to present to you. They are huge, but they are extremely skilful as well. Their players look functionally big and strong—not like the gorilla at the end of the bar downing beers. They tossed big, strong English players around like rag dolls and they blew away a skilful but much smaller Welsh team. The New Zealand management have gone away and thought about how to train smart. Their guys have worked hard, no doubt, but they haven't been flogged to death in the weights room or on the track. If you get the chance to see them play, do so.

Earlier on in this article I made reference to the physical culture apparent in parts of the US. This gives you a huge advantage in developing your game. That you are reading the Performance Menu would suggest you are on the right track. Take advantage of all the things you have read and the facilities you have available to you. Work intensely on your skills and structure your training to be manageable. Many officials in the Rugby world are very envious of the talent available in the US, all the guys who don't make it in the NFL, the NBA, track & field and so forth could easily be channelled into rugby. And those same officials are pretty fearful that one day that might happen. To quote one official: "If Americans will pay good money to see monster trucks smashing into other monster trucks, they're going to love rugby."

KETTLEBELL POWER METRICS
JASON C. BROWN

Kettlebell training purists (self included) like to point out the fact that many kettlebell exercises such as the Swing, Snatch and Clean extend the range of motion by allowing the kettlebell to float behind the hips during the lowering or eccentric portion of the drills. Kettlebell purist are equally as fast to point out that the extended range of motion and the eccentric or yielding contraction simply don't exist in barbell Olympic lifts, since the athlete usually drops the barbell under control once the lift has been performed successfully.

In fact, this one benefit of kettlebell training has been credited to improving deadlift numbers, increasing beneficial hormonal responses to exercise, and positive body composition changes. Pavel Tsatouline, the man responsible for bringing the kettlebell back to life in America, even has a program based around kettlebell quick-lifts such as the Snatch, Swing and Clean. Pavel calls his program "Fast Tens" and many athletes report dramatic changes in lean muscle mass and strength levels.

A similar phenomenon occurs with kipping pull-ups. Many athletes report that their strict pull-up numbers, weighted and non-weighted, skyrocket after focusing on a program based around kipping pull-ups.

What do kettlebell quick-lifts and kipping pull-ups have in common that illicit such positive training responses?

Before we get into details let's cover some basics. There are three types of muscular action, concentric or overcoming, eccentric or yielding and isometric. Concentric muscle actions are a shortening of the muscle to overcome an external resistance. Eccentric muscle action is a resisted lengthening of that muscle or simply a muscle exerting force while being lengthened. An isometric muscle action refers to a muscle exerting force without any actual movement or change in its length.

The focus of this article will be on the eccentric muscular action or, to be precise, a fast or over-speed eccentric action.

Below are a few reasons why we'll be focusing on fast eccentric contractions:
To increase Reactive Strength. Reactive Strength is a term used to describe how quickly you can shift from the eccentric portion of a lift to the concentric portion of the lift. Poor

Reactive Strength will increase the amount of time it takes you to shift from eccentric to concentric actions. This all translates into less force production and less power output during the concentric contraction, making you slower and less explosive.

To Alter Motor Unit Recruitment. Research shows that fast eccentric contractions recruit a greater amount of Type 2 (fast-twitch) motor units. The greater involvement of Type 2, higher threshold motor units translates into more explosive movement and greater power output.

To promote structural changes. Some researchers have also found a decrease in Type 1 (slow-twitch) muscle fibers after a period of training using fast eccentric contractions. Type 1 fibers are slow twitch, endurance fibers, and if you're a power/speed athlete, the fewer you have the better.

The Drills

We'll be using standard kettlebell exercises such as the Swing, but we'll be adding one simple twist—an environment of hyper-gravity. Instead of allowing gravity to bring the kettlebell back down on its own, we'll be actively lowering it either by our own force or through the use of a trusted training partner.

The Active American Swing

We use the term active to illustrate the fact that you are pulling the kettlebell back down and not gravity. You'll be doing this through powerful shoulder adduction and hip flexion. As the kettlebell reaches its peak height above your head, pull the kettlebell back down between your legs and hips using your upper back musculature and your hips flexors.

The Power-Bomb

For this variation you need a training partner that you trust 100%. Perform two standard kettlebell Swings to get set, and on your third repetition, have your training partner throw the kettlebell down as fast as you're able to handle. Change directions as fast as you can in the bottom position—touch and go!

The Power-Bomb Figure 8

Swing a kettlebell around your legs using a figure 8 pattern. Traditionally this is performed with a slight pause in the up position. For this variation however you'll throw the kettlebell back down between your hips as fast as you can handle.

Programming

The Active American Swing can be used within any metabolic conditioning workout to improve your time and power output. Simply replace your standard swing with this variation.

The Power-Bomb works best as a component of a power couplet. A power couplet is two explosive drills performed back-to-back for low repetitions. Power-Bombs work well with Clapping Push-ups and Clapping Pull-ups. Power-Bombs also work well within a complex using a plyometric drill or box jumps, again for low repetitions.

The Power-Bomb Figure 8 is simply thrown in as an active recovery drill or alternated with other less intense activities such as agility ladders or rings.

If you're not used to fast eccentrics, break into them slowly as they cause more muscle damage, particularly to fast twitch fibers. You'll be happy with the results regardless. Enjoy.

HORMESIS: A UNIFIED THEORY OF PERFORMANCE, HEALTH AND LONGEVITY?
ROBB WOLF

The Devil is in the details. Make no assumptions. These are good rules to follow in life and they are particularly good to follow if one delves into the action packed world of science. Why? Because "WE" have a profound ability to fool ourselves. Missing the obvious because it does not fit our expectations describes human endeavors as divergent as spouse selection and scientific data interpretation. Typically we see what we want to see but occasionally unexpected results pique interest and new avenues of investigation are born. In other circumstances we turn a blind eye to observations that get in the way of "further validating" a solid, trusted theory. When the situation is highly counterintuitive, we experience the greatest resistance and problems.

Take hormesis, for example. Never heard of it? Neither had I until recently, when I was researching new developments in intermittent fasting. Hormesis describes a favorable adaptation to low dose exposure to an irritant/toxin/toxicant. Hormesis is a tough subject to make sense of in many instances as low doses of a given hormetic agent create the OPPOSITE effect of high dose.

Hormesis is characterized by a graphical sign change as one moves from low to high dose in contrast to classic dose response curves.

Just to muddy the waters, not all agents are hormetic! Many agents follow a fairly simple dose response curve in their action, with perhaps a threshold of activity and then diminishing activity at higher levels. For the math geeks out there this can be described by a third order polynomial and is the backbone of modern pharmacology and toxicology. Let's now look at two interesting examples of hormesis: energetic or radiation hormesis and opiate-induced hormesis.

One might think radiation is a good thing if we can take a complete squid like Tobey McGuire "expose" him to an irradiated spider and find him later smooching on Kirsten Dunst… upside down…. in the rain…. Kreiki! Sign me up for the Hot Spider! Well, sequels are never as good as the original and it's likely not a surprise that radiation is not good for you… unless you are going to be exposed to a whopping dose of radiation. As far back as the 1950s, it was observed that a small exposure to gamma radiation could greatly enhance survivability of a later large dose. Incidence of DNA damage, cancer and oxidative damage were seen to decrease greatly in test animals. This was about the time major progress was made in the development of vaccines and thus an analogy between "vaccination" and radiation hormesis has been made and is perhaps not too far off. Consequently this flavor of hormesis has been thoroughly studied and is largely accepted.

The situation of Opiate hormesis is a bit different and has left everyone studying hormesis scratching their collective noggins. I'm sure you are aware that opiates produce a sedative and analgesic effect which follows a fairly typical dose response curve with the following exception: At very low doses opiates produce increased pain perception. No one knows why and mechanisms are not forthcoming. Some contend that a gene/opiate interaction occurs which up-regulates some aspect of pain perception/transmission, but again, no one really knows what is happening.

You may be asking what does ANY of this have to do with Performance, Health and Longevity ? Possibly everything. We have looked at the idea that pulsatile, random stressors such as ketosis, intermittent fasting and exercise may be integral to disease prevention, health and longevity. Folks like Art DeVany have talked about it and appear to "live it" to great success. My intention with this article is to place some of the mechanisms of intermittent fasting, exercise and CRAN in more prominent and accessible context. To do that effectively we need to delve into a little chemistry and physiology. All of this will certainly increase your Geek Factor, but I promise this will also increase your AKP.

A ROS by any other Name…

Fifty years ago a cornerstone of modern medicine was put forth: The Free radical theory of aging . At the dawn of the nuclear age it was postulated that the production of Reactive Oxygen Species (ROS) from ionizing radiation, hydrocarbon combustion (smoking, automobile exhaust) and bad Elvis devotionalscould damage cellular proteins and, perhaps more importantly, DNA, and lead to death and disease. Now the data on this was fairly conclusive in that if one exposed an organism to a given dose of gamma radiation, one could predict a given amount of DNA damage and associated ROS production. This early work inspired the notion that if ROS were "bad," squelching the activity of ROS should be "good".

An understanding of ROS prompted research into the therapeutic use of antioxidants as a means of slowing aging, preventing disease, and forestalling death. The hypothesis went something like this: Reactive oxygen species damage DNA and cellular proteins; this leads to disease and death. Therefore, any activity that decreases ROS production (antioxidant intake) should decrease ROS and consequently disease and death! Unfortunately, antioxidant supplementation never lived up to its expectations, and has actually proven to be deleterious to health and longevity in some cases . This is not to say, however, that antioxidants are worthless. Although supplementaiton with Vit

E and other antioxidants has not proven to be a cure-all, it is interesting to note that high antioxidant intake from food has shown benefits in both epidemiological and clinical studies.

This has perplexed researchers, as this does not follow linear reductionism. Why would antioxidants from food be beneficial whereas isolated antioxidants in the form of a supplement are not only unhelpful but also potentially harmful? Like I said in the opening, the Devil is in the Details. It appears that cataloging a given chemical as simply an "antioxidant" may be too narrow a term. In many instances location within the cell as well as types and concentrations of other chemicals will determine whether a given agent is an anti- or pro-oxidant. This is true not only of cellular material in our bodies but also the mix of chemicals we ingest via plant materials. These chemicals have complex roles both in the plant and our mammalian physiology, and these roles are often subject to change as cellular conditions change. In essence, something that was an antioxidant in one circumstance may become a pro-oxidant in another. Interestingly, this appears to be a good thing with regards to health as viewed through the perspective of hormesis.

As you will see, the topic of antioxidants and free radical/ROS damage has proven to be as if not more convoluted than the investigation of dietary fat in health and disease.

OK, we need just a little more background before we talk about the underpinnings of Hormesis. Put on your goggles and lab coat Poindexter! Time for a wee bit of chemistry and physiology.

Weird Science

When we talk chemistry, we are in fact talking about electrons and how they exchange between elements and molecules. Most chemical bonding involves electrons setting up in pairs; however, free radicals have an unpaired electron that makes these little buggers VERY reactive and potentially destructive. Do you need a thorough knowledge of radical chemistry to be a stud athlete or good coach? No, absolutely not. However, a steeping in terms and an understanding of the free radical theory of aging will help put some new material into valuable context.

Hang with me for one more geek-fest as we look at glycoloysis, and then, my friends, we can look at how hormesis may be the underpinning of intermittent fasting, exercise, CRAN, resveratrol and more.

The key point to get from the topic of glycolysis is that glucose is a substrate used in energy production. Through a series of enzymatically-mediated steps, glucose is cleaved into two molecules, each of which contains 3 carbons. These molecules are glyceraldehyde-3-phosphate (GA3P) and dihydroxyacetone-phosphate (DHAP). It is important to note that glucose, DHAP and GA3P are all potential glycating agents that can and do stick to cellular proteins creating what is known as advanced glycation end products (AGEs). Glycation can reduce the effectiveness of proteins or make them completely non-functional. Just a quick sideline. John Kyrk is the chap who created the animated glycolysis I linked to and he has a load of other cool animations on a range of biology topics. Check them out!

OK, you now have an understanding of what hormesis is and you suffered through a 101 course in chemistry and physiology and now grasp the finer points not only of the free radical theory of aging but also the reactive species produced in glycolysis. Let's look at CRAN, intermittent fasting, exercise and some phytonutrients—all agents known to improve health and longevity—and see if there is a common thread amongst all of them explained by hormesis.

Have A CRAN and a Smile

In earlier discussions we have looked at the similarities and differences of CRAN and IF. What has been postulated is that CRAN and IF work via similar but separate mechanisms1. In the case of CRAN we see a significant decrease in body weight, a slight increase in circulating ketone concentrations and some increases in cellular stress response mechanisms such as increases in heat shock proteins (HSP). In contrast intermittent fasting shows little or no decrease in body weight, significant increases in circulating ketone concentrations and significant increases in HSP expression. Our newfangled understanding of hormesis may offer some help in understanding what is happening in these two scenarios and why we might choose one over the other and how to optimize desirable results such as improved performance and a decreased rate of aging.

In the case of CRAN, we initially see an increase in circulating ketone concentrations and cellular stress mechanisms such as HSP expression; however, once the animal has reached a maintenance bodyweight (~40% of ad libitum weight), ketone concentrations and expressions of HSPs and other cellular chaperones are elevated compared to ad libitum animals but decreased compared to IF3. What may be occurring is an attenuation of glycolytic damage in both IF and CRAN and a potent hormetic effect in the case of IF3, 4.

If you recall from our previous geek-fest, glycolysis starts with glucose and ends in the production of GA3P and DHAP. All three of these agents, as well as the intermediates of glycolysis are potential glycating agents that can and do cause significant damage to cellular proteins. In the case of CRAN, glycolytic flux is reduced in total by overt caloric restriction. In simple terms, CRAN offers some benefits simply because less fuel is passing through metabolic pathways. It is intriguing that IF offers potential benefits in two ways. The first is transient and dramatic decreases in glycolysis during fasting. After a few hours the liver is typically emptied of its glycogen reserve and we see an up-regulation of gluconeogenesis from protein and a significant shift towards fat metabolism. How much of a shift towards either gluconeogenesis or fat metabolism appears to be a function of insulin sensitivity and up-regulation of fatty acid oxidation enzymes. It is important to note that at this point two separate but related elements of hormesis are at work: a reduction in glycolytic flux and an increase in fatty acid metabolism. The shift in fat metabolism actually produces a transient increase in oxidative stress in the mitochondria, which is likely responsible for the increased expression of chaperones, heat shock proteins and endogenous antioxidants. It is important to note, however, that excessive levels of antioxidants during this time will squelch this oxidative stress and stymie subsequent favorable adaptations5. It is also important to note that with re-feeding we witness a dramatic increase in glycolytic activity; however, in the adapted organism, this increase is quite short in duration and metabolism shifts to a fatty acid dominant, pro-ketogenic state5. OK that was a mouthful! Let's look at a diagram that covers the same information:

IF ➔ initial decrease in glycolysis ➔ increase in fatty acid oxidation/ketone production ➔ increase in transient oxidative damage ➔ increase in HSP/chaperone and antioxidant expression + transient increase in glycolysis after re-feeding.

Now here is something that is REALLY interesting... many of the characteristics of aging and disease include excessive oxidative damage and mitochondrial pathology6. It appears that the chronic oxidative stress of overfeeding either overwhelms an organism's adaptive capacity or never triggers the normal adaptive mechanisms that lead to health and longevity. This is the real importance of hormesis as a model for understanding IF, CRAN, exercise and phytonutrients that exert an anti-aging action. Ironically, we may need a pulsatile increase in oxidative stress to protect us from chronic oxidative damage, and, not surprisingly, chronic glycolysis may not be a great thing for aging effectively. Someone should let Dr. McDougal know his starch-based, 8-meals-per-day diet is perfect for accelerated aging!

We now have a much better understanding of the mechanisms that drive the results we observe with IF and CRAN. I want to look at one more concept that should help to put this whole process into perspective: Darwinian evolution on a cellular level.

That Which Does Not Kill You

All eukaryotic organisms have within their cells two information processing/storage centers composed of DNA. One is the nucleus of the cell and the other is mitochondrial DNA. The mitochondrion are thought to have once been free living organisms that became incorporated into larger, more complex cells and a symbiosis was established with the result being nearly everything on the planet that is not bacteria. A little reading on the endo-sympiotic theory of biology is sure to alienate you from friends and family, but leave you with a feeling of extreme hoiti-toiti-ness. So… metaphysical and political considerations aside, the accepted role of DNA, whether cellular or mitochondrial, is to replicate itself. You can get elbow-deep in information and game theory trying to describe the information processing elements of DNA and how this ties into Darwinian evolution… but that's a topic for another publication. Part of the replication scheme appears to be adapting to the environment to optimize survivability and continued propagation. How this works has shifted from a picture of purely random events leading to "lucky" adaptations that favor survival to the almost Lamarckian view of epigenics. Perhaps not surprisingly, both random chance and an awareness of the environment appear to drive both micro and macroevolution.

In the case of hormesis we see both DNA centers (nuclear and mitochondrial DNA) affected by environmental factors the lead to a selection pressure favoring healthy phenotypes. If you recall our interview with Dr. Seyfried and the discussion of metabolic control analysis, you are familiar with the concept that subjecting cancer cells to either a ketogenic and or IF/CRAN environment selects for healthy cells, effectively culling unhealthy cancer cells7. This is due to the fact that cancer cells lack the cellular machinery to use fatty acids as fuel sources and rely solely upon glucose metabolism (glycolysis). Another facet of hormesis appears to be a selection pressure on the mitochondrion themselves as the acute stress of IF creates an overwhelming oxidative stress that healthy mitochondria can withstand and unhealthy lines cannot. The effective result is a cell population that is comparatively healthy and adaptive. We also need to consider two other factors. IF and CRAN increase the activity of DNA repair enzymes, helping to keep cells healthy and normal. This slows the speed at which an organism moves through its pool of stem cells which are utilized to replace damaged/dysfunctional cells. It appears that chronically high growth factors, as is associated with chronic overfeeding, burns through the stem cell pool8,9. Here is the money shot folks:

The hormetic action selects for healthy cell lines, whether we are talking just the mitochondria or the entire cell. This occurs via transient stressors that increase cellular stress mechanisms, typically by production of ROS, in an adaptive manner that mitigates deleterious levels of oxidative damage. Concurrently we observe the mitigation of chronic stressors such as glycolysis, which if left unchecked, overwhelm cellular repair mechanisms.

Sorry it took me so long to spit that out! So what is the take-home message here? How does an understanding of hormesis improve Performance, Health and Longevity? For starters, it puts antioxidant supplementation into a very different perspective. I would be conservative and keep dosages at or near physiologic levels. Also I think this lends support to a nutritional plan that minimizes glycolytic flux by shifting metabolism towards a fat adaptive state. For the athlete who requires ample muscle glycogen to perform, I think this supports an argument for squirreling glycogen into the muscles during the post workout window. I'm still not sure if hammering a glucose polymer drink is a good idea, and prefer whole food consumed in a real meal format, but extreme situations may call for extreme measures. It would appear the post workout window would be preferable to spreading carbs throughout the day, and for certain it makes an argument to minimize carbs before bedtime to get some mileage from that period of "forced" fasting. This also squares nicely with previous discussions of seasonal eating and utilizing a period of purely ketogenic eating, perhaps with some intermittent fasting, to select for stress resistant, healthy cell lines (that means you).

Researching and writing this article has not moved me to change much of what I was already doing. I do, however, better understand what is happening on a cellular level when I choose a lower carb paleo approach to eating, with occasional intermittent fasting. I think this information is fascinating and real understanding is only beginning. Perhaps more than anything else, this paper has encouraged me to make no assumptions while keeping an eye on the details.

GRAPPLING AS A WOMAN
HEATHER GIBBON

When you find yourself down on your hands and knees in a room full of SWAT officers, you're bound to question some of the decisions you've made. When one of those officers is tucked in behind you and draped over your back, those questions in your head are asked more earnestly. For that split second five years ago, I questioned what I was doing in a Brazilian Jiu Jitsu class. Then I rolled him into a leg lock.

The truth is, man or woman, grappling can be awkward and that's something that you get used to early on and then get over. In my case, I didn't know much about the ground game when I started and so I didn't know enough to be apprehensive. I was usually the only woman in Marcelo Alonso's class, but nearly all the other students were police officers and were accustomed to working with women.

Like me, Jenika Gordon of Vancouver, BC is an accidental grappler of sorts and she could easily relate to the early discomforts. "It was a bit odd at first to be straddling some guy you didn't know. I mean you are rolling around and sweating and grabbing! However, I felt comfortable because each person would introduce themselves and we would do the "secret handshake" to lighten the mood before we started. Each person took his time with me and would guide me along the new skill we learned. I only had one uncomfortable experience with a new guy who got a little excited when we started grappling, if you know what I mean! I just made sure I didn't partner with him again."

Gordon, a white belt at Gracie Barra, is athletic, energetic and attractive. If you bumped into her in a bar, without even a scowl, she'd be the first to apologize and check that your drink didn't spill. When I asked her if she'd let me interview her about Jiu Jitsu, she immediately deferred to another female grappler expecting that I would want to talk to a more ambitious competitor.

Neither Gordon nor I went into the sport in the hopes of being the Million Dollar Baby of BJJ. Both of us are CrossFit trainers and couldn't afford injuries, so both of us trained on the cautious side. At the time, I was only looking for something that was challenging and would focus my training when a boyfriend said, "You'd be a great grappler" for reasons I still don't understand and based on evidence I can't even imagine. Without any other bright ideas, I decided to try.

Gordon made her decision in much the same way. "I wanted to try a new sport and learn something new," she said. "I was training the owner of a BJJ gym and he told me I should try it. I love sports and I thought it would be great to try something that is physical, mental and allows me to learn how to protect myself. My goal was to learn a new skill, get a good workout, and learn how to protect myself on the ground."

On the other side of the mat, Cindy Hale, now 32, is a well respected local fighter who started grappling in 2002 and won the US Open her first year, then went on to place second as a blue belt in the PanAm games. When I started in BJJ, she was training in Marcelo's Tacoma school and students often wondered who would be the dominant fighter between the two of us. I never aspired, talk soon faded and I only ran into Cindy in passing. When I heard she was going in for surgery, I felt the need to support her and I went to visit her in the hospital the day before her Cervical Disc replacement.

Cindy is lightening fast and talented, but that's in the job description of a 135-pound brown belt. When you're light-limbed and fighting in a rough neighborhood where egos are sometimes more savagely protected than major joints, you get stacked often. Cindy knew male fighters would ball her up in order to buy time and rest. She would just fight her way out and win. I asked her if she'd train differently now and she nodded: "I'd tap." It's not that she regrets it, exactly; she just doesn't want to trade years of training for those little victories.

Recently she joked with me on the phone about how she'd get paired with Army Rangers and local toughs as some sort of experiment by fellow classmates. They'd say, "Let's see what happens," and she'd laugh, "Yeah, won't that be fun for you." The fun of grappling got turned upside down and strangled for Cindy, until she returned from surgery ready to look at the sport from a less competitive perspective.

That wasn't a path I traveled, but I started in the sport when I was already 32—not that that has to matter. With a CrossFit foundation and years of work as a laborer on my father's farm, I was blessed with above average strength that I had proudly maintained. If there was something I was trying to prove in the sport, I suppose that was it.

That desire to showcase my strength was more of an obstacle than an asset since I tended to muscle everything and inadvertently frustrate my training partners. They proved more patient than me as I forged ahead with a "square peg, round hole" approach that prompted me to yank, pull and push even harder. It's a common mistake that usually gets you solidly submitted by the partner whose patience you've finally worn thin. Like all white belts, I was a bit frustrated, but unlike many new women in the sport, I didn't decide that I wasn't strong enough. I've seen women walk away from grappling making that mistaken assumption.

With greater wisdom, Gordon understood the part of the game I didn't. "I was quite surprised how technical it was. I was finding it more challenging mentally than physically. As I got better, I found it both mental and physical, which I liked. I fell in love with it. I don't know if I would compete, but I definitely want to learn more and more about it. You learn so much body awareness and how to move when pinned down. It is almost like dancing. It just felt good. And I want to learn more about how to get out of situations where my life might be in danger."

Gordon has reason to worry. At somewhere around 5 feet tall, she'd be easy prey without this sport. She explains, "The more skill you have in BJJ the more likely you are able to tap someone out, even if they're bigger than you. I thought that was kind of cool. It doesn't matter if you're small, if you have more skill you can get out of some pretty crazy things and still tap out a bigger, stronger guy. That felt good." And when all else fails there's always the bag of tricks Marcelo taught me called "No you friend" moves, mentioned with a finger wag and in your best Portuguese accent.

Though I now know how to manipulate a larger opponent, the most important thing I learned was to process panic. At first, grappling was a series of erratic movements followed by an on-the-ground assessment as I lay there checking my body for trauma. That was often frightening. Now I've developed an awareness that allows me to formulate a strategy even in the most unfortunate situations. The ability to sort what is actually lethal from what is either simply annoying or painful is at the very least empowering and something I feel all women should have experience with.

Perhaps this is the mental aspect that Gordon touches on in her advice to other women. "Be patient; it takes time to learn the skills. It can be frustrating, but once you get some of the moves down it feels really good. You can tap out anyone regardless of size. Also, it is a great workout both physically and mentally. I love that about it. Try it—it is FUN!"

Five years later and it's still my favorite part of the day four days a week. I train with Ben Blackstone, one of Marcelo Alonso's most trusted Brown Belts, for a one-on-one split Muay Thai and BJJ class where I get individual attention. He has the skill to roll without using his considerable weight and strength advantage and it's accelerated my game.

Blackstone's mantra of 'Position before submission' speaks to both a more traditional teaching style of Brazilian Jiu Jitsu and what I feel is a wise approach to training women athletes who will likely require precision to finish a move when potentially lacking the might to muscle it. Though I miss the broader class experience, I benefit from the ability to work through a move without getting stuffed from the start. It's not to say he lets me finish a sloppy move, he just lets me get farther so I see my mistake.

Gordon's coach seemed to understand this as well, pairing her with partners that could help her learn. "The coach almost always made sure I was paired with the other girl or with an experienced athlete in BJJ. That way they could coach me through the skill we just learned," which shows that in the right environment and with the right coaching, women will be cultivated and successful, regardless of their goals.

FROM GLYCOGEN TO COSOMOLGY: NOTHING NEW UNDER THE SUN
ROBB WOLF

Have you ever-noticed how increasing variables increases the complexity of a situation? Physicists have struggled with this increase in complexity of seemingly simple systems for several hundred years in the three-body gravitational problem. For those of you who get out a lot more than I do you may not know that it is a fairly simple matter to model how gravity and movement mutually influence two bodies, say the earth and moon. Now, if you add a third body to the system, like the Sun, things get VERY complex and we must rely on approximations to model these systems and quite quickly these approximations introduce enough error into our calculations to make the system largely chaotic and unknowable. Professor Peit Hut has a fantastic site that introduces the three body gravitational problem and he has a description of solar behavior that is essentially fractal in nature i.e. self-similar at all scales:

"The sun can shine for billions of years because nuclear reactions deep in its interior generate the energy that is lost through the sun's radiation at its surface. On a completely different scale but in an analogous way, stars are lost from the `surface' of a star cluster by `evaporation', and there is a similar need to replenish the energy in the central regions. In fact, the mechanism is remarkably similar in both cases: the sun burns hydrogen through slow nuclear fusion into helium, while star clusters `burn' single stars through a kind of gravitational fusion into binary stars."

I guess it's a sign of my extreme geeky-ness but I find this fascinating. The same processes that govern how a cup of coffee cools are at play on the surface of the Sun and heart of the galaxy. I need to expand on this dork-fest just a bit more but I will make this pertinent to you folks who are interested in performance health and longevity and did not subscribe to the Pmenu with the intentions of learning about sciency stuff! So back to this three-body problem... the difficulty with this scenario is keeping track of HOW the elements in the system influence each other. Imagine two particles, or planets or perhaps magnets, whose gravity, charge or magnetism affects each other. We'll call one A and the other B (catchy, I know). In this pared down system if something happens to A it has an effect on B and vice versa. This is pretty straightforward and easy to predict and track. Things get spicy when we introduce another element... in avant-garde fashion we shall call this interloper C. So now we have a system in which A influences B&C, B influences A&C and C influences A&B. This may not look like much more complexity but this creates a situation in which it is almost impossible to know exactly how a change in one element will influence the other two elements—because simultaneous to let's say a change in A, B is being altered, which changes C... which is feeding back on the original change in A... which influences B... and on and on.

To make a little more sense of this check out this handy three-body gravitational model from the University of Toronto. First just press play for the single planet scenario without changing any of the controls. Pretty cool, eh? Now choose the "three planet" option. Things get chaotic pretty quickly. So what you might ask? Well, let's call Sun 1 insulin, Sun 2 glucagon, planet 1 protein, planet 2 carbohydrate and you guessed it, planet 3 fat. Although far from perfect I think this is a compelling analogy of the interplay and complexity of our hormonal system—and in an amazingly paired down format no less.

We are not looking at other hormones or environmental issues that change the "settings" on our simple model. Try this: Set up the three-planet run as before and open that same page in another window. In the second window set the mass of Sun 1 to "two" and start both animations. Two things should grab your attention. The first is that the two scenarios play out very differently with the increased influence of Sun 1 (increased insulin) and the second is that the animation looks like something you saw after eating several of Yael's "Magic Brownies".

All of this was a lead in for a "How To" piece on glycogen repletion. Sorry if that's an abrupt lane change but that's where this ride is heading! I'm obviously going to talk about that a bunch but I want to tie all this together first since you might be wondering why the analogy using the three-body gravitation problem? Well... it may be a stretch, but I think this illustrates how incredibly complex some of these systems can become with only a few variables and this pales in comparison to the actual complexity of living systems (us). A sub-point is the complexity of these systems is an outgrowth of the interaction of the various elements and how said interaction can change the state and or outcome of the system and its constituents. For example if we increase insulin, how does this affect protein, carbohydrate and fat metabolism? At the same insulin level how does various mixtures of macronutrients, and amounts of macronutrients, affect things like performance, health and longevity? If performance, health and longevity are affected by gene transcription as a consequence of insulin levels and macronutrient amounts and ratios (which is absolutely the case), how does this then feed back and affect hormone levels and how macronutrients are metabolized? Obviously this scene can get very murky and I don't want to befuddle you with minutia and imponderables, but I do want to analyze all this information critically and remain just a bit skeptical about ANY conclusions.

We can draw some sound deductions from much of this material, but it's always good to remain open to later modifications and better information. With all that said

I want to look at the reasons WHY we might want to approach glycogen repletion in different ways... and if we have different methodologies that must mean we have different goals we might be considering. Why would one want to replenish glycogen stores AT ALL? Much has been written on this topic from a number of very bright people, who appear to split into two camps.

The first camp advocates aggressive post workout glycogen replenishment with the argument being that this activity will enhance both recovery and performance. There is no doubt this approach has merits but the methods for determining how much glycogen needs replenishment have not been well developed. Hopefully this article changes that.

The second camp advocates no aggressive post workout glycogen replenishment, arguing that this will impair health and longevity due to the deleterious effects of insulin spiking. These folks may be onto something, but they might also have something to contribute to enhanced performance oddly enough.

Performance, Health, Longevity-One More Time

I've kicked the concepts of performance, health and longevity around for a couple of years now, but I have never tried to define what these terms mean. I think this is due to the fact these are common usage words. It's not like running across procrustean. Great word by the way. This lack of clarity is sloppy and frequently I find that a tight definition of a word or concept can help focus my usage and understanding. I'm not shooting for Webster-type definitions in this case—those are easy enough to find—I want something that just fleshes out meaning a little and shows our nutrition and athletics bias.

Performance: How well something does at a given activity. This could be anything from free kicks in soccer to a stock portfolio but for our purposes it is certainly more athletics and training oriented. Typically we are keeping track of some numbers; otherwise we are dealing with opinion. We need some data and comparisons to move into the realm of facts.

> **Health:** I'd like to define health as one's biological status... perhaps even "fitness" in a Darwinian sense, right now. Today.

> **Longevity:** For our purposes at the Performance Menu I'd like to think about longevity as health over a period of time.

Now a few points need to be made. The first is that these concepts are interrelated and at some points mutually supportive, and at other points mutually exclusive. Said another way we see both convergence and divergence in these concepts. The second point is that these definitions are not perfect. One could experience longevity in that one lives to be

90 years old... but one's health may have been terrible for 30 or more of those years and it was only a miracle of modern medicine that one got to lie in a bed and contemplate eternity... for nearly that long. Alternately you may have rocking performance and stellar health but you make the mistake of wearing a T-shirt that says "I Support Title IX" into an Iowa wrestling tournament. There goes your longevity.

Now that we have better defined the terms performance, health and longevity, I'd like to put forward the notion that we have a few different glycogen reload options, each of which will play to a bias of performance, health or longevity.

Performance Bias

The performance bias prioritizes recovery and high intensity training above all else. That said, glycogen recovery needs will vary from situation to situation. A hard training Olympic weightlifter may have very modest glycogen replacement needs due to the demands of that sport and the associated training. For example heavy 1-2 repetition sets with long 2-5 minute rest periods will be remarkably taxing on the nervous system but create little inroads with regards to glycogen status. In contrast, a wrestler or MMA competitor who is living in the lactate pathway for multiple 3-5 minute bouts in addition to specific strength work and adjunctive anaerobic/GPP sessions will have significant replenishment needs. A triathalete in race preparation will likely have needs more in common with the fighter than the weightlifter but that will depend upon how the triathalete structures training. Forty minutes spent at or near the "lactate threshold" will require far more glycogen for recovery than 40 minutes spent at 70% VO2 max. Keep in mind different situations and goals require different and sometimes antagonistic approaches to achieve the desired result.

Something I have found frustrating is the lack of precision in glycogen replenishment. Most studies simply quote a formula that consists of a 4/1 carb/protein mixture with the carbs weighing in at about 100g. That is a pretty big whack of high glycemic load carbs, and although at times it may be completely appropriate to use this formula, we must also ask are there times when smaller doses are more appropriate? The best thing I have seen was generated by Charles Poliquin and it correlates total volume of work performed to the glycogen repletion need. Here is a snippet from that:

> 12-72 reps per workout: 0.6 g/Kg/LBM (Lean Body Mass)
> 73-200 reps per workout: 0.8 g/kg/LBM
> 200-360 reps per workout: 1.0 g/kg/LBM
> 360-450 reps per workout: 1.2 g/kg/LBM

Now I really had a bug up my fanny to construct a glycogen repletion strategy that was much more detailed. I wanted this to look at total work performed during the workout, factor in some intensity elements such as work-rest pacing to take account of elements like the Cori Cycle in which lactate can be regenerated to glycogen. Well... I discovered why no one else has this information figured out! There are more variables and more errors involved with trying to tie things down than one can imagine and it's interesting that an eyeball method can provide some pretty remarkable results.

Here is something I noticed: In the above example the relatively low volume workout, 12-72 reps calls for about 43g of carbs (0.6x73kgLBM). That's about 5 Zone blocks. At the top 360-450 reps workout I'm looking at about 87g, or about 9 blocks. If one is following an Athletes Zone diet it simply means shifting somewhere between 25-66% of ones daily carb allotment to the post workout window. This is all based on my 16-17 block daily allotment and it REALLY simplifies things. If my training session was very intense, I could shift nearly all my carbs to that post workout window. Keep in mind that as total activity level goes up, so does block level.

Some special circumstances may necessitate more carbs in total to facilitate full recovery, but this is pretty manageable as one simply deletes fat blocks and ads additional carb blocks like this: For every 3 fat blocks deleted, add one carb block. If the initial large post workout carb meal is sufficient for recovery I would then recommend as many of the remaining carbs as possible come from low glycemic load veggies, and if you cannot fit in all the veggies, add 3 blocks of fat for every carb block deleted. If one is following a seat-o-your pants method, this boils down to Protein and carbs post WO, protein and fats most other meals. Pretty simple, No?

Health and Longevity

Since we are looking at longevity from the perspective of "health over the course of time" the approaches to optimize health and longevity are likely similar. In this scenario we are looking at nutrient intake, both with regards to composition and timing, as TOOLS to optimize health and longevity. This may be in stark contrast to the performance approach on a mechanistic level but we may also have something to learn from the performance mindset with regards to enjoyment of life, not just quantity.

If we adopt a health and longevity bias, we will rely on hepatic carbohydrate production and VERY low glycemic load carbohydrate for our glycogen repletion. Obviously this will limit our CrossFit-style metabolic conditioning sessions, but we can still be plenty active and develop attributes like strength, joint mobility and skills on a nutritional approach such as this. I'll touch on some potential programming to complement the nutritional recommendations that carry a health and longevity bias. Why not the performance? Hopefully you have your performance training figured out!

Back to nutrition. If we are taking in mainly nutrient-dense, low-glycemic-load carbohydrate like greens and multicolored veggies, we will receive a very modest amount of carbohydrate to replenish glycogen. We can also manufacture glucose, or at least our livers can, from amino acids and the glycerol back bone of fats via gluconeogenesis. Glycerol will contribute relatively little to this process but it does help. Amino acids from our dietary protein will supply the carbon backbones necessary for the liver to manufacture glucose; however, gluconeogenesis is dependent on what percentage protein accounts for in the diet and overall energy balance. If one is following an Athletes Zone protein intake is quite modest, only about 15% of calories. However this should be adequate to replenish glycogen to a level that allows for about one hard metabolic conditioning session per week. Our key goals with this approach are to minimize glucose flux and, if possible, to induce a state of ketosis as this appears to confer potent adaptive and cellular protective properties via hormesis. You might be tired of hearing this, but including intermittent fasting in this protocol may be an easy way to accentuate the effects of the hepatic-driven glucose production. Intermittent fasting, as I've talked about elsewhere, may offer a route to straddle the worlds of performance and health/longevity by increasing insulin sensitivity, allowing for increased muscle glycogen stores which facilitate training, while simultaneously minimizing our exposure to the complications associated with constant glucose intake.

Training to optimize health and longevity should, not surprisingly, be a balanced affair. Something akin to the ME-Black Box template is very good so long as potent metabolic sessions are kept to around once per week. Now this is dependant on the situation as a short workout like Fran, although demanding, is not the glycogen depleter that a 400m run, 30 box jumps and 30 wall-balls for 5 rounds (Kelly) will be. Something else to keep in mind is that activities can be more or less glycogen dependant depending upon how you approach the activity. For example boxing or kickboxing is typically a very glycogen intensive activity; however, one can approach that activity by minimizing how many strikes are thrown in sequence and mixing fairly long rests between efforts. This may look like a jab, cross, round kick and then 5-10 seconds of foot work and movement to allow ATP/CP to be replenished via aerobic metabolism and fat stores. Sledge hammer GPP, wheelbarrow work and sled drags can all be approached in this beneficial but less glycogen-intensive manner. This is much like the training Scotty Hagnas has reported doing at various points of the year when he is eating a lower carb diet.

In closing, I think it's important to remember complexity can be better managed with a clear plan and focused desire. The concepts mentioned above should provide a framework from which you can optimize your glycogen repletion strategies to suit YOUR needs. Also, some woo-woo physicists think our thoughts can actually organize and shape reality. Whether you buy into that or not, clear focus and an understanding of where you want to go and why you are doing things can help to remove you as a confounding element in an already complex situation.

FIGHT!
ROBB WOLF

Five years ago if you asked most people who Chick Liddell was or showed them a photo of the Ice Man he might have been mistaken for a NASCAR fan, not a world champion athlete. Obviously much has changed. Now mixed martial arts (MMA) along with the attendant sports of wrestling, Brazilian Jiu-jitsu, Thai boxing and even stuffy old boxing have witnessed an up-tick in popularity and participation. Unless one lives in a backwater town like Chico, CA it's an easy proposition to find a good school to train any or all of these arts. The result has been an explosion in the skill sets of current competitors and an amazing acceleration in the development of MMA. However, one component has remained elusive and fairly steeped in voodoo: strength and conditioning. A quick perusal of some of the more popular MMA sites leaves one with the impression that a day of Back & Bi's followed by Chest & Tri's with a "little cardio" is the route to optimum fight performance. There are some exceptions like Ross Enamait's phenomenal work and some material from Parisi. That's about the extent of what I would tip my hat to.

What's the best approach? It's tough just looking to the competitors of this relatively young sport. Win/loss has historically been an extension of technical proficiency, particularly in Brazilian Jiu-jitsu (BJJ) however that story has changed in recent times as we have witnessed wrestlers who possess phenomenal conditioning, heart and aggression winning many events and titles with only a modest understanding of BJJ and stand up skills. Thinking back to the beginnings of the UFC this was obviously not the case as smaller, weaker individuals could consistently win against larger stronger opponents, even wrestlers, given adequate technical advantage. Like I said however, times have changed! Now everyone at A-level competition has at least a working knowledge of take downs, submissions and their respective defenses. When the technical field converges upwards what then are the determinants of success? Louie Simmons has made the point that on average when two individuals of equal skill-set compete, the individual who is stronger will prove victorious. Some seem to interpret this to mean start a cycle of anabolic steroids in conjunction with a double split bodybuilding routine. That approach worked for some top-level competitors; however, the evolution of the sport is calling into question bodybuilding as an effective approach to Strength & Conditioning, even with the advantage of anabolics. I'd like to look at some integrative approaches and help to drag strength and conditioning for combatives out of the dark ages. This is not intended to be an exhaustive "How To" guide… that will come later! This is more an open communication of one fighters preparation for competition and what our strategies were along the way.

At NorCal S&C we had the good fortune of prepping a fighter for the rigors of MMA competition, one Glen "The Mad Man" Cordoza. Glen is a phenomenal athlete and coach and will be a major force in the lightweight MMA scene… trust me! Glen was a client of ours several years ago and proved to be a tough and supremely coachable athlete. He worked with us for about five months and then spent the better part of two years in Thailand wracking up an impressive professional Muay Thai record. In addition to Glen's Thai boxing he had (at the beginning of our training) a blue belt in BJJ under John Frankl and a mountain of experience working with such fight luminaries as Randy Couture, BJ Penn, Marcello Garcia and Eddie Bravo to name a few. Glen's day job is the role of author for Victory Belt publishing, so he gets to fly to exotic locations, interview the best fighters in the world, and help to write instructional books with these folks. If you like to dismantle people or write and read about the dismantling of people as Glen does, this is a pretty kick ass job.

Before we jump in I want to mention that whenever a client approaches me for help with an element of their performance it's usually with a specific goal in mind. For some it may be an athletic event like Glen's fight. For others it may be weight loss or working with a family doctor to reverse hypertension. Whatever the case it's important for me to thoroughly inventory not only what the person wants or needs to accomplish but also to honestly evaluate where they currently are. From this we can engineer a plan that will address weaknesses and build on strengths to reach a mutually agreed upon goal. This may be obvious for many and I apologize if it seems trite or remedial, but it has been my experience that good coaches have sophisticated means of assessing a client's status relative to a projected goal. With this information, rational planning can follow. This method also lends itself to cost/benefit projections of the form "Given our current set of circumstances this is how much suffering you will need to endure to get this desired outcome."

With the above in mind, here is the scenario I faced for Glen's fight preparation: Glen came to me interested in help with his strength & conditioning for a fight in late March. This was in early January and it seemed we had more than ample time to get Glen in top fight shape. I knew that Glen had excellent stand-up, clinch and ground games and he always took his conditioning seriously. We did, however, have a few interesting twists to this story from day one. The first was that Glen's normal fight school had closed about three months previously. What this meant was that Glen had very little hands on sparring, rolling or drilling. The second issue was that Glen was in the middle of writing several books, including one with BJ Penn and another with Randy Couture. In essence big, important, time-critical books. The demands of book writing placed Glen in front of a computer for upwards of 10 hrs per day writing, editing and working on page layouts. Glen was stiff, moderately deconditioned (for him) and had a bit of rust on his game… and we had no legit fight school. Hey, we didn't want this to be a cakewalk!

Once we established where Glen was and where we needed to take him the following points helped to focus our training:

1. Establish an objective measure of sport-specific conditioning.
2. Restore and expand Glen's fighting skill sets.
3. Implement an effective S&C protocol.

Objective Measures

For an objective measure of sport specific conditioning I chose to use the CrossFit classic Fight Gone Bad. Glen had experience with this workout both from working with us in the past and in his time with BJ Penn. FGB is time indexed to match an MMA fight (three 5 minute rounds) and since Glen had familiarity with the test his improvements would accurately reflect performance improvements and not test improvement. In sports science language, Glen had gone through his acclimatization phase with the FGB test. Glen did however display significant muted hip function on several of the movements, perhaps most notably the push press. This improved over time and correlated nicely with improved scores on this activity. Glen's first exposure to FGB produced a green, but not unimpressive 276. As we will see later, this number improved dramatically in the weeks to come and by somewhat surprising means.

Fight Skills

We began restoration of Glen's stand-up, clinch and ground skills. I had a decent Thai boxing game at one time so we started working light, technical sparring to re-establish distancing and timing in stand up. Positional sparring was used in BJJ. We started work on the heavy bag and Thai pads. ALL sessions were videotaped and analyzed during flexibility training to make plans for the following day and shore up any weaknesses in the game.

Strength & Conditioning

Integrate effective strength & conditioning. Glen had never followed a specific strength training program. In the past he had used track intervals, dips, pull-ups and some band work for his training with quite good results; however, I wanted to bring up his absolute and relative strength without increasing his weight. Glen fights in the 155 class and runs right around 165. This is not a huge drop to make, but neither of us wanted to push that margin. This considered we started Glen on the deadlift, ring dips and pull-ups. Initially the dead lift was an awkward and challenging movement that exposed a surprising degree of hamstring tightness and what I call a "glassy" lower back. Tight hamstrings and hip flexors appeared to contribute to lower back pain from flexion at the hips. This alleviated with strength and flexibility work. I kept Glen very light and conservative on the strength movements, hammering form while keeping the rep range below 3 to minimize hypertrophy. Even at the light initial loading on the deadlift (62 kg) Glen noticed an immediate improvement in his game. We never maxed Glen but over the course of several weeks we worked him up to very comfortable sets with 100kg in the DL. I will detail this more later; however, it is stunning how much this improved strength added to Glen's already formidable game. It is important to note also that this strength circuit of deadlifts, weighted pull-ups and weighted ring dip, required less than 15 min to perform and made virtually no inroads into Glen's recovery capacity. This is a huge consideration when we are pushing the envelope of human performance.

With our objectives in place we started with 2 weeks of general "pre-season" work structured as such:

Warm-up including light shadow boxing, dynamic range of movement and 1K on the concept 2 rower. Next we either worked sport specific activities such as Thai pads, clinch work, BJJ positional sparring and heavy bag work OR we put Glen through his strength circuit comprised of the deadlift, weighted pull-ups and ring dips. I alternated these days so Glen would occasionally do his strength circuit in a fairly fatigued state.

Sets and reps on the strength circuit were 3-5 sets of 2-3 reps. As I mentioned previously, Glen had some difficulty with the deadlift in the beginning. Tight hips made proper position in the beginning of the lift a challenge and it was common for Glen to lose his lordotic arch upon initiation of the lift. Using dynamic range of movement and the Potato Sack Squat (© Dan John Inc) we were able to get Glen into a safe, ergonomically sound position for pulling. It is interesting to note that once we addressed positional/structural integrity, small technique errors in Glens pulling immediately improved. Similar to a math problem, the set-up proved to be all-important. I started Glen very conservatively on the DL with 62 kg and kept him there for about two weeks just hammering form. The ring dips and pull-ups were un-weighted for two weeks, then I began wave loading all the movements, adding a little weight for 2-3 consecutive workouts, then dialing back 1-2 steps. This may not seem to be very aggressive but amidst the rest of Glens training I wanted this strength circuit to be safe, productive and non-taxing. I had Glen move from one movement to the next, with about one minute rest between stations. This allowed for quick completion of the circuit but allowed for 3-4 minutes recovery between each station.

Once the strength circuit or sport specific practice was done we used some form of a mixed modal, CrossFit style circuit. We time indexed efforts to match about five minutes of work and one minute of rest for most workouts; however, I did play with shorter intervals to emphasize power. We also worked hybrid sessions in which Glen wore MMA gloves and included Thai boxing work on either pads or the heavy bag in addition to movements such as running, pull-ups and thrusters. We wrapped up the day with foam rolling, stretching and the daily plunge into the ice bath. Total training time ranged from 1.5-2.5 hours.

This initial two-week period of training brought Glen's work capacity and anaerobic conditioning up pretty dramatically as evidenced by his 310 FGB score. This was certainly a plus; however, Glen often experienced extreme soreness from the metabolic sessions to a degree that made SSP work vary from unappealing to impossible. As I mentioned before, Glen has a solid MMA game, but we needed to cover many aspects of the fight preparation beyond just S&C. This was late January and a few of the people from the old MMA school in Chico put together a quasi-functional operation about 15 minutes outside of town. Glen could train here and get some reasonably good sparing, BJJ and expert pad work. At this point I wanted to accomplish the following:

1. Shift most conditioning to sport specific work. As the saying goes, the best way to prepare for a sport is to DO the sport. That considered, however, more and more of the same activity will lead to burnout unless volume, intensity and variety are managed effectively.
2. Increase the amount of skill work Glen performed.
3. Continue strength circuit work.

The schedule we developed allowed for a large volume of high quality work that accomplished both the above objectives. Here is what most days looked like:

8:00 am

Glen arrived at the gym and performed 15 minutes of shadow boxing for a warm-up. We developed call-outs that drilled certain combinations and responses. For example sprawling, counter-punching, circling, etc. Once Glen was warm we worked light, technical sparring with MMA gloves. We again worked many scenarios establishing "A" game combinations and then transitioned into open movement. Contact was quite light but movement was alive and spontaneous. We videotaped and analyzed each session. From this we planned the curriculum for the noon session, Glen's evening sparring, and the following morning session. This process was remarkably productive, but the key to the efficacy lay in focusing on one or perhaps two elements to improve in the following sessions. It was tempting to try to fix everything at once, but by isolating one element, such as footwork during a combination, we were able to fix minor technical elements of Glen's game that might otherwise go unnoticed. It may be tedious and a bit boring, but it is absolutely crucial to make significant technical progress. We concluded this session with foam rolling and light stretching.

12:00 pm

Glen went home after the morning session to eat and work on his writing. He then returned to the gym to work the intense skill/conditioning session for the day. This second session involved time-indexed fight training structured in one of the following formats:

Working with five different people for one minute each then a one-minute rest or an on going rotation of people lasting 15-20 minutes. In the case of the five-minute rounds we typically worked up to six rounds whereas the longer, continuous sessions lasted up to 40 total minutes in 15-20 minute increments. We utilized stations such as the following:

1. Thai pads. Mainly "A" game combinations attempting to pack as many into one minute as possible. This station was a pre-fatiguing technique that put Glen into a significant oxygen debt and consequently at a disadvantage for the following stations in which he faced a fresh opponent every minute while his fatigue mounted.
2. Single leg takedown defense. Glen started with his leg in his partner's hands and then fought to avoid the takedown. If a takedown occurred a five-second scramble was allowed before breaking and resetting. This is an isolated drill and we wanted to emphasize the takedown defense, but we did NOT want to ingrain a sense that if Glen was taken down he could give up. Jeff Martin of Brand X Martial Arts relayed a story to me of police officers who have handed weapons BACK to assailants after disarming the individual because that is what the officers have done thousands of times in training. This five-second scramble allowed for a real sense of flow from clinch to ground as it would happen in a fight, but allowed for a great deal of focused work.
3. Escape from guard, mount, side control or similar position. Glen's partner would start in one of these positions and they would reset if Glen managed to make it to his feet.
4. Thai and Greco clinch. We sometimes isolated the two styles of clinch work and sometimes integrated them. We worked to takedown, occasionally with unforeseen results such as my separated shoulder during one session. But hey, I got the takedown!

The above sessions allowed for fight specific anaerobic training and constant technical improvement. The anaerobic conditioning was brutal as Glen was forced to work against fresh opponents round after round. Most of his partners outweighed him by a significant amount. A highly objective measure of Glen's metabolic conditioning was his eventual FGB score of 360 at a body weight of 165. It is interesting to note that Glen performed no other conditioning workouts besides evening sparring and these mid-day SSP sessions. I think that is interesting and quite validating of CrossFit's insistence on "Constantly varied, functional movements, performed at high intensity." At first glance this may not square with one's notion of thrusters and pull-ups, Frans and Helens, but really what is more intense and functional than fighting? Where people can miss an opportunity for improvement is in a lack of variety in training. Sparring at too high an intensity for too long will lead to mental and physical exhaustion. With the above format we were able to dramatically improve Glens sport specific conditioning AND his general anaerobic conditioning. Although we used mixed modal workouts for Glen's "pre-season" we could not afford the lack of specificity as fight time neared. There are other routes to get to a 360 Fight Gone Bad score but they will not provide both improved metabolic conditioning AND improved skill sets in stand-up, clinch and ground.

The above considered, we attempted to balance two mutually exclusive training adaptations: improved general conditioning and sport specific efficiency. Greg Glassman first exposed me to the work of Stephen Seiler and his Time Course of Training Adaptations. In essence one must become very efficient at a given activity to reach the highest levels of performance possible, yet one must also augment sport specific conditioning. This is the conundrum many face in that simply doing more of the same sport eventually leads to stalled or diminishing returns. We employed the above sessions such that the longer continuous sessions forced efficiency of movement on Glen's part. All extraneous movement was polished out of his game and Glen became VERY adept at reading his opponent, thus allowing for economy of movement and conservation of energy. The short intense sessions imposed extreme demands that allowed continuous progress due to the unlimited variations in the sport specific conditioning. We could alter station order, who performed at the given station and of course the time variables. We were working five one-minute intervals. We could easily have worked 10 thirty-second intervals. These other sessions would be sport specific yet variable enough to ease some of the mental and physical stress of training while allowing for continual progress.

If Glen proved to be especially tired or beaten up, we dialed back the intensity or called that session altogether. In either case if the sport specific drilling looked like too much work, we put Glen through an easy session on the C2 rower, stretched, foam rolled and looked at video from previous sessions and discussed strategy. It is important to have a general guide and plan but it is equally important to be flexible and know how to keep the whole operation moving forward by taking a few steps back. This is of particular import for the S&C coach who must monitor recovery and decide when to dial back and when to push forward, all with the fight date looming in the near future. This process is often at odds with the desire of the fighter to go 100% all the time. Although this mindset and mental toughness is requisite to achieve the highest level in sport, so too is the ability to save a little for another day and bag the operation altogether if need be, to ensure forward progress.

The noon session always wrapped up with foam rolling, stretching, ice baths and review of that sessions video. Glen then shuffled home to eat, work and revive for his 5:00 pm session in Oroville.

5:00 pm

Glen's 5:00 pm session involved no-Gi BJJ, sparring and mitt work. I did not participate in these sessions, but Glen took video and we discussed performance and strategy the following day.

Bravo?

As I mentioned previously, Glen writes for Victory Belt Publications and he occasionally flies to a location to shoot video or work with an individual on a project. About 18 days before Glen was to fight, he went to Legends Mixed Martial Arts Training Center to work with Eddie Bravo. In the course of training with Eddie and his students Glen was awarded his Purple belt from Eddie… and managed to tear his ulnar-colateral ligament. One "hurrah" and two "Oh Shits". Glen was scheduled to fight March 31st and then four days later fly to Thailand to train and get in two or three pro fights. Due to the severity of Glens injury we pulled him from the March 31st card and shifted gears to rehab/maintenance mode so his Thailand trip would not be a complete wash… other than partying down for Songkhran! I'm not going to go into the rehab here, but I do want to highlight some of the improvements and subjective/objective measures of success we had for this fight preparation.

Objective Improvements

1. Improvement of Fight Gone Bad score from 276 to 360 in six weeks. Glen progressed from 276 to 310 during two weeks of CrossFit style programming. He then progressed from 310 to 360 only as a consequence of his strength circuit and MMA specific training. I find that very interesting.
2. Increased deadlift working weight from 62 kg to 100kg. This may seem a very

insignificant increase and not an "impressive" weight overall, but this was Glen's first exposure to these movements. I wanted to establish a base of technical proficiency while minimizing injury risk and recovery demands. I think Glen will easily achieve a 2.5-3.0 times bodyweight deadlift within six months of training once he returns from Thailand.

3. Decrease in body fat of about 5% while maintaining bodyweight at 165. This translates into in increase of about eight pounds of muscle while maintaining bodyweight. This objective measure squared well with a dramatic increase in Glen's sport specific strength.

Subjective Improvements

1. Glen's recovery ability, both within a session and from day to day, improved remarkably. Minor bumps and bruises healed seemingly overnight.
2. Glen's stand-up clinch and ground improved dramatically, both in technical execution and aggression due to improved conditioning and skill refinement. The initial conditioning circuits witnessed Glen quickly fatigued and more often than not fighting from his back. In subsequent weeks however it was Glen's partners who needed a break! It was rare that Glen did not have the upper hand during a session. Keep in mind Glen's training partners were all experienced fighters and wrestlers.
3. Glen received his purple belt from Eddie Bravo. Glen was working essentially in isolation and is easily the most technically proficient BJJ practitioner in the Chico area. By analyzing tapes to pinpoint and fix technique flaws and by increasing his overall strength and conditioning, Glen was awarded his next rank in BJJ from one of the sport's most respected instructors.

Nutrition

Glen followed a Paleo diet with no real restrictions on intake other than he consumed protein and carbohydrate meals post workout, typically chicken and yams. All other meals were protein, greens and good fats. These meals were typically salads with canned wild Alaskan salmon, veggies and olive oil. The only supplement Glen used was Kirkland fish oil at 10-15g/day of EPA/DHA. We used this loose, unweighed, unmeasured approach as it simplified the nutrition side of the game without introducing more time demands on Glen's already busy schedule.

I was initially concerned that Glen might gain too much weight on this program. We monitored Glen's weight daily and we were prepared to implement a weighed, measured Zone if Glen's weight began to creep upwards. We simply kept portion sizes reasonable and used rough measures such as "a lot" of sweet potatoes after a very demanding training session and much smaller portions after relatively easy sessions. This allowed us to take advantage of the post exercise non-insulin-mediated glucose transport which minimizes insulin secretion. Since Glen had multiple training sessions this allowed for immediate, reasonable recovery that accentuated our body composition goal: Lose body fat, maintain bodyweight. I think this puts to bed the notion some in strength & conditioning put forward that the Paleo diet is sufficient to avoid the scourges of metabolic syndrome but not up to the task of fueling elite performance. And of course, it would be impossible to eat Paleo foods in a 40/30/30 ratio (wink)!

Acknowledgements

Thank yous are in order as many people gave in various ways to help Glen prepare. Dr. John Fragoso was our fight Doc and managed to keep Glen bouncing back from most of his bumps, bruises and contusions. Dr. Fragoso is also an excellent wrestler and a savage athlete. He helped in some of the fight prep circuits and had some of the best success of anyone at taking Glen down. Jason Pietz and Cedric Schwyzer are both accomplished MMAs and they were instrumental in helping Glen refine his technique and timing. Shawn Gower paid the ultimate sacrifice and met Pukie during one conditioning session. Also, NEVER give Shawn tequila when he stays at your house. Finally thank you to Nicki and all the NorCal S&C clients who put up with loud, sweaty guys thrashing about the gym at all hours. Shoot Glen an email if you have any questions about his training, Victory Belt projects, or how to survive Songkhran!

BODYWEIGHT SKILL INTEGRATION
JIM BATHURST

I admire the strongmen and women of old. Here were people who could move a mountain of iron yet could also control themselves in various bodyweight strength, acrobatic, and balancing skills. And why shouldn't they (and we) be proficient with both the weights and our bodies? As it's been said, "Handbalancing to a bodybuilder, a weightlifter or any barbell man, is as natural as a duck taking to water."

Both weight training and bodyweight skills create muscular tension and test the body's ability to coordinate itself in a single task. Yet I feel being able to move and control your body builds a unique strength and coordination that weights can't quite match, and vice versa. This is the reason I've included various bodyweight skills alongside my weight training for quite some time. I also include both in my workouts because I enjoy training each one. Is any other reason really needed?

Now when I talk of bodyweight skills in this article, I'm talking of both static positions (e.g. planche, handstand) and those requiring joint movement and range of motion (e.g. one arm chin, one arm pushup). The term skill also assumes an above average amount of strength and/or balance to perform.

When I name a skill, I'm also referring to any lesser progressive skills and exercises. So this means easier skills that match one's current strength level as well as any other work one might do to achieve the named skill. I have not elaborated greatly on all these progressive exercises and skills, though, as it would turn this article into a very long list of tutorials.

Strength Skills:
Complementary Combinations

When attempting to integrate bodyweight skills into your workout, the first inclination is to continue your regular weight training routine and tack on the various skills wherever you see fit. Problems often arise, as you may do too much work during the week and not allow the body to properly recover. You may also fatigue the body too much during a workout and interfere with other exercises in your program. Another problem is the lack of focus you'll feel when trying to cover several dozen different exercises in the same training week.

A better alternative comes in understanding how various bodyweight skills and weight training exercises complement each other. Working on one will show a carryover and improvement in the other. Instead of including both during a training session, you can switch back and forth as needed. It's the concept of "same, but different." The same general movements and muscles are worked, but in different ways. You'll still need to spend time practicing the skill, working through its various progressions, and learning its subtleties, but now you won't feel that you're completely neglecting a skill as you work on a complementary weight training exercise.

This is by no means a comprehensive list, but should get you thinking about the various combinations you can put together. I'll elaborate how to work these combinations into your training routines later in the article.

Planche:
Weighted dips, weighted pushups, decline and flat bench pressing (barbells and dumbbells)

I've found working weighted dips to be one of the best exercises to compliment planche work. The dip builds up the strength in the pressing muscles of the chest, shoulder and triceps at a similar angle. Also important is the fact that the scapulae can move freely during the exercise. In fact, I find it essential to make sure to press up as much as possible at the top of the dip, mimicking the press needed when holding the planche.

Working on weighted pushups also allow for scapular movement, as well as the added challenge of keeping the midsection tight. They generally don't allow for as much added weight as a dip, though.

The decline and flat bench press are included because they will improve general pressing strength. In fact, it's often said that some Olympic gymnasts who posses a high level of planche strength can bench-press nearly twice their bodyweight the first time they try. While this may be just an urban legend, the exercises should help the planche to some degree. They do not allow the scapulae to move as freely as in the weighted dip, though.

One arm pushup
One arm dumbbell chest press, weighted dips, any bench press (especially close-grip)

The one arm pushup is a skill requiring good horizontal pushing strength and the ability to generate tension through the body. The one arm dumbbell chest press accomplishes both of these things. There is a difference, though, in the exact tension needed throughout the body. The one arm pushup requires cross-body tension from the pressing hand to the opposite foot while the one arm dumbbell chest press requires tension from the pressing hand to the same side foot. Despite this, learning to keep a unilateral tension in the body while pressing will help the one arm pushup.

The bench presses and dips are again included, as they will increase general pressing strength in the horizontal direction. The close grip bench press is particularly recommended, as the arms are close to the sides, just like the one arm pushup. Such a position focuses on and helps strengthen the triceps.

Front lever, Back Lever, Muscle-Ups, One arm Chin-ups/Pull-ups
Weighted Chin-ups/Pull-ups, One Arm Rows, Weighted Rack Rows, Bent-over Rows, Pullovers

The common factor among all these skills is the need for a high level of back strength. While the weighted chin-ups and pull-ups seem to be the most complementary to other vertical pulling skills (such as the one arm chin-ups/pull-ups and muscle-ups), one should not discount heavy rowing to help these skills as well. Rowing will especially help you pull the elbows back and finish strong and high above the bar for the one arm chin-ups/and pull-ups.

The front lever is a skill that requires a great deal of upper body tension and a lot of back involvement. It is often said that the skill doesn't even need to be trained; that heavy pull-ups will be sufficient to build the strength. I've found this to be true to a certain degree. You'll still have to practice the front lever, but once you can do a pull-up with 100 extra pounds around your waist, you'll find the front lever much easier! The pullover is also included in the list as a complement to the front lever. Muscle recruitment is very similar, even if the midsection is not stressed to as great a degree.

The back lever will also come about with heavy weighted pulling and rowing exercises, even easier than the front lever in my experience.

Now in the choice between chin-ups and pull-ups you should definitely work both, but I've found a better carryover to the front lever with weighted pull-ups due to the similar line of pull and muscular recruitment of the back and biceps. Specifically, I keep my elbows about shoulder width apart when I pull instead of flared out to the side. This feels remarkably similar to a front lever.

Pulling in this manner will also carryover very well to the muscle-up (on the rings or a bar). The muscle-up is another skill that some may find doesn't need to be trained often (or at all) if one is doing heavy pull-ups. Building up your maximal strength through weighted pull-ups will allow you to fly through the sticking point of this skill—the point where one transitions from pull-up to dip.

Handstand pushups, Simple Handstand Press
Military press, Push press

The military press and handstand pushup are perhaps the most obvious of the skill-weight training combinations. Each is going to increase your vertical pressing strength in a very similar way. Make sure to work the handstand pushups in a full range of motion with shoulders lowered all the way down to the hands in order to see the greatest carryover to the military press.

The biggest difference to point out is a greater demand for torso stiffness and stability with the military press, while the handstand pushup, especially freestanding away from a wall, will require a greater sense of balance.

The push press has the advantage of putting the weight over the head with help of the legs, then lowering it down slowly. This is quite similar to the progressive means of learning a handstand pushup where one lowers oneself down from the top of a handstand to the floor.

The simple handstand press, where one presses into a handstand from a squatting position, will greatly benefit from the increased shoulder strength that the military and push press provide. Practice will still be needed though to learn the balance for this skill.

One arm handstand pushup
One arm shoulder press, One arm push press

Both the one arm versions of the handstand pushup and overhead press have different techniques then their two arm brethren. Most notably is the ability to "press off the lat." By flexing the lat you can create upper body tension and control the movement better.

With any one arm handstand pushup work, you have the advantage of using the other arm for assistance - something that is too awkward to do smoothly with the shoulder press. But with the one arm shoulder press, as with the two arm version, there's the demand for greater muscular tension through the midsection.

The one arm push press will also allow the arm and shoulder to experience a higher load and degree of tension, which is essential for controlling the negative motion of any one arm handstand pushup work.

Pistols
Weighted squats, lunges, step-ups

When learning how to do a one legged squat, I have found the biggest limiting factor to be strength, not balance. And the more strength one has in their legs, the more one can focus on the balance. With that said, deep, weighted two legged squats are arguably the best exercise for the quad-dominant one legged squat. It should be noted that I'm referring to high-bar Olympic squats and not low-bar squats, which are hip dominant.

Just about every other heavy, weighted exercise you do for the legs is going to help the pistol along in some way. Unilateral work such as lunges, especially overhead versions, will work to build up stability in the frontal plane. This should prove helpful if side-to-side balance in the pistol is a problem.

Iron Cross
Straight Arm Cable Pull-downs, Weighted Chin-ups/Pull-ups, Weighted Dips (especially on rings)

Of all the skills discussed so far, the iron cross will be one that requires the largest amount of specific skill training in comparison to its weight training complements. This is due to the highly unique activation and synergy of the muscles of the upper body.

Straight arm cable pull-downs to the side of the body most closely mimic the motion and unique muscular stress of the iron cross. Even still, there are ways to cheat the movement and give a false sense of progress towards the iron cross. In addition, shoulder positioning and balance on the rings still needs to be learned.

The other complementary weight training exercises listed will help to build up general strength in the chest and back, which are the two largest muscles activated during the cross. Exercises such as weighted ring dips, especially focusing on the hands turned out, offer a close approximation of the muscular stress of the iron cross.

When talking of balancing skills, I include such skills as the handstand, the headstand, and the two arm elbow lever. These are skills that require one to learn a delicate balance while inducing relatively minimal fatigue of the body during each attempt.

I also include one arm variations such as the one arm handstand and one arm elbow lever. These tend to be more strenuous though, so one should take note of the accumulating fatigue and plan accordingly, whether in less volume or different placement in one's training, to prevent them from interfering with other workouts.

I do not include such skills like the planche in this group. Although it requires balance to perform, it is very fatiguing for most. You may reclassify certain skills based on your strength level, though.

I find one can include these types of skills in their workout at the very beginning when fresh. Training the skills for just a short period of time at the start of each workout will help to keep the skill familiar, yet prevent excess fatigue for the rest of the workout to follow.

You may also practice these skills on the off days for 10-15 minutes. I've found that such small blocks of time taken on your rest days to mesh well without interfering with recovery.

You can also integrate the skills in short amounts of time throughout the day—a method commonly referred to as "greasing the groove". Here you try to get as much quality work done throughout the day while staying as fresh as possible.

Remember that we are trying to teach the body to how to delicately balance, so the quality of the practice is diminished when overly fatigued. So whichever method you choose, stop practice when you become tired and your form becomes consistently worse.

Integration and Periodization of Skills

I don't write this section to fully explain the various forms of periodization; there are numerous articles written on that already. I am also not giving complete sample programs. In an article that already presents the reader with several options to think about, I would like to continue by offering several more ideas.

Basic Integration

Let's look at a simple four-day M-Tu-Th-Fr, upper/lower body split. Let's assume we are able to both a front lever and a planche at this point and would like more proficiency at a handstand.

Monday – Upper
Weighted dips
Front lever

Tuesday - Lower
Handstand work
Weighted squats
Weighted lunges

Thursday – Upper
Planche
Weighted Pullups

Friday - Lower
Handstand work
Pistols
Deadlift

Notice how planche holds have taken the place of weighted dips as we moved from Monday to Thursday, while the front lever is replaced with weighted pull-ups. Handstand work is placed at the beginning of lower body workouts, but again may be placed just about anywhere if the volume is monitored.

Or perhaps we're working a M-W-F, total body workout. A sample routine might look as such:

Monday
Bench press
Chin-ups
Lunges

Tuesday
Handstands throughout day

Wednesday
Military Press
One Arm Rows
Deadlift

Thursday
Handstands throughout day
Friday
Planche Holds
Muscle-Ups
Front Squat

You can devote as much or as little time to the bodyweight skills as you want. In the example above, there's only one workout containing bodyweight skills, with handstand work done on the off days. You could just as easily include different bodyweight skills in two workouts, or even once every two weeks. The decision will be based on your goals.

Olympic Lifting and High Intensity Interval Training

When working the Olympic lifts, High Intensity Interval Training, or any other training modality that stresses the whole body at once, the bodyweight exercises can be integrated in several additional ways. Whichever you pick, care must be taken to track total volume and allow for adequate recovery.

One way to handle things is an AM/PM split where the total body workout is done in one half of the day, and the bodyweight skills done in the second half. This will allow for sufficient time to rest and recover between sessions. Keep in mind, though, that some level of fatigue will still exist. Placing an Olympic lifting session as the first workout in the day will help prevent any bodyweight skill work (done several hours later) from fatiguing the muscles and affecting power and technique. On the other hand, a high intensity interval training session may be best placed as the second workout in the day, so that strength is not compromised for the bodyweight skills. One can then just grind through the interval session with minimal compromise of training effect.

I would recommend only working two or three skills a day in this way in order to control fatigue. For example, work one pushing skill, one pulling skill, and a lower body skill. Alternate the different skills practiced throughout the week if needed.

Undulating and Conjugate Periodization

In a training program where the intensity and reps change often, or one that calls for both dynamic and maximal efforts, the bodyweight skills are easily adjusted. Rather than working at your maximal level for the skill, use an easier progressive exercise and change the repetitions or the speed at which the exercise is performed.

Let's look again at a four-day, upper/lower split, this time the max effort days have a greater recovery surrounding them. We'll assume again that the planche and front lever are maximal efforts. Pay particular attention to the fact that the muscle-up is used for a pulling motion on the upper dynamic day.

Monday – Lower Max
Pistols
Deadlift

Wednesday – Upper Max
Front Lever
Planche

Friday – Lower Dynamic
Jump split squats
Speed box squats

Saturday – Upper Dynamic
Tuck planche pushups
Muscle-ups

This particular routine happens to be fairly heavy on bodyweight exercises for the upper body, but one could just as easily substitute a speed bench on Saturday for the planche work.

Of course, one can have maximal and submaximal bodyweight skills in the same workout. For instance, working the planche as a maximal effort, and adding tuck planche pushups at the end for higher repetition, accessory work.

While this guide is not perfect for instances where one uses a dynamic exercise (pushups) to work on a static position (planche), it at least helps quantify the difficulty of progressive exercises.

When dealing with time-based skills, such as how long one can hold a planche or a front lever, simply take the percentage of maximal time held. Again, it's not perfect, but it will give you something to measure if you so choose.

Deloading
(Back Off Periods)

When taking extended time to fully recover, simply pick an easier variation of the bodyweight skill you are working if you want to decrease the intensity but maintain the same volume. You can also decrease the number of repetitions or total number of holds for the skill if looking to maintain intensity but decrease volume.

If your maximal effort for a skill is one of the most basic progressions, it would be wise to pick an easier bodyweight exercise (pushups, chin-ups) or light weight training exercise to work.

Conclusion

The decision to start training for various bodyweight skills is completely up to you. I' recommend them for the variation they provide, the well-roundness they can give to one's athleticism, and just for the fun of them. Whether you're just adding these skills into your routine, or have been working them for years, proper planning and integration will help to maximize the efficiency of your training and prevent overtraining, stagnation, and frustration.

42 WAYS TO SKIN THE ZONE
ROBB WOLF

Have you ever heard the term "If all you have is a hammer all the world looks like a nail"? How about "You can put lipstick on a pig…but it's still a pig"? How about "Joey… do you like movies about Gladiators?" Two of those statements are analogies and one is a classic movie line…all are an attempt at an interesting introduction to all things Zone. The intro is always fraught with danger and difficulties. Much like stealing food from an O-lifter or bare-back sex in the Mission District…I hear both are VERY dangerous. Anyway…I've noticed on the CrossFit message board and a few other locations, confusion on how to make the Zone work. Some of the well-intentioned advice is similar to the analogies above. Trying to make one flavor of the Zone work for everyone and or making the Zone something it is not. Both activities have caused me to resort to Gladiator movies, which my Parole Officer has strongly recommended against. Hence this article. Much in the vein of Freud and Jung I want to look at a few archetypes that constitute most of the questions surrounding the Zone. Let's take a look at these folks.

The Gyro With A Thousand Faces

Before we really jump into this I need to point out that I am assuming a basic comprehension of the Zone. You have read and understand some resources like the CrossFit Journal issue 21, the witty and reasonably priced Performance Menu issue 2 which received the accolade "It didn't suck" from some guy on MMA.tv, or even the holiest of holies, the book that broke America's carb addition…until Ornish and McDougall got them back on the crack…Barry "I can't follow my own diet advice" Sears' Masterpiece… that wrongly states protein is the cause of ketosis… Enter the Zone. If you have not read these things, can't figure the block method…Christ, you are beyond help. Just do what Oprah is doing…it will be better that way. If you are past the training wheels stage but are not quite ready for the Huffy 10 speed…this article is for you. OK, back to the real fun. Let's look at our first Zone contestant: "Do I have to eat ALL of that?!"

DIHTEAT

Yes...DIHTEAT has figured out blocks, how many he or she needs and is chugging along nicely. DIHTEAT is dutifully eating all carbohydrates in the form of low glycemic load veggies...and this individual devotes more than 10 hours per day chewing food but only 2.8 nano seconds dropping stool in the LOO. Solution? It seems pretty obvious to use some dense carb sources like fruit or yams but this may not be an easy or straight forward thing. Dense carb sources can turn one into an Always Hungry Carb Crash Zombie (AHCCZ...see below). Nobody likes that so one must do one of several things:

1. Ratchet up the dense carbs slowly. For example if you have historically choked down 3 blocks of carbs in the form of broccoli, try swapping in one block of apple or yam for a block of broccoli. See how you feel. If you are "OK" try 2 blocks of apple or yam. Still "OK" or do you need a binky and a nap? We certainly want to solve the problem of too many veggies to eat but not at the expense of loosing glycemic control. Tinker and see what happens. Perhaps you need to use option 2.

2. Eat some dense carb sources in your post workout meal. I have used this method with much success and it really streamlines my eating as I only require one meal with dense carbs and then my subsequent meals are protein, veggies and good fats. Taking advantage of the post workout window enhances insulin sensitivity and allows one to skirt some of the issues of a carbier meal. I use about 50% of my daily carb allotment in post workout meals that follow a very demanding training session, about 8 blocks, or it may be as small as 4-6 blocks for a lighter workout. If I have not trained in a given day or if I find it impossible to get in all my carb blocks I employ option 3.

3. Just delete some damn carb blocks! It is complete crap that you need to balance every Zone meal...or even keep the original 40-30-30 ratio intact. The Athletes Zone in which one increases the fat by as much as 5 times is testament to this fact. The Athletes Zone changes the ratios to ~ 25-15-60! The Zone is effective in that it introduces a caloric deficit yet provides adequate protein for muscle maintenance and just a smidge of fat for hormone balance. On a ramped up Athletes Zone one consumes a high fat diet that promotes fat as a primary fuel source. That's it. There are other methods that provide similar results but the Zone is nice due to its block system and ubiquitous societal exposure...but don't turn it into magic folks. You CAN delete carb blocks depending upon your needs. Like in one of the above situations if you are having problems with either glycemic control or just packing in the carb blocks, just delete a given number of carb blocks and add 3 fat blocks for each barb block deleted.

Let's look at a typical day for me:

16 blocks at 5x fat. That means 16 blocks of protein, potentially 16 blocks of carbs and at least 80 blocks of fat (16 x 5). Let's say I do a hard workout and take in a 4 block protein meal, 8 blocks of carbs and 0 blocks of fat. In the later meals I want to keep things simple and remain with 4 block protein meals and only 2 blocks of carbs at each meal…things look like this:

>   4P 8C 0F
>   4P 2C ?F
>   4P 2C ?F
>   4P 2C ?F
>   Totals: 16P 14C

How much Fat? Well, at the 5X level I need 80 blocks of fat, that's a given. Since I will finish out the day with only 14 blocks of carbs I need to add 6 blocks of fat to make up the caloric deficit. So I need 86 blocks of fat for the day. Since I have one protein and carb meal with essentially no fat I have 3 remaining meals to get those fat blocks in. Obviously you can break things into smaller, more frequent meals if you like…I'm trying to minimize my time in the kitchen so the 4 meals works for me. I need 86 blocks of fat to reach my days allotment and stay in the quasi-erotic Zone Bliss state. It might be nice if 86 partitioned easily into 3 equal pieces…but alas it does not. 86/3=28.6. Being the rebel that I am, however, I'd recommend 29 blocks per meal. In that case things look like this:

>   4P 8C 0F
>   4P 2C 29F
>   4P 2C 29F
>   4P 2C 29F
>   Totals: 16P 14C 87F

Pretty Fracking close. Not just that but for me this is sooooo much easier than trying to balance every meal. I'm fairly organized but one of the things that has killed the Zone for me in the past was trying to adhere to the same macronutrient ratio at EVERY meal. What if I run out of apples? What carb source can I get while eating out that does not require a trough to eat from? With the above method I can get 4 oz of chicken or meat, a salad and ask for extra olive oil. Easy meal, good glycemic control and no bullshit. Ok enough of that noise. Let's go talk with the Always Hungry Carb Crash Zombie.

AHCCZ

One must approach the AHCCZ with caution. This individual has typically just started the Zone and may feel like they are being both starved and abused. It would not be a good idea to tie pork chops to oneself while near this person. Now that the safety issues are covered let's talk about what the deal is with the AHCCZ. In a nutshell this person is getting too many carbs, too often. Many people who adopt a very low carb diet notice no hunger AT ALL. One may not be able to be a CrossFit Rock Star on Atkins carb levels but one will also not turn into the AHCCZ. Typically the AHCCZ is eating dense carbs sources like fruit, yams, bread and the like at EVERY meal and it is not working out well. Barry Sears offers a flow chart in Mastering The Zone that recommends deleting one carb block from a meal if one is hungry and foggy headed a few hours after a meal. Sage advice...I'd recommend replacing that carb block with 3 blocks of fat as we talked about above. One can also shift towards less dense carb sources but that can be a slippery slope towards DIHTEAT.

Let's suppose you are a female on 10 blocks and you are trying to lose a fair amount of body fat. You have just started exercising, so your intensity is pretty moderate. You have dutifully followed the Zone and you are an AHCCZ. Here is something you might try. Shoot for 4 meals. Only have a block, perhaps two of carbs in the form of low carb-density veggies like broccoli, kale, spinach, etc. The day might look like this:

3P 2C ?F
3P 2C ?F
2P 1C ?F
2P 1C ?F
Totals: 10P 6C ?F

In this scenario we are looking at 10 blocks of protein, and an easy to chew, non-insulin spiking 6 blocks of carbs...but how much fat does our recovering AHCCZ need? Since this poor soul is still on the base Zone she would need only 10 blocks in the normal Zone world, but we are a bit more sophisticated than that. Since we have deleted 4 blocks of carbs we need to add 12 blocks of fat for a whopping total of 24! This can be partitioned any way we like but 6 blocks at each meal makes sense:

3P 2C 6F
3P 2C 6F
2P 1C 6F
2P 1C 6F
Totals: 10P 6C 24F

Won't the Zone Police come and haul us away? Isn't this some violation of the Patriot Act? Why is Allan Thicke still one of the most recognizable Canadian actors to US citizens? The answers in this order: 1. No. 2. Probably not but if I disappear we know I pissed someone off "real good". 3. Ds Gustibus non est disptandum.

What I'm trying to get across is that you have some serious flexibility with how you implement the Zone and instead of trying to make this a one-size-fits-all affair we can customize The Zone to make it YOUR Zone. Nifty, eh? In the above example we have established BETTER glycemic control than the standard Zone offers and our former AHCCZ will not become a DIHTEAT. Once the FAHCCZ (former always hungry carb crashed zombie) has reached a desired level of leanness the fat blocks will be ratcheted up to somewhere between 3 and 5x the base level...but that was discussed in the PM issue 2! What if this individual is ramping up the intensity of workouts and is not feeling recovered? Use the post workout carb method as mentioned above adding some dense carb sources...adjust fat blocks accordingly.

I just want to do a teensy digression here and talk about the Black Box and empiricism. It is righteous to base decisions on empiricism and not get hung up on theory. Experiment, observe, experiment, observe...that's the schiznitz but occasionally some understanding of how things work can help to direct our efforts. If for example someone is not feeling good on the Zone it's neither elegant nor educated to simply say "hang in there, things will get better". Yes people botch the Zone but if people are having glycemic control issues (some obvious signs like hunger and foggy headed-ness) we have some easy ways of dealing with this IF we have not turned our Zone experience into a religion. Related to this is the assertion that anything goes with regards to food quality so long as it fits into a 40-30-30 ratio. That's retarded. No one should use Seitan (concentrated wheat gluten) as a protein source. Similarly some coaches seem to think it's impossible to eat "Meat and vegetables, nuts and seeds..." in Zone proportions.... come again? When a tool ceases to be a tool and becomes and end unto itself...squirrelly crap can happen. OK. Back to our Zone fun...let's look at our next archetype "skinny but want to be heyuge" (SBWTBH).

SBWTBH

SBWTBH...typically a white male, 18-30 years of age, 5'9"-6'0", 140-160lbs. Known to train up to 7 days per week, often in double sessions. Chronic under-eater...yet finds gaining quality muscle mass a problem. Shocker. SBWTBH has landed on a message board near you and wants to know the secrets of being a sculpted Greek God...much in the likeness of Greg Everett. Well the solution to this problem is one word: EAT. OK, I'll flesh things out more than that. SBWTBH will need to engage in some smart progressive overload training, a minimum of extraneous activity and an acceptance that he may not be able to see all 8 of his lower abs for a period of time. This will necessitate a significant financial outlay not only for the food to fuel this endeavor but also the therapist to hand hold Lil' Jimmy through his loss of abs status. Once SBWTBH has funneled all of his financial aid money into groceries it's time to get down to some serious eating!

Similar to progressive overload we will employ a progressive approach to eating to allow the digestive system to adapt to larger meals and more total volume passing through the system. Start things at a base Zone for one week, then ratchet up to 5x fat and maintain this level for one week. This will initiate a protein sparing state in the body we will take advantage of periodically on the quest to gain a few kilos. So the above might look like one week at 16 blocks then one week at 16blocks and 5X fat. Now every two weeks add 2 blocks at the 5x fat level until you have added 4 blocks. Hold this level for 3-4 weeks, then ratchet things up again. Approximately every 6th day go back to your ORIGINAL base Zone. Yep, all the way back to 16 blocks. Do this on a non-training day and try not to eat off your own arm. This practice will re-set your protein utilization AND your metabolism overall. Just a little tweak to keep the body efficient with calories and not shift towards frittering away all those pricey food calories by decoupling mitochondrial REDOX.

Cycling nutrient intake is nothing new. From Fred Hatfields Zig-Zag diet to Anabolic Burst Cycling to the Metabolic Diet, people have noticed that eating the same thing, day in day out is not the best way to gain muscle. We presented an exhaustive approach to Mass Gain in Issue 17 of the Performance Menu. I suggested the inclusion of intermittent fasting to achieve metabolic changes favorable to mass gain. That's one approach but I think simply dialing the calories back significantly may be an easier solution. Let's see how all this plays out over a month or two:

Week 1 16 blocks
Week 2 16 blocks @ 5X fat
Week 3-4 18 Blocks @5X fat
Week 5-8 20 Blocks @5X fat
Week 9-11 22 Blocks @5X fat
Week 12-15 24 Blocks @5X fat
Week 16-17 26 Blocks @5X fat

Keep in mind that every 5-7 days drop things back to a base 16 blocks to give the digestion and metabolism a rest. The above approach SHOULD allow your system to adapt to the increasing food intake and will provide adequate calories (over 4K at the 26 block level) and protein (182g) for growth. This may appear to be on the low end of the protein scale for mass gain but I want to encourage the body to use fat as a fuel, not protein. If you are finding that you are simply not gaining weight you might try adding an additional 50% of your daily blocks in your post workout meal. So if you are at 26 blocks @ 5X fat try getting an additional meal of 13 blocks of protein post workout. What this effectively does is increase your protein blocks significantly. Under this scenario on training days you would consume 39 blocks of protein, 26 blocks of carbs and a stool loosening 195g of fat.

It is almost a certainty that you will need to use copious amounts of shakes, olive oil, coconut milk and nut butters to stuff down all these calories. Take pro-biotics daily and digestive enzymes with EVERY meal. Chew your shakes. Try not to delete carbs on this plan; however, you may benefit from partitioning more carbs into the post workout period, along with the increased protein. For more details and a training program to accompany this hog-fest, read the mass gain issue.

All right folks! I think we touched on the main issues I see crop up with regards to the Zone. I just want to make the point again that it's important to tailor any program, whether it's CrossFit, BJJ or the Zone to meet YOUR needs. A little understanding of how these technologies work makes this easy to do.

THE PATCH: FUNCTIONAL TRAINING AS NATURE INTENDED
JOSH EVERETT

"The Patch" (registered trademark by Pete Egoscue and The Egoscue Method) is a very unique obstacle course with drills designed to enhance all areas of fitness. You name it, you can train it on the patch... cardiovascular endurance, stamina, strength, flexibility, power, speed, coordination, agility, balance, and accuracy are all required during a workout on the patch. For those that are unfamiliar with the patch, it's basically a combination of plyometrics, Parkour, gymnastics, military obstacle course, and, as Coach Mike Burgener calls them, body-hardening drills". Later in this article you'll see just a small sample of what you can do on the patch.

As a college strength & conditioning coach, the big plus of training on the patch for me is these exercises bridge the gap between strength gained in the weight room and the strength that athlete will need to use in their sport. On the patch, the athletes not only gain strength but they also learn to use that strength in a functional way and learn how to control their bodies. The patch helps teach them how to put to use the strength and power gained from Olympic lifts and squats done in the weight room.

I first discovered the patch while reading some of Pete Egoscue's material while working on my master's degree. Once I moved to California, I knew I had to check out the Egoscue clinic down in San Diego and get some hands on experience with the patch. My first visit I fell in love with the patch and the training done on it. I knew I had to find a way to get one on my own campus. Then when Coach Burgener beat me to the punch by having on installed at his high school I was even more determined to get the project done at UC Riverside. Finally, thanks to many people, but especially UCR Athletic Director Stan Morrison, we were able to have one built by patch expert Danny Wright and his Fast Aggressive Sports Technologies company in March 2007.

Along with what will be visibly obvious from the following video clips, the patch really works the abs, low back, and is unparalleled in the shoulder stability work it offers. For athletes in baseball, softball, tennis, swimming, volleyball, etc., the shoulder stability work alone is worth the workout.

There is some great psychological training going on here as well. There is a certain amount of fear (very justified and for my job security reasons, we have chosen to edit out that footage) associated with some of the drills. Overcoming that fear, gaining confidence, and just plain being tougher are some of the mental improvements I've seen our athletes make on the patch. Life is all about getting back up when you fall down, finding a way to overcome obstacles you never thought you could get past, and eventually having the ability to take those obstacles in stride. The patch teaches those very real life lessons in a tangible, physical way.

The Workout

- LateralHurdle-unders: Basic hip mobility/flexibility drill
- Lunge-unders
- Hindu pushup + crawl-through: Getting the upper body & low back warmed up
- Step & land: On our drills we place an emphasis on landing properly. The goal is to land with soft/quite feet in the athletic position with a lot of give by the hips, knees, & ankles. The ability to make this your natural landing pattern will reduce injuries to the knees, ankles, and back.
- Jump up & Land: Again quiet and soft and in proper position.
- Over the stumps
- Lateral bear crawl & Dismount
- lateral crab crawl & dismount
- Forward bear crawl & dismount
- Side shuffle
- Stork walk
- Donkey kicks
- Hip-ups
- Over the vaults + decline push-ups
- Speed runs

There are literally hundreds of other drills you can do but this is our basic routine at UCR for now!

After watching the video clips you may be thinking to yourself, "I can do that in my own backyard." Yes you can! That's the point—take hat nature has given you or what the local park has to offer and find a way to train. Get back to your childhood where the line between play and functional training was blurred. Another great thing about the patch is everyone can do these exercise—everyone can find a way to get over a vault or onto a stump. Everyone from world-class athletes to unathletic fatties can do this stuff.

An added bonus for P.E. teachers & coaches is it is so simple to teach. It is much easier to teach than a deadlift, squat, or snatch. There should be a patch at every high school in America. The patch and CrossFit is what every PE program should look like, but that's a whole other article.

The patch is simple, effective, functional, and fun! If you're ever in the neighborhood, you're invited to come watch one of our teams train on it, or, if you're game, I'll even put you through the paces!

AN INTERVIEW WITH JOEY MILLER
NICKI VIOLETTI

At eighteen years old, Joey Miller is one of the most accomplished high school female wrestlers in the country. She has been named not once, but three times to the ASICS Girls High School All-American wrestling team. Her website www.wrestlegirl.com provides a wealth of information, including photos, videos and links pertaining to all things girls wrestling. Together with her father Jerry Miller, she has made it her mission to promote girls wrestling with the ultimate goal of girls wrestling girls in high school in all 50 states. Joey recently signed with Oklahoma City University to wrestle in 2008-09.

Joey, please tell us a little about yourself. How did you first get into wrestling? In what weight class do you wrestle? What is your current win/loss record?

When I was six my brother wanted to buy me a cheap Christmas present. He went to a local shoe store that was going out of business and found a size 10 wrestling shoe for $5.00. Since he wrestled he thought that would be a great present for me. I went to my first tournament a week later even though I had never practiced with a team. My Dad showed me some moves. I made it to state that year and won state the next year. I only lost four matches that year.

In High School I wrestle at 119 lbs, and in the Women's senior division I wrestle at 55kg (121lbs).

My win/loss record this last season was 38-25. This was my worst season since I started wrestling. I went from 103 to 119 and the strength difference of the guys jumped dramatically. I welcome the challenge and think it will pay off in my wrestling future. I have only been beaten by one girl in folkstyle since I was eight. I lost to Michaela Hutchison two years ago by a score of 0-2. Michaela was the first and only girl to win a High School state championship against boys. I have won girls nationals four times and hope to get my fifth next year.

Please explain to our readers the difference between folkstyle and freestyle wrestling.

Freestyle is the college, Olympic, and international style. In Freestyle you can throw, lock hands, and have a tie score and win. You have to win two out of three periods. The last point scored wins unless the other wrestler scored points by a two or three point move. If you push a wrestler out of bounds you get a point if you both are on your feet.

Folkstyle is elementary through high school. It is also the style for college in the men's league. You have to win by one point or pin in three periods. The first period is on your feet and the other two are choice of up, down, or top. Each wrestler gets choice of one period unless he gets pinned. A pin ends the match. You do not get a point by pushing the opponent out of bounds, but you can lose a point by stalling.

You have a great mission statement!

"It is our goal for girls to wrestle girls in high school in all 50 states. We realize that it will not happen anytime soon, but with every girl striving for that goal the competition will get better. The only way for girls to get better now is to wrestle boys."

There are many people who are quite vocal in their opinion that girls should not wrestle boys for reasons ranging from the fact that it's humiliating to boys if they get pinned by a girl, to strength inequalities due to girls maturing faster than boys, and others saying that it's dishonorable to both genders. Talk a little about this gender issue. Most importantly, do you or any of your female or male wrestling friends find there to be anything awkward about mixed wrestling?

I really don't get caught up in the so-called debate. Everyone has his or her opinion and I respect that, but if I want to get better I have to wrestle the guys. I don't do it to humiliate a guy or prove anything. I just want to be the best I can so I can compete in college and the senior women's tournaments and be prepared to wrestle the best the world has to offer in the future. Here in Oklahoma I have been wrestling for over 12 years and am regarded as a wrestler, not a GIRL wrestler. That is the way I like it. I hate it when a girl wants special treatment or a guy wants special treatment. I tell them, Just wrestle. I would rather lose a tough, hard-fought match than win by forfeit or an easy match. I still wrestle some of the same guys that I used to 10-12 years ago. Some of them I used to beat, but they beat me now. It gives me a goal to shoot for. I want to beat them the next time I wrestle them. Most of the complainers are parents of the guys that have lost to a girl. I say to them get over it and get better or it will happen again. You get out of wrestling what you put into it. This is just my opinion.

How close do you stay to your competition weight? Do you have any tips you'd like to share about safely cutting weight?

I walk around at a weight that I know I can safely cut and can handle. I eat healthy and don't take any pills. I cut weight the right way. You don't have to starve yourself to lose weight. You can cut and still eat.

What do you do for strength and conditioning? Do you do any of the Olympic lifts? Which aspects of conditioning do you like the most/least? Is there any one thing that you do that you feel gives you an edge over your competition?

I run and lift everyday. I run a couple of time everyday and lift every other day and the days I don't lift I do cardio, abs, and legs lifts. I spend a lot of time in the gym. I have a copy of the workouts the Olympic and world team uses. I use it sometimes for a change of pace and use it when it gets closer to tournament time because it is a complete workout. I love any kind of running and I jump rope a lot. I don't like the stationary bike because it bores me. Sometimes I play games in the wrestling room for conditioning. It makes the workouts a lot more fun and really works you out. I learned this at the Olympic training center at one of the camps I went to. There isn't just one thing that gives you an edge. It is a combination of time, dedication, and commitment.

How do you prepare yourself mentally before your matches?

I have to listen to my music so I don't have any distractions. I think about my next match and what I need to do to be successful. I also watch the matches before me so I can see different situations and think about what I would do if I were to be in them. They might come up in my match. I also move around a lot to get loose.

What female wrestler do you most respect? Why?

Toccara Montgomery, because she had a rough life and kept going... all the way to the Olympics. She never gave up, stayed focused, and did what she had to do to be the best. She is a friend of mine and I respect her.

You'll have to forgive me for this very un-warriorlike question, but are you concerned about getting cauliflower ear?

No, I always wear my headgear and always have. My Dad made me when I started wrestling and I never stopped. I am glad he did. I have some friends that have cauliflower ear and it is painful.

Mixed Martial Arts is one of the fastest growing televised sports. Many of the fighters that dominate this sport have collegiate wrestling backgrounds. Do you watch MMA? Could you ever see yourself as a professional fighter?

No I have never watched MMA other than the UFC and would like to try it but my parents will not let me. For now I would have to say no, but who knows what the future holds.

What are your long-term wrestling and career goals?

I would love to go to the Olympics and place. That is my biggest goal. My next goal is to graduate college and be a chiropractor or a physical trainer. I also would like to coach a wrestling team someday.

STAYING FIT DURING AND AFTER PREGNANCY
LAUREN BROOKS

Getting pregnant is a wonderful experience but it can be accompanied by an extreme mix of emotions. The thought of having a baby growing inside of you is very exciting, while not knowing what to expect can be very scary. Questions that may run through your head will be: Will I ever look the same after pregnancy? How am I going to stay in shape? Is exercise safe for my baby? As living proof, I can assure you the answer is Yes. In this article I will discuss how I exercised throughout my pregnancy and got my body back in record time after a Caesarian section, which is major abdominal surgery.

As a fitness trainer and nutritionist, living an active healthy lifestyle has always been important to me. Prior to my pregnancy I worked out regularly with kettlebells to stay strong and lean. It is definitely beneficial to be in the best shape possible before becoming pregnant. You can still start exercising during pregnancy even if you have not been active prior, but I would recommend easing in to a safe program with a doctor's approval.

During my first trimester of pregnancy, I felt very sluggish at times and had horrible cravings for starchy carbohydrates, although I luckily never felt nauseas. I noticed that when I did exercise my energy and mood increased tremendously. Even if it was just a 20-minute walk, my mood and energy would improve. My workouts during this time were very similar to what I had been doing before getting pregnant, except I took more rest and closely monitored my heart rate with a heart rate monitor. Here is a sample program of what I did during my first trimester with kettlebells. I would only recommend someone to follow this if they were already doing a workout that was at this level and experiencing no pregnancy complications.

Swings 12kg 30x3
Single Leg Dead Lifts 2 12kg's 6x3
Over head press 12kg 8x3 on each arm
ush ups on Kettlebells 10x3
Lat Pull Down 60lb 10x3
Snatches 12kg 15x3 on each arm

I would take rests as needed if my heart rate got exceedingly high. Normally if I do snatches or swings my heart rate gets between 160-180 bpm. As long as it came down quickly I would continue with the workout.

In my second trimester I had to lower the intensity of my workout program. Pressurized breathing is unsafe for the baby, so I needed to start going a little lighter with my workouts. I had to convince myself that my goals were different at this time—I had to stop thinking about getting stronger and focus on maintaining and moving regularly. After 20 weeks of being pregnant, doing any exercises on your back can be very unsafe. Turkish Get Ups and Floor Presses were definitely out of the question. Here is an example of the type of workout I did during my second trimester. I went through each exercise and rested as needed. I did this about twice a week and walked 45 minutes three times a week. Towards the very end of the second trimester I was lucky if I could get through 2 sets.

Front Squats 12kg 10x3
Overhead Press 8kg 8x3 on each arm
Push ups on KB's 5x3
Swings 8kg 20x3
Lat Pull down 50lb 10x3
Snatches 8kg 15x3 on each arm

During the third trimester, I was extremely impatient as were most of the women I've spoken to. I just wanted it to be over with. I was anxious to meet my baby, get my body back, and start my workouts again. With my stomach expanding like no other, I had to adjust my training completely. Around my 30th week, kettlebell snatches, swings, and squats were all I was safely able to do. I would keep kettlebell exercise reps under 5 and would use nothing heavier than the 8kg kettlebell. My main exercise at this time was walking. I found at this stage that listening to my body was the most important thing to do, and all I felt it wanted me to do was walk every day up and down hills at a comfortable pace.

By remaining active during my pregnancy I gained roughly 23 pounds while carrying a 7-pound 9-ounce baby. After giving birth, I lost 27 pounds in 4 months, and I'm now 4 pounds lighter than I used to be. The first 20 pounds came off within days of having my daughter, but I didn't look the same as I did prior to pregnancy. My abdominals were stretched and loose from carrying such a large baby and my muscle tone was gone. My body composition had definitely changed.

In order to really get back to a physique I was happy with, I had to be very disciplined with my entire lifestyle. The last 7 pounds of fat loss were what I had to work hardest for. Since working out was not an option for 6-8 weeks after my C-section, I had to really pay attention to my nutrition. The only activity I was able to do at first was walk extremely slowly. Every step I took was very painful. I refused to take any painkillers, due to the fact I was breastfeeding and I do not like drugs in my system. As the pain in my abdominals decreased, I tried to add a couple minutes to my walk every week while slowly increasing the pace. After the first 6 weeks, I was able to gradually start a safe workout program and I was walking over a mile a day.

Below is a sample nutrition program from my first 6 weeks following giving birth. Keep in mind I was breastfeeding every 2 hours and my appetite was enormous. My body required many more starchy carbohydrates during this new lactating stage in order to get my milk established, which was the first priority. Once my body adjusted to taking care of a newborn and breastfeeding, I was slowly able to reduce the starchy carbohydrates. I now follow mostly a gluten- and diary-free diet. I am still breastfeeding, but my body has learned to regulate itself now that my milk has been established for over 6 months.

Breakfast
- ½ cup of Oatmeal
- 1 serving of a Protein Shake. (either Jay Robb or Fit 365)
- ½ Tbs of Flaxseed Oil
- 1 Cup of Green Tea

Snack
- 1 piece of Ezekiel Bread
- 1 Tbs of Almond Butter

Snack
- Handful of Nuts
- ½ of Banana

Lunch
- 2 cups of Spinach
- 4oz of Grilled Chicken
- 1 tbs of Gorgonzola Cheese
- 1/8 cup of Walnuts
- 1 Tbs of Balsamic Vinaigrette

Snack
- 1 serving of Dried Mango Slices
- Cup of Herbal Tea

Snack

- 1 piece of Ezekiel Bread
- 1 Hardboiled egg

Dinner

- 6oz of grilled Wild River Salmon
- 4-6oz of Sweet Potatoes
- 1/2 cup of grilled Asparagus

Snack

- 1/3 cup of Unsweetened Apple Sauce
- 1/3 cup of Nonfat Cottage Cheese

Snack

- 1 cup of Red Tea with a splash of Milk
- 1 small Apple

All the meals were roughly spaced 2 hours apart. I was hungry at every meal and felt satisfied until the next snack. By keeping the portions small I was able to help shrink my stomach down and keep my metabolism high. I also drank around 8 cups of water a day, not including tea.

11 weeks postpartum

As anxious as I was to jump right back in to my kettlebell training, I had to take a different approach due to my lack of strength and the fact that I was recovering from surgery. I would only recommend doing isolation or machine exercises for women who have had a C–section. I was still feeling a lot of discomfort in my core and was not sure if it was completely healed. In order to stay safe, the first week I focused on simple, traditional weight training, which is definitely not my favorite. By the third week back, light kettlebell training was added to my regimen. Here is a program that I felt was safe and effective for the first several weeks back. As I felt more comfortable, I would add a set and gradually decrease the rest.

Traditional Weights and Machine Day

Monday and Thursday

1. Leg Press
   Assisted Pull up
   Cable Flys

2. Leg Ext
   Leg Curls

3. Bicep Curls
   Tricep Pull down
   Military Press

4. Back Extension
   Plank 60 sec (1 set, due to pain near incision)

Did 2 sets of each twice a week for the first several weeks.

Kettlebell Day

Tuesday and Saturday

Sequence 1

Turkish Get Up 2 reps
Alternating Back Lunges 10 reps per leg
Clean and Press 6 reps each side

Sequence 2

Renegade Rows 3 reps (felt C-section incision so kept the reps low)
Kettlebell Push ups 6 reps
2 Handed Swings 20 reps

Began with 2 sets of each twice a week for the first several weeks.

By 3 months I was almost feeling and looking like myself again. My strength was coming back rapidly, but not to its former level. I used to be very strong for my size, but I worked very hard to maintain my strength. Due to lack of sleep and frequent breastfeeding, I did not have the energy to go as heavy as I used to, and I had to be realistic with my short-term goals. When just starting again, the best goals are strength, conditioning, and having more energy. You will lose weight when doing efficient fat burning workouts and eating properly. You just have to stick with it.

After the first month of working out, I was able to safely move up to the 12kg kettlebell. Here is an example of a short but challenging workout I did with kettlebells 2-3 days a week. I was also walking 2 miles while pushing a stroller up and down hills about 4 times a week.

Sequence 1

Double Suitcase Deadlift 12 reps
Push Ups on Kettlebells 10 reps
Snatches 10 reps per side

Rested at the end and repeated 3 times.

Sequence 2

Squat and Press 5 reps per side
Swings 20 reps
Plank Hold 30 seconds

Rested at the end for 1-2 minutes and repeated 3 times.

Here is an example of a workout I was doing between 4 and 5 months postpartum. I was able to do this in my backyard which made things much more convenient. All you need is a kettlebell and a jump rope to do this workout.

Sequence 1

Turkish Get Up 12kg 3 reps per side
Double Front Squat 12kg's 5 reps
Clean and Press 12kg 5 reps per side
Swings 20kg 15 reps

Rested at the end for 1 minute and repeated 3 times

Sequence 2

> Jump Rope 1 minute
> Snatches 12 kg 1 minute
> Swings 20 kg 30 sec

Rested at the end for 1 minute and repeated 3 times

I am very content with my physique now, considering I am still nursing. While you are breastfeeding you will lose weight, but I have discovered that the body likes to hold on to a small amount of fat in order to continue making quality milk. As of now my body weight is 111 pounds and I fluctuate between 16-18% body fat. When I stop breastfeeding it will be interesting to see how my body continues to change. For the time being kettlebell workouts, walking, and proper nutrition will be my way of continuing to improve myself.

DEVELOPING THE IRON CROSS
STEPHEN LOW

Training for the iron cross is no joke. The long-term difficulty of attaining this move is similar to the time it takes to acquire strength moves like the planche. It is very hard to see consistent progress over a couple of weeks; however, looking at the big picture the strength gains are incredible. Thus, it is recommended that iron cross development should only be undertaken by very motivated athletes who can dedicate enough time.

The iron cross gives an enormous amount of brute pulling strength. From my experience, training the cross is the pinnacle of upper body pulling strength—much more so than working the back lever, front lever and rowing variations. There are only a few pulling exercises that may provide more benefits, such as deadlifts and the Olympic lifts.

Judging from said experience, developing the cross should take a person with average pull-up strength of about 8-10 repetitions, good conditioning of the elbows and shoulders, and a light body frame—150 lbs or less—around 9-12 months. It will obviously take more or less time depending on the level of training beforehand as well as how well the athlete's genetics tend react to strength training.

Exercises

Unfortunately, not all exercises are created equal. This being the case it is imperative to seek out the best exercises to use to progress with the cross. There are some similar to pull-ups or dips in which the user pulls or lowers respectively to shoulder height with the rings and one arm can go out to the side. Likewise, in some gyms with machines, it is possible to set up cable pulleys that are used for crossovers to

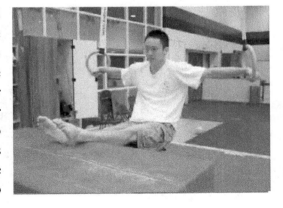

simulate the cross. While these exercises do work the muscles, it is much more important to be on the rings as much as possible to develop the necessary stabilization muscles and to simulate the cross position as close as possible. The following can be used to maintain and even gain strength—these are the recommend exercises from best to worst:

- Assisted crosses with a spotter
- Weighted progression therabands cross pullouts or "dream machine" pulley system cross pullouts (see references for more details).
- Cross pullouts with block with weight added
- Theraband cross pulls

1. Assisted crosses are, without a doubt, the best. They require muscles to be at or near maximum effort the whole time, which is extremely good for developing strength and muscle mass provided you eat enough. In addition, a training partner makes workouts more effective through competition and encouragement.
2. Theraband cross-pullouts with weighted progressions or a dream machine type device with pulleys which can be connected to weights or your bodyweight are second preference. This is because it simulates the cross position very well as well as gives a means by which to measure strength gains.
3. Block cross-pullouts tend to put a bit more stress on the lats as opposed to the pecs. For this single reason they are rated below the above exercises in which you can achieve the actual cross position. On the other hand, these are good because progress can be measured by how much of the legs are on the block as well as block height. More about this will be posted in the technique section.
4. Last but not least is the Theraband-assisted cross. The assistance force is less measurable—pick something that makes you struggle but allows you to eventually push through. The reason this exercise is rated below block cross-pullouts despite its being a more effective exercise in terms of stimulating the muscles in the right position is that measurement of progress is very difficult. Consequently, if using a block feels unnatural, switch to these instead, but make sure that there is constant progression.

Technique

Technique is extremely, extremely important for the cross. It is easy to develop shoulder problems due to a lack of scapular stabilization and external rotation as well as tendinitis in the elbows. In fact, it is entirely likely most people will encounter these to at least some degree even with perfect technique. Having the right technique will help reduce injury chances, making the user stronger

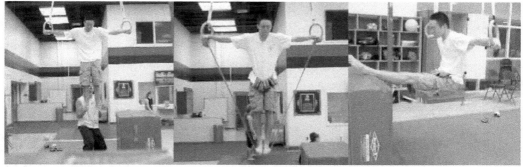

From left to right: Partner-assisted cross, Theraband cross pull-outs, Block cross pull-outs.

overall and will also lead to a cross position that looks crisp and clean.

Starting from support, rotate the rings out so that the palms and elbows are facing forward; when starting to lower yourself, the shoulders should be rotated so that the inside of the elbows start to point down and forwards instead of just purely forwards; and the shoulders should be pushed down as hard as possible to avoid scapular and shoulder destabilization.

The elbows MUST be locked at all times. This is the number-one bad habit encountered because it makes the exercises easier by placing more emphasis on the lats. Do not give in. After developing this bad habit it is extremely hard to correct because the body learns that movement neurologically and the lats are too heavily stimulated at expense of the chest.

There are a couple things to keep in mind here because there are different accepted variations of the cross.

1. The current official gymnastics code requires that you have no false grip although it is easier to obtain the cross position with one. The false grip can be slid into while turning the rings out and lowering if preferred.
2. Rolling the shoulders forward is not necessary although doing so it will allow the shoulders to 'lock' into place by moving them to the limit of their range of motion. Thus, rotating the shoulders forward is a good marker to ascertain a good cross depth.
3. If block cross-pullouts are chosen then correct technique with them is imperative. Since the exercise tends to push the arms back behind the torso, it must be fixed to get the correct amount of stimulation to the cross muscles. Similarly, as fatigue sets in, the hands tend to drift backwards which results in a suboptimal position. This can be corrected by emphasizing the arms to be slightly in front of the torso or within peripheral vision at the very least. This will keep the chest properly stimulated.
4. Proper block progression is fairly simple. Starting from the back of the knees first, try to move to the ankles as quickly as possible. Next, start adding weight, preferably in the form of a weight belt or vest but a loaded backpack put on in front can also be used. Weight should mainly be located in the front because weight in the back will make

the exercise more lats-centric, which it already will be with the block progression. One other optional way of increasing the difficulty is lowering the block height.

The L-cross has not been mentioned and will be discussed only briefly here. The move itself is considered to be at the same skill level in the code as a regular cross (B rating). The correct technique is exactly the same as the regular cross except the feet are brought up into an L position such as in the L-sit. Since this forces the body's center of mass forward, the arms are inclined to move forward relative to the torso (transverse flexion). This puts more stress on the pecs as opposed to the lats, which is great for training if the pecs are lagging behind in strength.

The best method with this is a pulley system or Theraband-assistance. If Therabands are used, looping the bands from the rings around underneath the butt and legs where the hamstrings meet the glutes is approximately where the center of mass is moved forward. This would be the optimal placement, and if it does not feel centered, some adjustment may have to be made. The assisted cross method is generally hard to do with this because the rings need to be sufficiently low to allow spotting at the waist, which may be hard to grip.

Training & Programming

The following training and programming will be at the very least a good template— variations will often be necessary based on each individuals training background, diet, genetics, sleep schedule, and various other factors such as stress levels.

Warming up for the cross is not at all complicated and should take fairly little time to accomplish. Any type of skill training for at least 15 minutes beforehand should be enough to warm up the body. On that same note, any warm-up that builds up a light sweat or at the very least warms up the pulling muscles such as the pecs and lats is fine as well. The most important thing is to just get blood flowing to the muscles to prevent the first few sets from being weaker and thus contributing less to strength gains.

Warming up specifically for the cross is optional, especially if the muscles are warm already, but it also does not hurt to do a cross-specific warm-up as well. For this it is advisable to do a couple of medium intensity isometrics or eccentrics. For example, if one Theraband is being used during the work set, the cross-specific warm-up may be with two Therabands, or if the ankles are on the block in the normal workout, the warm-up reps would be with the back of the calves or ankles on the block. If the muscles are already warm, one set of 3 eccentrics or isometrics of 3-5 seconds each is generally a good way to prime the muscles for working the cross. This is, of course, with reduced difficulty as described previously.

Pain in the elbows, shoulders and scapulae will hinder your training. If it is just at the edge of pain and it goes away during training, it's fine. On the other hand, if it is a persistent pain and it is sticking around even after workouts and during off days then you have a significant problem. In this case, it is advised to just rest and let it heal. The more the pain is trained through, the greater the potential for injury and setbacks that could take weeks or even months to heal. See the references section at the end for more details on elbows and shoulder conditioning.

Phase I
3 days/week, rest 3-5 minutes between sets

Cross pullouts

- Start with 3x5 with the block as far out as possible while allowing all prescribed sets and reps to be completed.
- Progress with 3x5 until only the heels are on the block.
- Start increasing the sets to 3x5 to 4x5 to 5x5.
- Start increasing the reps to 5x5 to 5x6 to 5x7 to 5x8.

First, the block cross-pullout workout is actually a good program setup even though it is probably one of the least recommended exercises to do now. With a partner or a Theraband, the training will be essentially the same except without the block progression. As the body adapts, the muscles are capable of handling the increased amounts of volume. Repetition cadence should be a slow controlled descent with the ascent performed as quickly as possible. This applies for all phases of training.

The initial 3x5 is a good balance of intensity and volume to allow any beginner to elicit good strength gains. The progressions from 3x5 to 5x5 to 5x8 allow the body to adapt to the rigorous nature of training the cross. In particular, the increase in number of sets and repetitions help to (1) increase muscular conditioning to eliminate soreness when starting to progress to more difficult exercises or weights, (2) to acclimate the central nervous system (CNS) to the exercise which results in increased efficiency in the movement, allowing heavier weights to be used, and (3) the higher volume will serve to help to condition the elbows and shoulders for the intense strength training that follows.

Planned rest is extremely important for full recovery from accumulative fatigue. It would be advisable to take a rest week or at the very least a half-volume week after every 5-6 weeks. This applies for both this phase of training and the rest of training.

Cross isometrics are not necessary in the actual workout. If the rolled forward shoulders technique is being used and enough concentric strength is acquired the cross position will click into place after the descent from support position. Nevertheless, if these are built into the program just to get a good feeling for the position, they can generally be practiced normally as any isometrics would be practiced. Put them into the beginning of the training session or have them replace the exercises for the day. A good rule of thumb for isometrics is that every repetition in the workout counts for 3 seconds of isometrics. For instance, a total of 6 sets of 5-second isometrics holds (30 seconds total) would be equivalent to a set of 2x5 pullouts (10 repetitions multiplied times 3).

Phase II
(Optional) 3 days/week, rest 3-5 minutes between sets

- Increase the repetitions and drop two sets to 3x10.
- Increase the weight each workout as you move from: 3x10 to 3x7 to 3x4 over the course of a week.
- Reset to 3x10 the next week and then work back through the progression again.
- Rinse and repeat steps 1-3 for additional weight

In my opinion, this phase is optional. If progress is starting to plateau, this is a good way to get it jump-started again. As strength increases towards its genetic limit, greater complexity in programming is needed to compensate to keep progress with strength gains. That is why instead of just looking at gains from workout to workout, you'll need to focus on progress from week.

This type of program is a variation of daily undulated periodization (DUP), and it seems to work very well. In the suggested rep scheme, the volume decreases as the week goes on while intensity increases. This allows a good rate of recovery between workouts as well as modulation of intensity to stimulate a range of motor units. DUP can be modified to fit different variables depending on need. For example, something like 3x8, 4x6, 8x3 would also work emphasizing strength a lot more than the suggested variation.

Phase III
5 days/week, rest 3-5 minutes between sets

- Start with very low volume in the 10-12 total repetition range per workout – (from best to worst) 5x2, 4x3, 3x4, 2x5.
- Increase the volume into the 15-18 range – 5x3, 6x3, 4x4, 3x5
- Increase the volume even more to the 21-25 range – 7x3, 8x3, 6x4, 5x5.

Since this phase of training is frequent, the Therabands along with a weight vest to gauge progress is probably the best method. It will be hard to obtain a training partner who is both near the same level of development and willing to devote the necessary time for multiple days and numerous sets.

With the previous training of up to 40 repetitions per workout (5x8) or 30 repetitions from DUP (3x10) a sufficient level of conditioning should be reached in the muscles that an increase in training frequency can be handled. From here on out it is going to be a lot of very frequent training with large amounts of strength work. High frequency training has the tendency to produce extremely fast CNS and muscular strength gains provided the volume is managed well enough that the athlete can recover during the two rest days.

If when starting with the very low volume overreaching becomes apparent even with these rest days, it is recommended that 1-2 of the workouts be made into "light" workouts in which the intensity of the exercises and the number of sets are reduced and repetitions increased. For example, instead of 5x2 go to 2x5 with lower intensity, or if in the third step, go from 8x3 to 3x8. During this phase, it may be optimal to take a light day here and there during the week especially if one is feeling run down or fatigued. The lower repetitions and higher intensity the better, but it will have to be offset with more sets. If there are significant time constraints such as working the cross in conjunction with other training or just not enough time in the day, it may be better to stick with a higher amount of repetitions and fewer sets.

In the end, if the training is diligently performed without any major setbacks from the elbows, the cross should be obtained within a few months at the most after switching to Phase III.

Conclusions

The iron cross for me has been a long journey spanning a little more than a year and a half and various training modalities—some less optimal than others. A lot of time was spent just testing out different set and repetition schemes with and without weights just to figure out what worked and what did not. Interestingly enough, in the end the program is composed of many elements from various programs that work for weight training and bodyweight training. The key then is just to ensure progressive resistance exercises no matter what method is used.

I have enjoyed my time working with this strength move, and it has given me great satisfaction performing it in my rings routines in front of audiences. I wish you luck in your journey for the cross whether it be for gymnastics, increasing pulling strength, or even just bragging rights. Good luck!

Notes

Mark Rippetoe and Lon Kilgore, "Starting Strength" (Wichita Falls: The Aasgaard Company, 2005).

Department of Kinesiology and Health Education, "A Progressive Strength Program to Perform the Iron Cross," University of Texas at Austin, http://www.edb.utexas.edu/ssn/CCA%20PDF/Gymnastics-Iron%20Cross.PDF (2005).

Christopher Sommer, "The Iron Cross for Bodybuilders," Testosterone Nation, http://www.t-nation.com/readTopic.do;jsessionid=987BFDBC532F6A1BBF087E2F8A2D2826.titan?id=581914 (2005).

Mark Rippetoe, Lon Kilgore and Glenn Pendlay, "Practical Programming" (Wichita Falls: The Aasgaard Company, 2006).

Jacob Wilson and Gabriel Wilson, "Periodization Part 3 – Traditional and Non-Traditional Periodization," ABC Bodybuilding Company, http://abcbodybuilding.com/periodization3.php (2006)

Kelly Baggent, "How to Benefit From Planned Overtraining," Higher Faster Sports, http://www.higher-faster-sports.com/PlannedOvertraining.html (2006).

KYPHOSIS
ROBB WOLF

Working as a generalist strength & conditioning coach using CrossFit methodology appears to be a case of "Jack Of All Trades, Master Of None" and in some sense this may be accurate. I teach some gymnastics, but I am not a gymnastics coach and will never develop an athlete to even an "A" level gymnast. We play with the Olympic lifts and although I am a "USAW Club Coach" my list of '08 hopefuls is…um, skinny. For most endeavors I feel that I am adequate for the job but for some people this lack of specialization may be a bit buggaring.

I enjoy the challenge and the freedom this work affords me and I DO feel that I have attained a high level of understanding in one element of the generalist coaching: An eye for Good Movement. I've seen quite a number of cyclists, soccer players, stay-at-home-moms (both professional and amateur), ruggers…and from this experience I can spot "good movement" pretty quickly. Does someone have adequate hip and shoulder flexibility? Watch them overhead squat, even with just a broomstick, and you will know instantly. Shoulder mobility, flexibility and health are actually something I have zeroed in on lately as I have seen problems across all movement backgrounds, ages and in both genders. This has actually been surprising as folks can range from sedentary to athletic, obese to lean and they frequently have severe limitations in shoulder strength and mobility. These limitations not only impede progress in the gym but also frequently predispose the individual to further problems such as rotator cuff impingement and deteriorating posture. I've been tinkering with ways to address this problem but before we look at that let's look at what is going on with the shoulder girdle itself.

Kyphosis

In a normal spine we have a structurally sound curve in the low back, with a counter curve in the thoracic region, and a final counter curve in the cervical region. From an engineering perspective arches such as those found in the human spine are remarkably strong and are capable of bearing tremendous loads. Perturbing the structure of the arch however causes the integrity to plummet, thus increasing the likelihood of structural failure under load. In Brazilian accented English this could be described as "No So Goud". The most common shoulder problem I see is kyphosis or a rounding forward of the shoulders and over-accentuation of the normal thoracic curve. I have not noticed much if any lordosis of the thoracic spine however it's possible that this condition does not impede movements such as kipping and overhead squats and thus is largely ignored. Whatever the case, kyphosis appears to have a few different causes including: muscular imbalance and postural "failure". Muscular imbalance occurs between scapular protractors such as the pectorals and latisimusdorsi muscles (strong) and scapular retractors such as the rhomboids and lower traps (weak). Postural failure is not a value judgment but an acknowledgement that hunching over a keyboard, sitting in chairs that slump one forward, riding bicycles, boxing and a host of other activities tend to round one forward to a much larger degree than one is opened backwards. Just as an aside, this is not intended as an in-depth exploration of the anatomy of the shoulder girdle and the potential structural pathologies that may accompany this complex. If you want to get hoity-toity on those topics give Kelly Starrett of San Francisco CrossFit an email. That guy is a genius and he certainly has the gift-of-gab regarding all things rehab and training. Tell him "Gaius Baltar" sent you.

Das Fix

Putting all the anatomy dookie aside, what EXACTLY does kyphosis mean for the athletes I (and you) work with? Do you need to know that someone has an imbalance between pectorals and rhomboid? Well, no. It's great to know your anatomy but the issue with these folks is their movement is not right. This is how you discovered the problem in the first place. Tight shoulders that eventually lead to kyphosis are observable in two ways.

1. Overhead work such as pressing, jerks and overhead squats (OHS) is difficult if not impossible.
2. Kipping pull-ups are tough and lack the ability to store elastic energy in the shoulder girdle, particularly at the apex of the chest forward position of the kip.

In the case of the OHS an individual with tight shoulders is incapable of a normal squat even with an inconsequential load such as PVC. The individual pitches forward and additional loading is all but impossible. With regards to the kip the individual is unable to bring the head through the arms into the frontal plane during the forward portion of the kip. This greatly limits maximum power generation and the ability to recruit the hips for this whole body movement.

I'm a bit dense at times however it may be obvious to you folks that the movements that cause the most problems should be the ones that are needed most. Along this line of reasoning, when it became apparent that our clients were not strong enough we instituted a strength circuit that kicks off virtually all workouts. We mix squats, dead lifts, presses and weighted pull-ups doing a Starting Strength type of progression before some mixed modal metabolic conditioning. The result has been dramatic increase in strength and proficiency for our clients. Shocker, practice something and get bEtter at it! I've known for some time that our clients have problems with shoulder mobility yet it only occurred to me recently that dedicated mobility work before EVERY training session might be of benefit. The approach we have used is simple yet it has proven to be remarkably effective. Mixed into the strength work our clients have added 3-5 sets of 10 repetitions of: Shoulder dislocates, OHS and glide kips.

Shoulder Dislocates This movement is likely familiar to anyone with a pulse however there are some fine points that are frequently missed. One should start the dislocates using a dowel or piece of PVC and start at a hand width that is easy to pass the bar from the hips all the way to the back with a firm grip on the dowel. For some people this may be impossible to accomplish at any hand width. This crisis prone situation should invoke the Magic Coaching Spell "do your best". Something that may shift this movement from impossible to doable is a fully active shoulder (shrug the traps HARD!), both when passing forward and backward. Do not explode through this movement, go easy and be persuasive. Look at this more like a long-term relationship that requires diligence and patience, not a one-night stand.

OHS For the purpose of shoulder mobility one should use as narrow a grip in the OHS as allows for the best form with regards to an upright torso and keeping the dowel over the ear and the heel. The feet should be between hip and shoulder width. For some this is not possible at present, and thus the need to do it to the best of ones ability. The chin should be neutral if not slightly down and forward. This will allow one to once again, fully activate the shoulders and drive the dowel up as much as possible. For the mobility challenged, descending into a full ass-to-ankles squat may produce extreme discomfort in the spinal erectors and mid-back. Good, there is hope. A key point is that EVERY repetition of this exercise can and should be uncomfortable. This should require focus and patience to execute correctly.

"Glide" Kip This is not technically a glide kip as it is known and performed in gymnastics. The movement we are looking for generates power in a similar fashion to the gymnastics glide kip however it is only a fraction of the power. That said, Greg Everett's Big Fat Pull Up is a perfect illustration of the mobility necessary to generate an impressive amount of power in the kip. For some basic mechanics check out this video from CrossFit. The point of the glide kip in this context is to mobilize the shoulders. This may necessitate a very small movement in the beginning but it will allow for greater movement with practice. Individuals with tight shoulders are frequently reduced to dead hang only pull-ups or greatly muted kipping power due to a lack of flexibility. Adequate mobility allows for the storage and release of energy in the shoulder girdle. This is not only advantageous for sport and training but I think a lack of kipping leaves one open to shoulder pathology over time.

A basic coaching cue to initiate the kip: Starting from the dead hang position have the client simultaneously drive the bar away with the hands, and with a straight body elevate the toes forward. This should place the client in a suspended hollow position. One should now pull forward and drive the legs back. In quick Coach Speak this is "Push away, raise the toes! Pull under the bar!" Corny, but it works. The forward position will be the tough portion of the movement for the mobility challenged. Ease into this and do not over kip.

This whole sequence has proven effective for improving static and dynamic shoulder flexibility. Folks are OHS better and heavier and the mechanics of kipped pull-ups have improved. Overhead movements such as push presses and push jerks have also improved nicely. At what point should you discontinue this work with a client? If the individual is strong in OHS (5-10 reps at body weight), L-sit pull ups (10-this a great developer of scapular retractors) and kipped pull ups (30+) the individual likely has all the mobility necessary. So long as these movements make up a significant portion of the S&C curriculum they should maintain and even advance what is now a healthy shoulder.

MIND FREAK: PART 1
AIMEE ANAYA EVERETT

Fear will beat down years of training in a matter of minutes. It will trap you in a corner and cause you to lose all recognition of yourself, your skill, your strength, and your will. Fear's best friend is doubt. Together they can destroy your confidence and wrangle your strength until you feel as if you have none. Fear, if you let it, will destroy all you have worked for—it is an athlete's worst enemy. Because of this, it is important to learn to get your mind as strong as your body. You accept that fear lingers and you control it. You face what you are not getting and what you are truly hungry for. You get serious about what you're missing in order to motivate yourself to make the changes necessary to start getting it. You live in the moment of truth as an athlete who confronts your fears instead of allowing them to break you down. You become mentally strong. As much as I try, I cannot describe the success of mental training better than the great Tommy Kono: "Successful weightlifting is not in the body, it's in the mind. You have to strengthen your mind to shut out everything—the man with the camera, the laugh or cough in the audience. You can lift as much as you believe you can. Your body can do what you will it to do... I don't think of my opponent, even in a close contest. I never would say to myself, 'I hope he slips.' That's a negative attitude. Saying that, you're relying on outside help to win. Prayer doesn't help, either. That's also relying on outside help. The will has got to come from me. It's all up to me."

Obviously I will apply the mental game to weightlifting because that is what I do, but being a mind freak applies to all aspects of life with all sports. Not just lifting heavy things only to put them right back down.

The Mental Breakdown, AKA freaking out

Ahhh yes. The freak-outs. A result of fear of failure, freak-outs produce tension in our bodies that slow reflexes and neurological movement, which then causes our breathing to become short. Short and irregular breathing patterns causes a contraction in opposing muscle groups, which then reduces the quality of our technique and coordination.

So, freak-outs due to fear of failure ultimately create an ugly cycle that causes what we most fear. It is when you clench your hands because you can't stop shaking. Tears are streaming down your face, you can't see yourself performing in your head, and you have lost all sense of reality. You stand up from your chair, chalk your hands, and walk on to the platform afraid of the bar. The weight feels heavy; you can't remember how to snatch. You start thinking too much, you get trapped in confusion and you miss. And you miss again. Your coach is yelling at you to just lift the weight. The more you try the more you fail. The look on your coach's face reminds you of your despair. Your technique is lost, and the misses have damaged your ability to relax. In these five minutes, your months of training have become meaningless. Your breathing is no longer controlled. You become broken, and your effort is destroyed.

Fear comes out of nowhere sometimes, blindsiding you when you have let your guard down and have forgotten to focus. Perhaps something is on your mind, maybe you don't feel like training, or you are just simply afraid of a number. Fear sneaks in at the very moment you think you are in a position in which you don't need or want to focus. At this time, the freak-out has won, and there is little opportunity to turn it back around. Then you remember you are an athlete. And you need to get things done. This is when you recognize that you need to keep fear out before it defeats you and your ability to focus. You are given a talent as an athlete. It is your job to develop it and watch it thrive by combining your physical strength with your mental strength. Don't let fear of failure create a pattern in your training. Break the cycle, appreciate failure and use it to make you better. If your mind has the power to make you fail, then it definitely has the power to make you succeed.

As I have recently discovered, your physical strength can only get you so far. I had yet to tap into my mental strength and said freak-outs occurred in training more and more until I started to understand that something needed to be done. Unfortunately it took me going to a National competition and freaking out in front of hundreds of people to realize my mental stability as an athlete was a little underdeveloped. Fear and I had become great friends, and according to those closest to me, it was time I found a new friend.

Confidence

It is important to identify the need to understand your own purpose and your own goals and not someone else's. You shouldn't train everyday for someone else's dreams, or for what someone else can snatch, or for how good a fighter someone else is. Instead have confidence in your own abilities. Have confidence in your improvement. Have faith in your skills as a great fighter. For how great your snatch is. For what an awesome floor routine you have. We can only ask to be the best that we can be with what we have to work with. We cannot be as good as someone else with what they have to work with. This continuous comparison can cause a lack of confidence in your own skills and potential. Now, this isn't saying to not be competitive, or to not have goals and desire to be better than another. I am simply saying that you need to train for you. You need to beat your own best, you need to compete the best that you can and hope that your best is better than another's. You cannot control what they do; you can only control what you do. When athletes lack confidence, they can never reach their full AKP.

I have learned that my fear took over because I lacked confidence in myself. My coach knew I could do it. My boyfriend knew I could do it. Everyone knew what I had before I knew what I had. I had to find my belief. I had to quit searching for my skills in my head, and realize that they were already embedded in my every move. I had to become confident in my strength, my technique, my talent, and myself so that I could move forward in my training. Once I faced fear, kicked its ass, and found that confidence, I finally realized my AKP. With confidence you are able to beat fear, overcome doubt, and start achieving your goals.

Mohammed Ali was known for his confidence. He was the greatest. He walked and talked his greatness. Everywhere he went, everything he did, he rapped how he was the best. He believed it. He knew it. He would shout to his opponents that he was the greatest, and he created a showboat of confidence. He never let fear overcome his poise, but rather would use it to put doubt into his opponents. Those he fought would be shadowed with doubt due to Ali using his overwhelming display of confidence to get under their skin. He was great not solely because of his skills as a boxer. He did something other boxers didn't do—he mastered his mental toughness, assumed the highest degree of confidence, and in doing so, completely set himself apart from the weak-minded. His confidence enabled him to obtain the level of greatness that other boxers with equal strength could not achieve. With his mastery of confidence in his talent and endless hours of training came the ability to relax. Ali was so confident in his fighting and in himself that when it came to step into the ring, he was able to relax and do what he knew he could do. This is why he said he could float like a butterfly but sting like a bee. Appearing as a powerhouse of strength and confidence is all part of being an athlete, even when and if you don't feel that way. 1

Relax

When you learn to master the ability to relax, it will enhance your strength, flexibility, energy, and focus. When you are tense, you waste energy and effort in even the simplest movements; your body becomes tense and you exert energy from muscles that aren't even needed for the movement being made. If you have trained your body for a particular movement, then neurologically you should be able to repeat that movement over and over again without flaw. However, tension in the muscles, stress, and the inability to focus create obstacles, which decreases your ability to replicate the movement with ease. Once you have learned to control your degree of relaxation physically, mentally, and emotionally, you can notice when tension is developing and take the steps necessary to release it. Relaxation allows you to trust your strength, your skill, and your power. With this, the mind can rest, you can let go of clouding emotions, and you can surrender yourself to your athleticism and the movements already embedded in you.

Someone said (I don't know who said it, but it wasn't me), "Your ability to relax reflects your willingness to trust." Trust in your abilities. Trust yourself. In doing so, you are not repressing your feelings, denying the anger, hurt, or whatever it is you may be feeling. Instead you are simply learning to maintain a level of physical relaxation in order to train and compete even under the most stressful conditions. Because you have much more control over your behavior while training than any emotions or thoughts you may be experiencing, it is better to accept them, understand they are lingering in your mind, maintain the highest level of relaxation possible, and focus on whatever it is you are doing. Keep your body relaxed so that said feelings cannot take over physically. Athletes, especially strength athletes, often have weakened effective strength due to their continuous muscle tension throughout their bodies. Effective strength comes when an athlete can relax certain muscle groups while simultaneously and consciously tensing only those needed to perform whatever movement they are trying to accomplish. If you have not mastered this skill, you have yet to tap into your full effective strength. As another anonymous person has said, "Greatness lies not in being strong but in the right use of strength," and Bruce Lee put it best when he said, "The less effort, the faster and more powerful you will be." 2

If you don't believe me, try this: You will need a partner. Stand with your feet under your shoulders. Stick your arms out to your side (forming a T). Close your eyes and think about something terrible. Conjure up a mental imagery of all that is stressful in your life, someone who has hurt you, something that causes you pain, or the most heinous thing you can imagine. Basically fill your head with all that has been bothering you lately. You get the idea…

Before starting, tell your partner that you will want them to push down on your arms with as much force as possible, once you have told them that your mind is clouded with the bullshit, but at some random time so that you will be caught by surprise. What happens?

Next, do the same thing, but this time put your mind at ease. Think about things that make you happy. Imagine times where you are most relaxed and where you feel most comfortable. Fill your head with all the good things in your life. The things that make you elated.

What happens?

Let me tell you what should happen. As your body becomes tenser due to the images clouding your mind, you have to apply more effort and your partner should be able to defeat you. Your arms will collapse, and you will lose your balance. However, when your mind is not clouded and your body is not tense with frustration, anger, or stress, you will be less likely to topple. Your strength will withstand.

Remember, when doing the exercise you cannot think about your partner who is about to push down on your arms at any second. You need to focus. As cheesy as this exercise may seem, it is a great lesson to show you the less effort, the faster and more powerful you will be.

1. Despite what you may believe, I did not discover the greatness of confidence. Fortunately, I stumbled upon Dan Millman's book, Body Mind Mastery, in which these ideas and thoughts came after reading it. Twice.
2. Again… I do know my stuff (now). But I did not know the importance of relaxation until Dan Millman came into my life. Credit goes where credit is due. The quotes were taken from his book as well, although I wish Mr. Lee had told me that himself.

INTERMITTENT FASTING:
NO QUESTIONS NECESSARY! (PLEASE)
ROBB WOLF

If you poke around the CrossFit message board, Performance Menu forums or a few other enlightened locales, you are likely to see a few questions regarding intermittent fasting (IF). Some of the questions involve the theory behind IF… what one might expect to gain from tweaking nutrient intake in specific ways. The other questions involve HOW to actually do IF. Theory is great but the how-to is really where it's at if you want to gain the benefits or simply scratch this nutritional approach off your list of potential Holy Grails. I want to walk y'all through a reasonable progression for integrating IF into your training program and address some common questions. We will not consider the theory in this article (much) as we have peered inside the Black Box of IF in previous issues. This article will just get you up and running while assessing whether or not IF is right for you and YOUR goals.

Why Am I Doing This?

Even though we are not going deep into the theory of IF, it might be helpful to review what benefits one might expect from tinkering with this stuff. Assuming we are correct regarding IF we might see the following:

Increaseed Lifespan. Or, more specifically, effective lifespan. I don't think anyone is interested in living 150 years with 75 of those years spent on life support looking at hospital walls. We want to live long and well and IF might help us do this.

Improved performance and recovery. Run faster, jump higher, lift more… come back and do it again sooner. Intermittent fasting might help

Simplification. If intermittent fasting provides no other benefit than simplifying one's life, it may be enough to warrant at least occasional use of this technique. The bodybuilding turds would have us believe we will waste away in a cortisol hell if we miss one meal. Bullshit. Our bodies are a little more complex than that.

Be Critical

I don't know about you but I'm pretty busy and I don't like to fritter away my time. That said, if I try something, be it a new approach to training or nutritional supplement, it's pretty important to run a cost-benefit analysis. In the case of IF there is a beautiful way to assess efficacy. Do you see improved, decreased or no change to your performance? CrossFit has four related definitions of what constitutes fitness and part of that involves this notion that anything that brings about retrograde performance, anything that decreases your work capacity across broad time and modal domains is bad. Lack of sleep, too much booze, missing an episode of Family Guy... this can all damage you in profound ways. Intermittent fasting should (in theory) improve work capacity, but if it doesn't, DON'T DO IT! Give it a go if you want, hang in there for a good month, but if it does not work for you we can find an approach that does. Be critical and miserly with your time and efforts.

Bang Fer Yer buck

Before we get into the specifics of how to incorporate intermittent fasting into your program I'm going to share with you a power progression to unleash your genetic potential and realize 99.99999876% of the benefit possible from nutrition... something so powerful you will need to know a secret handshake and recite lines from various Mel Brooks movies just to contain it's power.

Sorry, I wanted to get your attention and I thought some ridiculous, over the top claims might do it. It is true, however, that the HEIGHT of nutritional science involves a Paleo diet (meat & veggies, nuts & seeds, some fruit, little starch, no sugar) sliced into Zone proportions. One will follow this base Paleo/Zone until a desired level of leanness is met OR retrograde performance occurs. Then one will increase fat intake between 2-5 times that of the base Zone (this is called the Athletes Zone).

This is the buy-in for the big leagues. If you want to get your food dialed, this is where you need to go and you have NO business messing around with intermittent fasting until you get this stuff squared away. I'll touch on this topic a bit more later in the "Damn Stoopid Questions" section. For the visual learners here is a schematic:

Paleo diet ⟶ Zone ⟶ Increase Fat (Athlete's Zone) ⟶ Intermittent Fasting (Maybe)

Do y'all have that? Food quality, then food proportions, then we can start thinking about food timing.

Doin' The Deed

I'm going to look at two different methods of applying IF to a Paleo/Zone diet. The first is the simplest to describe: Eat one day, don't eat the next day. Kurtis Bowler of Rainer CrossFit has eaten this way for over two years. He competes in strongman competitions, is a cop, dad, husband and business owner. The key is that Kurtis eats the same amount ON AVERAGE in a 2-day period as he would if he was not intermittent fasting. This allows him to maintain activity level and muscle mass. Frankly I'm surprised this works so well for Kurtis, but he experimented, liked the results and has stuck to the program. Genius!

The second method to implement IF into your schedule is what I call the compressed feeding window. Hold on to your hat: You limit the time you have to consume your normal amount of food. A simple way to do this is to make your last meal finish an hour earlier than normal, let's say 6:00 pm and make your first meal happen a little later than normal, lets say 9:00 am the following morning. That's 15 hours and a great place to start things off. If you feel good, try pushing this up to 12:00 pm, which will make it 18 hours. Start small and work your way up if you like the results and how you feel. Give each transition a good week to see how it feels. Tinker, observe and keep in mind the idea that performance and work capacity should increase!

Damn Stoopid Questions

Not all of these questions are stooopid, just most of them. Be that as it may, they are still frequently asked, so here are a few pithy responses.

How many days should I intermittent fast each week?

This is actually a pretty good question but my response may not be uber-helpful Implement IF as much as YOU want. Kelly Starrett of San Francisco CrossFit reported benefit (improved body composition and recovery) from a Tuesday/Thursday fast that lasted 15-18 hrs. Scotty Hagnas does fasts of varying lengths and does it nearly every day to great benefit. There are no set answers on this. Do what works for you.

I want to get HEYYYUGE! Can intermittent fasting help?!

Easy tiger! Step away from the Myoplex and let's talk. You need to be really clear about your goals here. If you want to gain weight, you need to eat… possibly disgusting amounts of food. If you want that composition to be good you will need to be particularly diligent with regards to food quality. Most people have no idea how hard it is to eat the food necessary to affect a good upwards scale shift. All that considered intermittent fasting might be something you use very sparingly, one to two days per week at most to enhance insulin sensitivity and to encourage your body to be miserly with calories.

The literature clearly illustrates that a post-workout meal with a high glycemic carb sources in conjunction with a micellular processed casein-whey-aqueous solution…

OK Poindexter, I got'cha. Post workout nutrition is important. Want a million dollar solution for just a PMenu subscription? Make your post workout meal like thus: normal large-ish protein meal (3-5 blocks) and ONE HALF of your day's carb requirements. Just shift the carbs and fat from your other meals to adjust for this. Make the carbs for the post workout meal consist of non-fructose containing items like yams and sweet potatoes. If you want the whys to all this, dig through my previous writing, it's in there. Oh, and Poindexter, why don't you ditch the casein, whey, albumin shake and drink some whole milk. You knuckle head.

I feel REALLY Dizzy when I do intermittent fasting… my chakras were misaligned… (or, in a similar vein) I want to fast for 22 hrs each day because I'm fucking neurotic with my food! But I can't fit all my food in during that 2-hour window and I keep passing out in the elevator…

Do this stuff to the degree it works for you. If you missed a bunch of sleep, have major stress in your life or are passing out at hour 12 of fasting, then eat something! Remember that Paleo/Zone progression? Default to that and stick with it. Intermittent Fasting should be a FAVORABLE stress, not something that makes you incapable of driving.

I'm skinny and I wanna be BIG! Do I train while fasted? Do I continue my fast after training? If so, how long?

Priority and focus should provide some answers here. If your priority is gaining muscle mass you need to EAT. Like I mentioned above, a few days per week of IF may help with insulin sensitivity, but I think a little food pre workout, say 10-15g of protein and a similar amount of carbs, should really help mental focus and keep intensity high. Post-workout, strap on the feedbag and take in the lions share of your carbs and a good size whack of protein. Capich? Oh yeah, steer clear of shakes and crap like that... just eat food.

I'm a little portly... Well, my step daddy called me "lil' Shamu"... but I'm mainly just big-boned... and i really want to get below 28% body fat... should I eat before and after my training... and before I go to bed? I'm a big guy and i need a lot of fuel to fire the furnace!

I think I may need a shot of tequila... So if your issue is too much body fat we need to bring insulin levels DOWN. Start with Paleo and keep the carbs on the low side—less than 100g per day. Do your training fasted and don't eat for at least an hour after you train. You will lose fat at a stunning rate AND folks will quit calling you Shamu.

Additional Resources

If you have more questions I recommend you direct them to Greg Everett. He is a world-renowned expert on intermittent fasting, Chia-pet landscaping and Mexican food in the greater San Diego area.

MIND FREAK: PART 2
AIMEE ANAYA EVERETT

Let's begin with our friend, Fear. We met Fear as a small child. You may not remember the initial meeting, but Fear was there all along. Fear started out a small part of our life. Simple Fear, we shall call our friend. We started out being afraid of the dark, afraid of our parents, afraid our friends wouldn't play with us, afraid our mom wouldn't let us by a new GI Joe. Simple Fear was there the whole time, silently waiting and growing into what we know as Fear today. As a child, Simple Fear rarely presented itself, and we were able to climb the highest trees, jump off the highest points, ride our bikes down the steepest hills with our eyes closed and our hands off the handlebars. We would fall on our faces and take all the skin off our knees, but we would stand up and do it over again. We weren't afraid of anything beyond such simple fears because we hadn't yet met Fear. I see my daughter practicing gymnastics, flipping all over the place and trying new tricks, falling over and over and over again—she is never afraid of her misses and always attacks each trick as if she hadn't just missed it 23 times. Why? Well, because she doesn't know my best friend Fear. I miss and I am suddenly afraid of the next lift. I miss and I remember it for days. I miss and Fear taunts me. How do you control Fear? Baby steps…

Relaxing and Breathing

As touched on in the first part of this series, when you learn to master the ability to relax, it will enhance your strength, flexibility, energy, and focus. When you are tense, you waste energy and effort in even the simplest movements; your body becomes tense and you exert energy from muscles that aren't even needed in the movement being made. Relaxation allows you to trust your strength, your skill, and your power. The inability to relax disables your thinking and focus, and delays clear and stable breathing. Your muscles lose flexibility and fluidity, and your performance is hindered. You become anxious, tense, and your body and mind is suddenly stressed. When you practice and master physical and mental relaxation, your heart's arterial pathways open up for better circulation, and your lungs are able to expand to increase oxygen consumption. With this, your muscles are able to lose the tension, your mental approach can be more tranquil and your performance improves.

In order to put a stop to the things that can inhibit your success, you need to learn to focus your breathing and relax . Only then can you see your way clearly in order to establish a firm balance for success in approved performance. Once you have learned to control your degree of relaxation physically, mentally, and emotionally, you can notice when tension is developing and take the steps necessary to release it. Newton's third law of motion states that for every action there is an equal and opposite reaction, and this applies to us in sport. As you train, relax—don't force your muscles or your mind. If our mind and body's action is that of tension and stress, than that is what is going to come back to us as performance results.

Bud Winter is known as one of the greatest Track Coaches of his time. He produced 102 All-Americans and 27 Olympians by diligently following, and enforcing, the Taoist paradox, soft is strong. He believed that keeping your body soft (or relaxed) would give you the most strength. He expanded this paradox, developing the "ninety percent law" in which he believed that running or performing at ninety percent effort stimulates relaxation and results in faster and snappier movement, more strength, a much sharper vision, less fatigue, and an improved sense of well being in competition. He believed that relaxation is the most widely ignored aspect of athletic training programs in the United States, and yet the most crucial . You can read more about his tactics in his book, Relax and Win: Championship Performance in Whatever You Do. Supreme performance occurs in an athlete when they are able to mentally, emotionally, and physically relax and harmonize before and throughout a competition.

So how do we do this? I like to start with breathing.

Vengeance. When I start to get myself all worked up in a frenzy of doubt, I think of vengeance. I treat my breathing patterns as an illusion of revenge against what it is I am afraid of. It is sort of like having something tear you down—you want to do everything to prove you can stand up again and keep going, right? The first step is to try to control your breathing so that your body can relax. Of course it is always ideal to monitor your breathing patterns from the minute you start whatever it is that you are doing, but because this isn't always the case, sometimes you have to work twice as hard to return to normalcy in your breathing. Here are several different techniques that I use to regulate my breathing in order to find optimum control.

- Sit with your head in your hands and eyes closed so that you can only focus on your breath. Breathe in through your nose and exhale through your mouth. I like to count to 7 when you inhale and exhale. Slowly breath in through your nose...

1-2-3–4-5-6-7. Slowly exhale through your mouth… 1-2-3-4-5-6-7. Do this for about five to ten minutes to get you relaxed. Do not think about anything during this time except the air and the numbers.

- Lie down or sit in a dark room. This one works well in the evenings before bed, or in a room before training or competition. Similar to above, you want to breathe in through your nose and exhale through your mouth. This time, when you breathe in, count… 1-2-3-4-5 then hold it for five seconds. Exhale forcefully then hold for five seconds. Repeat until you have calmed down. Once you feel like your breathing is controlled, continue to breath in through your nose, exhaling through your mouth. What I then like to do is relax my whole body. I focus on one body part at a time, my feet all the way to my head. While focusing on the individual part, I repeat to myself, "You are relaxed, you are strong… your feet are relaxed, your feet are strong." Then I move to my calves, my knees, my quads, my hips, my butt, and so on. Don't forget to keep your breathing regular! This normally takes about 15 or 20 minutes..

- This is the one I use most often, especially when I am training—Breathe in through your nose slowly for as long as you can then hold it for about five seconds. Exhale as quickly as you can then hold it for about five seconds. While I am breathing in, I am repeating, "Strength, strength, strength," and while I exhale I repeat, "Relax, relax, relax."

The above tools will aid in your ability to relax. Please don't think that mental training starts and ends with breathing—it is one of the fundamentals you need to master before continuing on in training your mind. My breathing techniques may not work for you—alter them until you find something that fits you. That is what I did—I changed, adapted, cried, and screamed myself into a hysterical hyperventilating-type breathing frenzy until I finally found something that worked for me. There is something out there that will work for you—just breathe a lot until you figure it out!

Mr. Miyagi once said, "Wax on, right hand. Wax off, left hand. Wax on, wax off. Breathe in through nose, out the mouth. Wax on, wax off. Don't forget to breathe, very important…" It worked for Daniel-Son, right?

Awareness of our bodies is a crucial part of training and competing. The power of awareness, specifically whole-body awareness, is critical in finding the path of mental, physical and emotional weaknesses and strengths. If you are aware that your breathing patterns are unstable and fluctuate, then you must find the willingness to acknowledge this and fix it before continuing. Your breath is similar to wearing your emotion on your sleeve; it is a huge indicator of the way you are feeling or thinking at any particular moment. Because we identify more closely and easily with our minds and our emotions than with our bodies, we are more inclined to ignore any "mental problems" over physical problems. So, let's just pretend that those "mental problems" are there, even if we are choosing to ignore them, and practice our breathing. Learn how to calm yourself down so that soon a fifteen-minute breathing exercise only takes two minutes. Teach your body to respond to your breath in ways that benefit your training and everyday life. Let's not forget that although we often find our minds playing tricks on us, we too can trick our minds.

In the next installment of Mind Freak I am going to assume your are a Master of Breathing and can move on with mental training. With this, I will address one of the greatest lessons I ever learned from James Bauman: "Focusing on the past or future. "I can't believe I just missed that simple lift" (past) or "Now I have to be perfect to win" (future). Not letting go of a mistake or "poor" performance takes our thoughts and focus away from where they need to be—on the present! Physiologically and bio-mechanically these past, present, and future self-conversations clutter up the connection between body and mind. Our body functions in the present only... so our thoughts must align with that time zone (not the past or future)", and I will discuss in great length Mental Imagery and Preparation. With this, we will also learn about vision, finding the positive, and what works in order to DO IT. Someone in the Tao world once said, "Hold fast to the great image, and all the world will come" (Tao Te Ching).

In Part 4 of Mind Freak, I will be discussing how to avoid and/or deal with athletic injuries. Mentally. The fabulous Dan Millman said "Injury most often results from a fundamental flaw in our talent foundation (of strength, suppleness, stamina, and sensitivity), or from impatience, a lack of attention, or some combination of these. "Accidents" aren't really accidents... to avoid injuries, you need mental clarity and attention, emotional stability, AND physical preparation. They are the three best insurance policies you'll ever have- and they don't cost a cent. Injury is the price paid for insensitivity, impatience, or inattention".

Unfortunately, I now have learned this the hard way. If I would have only taken his words seriously...

BREATHING AND BREATH CONTROL FOR OLYMPIC WEIGHTLIFTING
GREG EVERETT

Breath control is critical for increasing and maintaining the structural integrity of the torso while under heavy loads. The supporting musculature is alone inadequate—in order to adequately stabilize the spine, the abdominal and thoracic cavities must be pressurized. Additionally, we need to create as broad of a base for the torso as possible—the rationale for this should be obvious if one considers the structural integrity of a pyramid versus an upside-down pyramid. Drawing in the abs may look nice on the beach, but it will dramatically diminish the ability of the body to support the kind of forces we intend to introduce.

The torso has only a single supporting structure along its height—the spine—on one side, and this structure articulates in all directions, requiring additional support to maintain rigidity. The weak point is the circumference below the ribcage in which there is no rigid structure tying the torso into the pelvis—this creates a compressible area into which the torso can collapse forward and to the sides.

This area is of course filled with organs, the tissues of which are relatively incompressible, but the space inside of which we cannot directly make more resistant to compression. Above this, separated by the diaphragm, are the lungs. This provides us a convenient way to reduce the compressibility of the contents of the torso. By filling the lungs, we increase the rigidity of the thoracic cavity, and we also force the diaphragm down, which compresses the organs of the abdominal cavity somewhat.

To improve further on this compression, we can tighten the musculature surrounding the torso, which prevents unwanted expansion of the container walls and the resulting reduction of the potential for the torso to collapse.

The athlete will need to draw in as much air as possible, allowing the abdomen to expand and the diaphragm to contract, ensuring the lungs are able to fill completely; filling the lungs partially by only allowing the chest to lift and expand is not adequate. Once this breath is taken, the lifter will tighten down the abdominal and back musculature to increase the internal pressure and reduce the potential for flexion or extension of the torso. This effort to tighten down around the pressurized torso will push air out of the lungs and up the trachea—the athlete will need to close the glottis in order to keep the air in (this should happen naturally with the effort to hold the breath).

It's important that the athlete not "hollow", or draw in the abdominals as many have been taught to do or believe is correct. If the abdominals are drawn in, the base of support is reduced in width, and this is obviously not beneficial. We want the muscles activated tightly while maintaining a broad foundation to support the load. It may help athletes having difficultly with this activation to think of pushing the abs down. (This does not mean that the transversus abdominis is not active; it simply means that it should not be the sole focus of the stabilization effort and should not be cinched in to a degree that limits the ability to fill the trunk adequately with air.)

Pressurization should be maintained throughout as much of the movement as possible. There will be times, however, such as during the recovery of a clean, that the lifter will feel dizzy and even near unconsciousness. This can be because the athlete is not properly racking the barbell and the pressure is compressing the carotid arteries and reducing blood flow to the brain, but it can also be from actually holding the breath and bearing down simultaneously; these actions, especially when combined, stimulate the vagus nerve and reduce heart rate and blood pressure (this can be easily demonstrated by feeling your pulse while breathing normally, then holding your breath—you will feel an almost immediate reduction in heart rate). In some cases, this can cause unconsciousness, but this can be avoided by paying attention and reacting appropriately.

If dizziness or light-headedness occurs during lifts, the athlete should release a small amount of air during the highest-pressure or highest-effort moment of the lift (e.g. the sticking point of the squat) by making some noise. This will release some pressure and prevent dizziness while maintaining trunk stability. Some athletes will be more comfortable, and even feel stronger, making a habit of always releasing air with noise during the recovery of the squat, as long as the release is controlled and minimal. If dizziness is considerable, it is always advised that the athlete drop the bar immediately and sit down safely to recover.

During the explosive second pulls of the snatch and clean, and even sometimes during the drive of the jerk, some lifters will make noise with an expulsion of a small amount of air. This is not problematic and is usually helpful in increasing the athlete's aggressiveness.

The effect of torso pressurization can be demonstrated easily with a new lifter with nothing more than un-weighted squats. The athlete can pressurize the torso properly and perform a few squats, utilizing the bounce to recover. Following this, the athlete will expel as much air as possible, and squat again with the bounce. Invariably the difference is dramatic enough to immediately elicit some kind of exclamation from the athlete.

Pressurize the trunk with all structural lifting, and learn to control that pressurization, and you'll be maximizing both safety and performance.

NIGHTSHADES PART 5: THE PROBLEMS WITH POTATOES
DR. GARRETT SMITH

Potatoes (Solanum tuberosum). They seem so harmless, right? Well, far from it! This month's article will be all about potatoes, mainly about their glycoalkaloids and the toxicity that has been demonstrated in human history, across multiple animal species and via multiple potential mechanisms. Sound familiar? Potatoes just may be the most dangerous food that westerners eat on a very regular basis. How is this so?

First of all, while not apparently related to glycoalkaloids, cooking potatoes results in high amounts of the carcinogenic compound acrylamide. In fact:

"According to FDA research, the top three foods with the highest mean acrylamide content were potato based. Products such as restaurant french-fries, oven-baked french-fries and potato chips could pose the highest risk to consumers."

The whole list of the foods the FDA evaluated is available online. As few folks are eating raw potato these days, the acrylamide issue (which is increased proportionally with higher cooking temperatures) is a pertinent one right off the bat. While this is not limited to potatoes only, as the FDA list demonstrates, it is very significant with potatoes in particular.

Solanine is the major glycoalkaloid found in potatoes, along with alpha-chaconine. A very important fact is that "the clearance of glycoalkaloids usually takes more that 24 hours, which implicates that the toxicants may accumulate in case of daily consumption." This fact alone puts a twist on acute (<24 hours duration) studies done on glycoalkaloid toxicity, as many people eat potatoes everyday, often multiple times a day when all potato-based food additives are accounted for.

Solanine is found in all edible members of the nightshade (Solanaceae) family—quick review includes tomatoes, potatoes, peppers, eggplant, paprika, Cape gooseberries, goji/wolf berries, and tobacco—and it is well researched and accepted that these glycoalkaloids are toxic to humans and animals in sufficient doses. Even the World Health Organization (WHO) has placed a "safe level" "limit" on the solanine content of potatoes at 20mg/100g fresh weight. Why did a limit on solanine content need to be created? Because of incidents like this:

"Seventy eight schoolboys became ill after eating potato at lunch on the second day of the autumn term. Seventeen of the boys required admission to hospital. The gastrointestinal, circulatory, neurological and dermatological findings and the results of laboratory investigations were in keeping with solanine poisoning."

And this:

"Death has occurred in previous outbreaks, usually within 24 hours; but those cases were mainly in undernourished patients who may not have received adequate treatment…Possibly unrecognized mild solanine poisoning may be the cause of many mild episodes of "gastro-enteritis."

Other references to this issue included Mass poisoning with solanine, Solanine poisoning, potato poisoning, and A small outbreak of solanine poisoning. So, chalk up a Black Box history of potatoes/solanine poisoning people.

What conditions create a situation where glycoalkaloids reach toxic levels? They are phutoalexins (defensive antibiotic compounds) that increase in concentration in response to real or perceived threat situations to the plant. These threats include:

1. Potato blight—Caused by Phytophthora infestans, an oomycete (water mold) that attacks potatoes and other nightshades.
2. Light and heat—As potatoes are tubers (roots) grow underground in the cool darkness, exposure is perceived as a threat.
3. Mechanical damage.

Glycoalkaloid content also rapidly approaches toxic levels once the potatoes are greening or sprouting(chitting). It is estimated that 60-70% of the total glycoalkaloids present in most varieties of potato are contained within the peel (aka the "most nutritious part!"). I doubt I was the only college student who cut the sprouts off of potatoes and eaten them just to save some money! The big question then becomes, how well do you trust your grocer and their produce department to protect you?

What are the systemic effects of the glycoalkaloids, besides acute poisoning, you ask?

Solanine and alpha-chaconine from potatoes have both been shown to disrupt cell membrane function (1, 2, 3). The negative effects of this disruption may manifest in multiple areas of the body.

In the gastrointestinal tract:

1. Studies on intestinal cell lines (Caco-2) have shown effects upon gene expression

and pathways related to cholesterol biosynthesis and growth signaling.

2. Exacerbation of irritable bowel disease (IBD) in Mice.
3. Necrosis of gastrointestinal tissue in Syrian hamsters.
4. Inhibition of human pancreatic proteolytic enzyme activity.

The irritation of the gastrointestinal tract is particularly important in those who are gluten intolerant. In many gluten-free foods, potato starch is a common "replacement" flour—this alone could possibly thwart much of the improvement that one expects when they go gluten-free!

Hepatic (liver) effects:

1. Reduction of liver weight in mice—"The significantly lower liver weights of mice treated with alpha-chaconine and alpha-solanine and the significantly lower %LW/BW [liver weight/body weight x 100, author] of mice treated with alpha-chaconine suggest that these effects may be due to hepatotoxicity."
2. Liver gene mutations in pregnant mice.
3. Inhibition of normal human liver cells in vitro
4. Destruction of normal human liver cells in vitro

Red blood cell effects:

1. Red blood cell disruption
2. Hemolysis

The relationship of glycoalkaloid teratogenicity has been relatively well studied in animals, including:

1. Frog embryos in vitro.
2. Chicken empryos
3. Mice:
   a. Low birth weight and fetal abortion
   b. fetal abortion, neural tube defects, growth retardation
4. Toxicity in pregnant rats
5. Birth defects in hamsters
6. In Vitro inhibition of pre-implantation bovine (cow) embryo development

As far as I can find, there are no direct studies on the relationship of potato or glycoalkaloid consumption and teratogenicity in humans. I wouldn't let my wife in that study! After looking at the data in animals, who would let a pregnant woman potentially do that to herself and her unborn child?

Important question—If potatoes were not already in the food supply and were introduced today, would you let them in based on those animal studies? I hope not! There have been enough reviews on the relationship of potato blight to human birth defects, particularly in Ireland during times of potato blight to give one serious pause in regards to consistent consumption of the glycoalkaloids in potatoes. It is quite amazing to me how much unnecessary fear is drilled into pregnant women over medicinal herbs of all sorts, many based solely on conjecture, while no precautionary advice is being directed toward potato (and other nightshade) consumption!

Being that I started this whole series of articles on the connection between nightshades and arthritis, I'll bring it back around to that point with potatoes as well as I can. The potato glycoalkaloids (remember, all nightshades share these compounds!) are potent acetycholinesterase inhibitors. This has been shown in:

1. Insects.
2. Rabbits
3. Horses
4. And finally, humans

Could this be the main cause of their toxicity and ability to cause physical discomfort? Let's investigate this further. What are some of the possible effects of acute (short-term) Solanine poisoning?

Gastrointestinal disturbances, nausea, vomiting, diarrhea, abdominal pain, hypotension (low blood pressure), rapid breathing, delirium.

What are some of the effects of acetylcholinesterase inhibition?

Gastrointestinal upset, nausea, vomiting, diarrhea, abdominal pain, hypotension, bronchoconstriction, dizziness, fainting.

Do those sound close enough for you? One other notable action of acetylcholinesterase inhibitors on the nerurmuscular junction is that they result in prolonged muscle contraction(s). I'm going to put out some conjecture that the typical "stiffness" found in all types of arthritis, especially osteoarthritis without inflammation, is simply prolonged muscle contraction(s)! Next, imagine what would happen in terms of mechanical wear to any system of moving parts that has increased friction (due to chronically increased muscular tension across joints). Mechanical wear would increase, correct? One mechanism can then explain two issues that are commonly found in arthritis.

For those who plan on eating potatoes (and the other solanine- and chaconine-containing nightshades) anyway, and you're wondering if there is anything you can do or take to reduce their impact on your system, here are your possibilities— probiotics (especially L. plantarum) and folic acid. A naturopathic physician colleague of mine who practices Appliet Kinesiology told me that whenever he found nightshade sensitivity in a patient he noticed that it was always accompanied by a vitamin B-6 deficiency.

On the vitamin note, folic acid is crucial in preventing neural tube defects before and during pregnancy. These malformations include spina bifida (open spine), meningomyeloceles, myeloceles, anencephaly (open skull), encephalocele (gap in the skull) and other anomalies. It also appears to be potentially protective against embryo damage from alpha-chaconine. So, a combination of a folic acid deficiency and a high intake of nightshade foods would spell real trouble for a developing fetus! If you missed the part regarding the documented history of potatoes and birth defects above, make sure to read that part again.

In conclusion, potatoes are just not worth the potential risk(s). If you are going to eat them:

1. Avoid eating the potato peel.
2. Do not eat greened, black, damaged, or sprouting potatoes.
3. If you have any doubt about the length of time (longer is worse) or temperature (warmer is worse) that the potatoes have been stored under, even if not green or sprouting, it is prudent to avoid eating them.
4. The more bitter the potato, the higher the glycoalkaloid content.
5. Pregnant women would do well to avoid all nightshades, potatoes in particular.
6. Realize that combinations of nightshades in dishes will increase the solanine content additively. Eggplant parmigiana with a side of gnicchi would be a bad idea.

Try switching to sweet potatoes (which unfortunately still carry an acrylamide risk likely higher than regular potatoes). Also try your old potato recipes with parsnips, as anything that can be done with a potato can and has already been done with a parsnip! Replacing mashed potatoes with steamed & mashed cauliflower equals no toxic glycoalkaloids, less carbs, and more nutrients!

All that and I never even went into the glycemic index and carbohydrate content issue…

MASS (A)GAIN
GREG EVERETT

Way back in June 2006, Robb Wolf and I collaborated on a mass gain training and nutrition program. That issue quickly became one of our most popular and has remained so since. After a couple years of reader feedback and consideration on all sorts of related items, I've decided an update was in order.

The Nutrition

The nutrition component of the program requires only a quick note regarding macronutrient composition. PM readers are of course familiar with our long-standing preference for diets comprised of as little carbohydrate as will sustain an individual's chosen activities. Accordingly, our recommendation adhered to this and achieved caloric surplus through elevated protein and fat exclusively. Since, more research and experimentation has suggested that in some cases individuals will find it nearly impossible to gain any considerable weight without the effects of insulin brought about by the consumption of carbohydrate.

The fundamental principle of bodyweight—and the one that is so frequently neglected—is the First Law of Thermodynamics: Neither matter nor energy can be created or destroyed. The two can be converted, but there is never any net change in the total quantity. What this means in terms of bodyweight is that weight cannot be reduced without a deficit of energy, and weight cannot be increased without a surplus of energy. No amount of heavy back squatting will make a skinny kid huge if said skinny kid refuses to eat more energy and material than his body is using simply to survive—as remarkable as the human body is, it cannot create muscle tissue from thin air. Likewise, no amount of physical activity will cause a reduction in bodyweight if the individual is consuming more food energy than is being used in a given period of time. These things seem obvious, but they're ignored to an exasperating degree. When evaluating a bodyweight plan, always return to and rely on this fundamental principle to guide your decisions.

The above said, it's unfortunately not such a simple equation—human metabolism manages to be remarkably complex. The first consideration is the second law of thermodynamics—entropy. Entropy is the transfer of a percentage of the energy during a chemical reaction to the realm outside the reaction—commonly this transfer is referred to as a "loss", but because, according to the first law, energy cannot be lost, it is simply being relocated, usually in the form of heat. Macronutrients ultimately provide different net calories because of the variation the efficiency of their metabolism. For example, protein has fewer usable calories per gram than carbohydrate because the greater number of chemical reactions required to use protein as energy result in a lower net amount of energy with the increased entropy. This of course does not alter the fact that a calorie is a calorie—it only forces us to consider calories in terms of net instead of gross. And it certainly does not change the fact that an individual cannot gain weight without a net calorie surplus, or lose weight without a net calorie deficit.

However, to complicate things further, it turns out that the basic energy balance equation that's relied on for most bodyweight recommendations is widely misinterpreted:

Change in energy stores = Energy intake − Energy expenditure

This is nearly invariably understood to mean that the change in bodyweight is entirely a product of the relationship between calories consumed and calories expended. In other words, it's assumed that by increasing energy intake, bodyweight must increase, and by reducing energy intake, bodyweight must decrease, because the equation has to remain balanced or the universe will fall apart—the calories in and calories out are the cause of bodyweight status.

However, real-world evidence demonstrates clearly that this is not in fact the case. Instead, the body apparently has a fairly well-established bodyweight set point that it attempts to maintain—changes in energy intake will cause the body to make changes in its energy expenditure in order to maintain that set point. For example, if an individual increases his calorie consumption, the body will find ways to expend more energy through largely unnoticed movement and internal heat-producing activity. This is precisely why dieting of the basic calorie-reduction form fails so much—the dieter's body simply reduces its energy expenditure to match intake.

All this said, pursuit of bodyweight changes is not hopeless, just more complicated. In the case of weight gain, it appears that the body can only increase its energy expenditure so much—this simply means that calorie surpluses will often need to be even greater than expected to exceed the body's ability to compensate. After existing at a greater bodyweight for a period of time, the set point seems to be adjusted upwards, making further gains easier. In regards to weight loss, the issue appears to be one largely of macronutrient composition and its effect on metabolic status. That is, management of insulin coupled with less dramatic calorie reduction seems to be far more productive than extreme calorie restriction. Again, with time at a new bodyweight, the set point seems to be readjusted. In all cases, slower changes are more effective than attempts at rapid ones.

While in theory gaining weight is no more complex than either maintaining or losing it, in practice it invariably proves difficult for a variety of reasons. Foremost of those reasons is that the discipline required by the pursuit of functional mass surpasses that of even aggressive weight loss. Nearly all will be quick to argue that the deprivation alone of weight loss eclipses weight gain in difficulty; these individuals have never attempted to gain large amounts of quality weight and have no basis for comparison, and consequently may be dismissed.

The fundamental principle of weight gain is merely the opposite of weight loss: create a surplus of energy and material while attempting to prevent compensatory metabolic adjustment by the body to maintain its set point bodyweight. In cases of aggressive weight gain, simply consuming the necessary quantity of food is uncomfortable at best and seemingly impossible at worst. Contributing to the difficulty is the great importance of food quality and macronutrient composition. A great enough calorie surplus of any composition will produce at least some weight gain—but the role of additional weight is to provide additional functional capacity, and body fat is incapable of contributing in any direct or significant manner to strength and power. The difficulty lies in encouraging the body not to simply increase its mass, but to do so through the hypertrophy of the functional components of muscle and connective tissue—this demands the control of food quality and macronutrient composition.

As is the case with weight loss, the longer the period of time over which weight is gained, the better the quality of the added mass can be controlled. There are limits to the rate at which the body's lean mass can grow, and reaching far beyond these limits will result in greater gains in body fat relative to muscle mass.

For gradual weight gain, the process is in essence no different than gradual weight loss, the difference being only that the daily calories will be incrementally increased instead of decreased. Accurate record keeping is equally important—the same ease of self-delusion during weight loss applies to weight gain. Protein intake can be adjusted up to around 1.5-2 grams per pound of bodyweight per day. How well this higher protein intake accelerates muscle gain seems to vary among individuals, but it has certainly never hurt. Vegetable and fruit consumption should be maintained, and fat intake can be adjusted to account for the necessary caloric increase after any increases in protein are considered.

For more aggressive weight gain, the rules must be changed somewhat. The rule standing high above all is eat more. More than you ate before, more than what you want to eat, more than what you think you can eat. Quality and macronutrient composition are irrelevant until quantity has been taken care of. This is by no means intended to dissuade attempts to maintain quality and composition, but to more forcefully underscore the importance of a large and consistent calorie surplus. In other words, if the only options are eating fast food and eating nothing, the choice must be fast food, and more than is appealing. Always remember—if you're not uncomfortable, you're not eating enough, and if you're hungry, you're failing miserably.

With gradual weight gain, the body is allowed time to adjust to progressively larger quantities of food; with rapid weight gain, there is no such luxury. In order to mitigate this problem, foods with the greatest possible caloric density will become necessities. Fats will be instrumental considering that a given quantity has over twice the calorie content of the same quantity of either protein or carbohydrate. Nut butters, olive oil, and coconut milk are relatively easily stomached but extraordinarily calorie-dense. For those who eat dairy, whole milk can replace its reduced-fat counterparts. In the same vein is supplemental protein, which will provide an extremely helpful service considering the physical difficulty of eating enormous quantities of meat.

Fitting in another meal in the middle of the night has been a successful tactic for many. Typically this meal is in the form of a shake consisting of supplemental protein, nut butter or coconut milk, and possibly fruit. This can obviously increase the number of quality calories in a 24-hour period, and will consequently be successful if eating the rest of the day is in order. However, the quality and quantity of sleep, particularly during times of weight gain, is of great importance. Because of this, the recommendation is to prepare a shake and place it in the refrigerator. If you wake naturally during the night, drink the shake. If not, you can drink it the next morning. Intentionally disrupting sleep is potentially more detrimental than night feedings are beneficial. If you're the kind of individual who can be awakened, drink a shake, and fall immediately back to sleep, this may not be an issue. But for some, a five-minute task can result in multiple hours of lost sleep.

Macronutrient composition in cases of aggressive weight gain does not necessarily need to be modified any further from the relative increases in protein intake described for gradual weight gain. Some have suggested as much as 3 grams of protein per pound of bodyweight per day and swear by its efficacy. However, real world practice of this for already large individuals is remarkably difficult and the effect is questionable. It can certainly be experimented with to gauge individual response; just be sure to continue consuming large amounts of fat and eating as much vegetable and fruit matter as possible to prevent any sickness from too high a percentage of calories from protein.

Just as with weight loss, individuals will respond very differently during weight gain. That is, with a given calorie surplus, athletes will gain different amounts of weight. Again—if no weight is being gained, not enough is being eaten. Individuals with extreme difficulty gaining weight will generally find that an increase in carbohydrate intake will help through the effects of insulin on the metabolism. This is not an invitation to put away a bag of Oreos each night—as always, higher quality food will translate into higher quality gains. Grains should remain limited as much as possible and yams, sweet potatoes and other tubers and starchy vegetables relied on as the primary dense carbohydrate sources. Milk can also be a source of carbohydrate in these cases.

Milk is commonly endorsed among old school strength coaches and athletes as the ultimate weight gaining food. There is no question that milk offers a generally easily consumed and inexpensive source of potentially enormous amounts of protein and calories, and consequently can help encourage rapid weight gain. Whether or not milk actually produces gains in muscle mass any better than the equivalent totals of quality protein, fat and carbohydrate is not as clear.

Recommendations tend to be between one half and one gallon of whole milk each day—this would supply approximately 1300-2600 calories. It's not surprising weight gain would be the result of this practice when supplementing continued whole food consumption.

For those unconcerned by potential but generally minor health drawbacks of dairy consumption, this is certainly worth evaluating. Even for those who normally wouldn't consume dairy, this can be considered temporary—adequate gains in weight will probably be achieved in several months, after which time, a return to a healthier diet to maintain the new weight will be possible. Lactose intolerance can be managed with inexpensive lactase supplements.

Raw milk is another option that will itself supply some of the needed lactase enzymes, as well as some colostrum, both of which will reduce the cost of supplementation for these two items. Whole milk with 100% of the lactose removed is also available.

The Training

The following program of course intends to help the athlete gain functional weight. For this it uses greater volume per session in the core exercises, but a lower frequency and overall lower volume to allow the greatest possible recovery. Instead of somewhat higher reps such as 5s and 6s, we're instead using 2s and 3s but with a greater number of sets to achieve the wanted volume while encouraging as much as possible myofibrillar hypertrophy.

The loading will be increased 2-3% per week (or less, according to each athlete's gains) for 4 weeks, then backed off for a week, the increases resumed for 2-3 more weeks as tolerated (starting at the weight used the week prior to the back-off), and the cycle finished with a taper week to allow 1RM testing of any exercises the athlete wishes.

Notation

Exercises are followed by the prescribed loading, reps and sets in that order. For example, Snatch – 75% x 2 x 5 would indicate snatching 75% of the athlete's 1RM for 2 reps for 5 sets. If a loading prescription is absent, the sets and reps will be in the reverse order. For example, Box jumps – 4 x 5 would indicate 4 sets of 5 reps. The prescription heavy single indicates that the athlete should take the weight up to the heaviest he or she can manage for a single rep without any misses, unless due to obvious technical mistakes. Max would indicate instead a genuine attempt at a 1RM, with an allowance for as many as 3 attempts to achieve it.

Core Training

Trunk stabilization training should be performed 4-5 days per week. This training should include isometric stabilization, trunk flexion, lateral trunk flexion, and rotation work. Each of these categories of movement require training with both heavier loads for stabilization and lighter loads with greater volume for stamina. Core training can be included on every training day provided the type of work is sufficiently varied among sessions. That is, it's generally best to alternate heavy and light emphasis training to provide recovery time for each. Additionally, more taxing core training is best performed during heavy lifting sessions to allow recovery and prevent reduced trunk stability in the next heavy session.

Monday

Weeks 1-4
Back Squat – 75% x 3 x 10
Clean & Jerk – heavy single
Push Press – 75% x 5 x 5

Back-off Week
Back Squat – 85% of last week x 3 x 6
Clean & Jerk – 85% of last week x 1 x 1
Push press – 85% of last week x 5 x 3

Last Week
Back Squat – 85% x 1 x 2
Clean & Jerk – 75% x 1 x 3
Push Press – 85% x 1 x 2

Tuesday

Weeks 1-4
Power Snatch – 60% (of snatch) x 2 x 3
Power Clean & Jerk – 60% (of CJ) x 2 x 3
Pull-ups – 3 x max

Back-off Week
Power Snatch – 60% (of snatch) x 1 x 3
Power Clean & jerk – 60% (of CJ) x 1 x 3
Pull-ups – 3 x 85% of last week's reps

Last Week
Snatch – 75% x 1 x 3
Bench Press – 75% x 2 x 2

Wednesday

Weeks 1-4
Deadlift – 80% x 3 x 3
Bench Press – 75% x 5 x 5
Pull-ups – 3 x 75% of Tuesday

Back-off Week
Deadlift – 85% of last week x 3 x 1
Bench Press – 85% of last week x 5 x 3
Pull-ups – 3 x 75% of Tuesday

Last Week
Power Snatch – 60% x 1 x 3
Power Clean & Jerk – 60% x 1 x 3

Thursday
Rest

Friday

Weeks 1-4
Front Squat – 75% x 3 x 5
Snatch – heavy single
Press – 75% x 3 x 5

Back-off Week
Front Squat – 85% of last week x 3 x 3
Snatch – 85% of last week x 1 x 1
Press – 85% of last week x 3 x 3

Last Week
Rest

Saturday

Weeks 1-4
2-position Snatch – 60% x 4 sets
2-position Clean – 60% x 4 sets
Push jerk + Jerk – 60% (of jerk) x 4 sets
Pull-ups – 3 x max

Back-off Week
2-position Snatch – 60% x 2 sets
2-position Clean – 60% x 2 sets
Push jerk + Jerk – 60% (of jerk) x 2 sets
Pull-ups – 3 x 85% of last week's reps

Last Week
Test 1RMs

Sunday
Rest

THE M.E. BLACK BOX FOR THE FAMILY MAN
MICHAEL RUTHERFORD

While I've had my successes with helping the aspiring athlete run faster, jump higher, and put more weight overhead, I derive the greatest pleasure from helping the family man or woman. He goes to work, he is likely in a relationship, has a family and probably volunteers in some capacity. These athletes have different stress and value systems. Elite performance and personal records are important but not at the expense of other values.

I recently received that following e-mail which was the genesis of The M.E Black Box for the Family Man.

> My name is "JASON" and I hope you are doing well today.
>
> I think I am experienced enough to answer my own question but wanted to see if you had 2 cents to add. I am going to begin the ME Black Box routine. (Thanks by the way!)
>
> However, as a devoted father of small children, a husband and coach of recreational Baseball, I will not be going to the gym on the weekends. I reserve those days for foam rolling, active BW recovery and family. So if I am trying to adapt the ME BB to a 5 day program how do you feel about Crossfit M/W/F and ME Total on Tuesdays and alternating Upper/Lower each Thursday? I know this does not fit the 3 on 1 off parameters so I may find myself needing a rest day towards the end of the week. I am looking for a starting point with the BB. If it makes a difference in your opinion I am 37 years old and have been doing Dos' Power training since it came out. And have been lifting for about 7 years now.
>
> Thanks for your time and I hope you have a great day.

The Nuts and Bolts

At this stage of the game I trust that everyone is familiar with the ME BLACK BOX and the variants presented thus far. The ME BLACK BOX will provide the necessary strength and power stimulus to accelerate your fundamental strength and propel your CrossFit WOD times and benchmark workouts.

The Family Man MEBB Rules

1. All training must take performed M-F
2. NO workouts are performed on Saturday and Sunday as these are reserved for the family and other pursuits.
3. No workout can exceed 45 minutes.
4. Other healthy practices should be in place.

	MON	TUE	WED	THU	FRI	SAT	SUN
WEEK 1	ME	CF	ME	CF	ME	REST	REST
WEEK 2	CF	ME	CF	ME	CF	REST	REST

The Family Man MEBB Training Template

This template is quite simple. The athlete will us an A/B split.

A = ME Day

B = CrossFit Day

Since there are five days for workouts and two primary focuses of training, there will be a week of 3 ME sessions followed by a week of 2 ME sessions.

I have included the ME Day tier rotation information below.

DAY	MOVEMENT POOL	ROTATION
MON	TOTAL BODY (T)	HIGH HANG CLEAN, DECK POWER CLEAN, CLEANS
WED	LOWER BODY (L)	ZERCHER SQUAT, FRONT SQUAT, BACK SQUAT
FRI	UPPER BODY (U)	PRESS, PUSH PRESS, JERK

Rep Rotations

Wk 1 - 5 x 5
Wk 2 - 5 x 3
Wk 3 - 5 x 1

The randomization of your program is completely your call. If your relative strength is the limiting factor then you should only incorporate short duration CrossFit workout challenges.

I believe this training template offers even the busiest of family folks an opportunity to maintain top tier performance while maintaining a balance of family time.

A CLOSER LOOK AT POSE RUNNING
BRIAN DEGENNARO

In the running world a "revolutionary" and "controversial" way of running, called POSE, was introduced by Dr. Nicholas Romanov. This approach, known as the POSE method, revolves around the notion that the runner is not actually propelling him- or herself forward, but rather allowing gravity to propel the body forward and changing support from foot to foot—"POSE-fall-pull," as Romanov states. No more than a controlled fall, this method is in stark contrast to the average runner's "heel-toe" method of running.

This has brought new attention to recreational and long distance running mechanics, which have devolved over the years since the advent of recreational running and the "innovative" running shoe that has resulted in misinformation. While the POSE method is functional for longer distances, its mechanics fail to meet the demands of sprinting.

Analyzing the Stride

Each stride of a run, whether it is the mile or the 100 meter dash, has three components: the support, the drive, and the recovery phase. All three phases occur within fractions of seconds and in quick, fluid succession.

In the support phase, one leg begins contact with the ground from the ball of the foot while the other is free and behind the body. The leg that is in contact with the ground remains underneath or slightly ahead of the center of gravity (COG) and flexes as it bears bodyweight, initiating a stretch-shortening cycle. The free leg is now in the process of swinging forward and the drive phase begins. The contact foot has now been loaded like a spring in the support phase and begins to extend from the ankles, knees, and hips. This action propels the body forward. The free leg, at the same time, is swung forward in order to add to forward propulsion. This push places the runner's body in the air and there is now no contact with the ground. This completes the drive phase. The recovery phase is when the body is airborne and the legs begin to cycle and change positions. The free leg, which had been driven upward, now begins to "unwind" and make its way down to the ground. Once it makes contact with the ground, the support phase begins all over again. What strides look like will vary from runner to runner and from distance to distance, but the basic components always remain the same.

POSE encourages running economy with its principle mental cues. These principles tell runners to "change support quickly… raise the ankle straight up under the hips… retain the support easily, effortlessly, light… to not try to increase stride length or range of motion to increase speed… to not fix on landing… [and] keep the knees bent on landing." All of these mental cues aid in achieving proper running mechanics. Many are the same points that track and field coaches use for their athletes.

The first step of the stride is the landing of the foot. Romanov reminds the runner to not fixate on getting the leg back down to the support phase in order to run faster. To run faster, one is covering more ground with each stride, not reaching for the ground ahead (resulting in overstriding). The runner allows the free leg to naturally drop to the ground rather than returning it by mechanical energy. Doing so, the runner prevents himself or herself from stomping the ground. A good runner does not run with "heavy feet," (caused by actively reaching the ground), but rather the steps are quick and light; there is only a light pitter-pat to each stride. If the foot stomps the ground, tremendous forces are sent upwards through the legs; these forces are much greater than what results if just allowing gravity to bring the foot back down. Also, actively reaching and stomping the ground reduces the hang time of a stride, which reduces the amount of distance covered.

Romanov states that with each stride the foot land—while keeping the knee bent—on the ball of the foot underneath the center of gravity, which is being displaced in a forward direction. Landing on the ball of the foot and under the center of gravity reduces the braking action, keeping the runner in motion. This landing also allows the lower legs to absorb impact much better than heel-toe running—the calf muscles are allowed to flex and absorb force. Landing on the ball of the foot and with flexed knees utilizes the stretch-shortening cycle, unlike heel-toe running, where the leg muscles are already in a stretched position, and must therefore generate more force to "toe off." The stretch-shortening cycle causes a recoil effect in the leg muscles, and the runner is able to use the body's natural reflexes in order to contribute power, resulting in more economical movement. The calf and hip muscles strike the ground in a semi-flexed position, immediately stretch, and contract, resulting in momentum forward only if there is a forward lean.

The runner's COG is displaced forward by leaning slightly from the ankles to facilitate forward motion by placing the runner's legs at the proper angle to push against the ground. If the lean is not present, the leg drive is straight down and propulsion is upwards. In order to move, the runner must "drag" the body across the ground or bounce, resulting in higher energy expenditure. Think of pushing a car. If you stand completely upright and try to push a car forward it will go nowhere. The body is not in a position to push against the ground or the weight of the car. However, if the body is angled only a few degrees then the legs can effectively push against the ground and move the vehicle.

POSE tells the runner to pull the ankle straight up instead of backwards in a pawing motion. This mental cue results in two things: a more efficient use of hip and knee flexion and a quicker change of support. This quicker change of support is important in running to ensure the entire system (the runner) is in constant motion and never decelerating due to the braking effect of remaining in contact with the ground for too long.

The reason it is more efficient to pull the foot straight up is because the runner performs the knee and hip flexion as one motion rather than as two separate motions. For example, stand on one leg with the free leg extended behind you, ball of the foot lightly touching the floor. Now, as fast as possible kick yourself in the butt and bring your foot underneath your body. Notice how long it takes to perform this and the momentum generated. Now, get back into that position once more, and this time bring your foot up underneath in one quick motion; imagine kicking a target underneath your butt. It was only a fraction of a second quicker but much stronger. The amount of force applied to the ground will change the amount of hip flexion, assuming the runner is reasonably flexible, because of the stretch reflex. The stronger the force applied, the more flexed the hips will be; this is why 100-meter sprinters appear to run with "high knees."

Most importantly, POSE reminds runners to just let it happen. If the body is strong enough and the motor patterns are well trained, everything just happens; the stretch-shortening cycle, the forward motion, the leg cycling, and all the other good mechanics of running. Often runners think of too many things to do at once. The mind can only process so many thoughts and perform so many actions at a time. Professional track athletes think nothing of form during a race; they allow the race happen and think about one thing, typically about running their own race. These athletes have drilled the form in their head and bodies at practice; what used to take dedicated effort to perform is now second nature. To quote Romanov, "Problems begin when we insist on controlling every aspect of our body moving… While we think about what we need to do to move our leg this way or that way and we think of what muscles should be working, our body and its constituent parts have already not only activated the necessary muscles, but might have already finished the job, too."

Analyzing POSE

Proper running form has been known since before Romanov introduced the POSE method. Gordon Pirie describes proper running technique in Running Fast and Injury Free in a very similar manner as Romanov. He touches on being light and springy, "landing elastically on the forefoot with a flexed knee (thus producing quiet feet). On landing, the foot should be directly below the body," and so on. Sound familiar? Romanov coined a teaching style. Just as there are several ways to learn how to do a back-handspring in gymnastics or clean a weight, there are several ways to teach a person how to run. The end result is essentially always the same; the teaching of such skills varies from coach to coach. Also, certain descriptions and teaching methods work better for one person than another. POSE's teaching method may not work for everyone. If running coaches can take anything away from the POSE method, it is that they should remind their athletes to let running happen. Drills done in practice are meant to create muscle memory so athletes do not have to think while competing, over thinking results in performance loss.

Runners often experience much ankle and calf pain once taking up POSE running. Romanov states that this is the result of the person "resisting gravity" and "tensing of the calves." As a quick fix, he says to focus on relaxing the foot on the support phase. This is good advice, but there are two problems. Firstly, many people who take up POSE are recreational runners who tend to have tight calf muscles and ankles to begin with, carry-overs from heel-toe running. So when running on the ball of the foot, these muscles are now stretched with forces exceeding three times bodyweight. This will cause slight tears and strains from repeated use. Secondly, running on the ball of the foot and utilizing the stretch-shortening reflex results in much more eccentric work being done by the lower legs. Eccentric movements are known to cause more muscle damage than concentric because the muscles are under greater tension. Now that the ankles and calves are supporting greater forces, the risk for tears is higher. It is obvious that adjusting running technique requires an adjustment of the training program as well. The body must be allowed time to adapt to the new stresses and demands, no matter the quality of the coaching.

Romanov touts that in order to run faster, all the athlete needs to do is lean more (displace COG) and pick up the cadence (change support quickly). Gravity is the "engine" that allows one to run and sprint faster and that muscular power and effort is of less importance. He states that because the contact time with the ground is so short that muscular strength cannot be expressed, even though the muscles contract once they are stretched. Romanov even cites a study linking muscular contractions in the quadriceps having insignificant input to running. Through this study Romanov concludes that there is no "push off" in running because the quads are mostly inactive in a stride. Voluntary push off is apparently nonexistent. However, this study analyzes the knee extension of the running stride and not the hip extension, which is where the "push off" comes from, or rather the "push forward." Running is about extending the hips and not the knees.

The biggest issue is the role of the hamstrings. POSE states that they are the only active component of running and their function is to pull the foot off the ground. Movement is caused by gravity alone and simply changing support at a faster pace results in faster running speeds. That is a great idea to have while running but you will not be a fast runner by just changing support quickly. You have to use the leg muscles to the best of their ability. Muscles are not meant to store large amounts of energy; they do a much better job at producing it. Here's a good analogy. Place two cars of the same model on a slight downhill. The downhill represents the forward lean of the body. Car A represents the POSE runner and will travel down the road by "gravity alone" while car B represents another runner with good mechanics and utilizing his leg muscles. At the start of the race A is shifted into neutral while B is shifted into drive and the pedal is pressed to the floor. A gradually picks up speed and tops out around several miles per hour while B has taken off into the sunset. POSE is an efficient way of learning to run, but not the best way to run. You can run utilizing all of POSE's concepts to the maximum, but in order to win the race you will have to run hard and use energy; you must use your internal engine. Muscular power must be exerted in order to run fast and run personal bests. No runner crosses the finish line without exerting most of their energy to win and run personal bests.

Regarding the lean, the human body can only lean so far before balance is completely destroyed and the runner lands on his or her face. The runner leans in order to effectively push against the ground, not chase their COG. Often when a runner attempts to pick up speed, he or she will over-stride or will thrust the leg to the ground. As stated before, thrusting the leg down to the ground results in greater forces generated in the legs, and almost definitely longer contact times. When over-striding, the runner will not only land ahead of the COG, but also create higher breaking forces by landing closer to the heel if not on the heel with straight leg. The runner must drag himself forward in order to position himself in the proper pushing position. Runners do not want to reach out with their legs but rather create a "piston-type" movement. This allows runners to run most effectively because they are striking the ground in the perfect position to push off. In a perfect world this is the most efficient way to run.

Also, the body can only take so many steps per second; in order to cover more distance there must be more power produced. Elite 100-meter sprinters take approximately 50 or fewer steps to complete the race—around 5 steps per second—but even average runners can achieve a cadence matching those of high-end level sprinters. The only difference is the amount of distance that is covered between the two runners.

In order for the elite sprinter to cover 100 meters in such a short time, there must be more distance covered per stride. A study by Dr. Peter Weyand at Harvard showed that force production per stride results in higher top speeds. Additionally, the higher the force applied the shorter the contact time, regardless of maximal speed. Power separates the great from the average. The more powerful athlete will always win in a sprint because the leg muscles are able to generate greater force against the ground. This athlete can generate a greater percentage of their max strength in the short time of contact. The greater this power is in relation to bodyweight, the more distance covered per stride.

For example, examine the dip of the jerk and the support phase of Michael Johnson's stride in these two frames. With the dip of the movement, the body assumes the same position as the support phase. The hips, knees, and ankles are all flexed and loaded. There is minimal flexion in this position. Any more flexion reduces the effect of the stretch-shortening cycle because the muscle contraction is delayed; energy will be released as heat if the change from eccentric to concentric is not immediate. The faster application of power allows the weight being heaved or Johnson moving forward. If the weightlifter were to slowly apply his force, the lift would be a missed attempt, and if Johnson were to not quickly apply force he would not have any world records.

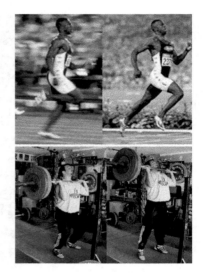

In the next frame the legs are in triple extension. Here the body exerts maximal force against the ground, resulting in a heavy load being heaved and Johnson's bodyweight propelled forward. The difference is the positioning of the bodies. Because Johnson is positioned a few degrees forward, the force generated by his legs drives him forward, while the weightlifter is as vertical as possible so the force generated drives the weight upward. One must note that the more powerful the muscles, the more powerful the stretch-shortening cycle, and therefore the faster the running. Form and technique aside, the most powerful will always win.

The problem with Romanov's assumptions is that running (more specifically sprinting) is about displaying maximal strength, which takes at least .4 second to achieve peak force development, when in fact, sprinting is a runner's attempt to express explosive strength. Athletes are constantly attempting to improve their explosive strength in order to gain the edge needed in sport. POSE running overlooks the importance of rate of force development and its application to running faster. Also, runners never exceed a lean of more than a few degrees (except for a sprinter coming out of the blocks), so greater leans do not necessarily translate into greater max speeds. Maximal strength is the key for force development but because of the short contact time maximal force cannot be expressed with each stride. Trying to exert maximal strength against the ground results in a longer than wanted or needed contact time, and the person you race against could be two or three strides ahead now, just as the weightlifter has to quickly drive out of the very brief dip in order to drive weight overhead. To solve this problem, the runner must be able to condition the muscles to increase the rate of force development. By training to increase the rate of force development, the athlete will increase the amount power in each stride and therefore distance traveled.

It's the Shoes

The average person fails to run with proper form because of being misinformed and having the luxury of cushioned running shoes; even current track coaches often fail to instruct running form well because of shoes. This trend started in the 1960s and 1970s when running started to become popular among recreational athletes. The shoes worn by elite runners such as Roger Bannister (top), Jesse Owens, Michael Johnson (middle), and Haile Gebrselassie (bottom) were nothing more than a protective slipper, in stark contrast to the modern, stylish shoes of today with all the padding in the world to "protect" the feet and "correct" running issues. If the average person attempted to run wearing these slippers or even barefoot, the first thing that would happen is they would strike with the heel and send a shooting pain up their leg. In order to prevent such pain while running barefoot or in these thin shoes, one learned to run properly. Besides Johnson, all these runners grew up running with lightly cushioned shoes or even barefoot, resulting in excellent running form, and few injuries, all because a thin protective layer separated the foot from the ground. These light shoes allow the body to apply the power needed during runs while reinforcing proper technique with each stride. Thick, soft heels disperse this energy.

Modern running shoes change the athlete's mechanics with each stride unless he or she is conscious of form or has correct mechanics ingrained in his or her muscles, but even then "to run in shoes was OK... it's better to have no shoes than not the right ones," to quote Gebrselassie. Shoes tend to be designed in labs based on testing and observation of the average person, who lacks correct running technique. This runner strikes heel to toe, landing with a fully extended leg, and pounds the ground or shuffles along amiably. Take a look at recreational runners at a park, and you'll find that 99% of them run in such a manner; the shoes promote terrible form by allowing people to run poorly.

Look at track flats or racing spikes and see that there is extremely little padding, and that the spike plate is on the midfoot rather than the heel. That ought to tell you something about how you should run. To quote Gordon Pirie, "Instead of looking for padding, learn to run properly, so that you stop punching holes in the ground with your feet... I have run more than 240,000 miles without any major problems, and more than half that distance covered on so-called hard pavement." The problem lies in the widespread ignorance of the running community and shoe companies promoting products that allow improper technique.

Conclusion

POSE running shatters the average person's notions of how to run, claiming to be "first official and complete running technique on the market" and that it cures "running related problems" such as shin splints, plantar fascitis, knee and hip issues, and other similar types of injuries. For years track and field coaches have known the proper mechanics of running, and good coaches and experienced runners implement much skill work into their training; Romanov simply invented his own method of coaching proper form, just as Dan John's method for teaching the snatch is different from Mike Burgener's method. However, the end result will look the same. What goes through the athletes' minds will differ.

Romanov is correct in stating that running is a learned skill, and POSE is a good teaching method because it is very simple to teach. No weightlifter just does snatches in order to practice, just as no runner just runs in order to practice. There are drills that are done in each session that aid in the development and perfection of skill. However, one must keep in mind that POSE is a method of teaching proper running mechanics and not its own biomechanical model of running. It is simply one method of learning the proper mechanics of a technical skill.

Notes

Chu, Donald. Jumping into Plyometrics. Champaign: Human Kinetics, 1998.

CNN. "Q & A with Haile Gebrselassie." November 9. 007. Retrieved April 24, 2008 from http://www.cnn.com

Ebbets, R. The Art of Running. Retrieved May 18, 2008, from http://www.texastrack.com/

Farrell, J. STRIDE LENGTH ANALYSIS. Retrieved May 18, 2008, from http://www.coachr.org/

Newton, R. The Great Stretch Shortening Cycle Debate - Why is a counter movement jump higher than a concentric only jump. Retrieved May 18, 2008, from http://www.innervations.com/

McGinnis, Peter M. Biomechanics of Sport and Exercise. Champaigne: Human Kinetics, 2005.

Pirie, Gordon. Running Fast and Injury Free. Ed. John S. Gilbody. John S Gilbody, 1996. Gordon Pirie Resource Center. <http://www.gordonpirie.com/>.

Romanov, Nicholas. Dr. Nicholas Romanov's POSE Method of Running. CoralGables: POSE Tech Press, 2002.

Romanov, Nicholas. Dr. Nicholas Romanov's Training Essays Volume I. Coral Gables: POSE Tech Press, 2006.

Romanov, Nicholas. "THE EXTENSOR PARADOX IN RUNNING." November 1, 2005. Retrieved April 24, 2008 from http://www.POSEtech.com/

Romanov, Nicholas. "FAST RUNNING with POSE Method." May 30, 2006. Retrieved April 24, 2008 from http://www.POSEtech.com/

Smith, Mike. High Performance Sprinting. Ramsbury: Crowood, 2005.

Weyand, P.G., Sternligh, D.B., Bellizzi, M.J., & Wright, S. (2000). "Faster top running speeds are achieved with greater ground forces not more rapid leg movements." Retrieved April 24, 2008 from Journal of Applied Physiology, 89 <http://jap.physiology.org/cgi/content/full/89/5/1991.>

Zatsiorsky, Vladimir M., and William J. Kraemer. Science and Practice of Strength Training. Champaign: Human Kinetics, 2006.

MY PRESEASON TRAINING TEMPLATE FOR GRAPPLERS
MICHAEL RUTHERFORD

As I scan the roster of my high school and collegiate clients over the last few years, I find the majority are from the ranks of wrestling. While I have enjoyed all the young athletes I have tutored, I consider these wrestlers some of the most focused of all athletes that I have had the pleasure of coaching.

For this month's column, I would like to present a training template I've used successfully for the last two seasons with my wrestling clients. This is the programming used for the final 12 weeks prior to start of wrestling practice in November.

NUTS & BOLTS

This August—November template is a three-day per week training program. The training phase preceding this is typically a four day per week training program of heavy pressing, squatting, pulling. I have used modified Westside Programs, Mark Rippetoe's Starting Strength and the Wolf/Everett Mass program. Very little if any metCon and lots of massing up!

While a part of me despises the weight-cutting aspect of the sport, there appears to be some win/loss support for being as strong as possible at the lightest weight possible providing the health of the athlete is not compromised in the process.

This lead up phase includes the following objectives.

1. Maintaining training qualities from the mass up phase
2. Introduce higher repetition/shorter rest interval
3. Lactate tolerance
4. Unilateral and contra lateral loading with my favorite tool—the dumbbell

Programming

The program has a movement from the weightlifting world followed by a superset combination. This is then followed up with a limited CrossFit challenge. Since the majority of wrestling coaches include running as a conditioning move, support for more interval running work is warranted. If an athlete has any injury history, prehab moves are done prior to any focus work.

Weightlifting Moves

Day 1
Push Press or Push Jerk (3-5 sets x 3-5 reps)

Day 2
Hang Snatch or Snatch (3-5 sets x 3-5 reps)

Day 3
Hang Clean or Clean (3-5 sets x 3-5 reps)

The second phase of the training day involves a number of supersets. These are 3 supersets of 8-12 reps. The rest interval is between 30-60 seconds between combinations.

Day 1

1. Alternating supine dumbbell press
2. Single leg squat or step up
3. 1:00 rest
4. Alternating dumbbell incline press
5. Single leg contra lateral dumbbell RDL
6. 1:00 rest
7. Dips or decline alternating dumbbell decline Press
8. Chin-ups (Supine Grip)

Day 2

1. Dumbbell rack front squat
2. Push-up (Cables)
3. 1:00 rest
4. Dumbbell contra lateral lunge and press
5. Dumbbell alternating bent over rows
6. 1:00 rest

Day 3

1. Pull-ups (Pronated grip) Strict form add weight if 12 reps are surpassed
2. Single leg contra lateral dumbbell RDL
3. 1:00 rest
4. Dumbbell Snatch from Deck or single dumbbell contra lateral overhead squat
5. Push-up (Cables)
6. 1:00 rest
7. Dumbbell alternating curls
8. Dumbbell standing triceps extensions

CrossFit METCON

Rather than limit the CrossFit METCON selection, I would rather give time guides for each day.

Day 1

8 Minutes: Something on the order of X number of reps in 8 minutes or 9 minutes of 2:00 sprint/1:00 Rest

Day 2

10 Minutes: I like Helen on this day. You could do worse than Helen once a week to see how you are progressing or, more importantly, overextending and regressing.

Day 3

5 Minutes: Something on the order of how many dumbbell Get-ups can you perform on 5 minutes? Or a timed mile.

While this template is a bit more traditional I believe your grapplers will perform very well that first month in the wrestling room.

TWO ROADS DIVERGED: A LOOK AT THE CONVERSION FROM POWERLIFTING TO WEIGHTLIFTING
MATT FOREMAN

Powerlifters and Olympic Weightlifters love to engage in verbal brawls. These brawls are almost always centered on the question of "Who is really stronger…powerlifters or weightlifters?" No matter how many voices of reason attempt to intervene with the idea that the two sports are simply quite different and difficult to compare, most coaches and athletes in both sports will throw rational thinking out the window and dive into a conversation that closely resembles two cavemen clubbing each other in the head with dinosaur bones. These exchanges pop up in articles and internet message boards quite often. But despite the fact that these arguments are frequent, it is noticeably rare to see athletes from powerlifting or weightlifting actually attempt to cross the great divide and convert from one sport to the other. Most powerlifters never try weightlifting, and most weightlifters never try powerlifting.

However, there have been some amazing examples of crossover success. The two most popular case studies in this department, and the favorite arguments of the powerlifting faithful, are the accomplishments of Mark Henry and Shane Hamman. Both Mark and Shane were record-holders in powerlifting with some behemoth numbers to their credit. They both left their squat/bench/deadlift days behind and became Olympic Weightlifters, and they both won multiple national championships on the way to becoming Olympians. So, does this mean that every strength athlete who attempts to convert to a different sport will have the same success as Mark and Shane? The answer is clearly "NO" because not every athlete has it in their destiny to make an Olympic Team. But the question remains, "If lifters decide to convert from one sport to another, can they expect to have success?" The answer is a complicated one with several variables to consider. This article will examine my own personal experience in this area along with some analysis of the basic challenges associated with jumping the strength sport fence. The Reasons for Converting.

Why would an athlete want to walk away from a sport they have trained seriously and competed in, especially if the athlete is talented and has tasted success? Furthermore, why would an athlete leave a familiar sport to move into a new area where he/she has to go back to being a newbie and start from the bottom again? Each individual has their own reasons and they are all unique, but my personal journey from powerlifting to weightlifting began with some internal conflicts about what I wanted to accomplish as an athlete. First, a little background information is needed. I began competing in powerlifting when I was fifteen years old and, fortunately, I experienced quick success. Less than a year after my first competition, I won the high school national championship and broke several state records in my age division. I continued competing and training for two years and I was able to make significant progress with no real coaching or training partners. However, there were certain elements of powerlifting that I could not get comfortable with. These issues become the foundation for my move to Olympic Weightlifting.

First, I was bothered by the supportive gear used in powerlifting. I competed in the late 1980s, long before the use of support gear was the complex science it has become today. But even back in those days, lifters were using squat suits and bench shirts to add huge numbers to their competition lifts. I used this gear myself. And even though I wore my suits/shirt loosely, I still knew that there was absolutely no way that I would be able to squat or bench the same weights if I was wearing shorts and a t-shirt. For whatever reason, this bothered me extensively and I considered it a shot to my pride. The second major issue in powerlifting that I could not swallow was the existence of multiple federations in the sport that all conducted their own state, national, and world championships. In my opinion, this situation cheapened the title of "National Champion" or "World Champion." If there were six or seven other lifters in my weight class who had also won national championships in different federations, how could any of us legitimately state that we were the best in the United States? At one point, my deadlift was an official national record in my age division and bodyweight class. But I knew that there were other federations where athletes of my same age and weight had deadlifted more than me, so the record was a hollow one. All of these factors might not have been bothersome to most athletes, but they certainly did not sit well with me.

However, I gradually began learning and reading more about the sport of Olympic Weightlifting during my powerlifting years. All of the problems of supportive gear and multiple federations did not exist in weightlifting. There was one state champion, one national champion, one world champion, and these champions won their titles with their muscles and talent instead of using the newest triple-ply bench shirt that added thirty extra pounds to their competition total. In my perspective, the sport was a much more pure test of skill and a much more definitive test of who the best lifters really were. And as an additional piece of bait, the chance to compete in the Olympics someday was a magical thought. The Olympic Games are the most sacred sports event in the history of the planet, and powerlifting is not a part of it.

Therefore, the allure was there. The excitement and interest in trying to conquer a new area was in place. Still, the obvious question remained, "What does it take to convert from powerlifting to weightlifting?"

Mental and Physical Obstacles

When I decided to try Olympic Weightlifting, it almost seemed like it was going to be too easy. This idea started when I picked up a copy of IronMan Magazine in 1988 and read an article about how a weightlifter named Dean Goad had recently done a 365 pound clean and jerk in the 165 pound class, and that lift was a new junior national record. "365 pounds?" I thought. "I can deadlift over 500. I know it's tougher to put the bar over your head, like in the clean and jerk. But I'll bet I can do 365 because deadlifting 500 is easy!"

It is not difficult to see where this story is leading. The first time I attempted to do an Olympic Lift, it was all very simple. I went to the gym, put 135 pounds on the bar, tried to clean it, and fell over backwards with the bar landing on my femur. All of a sudden, that old bench shirt seemed very, very comfortable.

There are several obstacles involved in transitioning over from powerlifting to Olympic Lifting. One of the biggest and most important obstacles is simply finding a coach. Because of the relative simplicity of the powerlifting movements, I had been able to make fast progress in the sport without having a coach's eyes on me. Many successful powerlifters do not even use coaches. Weightlifting, on the other hand, is extremely complex and incredibly difficult to learn if there is no coach present to teach the basics of the snatch and clean and jerk. And even if a powerlifter is able to find a good coach to teach the Olympic movements, the mental battle is a fierce one. Going from being an athlete who can easily hit a 500 pound squat to being an athlete who is getting owned by a 150 pound snatch is humbling, to say the least. If the athlete is hungry and competitive, as most strength athletes are, the process can be maddening. The athlete has to have patience to learn the Olympic lifts. If the athlete has no patience, it will be force-fed during the learning process.

And then, if the athlete is persistent enough to find a competent coach, the physical challenges begin to surface. For most former powerlifters, flexibility is a problem. The usual culprit areas are the wrists, elbows, shoulders, hip flexors, and ankles. Because of the relatively short range of motion in the power lifts, the muscles and connective tissue often develop in a way that creates stiffness and, in some cases, prohibitive or "muscle-bound" lack of flexibility. The longer the athlete has spent intensely training the bench press and powerlifting-style squats, the more limited the flexibility is likely to be. I had two factors that benefited me when I converted: a) I was only 18 and had not lost my ankle flexibility yet and b) I was not heavily muscled in the upper body. This second factor worked against me as a powerlifter because I was a weak bench presser. But in weightlifting, it was a positive attribute because I had solid lock-out in the elbows and I was able to fix the bar comfortably over my ears when performing snatches or jerks. Any powerlifter who has a severe lack of flexibility prior to beginning weightlifting training will have to begin with an extensive stretching program. All of the stretching that is performed in this program should be directed towards attaining the positions of the snatch and clean and jerk. Generally speaking, pre-workout stretching should be more ballistic and post-workout stretching should be more static. The positives and negatives of both types of stretching are outlined in Greg Everett's *Olympic Weightlifting: A Complete Guide for Athletes & Coaches*. It is worth mentioning that I did a large amount of intense pre-workout static stretching in my early career, and I suffered frequent muscle pulls and partial tears during training. These injuries became much less frequent when I abandoned pre-workout static stretching and moved to more ballistic, movement-centered stretching.

Interestingly, the conversion process from powerlifting to weightlifting is when it becomes obvious that there are different types of strength involved in both sports. Here is an example. When I was a powerlifter, my strongest lift was the deadlift. It is clear that the pulling movement of the deadlift relies heavily on the back muscles. Because of this, I concluded that I had a strong back. However, when I began training the Olympic lifts, I had an extremely difficult time keeping my back flat and tight. Heavy cleans and front squats would put me in the "turtle-back" position where the spine is rounded and the elbows are collapsing forward. It made no sense to me because the turtle-back problem indicated that I had a lack of back strength, along with a weak overall core. How could I have a lack of back strength if I had an outstanding deadlift?

The answer is that a strong back in powerlifting does not necessarily guarantee proper positions in the Olympic lifts. The muscles of the spinal erectors, trapezius, latissimus, and infraspinatus have to be developed in a very particular way to keep the strict, flat-back position necessary for the Olympic lifts. These muscles are not going to be developed in the correct manner if they have been trained to haul up maximum deadlifts in a grinding, rounded-back fashion. The only way the transition can be made is through extended training where the athlete pays constant attention to detail and physically forces him/herself to maintain a flat back posture. After hundreds and hundreds of reps with light weights where the muscles are required to contract in a way that keeps the back as flat as a board, the athlete will eventually be able to maintain proper positions.

The Process of Training and Competing

To make the transition even more complicated, the issue of developing an effective training program must be tackled. It is worth mentioning that this was a much bigger problem around 1990 than it is now because of the internet. These days, a new lifter can Google "Olympic Weightlifting" and come up with a variety of sample training programs and message boards where there will be mountains of information. Twenty years ago, it was much more difficult. I can recall having to mail (no, not e-mail…MAIL) coaches around the state and ask for help with training programs.

Fortunately, there were a few good coaches who were willing to show me the bare bones of a training program involving sets and reps, pulling exercises, volume/intensity in the squats, etc. The routine I used in the early days was not terribly complex:

MONDAY	TUESDAY	WEDNESDAY	THURSDAY	FRIDAY
SNATCH	RACK JERKS	CLEANS	SNATCH	CLEAN AND JERK
CLEAN PULLS	POWER CLEANS	SNATCH PULLS	CLEAN PULLS	SNATCH PULLS
STOP SQUATS	PRESSING		FRONT SQUATS	BACK SQUATS
ABS	ABS	ABS	ABS	ABS

This was the general outline I used. I almost always did doubles and singles in the competition lifts and triples in the pulls/squats. However, the weights I used on a daily basis were problematic because my approach was very simple; I went as heavy as I possibly could in every exercise every day, often not stopping until I had missed several attempts or had a mental meltdown, or both. I still had no coach to work with me for the first two years and the idea of using light weights to improve my technique seemed morally wrong (remember, I was eighteen years old and on my own). Needless to say, minor injuries and failed attempts quickly became a consistent part of my training. It would have been extremely helpful to hold back on the weights in the early days and focus entirely on positions as opposed to poundage. Looking back now, I should have spent a great deal of time practicing snatches and clean and jerks with an empty bar or PVC pipe in the beginning.

Also, one of the notable problems from those days is that I spent a lot of time working on power snatches and power cleans instead of forcing myself to perform the full movements. I believed that power snatches and cleans would make me better at finishing the pull. And, of course, I was much more likely to miss a lift if I tried to perform the full version because of my inexperience and rough technique in the bottom position. As with many beginners, I could power snatch more than I could full snatch. With these two considerations, I probably performed 70-80% of all my training lifts as power movements. The obvious result is that I was very good at power snatches and power cleans, but I had shown little improvement in the full lifts. My idea that performing power movements would make me better at finishing the pull was partially correct, I believe. But the pull is obviously only part of the movement. The receiving position of a full lift has to be trained and memorized by the motor system as precisely as the pull does.

However, even with all these early mistakes, there are still a few positive ideas from the transition process that I would recommend to potential converts. One of these ideas is jump training. I did quite a bit of plyometric work during my first two years of training the Olympic lifts because all of the literature I read indicated that Olympic Weightlifters had tremendous jumping ability. I would usually finish each workout with a few sets of box jumps and depth jumps to improve explosiveness. As with anything else, it is entirely possible to do too much jump training and I definitely did too much. Patellar tendonitis was not far behind. However, the basic idea of using jump training in the early part of an Olympic lifting program is essential, especially if the athlete has a prior background in a sport that emphasizes slow movements like powerlifting. It simply has to be incorporated into the training program with some planning and common sense.

In addition to all of these training considerations, the questions of competition should be addressed. When is an athlete ready to compete, and how frequently should he/she compete in the early stages of training? Different coaches will obviously have different philosophies on this. My personal idea is that athletes should begin competing as soon as they have a strong command of the movements. When they can perform snatches and clean and jerks with a solid level of technical proficiency, let them enter meets and compete. However, beginners should have their attempts chosen very carefully. The competition goals of beginners should be A) go six-for-six and B) set new personal records. Winning trophies and medals should be emphasized less than personal performance, because most newcomers will likely be beaten by more experienced lifters in their early meets. Additionally, it is the coach's job to instruct the athlete on how to compete. No athlete should shy away from tough competition. If a rookie enters a first meet and happens to be competing against an experienced national level lifter, the rookie will be demoralized if the coach has emphasized winning as the primary goal. At my first competition, I competed against a national champion who beat me by 115 kilos. Instead of being discouraged, I was inspired by the huge weights I had seen this athlete lift. I walked away from the meet saying to myself, "I want to be as good as that guy some day." Newbies should be energized by seeing incredible performances, and it is the coach's job to teach that idea. I also believe that newcomers should compete frequently. It is essential that the athlete gains experience and develops a sense of being in control on the competition platform. This will happen if the athlete gets a lot of "platform time" and completes a lot of successful lifts.

Overall Perspective

After the swelling has been iced and the chalk has settled, the question remains; "If lifters decide to convert from one sport to another, can they expect to have success?" The answer is that it all depends on the athlete. As mentioned, there are a variety of physical variables that have to be examined such as flexibility, elbow lockout, coordination, agility, and others. Long-term powerlifting training can certainly put the athlete behind the eight ball when it comes time to convert to Olympic Weightlifting because these physical variables are developed so much differently than they need to be for Olympic success. Physically, there are some athletes that are clearly "naturals." Mark Henry snatched 150 kilos in the first weightlifting meet he competed in. That is a fairly strong indicator of physical potential.

However, as any weightlifter can tell you, having the body is only half the battle.

You also have to have the brain. After twenty years of competing, training, and coaching, I now subscribe to the idea that there are two types of talent: physical and mental. And no athlete can be successful without a long supply of both. Weightlifting will not forgive laziness or lack of discipline. Unfortunately, it will also not forgive a lack of athletic ability. The sport will strenuously test every physical and personality trait you possess. It is the individual journey of the athlete to make a complete commitment, press the gas pedal to the floor, and see how far the journey goes.

MY PREPARATION FOR THE CROSSFIT GAMES
JOSH EVERETT

Over the last few months since my second place finish at the 2008 CrossFit Games, I've been repeatedly asked how I trained for the Games—I get asked in person quite often whenever I'm at CrossFit-related events, and I receive regular emails about the subject as well. I guess people are really interested because I'm the only person, male or female, who has finished in the top three both years. I'm very proud of that accomplishment and very flattered that people are interested in what I'm doing. However, the short answer to the question is that I didn't train for the CrossFit Games… And the long answer isn't as nearly complicated or as interesting as most people are hoping for when they ask.

I'm actually having trouble getting started on this article because I'm about to take something simple—this article was originally a two-sentence email—and make it much more complicated than it actually is. Genius is found when people take the complicated and turn it into something simple and understandable… those who know me well no I'm no genius, so I guess I should be OK with what I'm about to embark on.

My training schedule:

Monday
Agility work for about 15 minutes followed by 1 sprint at each distance: 50 m, 100 m, 200 m, 300 m

Tuesday
Olympic lifting workout & squats for about 45 minutes followed by a 2-5 minute weightroom based met-con

Wednesday
Sprints: generally 10 x 40 yds or a hill about 30-40 yds—sprint up and walk down for 20 minutes

Thursday
Olympic lifting & squats for 45 minutes, followed by a 7-15 minute running-based met-con (think Helen-ish)

Friday
Off

Saturday
Olympic lifting workout followed by usually 1 x 40 chins

Sunday
Off

Why do I train like this? Because I enjoy it. I love the feeling of sprinting and what it does for my body. I enjoy being able to throw up heavy O-lifts. I could have skipped Mondays and Wednesdays all together and done just as well at the CrossFit Games. This is my workout regiment because it's the most volume I can handle at this age. If I could, I'd train 6 days a week, 2 hours a day like I did all through my late teens and twenties. I would train like this not because it would better prepare me for the games or give me better fitness, but because I love the O-lifts, kettlebells, the patch, strongman training, track workouts, etc., but I can't do it all anymore. I follow this regimen for three weeks then take a complete week off—three weeks on and one week off per month.

I make no claims that this is a superior training program to any other in developing fitness. This program allows me to practice my first and second modality loves (Olympic weightlifting & sprinting) at a high level (for me) while maintaining a reasonable amount of fitness (as defined by CrossFit). If your goal is fitness or your goal is to place as high as you can in the CrossFit Games, it's my opinion that you should be following the WOD on Crossfit.com. Those aren't my goals, so I don't.

The reason why this program works for me (work as in I can also be a top CrossFitter) is the past 20 years of my training. I started running competitive track at age 10... I began squatting in the gym at age 14... Ethan Reeve taught me how to O-lift at age 22, I've been training under Mike Burgener since age 24... proficiency of those elements combined with a certain mentality equate to a high level of fitness.

Before Mike Burgener introduced me to CrossFit my training looked like this. What allows me to not follow Crossfit.com and still compete with Khalipa, OPT, Speal, etc., is the fact that I've been practicing real fitness for almost 20 years with a level of dedication that, for the most part, only CrossFitters understand. I've been able to squat 400+ pounds and run a mile in under 5:30 for the last 15 years of my life with the only exceptions being a few months following surgeries from playing football. That type of rock solid fitness foundation and consistency allows me just to touch on certain aspects of my fitness and still maintain a fairly high level with them.

People also ask me about my diet as well since they have heard I don't follow the Zone. I'm not even going to go there because my diet is not designed to optimize health or performance. I eat healthier than 99% of the American public, but that's like saying I'm the smartest kid on the short bus. I choose a diet that I enjoy and that does not hinder my health/fitness… I'm a few small steps away from a diet that would optimize performance. If I were serious about my nutrition, I'd do paleo-zone.

Seems like boring stuff to me, but I hope you find it interesting & helpful.

PULLING, PUSHING, AND THINKING: EXTENDED CONNECTIONS BETWEEN OLYMPIC WEIGHTLIFTING AND POWERLIFTING
MATT FOREMAN

My earliest workout routines are very clear in my memory. I started lifting weights at the high school weight room when I was thirteen with some of the kids I played football with. We developed our own training program, based on some advanced scientific principles and theories. Here is a rough skeleton of our normal training week:

MONDAY	BENCH PRESS	CURLS	WRESTLE
TUESDAY	BENCH PRESS	CURLS	GO HOME
WEDNESDAY	BENCH PRESS	CURLS	HIT EACH OTHER
THURSDAY	BENCH PRESS	CURLS	WRESTLE
FRIDAY	BENCH PRESS	CURLS	GO SHOPPING

For better or for worse, thousands of young athletes in this country become enthusiastic about weight training because they are obsessed with the bench press. If the athletes are young and have no guidance from any coaches (which we didn't), it is an easy trap to fall into. However, I was lucky enough to learn squatting and deadlifting shortly after I started working out. It didn't take long for these lifts to replace my obsession with bench pressing. I did not learn the Olympic Lifts until the summer after my high school graduation.

This article will revisit the subject of connecting the power lifts (squat, bench press, deadlift) with the Olympic lifts (snatch, clean and jerk). There are millions of athletes who use a combination of these two disciplines to gain strength and overall athleticism. Likewise, there are millions of athletes who completely specialize in powerlifting or Olympic Weightlifting for competitive purposes. Converting from one sport to another has already been examined in a previous Performance Menu issue. However, there are many other nuggets of information lying in the dirt. My own personal experience and the experiences of other athletes will dust these nuggets off and give us a better look at them.

Pull for Your Freedom!

One of the simplest commonalities between Olympic lifting and powerlifting is the pull from the floor. The technique used in deadlifting and cleaning/snatching has several similarities and, admittedly, several differences. However, every athlete wants to improve his or her pulling strength regardless of the particular movement. Here is where we find an interesting truth: training the pull as an Olympic lifter can dramatically improve the powerlifting deadlift.

There are two personal examples that will better illustrate this idea. When I was seventeen, I had trained the deadlift specifically for four years. I had never done any Olympic movements. At this time, my best deadlift was an absolute gut-busting 535 pounds. Then, after I graduated high school, a coach taught me the Olympic lifts and how to train as a full-time Olympic lifter. I was hooked, so I completely abandoned powerlifting and concentrated on Olympic lifting. My training program was very basic. I practiced the competition lifts every day, did front/back squats, and did clean/snatch pulls three times every week. The heaviest pulling I ever did was around 150 kilos (330 pounds) in the clean pulls and 120 kilos (264 pounds) in the snatch pulls. And these weights were the absolute heaviest I would ever pull; my pulling weights were often lighter than these. My top squat workout weights during this time were usually around 400-420 pounds.

I had trained this way for ten months. I had not done a single deadlift during this time. Then one day I decided to do some deadlifts, just for the hell of it. I deadlifted 555 pounds easily that day, which was a 20 pound improvement over my old personal best from when I was focusing on the deadlift. I simply could not believe that my pulling strength had increased so much because I had not been pulling heavy weights for almost a full year. However, that was not the only time I saw this happen in my career.

After the day when I deadlifted 555 pounds, I went back to full-time Olympic lifting and did not deadlift again for ten years. During this decade, my Olympic lifting career moved forward steadily as I fought to climb up in the national rankings. I eventually achieved a 155 kilo snatch and a 185 kilo clean and jerk. My top back squat during this time was 245 kilos (540 pounds), and I continued to utilize clean/snatch pulls three times per week in training. The heaviest weights I ever used in the clean pulls were around 205 kilos (451 pounds) and around 165 kilos (363 pounds) in the snatch pulls. And again, my weights in these exercises were usually lighter than the ones I just mentioned. Then, just as I had done ten years earlier, I decided to pull a few deadlifts one day. I deadlifted 617 pounds that day (285 kilos), and then tried it again three weeks later and pulled 650 pounds (295 kilos). This was almost a one hundred pound increase over my previous best of 555 pounds.

Now, a one hundred pound increase in the deadlift over a span of ten years is not amazing. That increase is only an average of ten pounds improvement per year. But the interesting point is that I had not pulled anything, in any manner, over 450 pounds during that time. Added to that, I had only squatted with weights around 530-540 pounds at the most. All of a sudden, a 650 pound pull was possible. Therefore, the question that arises is, "How can an athlete develop the strength to pull heavy weights without pulling heavy weights in training?" The answer, although complex, mainly lies in repetition. Most powerlifters deadlift once a week, with some additional auxiliary pulling exercises possibly thrown in after the deadlifts are finished. However, Olympic lifters perform a pulling movement every time they snatch, clean, RDL, snatch pull, or clean pull. Knowing that a typical Olympic lifter's training program will include several of these exercises on a daily basis, the Olympic lifter simply does many more reps of some sort of pulling exercises than the powerlifter does. Even if the Olympic lifter does not pull maximum deadlift weights every week, the pulling muscles are still being strengthened through a daily, weekly, and yearly accumulation of thousands of repetitions. This accumulated strengthening effect is what makes improved deadlift maxes possible without specializing in the deadlift.

How much ya bench?

From examining the pulling connections between power and Olympic lifting, we can move to a look at upper body strength and the bench press. And the first point that must be understood is that many successful Olympic lifters have included bench presses in their training, contrary to the usual Olympic mentality that bench pressing is a tool of Satan. IronMind training videos are available and ready for purchase that clearly show lifters like Simon Kolecki and Evgeny Chigishev bench pressing around 200 kilos. Former Canadian champion Mark Cardinal once told a story where he missed some snatch attempts at a major international competition in the 1970s, after which David Rigert told him that his upper body was not strong enough to hold the weights he was capable of pulling and that he needed to start bench pressing in training. Former Soviet world champion Gennady Ivanchenko has reported that he benched throughout his career, and the physiques of most of the great Soviet lifters of the 60s, 70s, and 80s include impressive pectoral development. My personal coach, John Thrush, benched throughout his entire Olympic lifting career and was able to clean and jerk a collegiate national record of 187.5 kilos in the 110 kilo class in 1977 while also bench pressing 480 pounds. Now, it is obviously true that many of the world's top Olympic lifters do absolutely no bench pressing at all. Nicu Vlad personally told me that he never did them. But the point here is that bench pressing is a tool of many great Olympic champions and it can be incorporated into an Olympic lifter's program with success.

Still, there is a caveat to this point. It has also become clear that bench pressing and other power/bodybuilding exercises have the potential to negatively affect upper body flexibility. If bench presses are performed with partial lockouts, as many powerlifters do in training, the range of flexibility in the shoulder and bicep tendons will shorten and overhead lockout can suffer. I once trained a young lifter who competed in both powerlifting and Olympic lifting. With a 140 kilo clean and jerk in the 94 kilo class at eighteen years old, this athlete had obvious potential. However, he was a fanatic about the bench press and trained it much as a bodybuilder would: partial lockouts in the bench and auxiliary exercises that added tremendous upper body mass. He did go on to win a junior national championship in powerlifting, but subsequent attempts to regain his Olympic lifting skill were unsuccessful because he had simply lost his elbow lockout in the snatch and jerk. If bench pressing is going to be incorporated into an Olympic lifter's program, it must be done in a way that does not inhibit flexibility. Full elbow lockouts in the bench and additional stretching exercises for the upper body would be useful suggestions.

Interestingly, I have also seen examples where Olympic lifting training has improved benching ability. In 1995, I trained regularly with a world powerlifting champion who was interested in Olympic lifting training just for a little variety. This athlete competed in the 165 pound class and had a top official bench press of 425 pounds, a weight he had been stuck at for three years. He dove into Olympic lifting full tilt boogie and stayed with it for around six months, dropping the bench press during this time. A few weeks after he decided to resume his powerlifting training, he informed me that he had bench pressed an easy 450 pounds. He told me that he could feel an obvious strength increase in his triceps and deltoids, which he attributed to the jerks and push presses he had used during his Olympic lifting time.

One other important consideration is that Olympic lifters who decide to begin bench pressing should be very careful with their pectoral tendons. Here is a personal example: I stopped bench pressing for almost eleven years, from the time I graduated high school until around 2001. I did absolutely no benching in this time. When I decided to try bench pressing again, my overall upper body strength was significantly higher. I had only bench pressed around 280 pounds in high school and by the time I decided to try them again in 2001, I had jerked 424 pounds and push pressed 319. When I resumed bench pressing, I started performing sets of five reps at around 250 pounds, which did not feel heavy at all. However, I had a string of small injuries in my pectoral tendons, mostly strains and a few partial tears. These injuries all occurred in exactly the same area, near the shoulder where the pectoral tendon connects with the humerus. They usually took around three weeks to heal with icing and no benching at all. I used bench presses in my training for around two years and I probably had five or six of these injuries. That specific part of my upper body was simply not well developed. Eventually, through gradual progressive resistance, the strength of my connective tissue caught up with the strength of my upper body muscles, the tendon injuries stopped, and I was able to bench press a mediocre 391 pounds. Did this benching improve my Olympic lifting? I would say that I noticed an increased "snappy" feeling in the lockout of my jerks. The weights felt much easier to stabilize and control when they reached arms length; I was also able to push jerk 180 kilos, which I had never done before.

Squatting? Not this time, folks...

The connections and differences between powerlifting squats and Olympic-style squats will not be discussed in this article because this subject is big enough for an article of its own. Suffice to say that a powerlifter's squats and an Olympic lifter's squats are apples and oranges in most cases. Attempting to completely analyze this area, along with the ensuing conversation/bloodbath over whether Olympic lifters or powerlifters are stronger squatters, is like watching Chris Farley doing his Chippendale's dance on Saturday Night Live, with his fat rolls flapping everywhere. In other words, it can get ugly...

The great Tommy Kono once said, "If you want to be a better presser, then press." This simple statement boils down a great deal of strength training conversation to a basic truth; the best way to improve at a particular skill is to practice that skill. However, it must also be acknowledged that there are many creative variations that can enhance the performance of that skill. Vasily Alexeev used to perform clean and jerks while standing up to his chest in a river. What is the bottom line? Simplicity and specificity are golden rules, but innovative thinking also has a place in the training of the athlete. So before you run out and buy that "I'm an Olympic Weightlifter, so I don't bench press" t-shirt, remember that David Rigert said it was okay to bench press, and he was better than you. Many ways to skin a cat...

LESSONS FROM ROMANIA
MATT FOREMAN

Nicu Vlad is one of the greatest weightlifters of all time. The Romanian legend won the Olympic gold medal at the 1984 Los Angeles games when he was only twenty-one years old, and that was only the beginning of his amazing career. Vlad went on to win the silver medal at the 1988 Olympics, the bronze at the 1996 Olympics (when he was thirty-three), and three world championships in 1984, 1986, and 1990. However, the accomplishment that Vlad is probably most famous for is his all-time world record snatch of 200.5 kilos in the old 100 kilo bodyweight class. He is the heaviest lifter in history to snatch double bodyweight, and many weightlifting experts believe that Vlad is one of the most technically perfect weightlifters of all time. His snatch technique has been the learning model for thousands of young weightlifters over the last two decades. So you can imagine how I felt when I found out that I was going to have the opportunity to train with Vlad for three weeks at the Olympic Training Center in Colorado Springs during the summer of 1990.

Nicu and his coach, Dragomir Cioroslan, came to the United States in 1990 to spend the summer training at various locations around the country. They spent most of this visit in Colorado Springs, and the national junior squad training camp was held at the OTC during the same time. I was invited to train at this camp, which meant that I was going to be working out in the same gym with an athlete whose pictures I had taped up on the walls of the gym where I worked out at home. I was seventeen years old and Nicu Vlad had been my weightlifting idol long before I knew he was coming to the United States. This was literally the opportunity of a lifetime, and this article will examine just a fraction of the many lessons I learned during that memorable summer.

First, the formal details of training…

I recall meeting Dragomir and Nicu for the first time. Dragomir, who was one of the friendliest people I had ever met in my life, smiled broadly and shook my hand with gusto as he looked me in the eye and exclaimed, "My name is Dragomir, how are you?!" After that, I was introduced to the big man, who shook my hand with his thick paw and growled, "Nicu Vlad," as he glanced at me with the same interest he probably showed in his morning bowel movement. Nicu was polite and respectful, but he had a quiet intensity in his personality that was obvious. This man was a legend, and everybody knew it. You gave him a wide berth.

Nicu usually trained twice a day, and his workouts were broken up into short segments. He generally performed the classic lifts along with front squats, back squats, and RDLs (more on that later). I never saw him spend any time doing supplemental exercises such as push presses, overhead squats, etc. He often performed his squats in the mornings and his competition lifts in the afternoons. In a typical afternoon session, he would train one of the competition lifts (snatch or clean and jerk) for around thirty minutes and then go outside the gym to lie down in the grass and relax for a while. After twenty or thirty minutes, he would come back in the gym to train again, often hitting the other competition lift. After this second session, he would sometimes go back outside to take another relaxation break before the next segment or sometimes he would go straight into a squatting or pulling movement, depending on which lifts he had trained that morning. Basically, Dragomir had him on a European-style program that combined many of the Russian and Bulgarian principles that we have all studied over the years. He was training around seven to nine times per week, with the morning sessions usually taking place around ten o'clock and the afternoon sessions around three or four. It's important to note that Nicu was twenty-seven years old during this time, which is generally considered a little old for most hardcore European training systems. I believe his volume and exercise selection had been narrowed to accommodate his age.

Nicu was training to compete at the 1990 Goodwill Games in Washington at the end of the summer, so I was able to see him train when he was around six weeks out from a meet. The top lifts I saw him perform in training during this time are as follows: 185 snatch, 210 clean and jerk (he clean and jerked 210, brought the weight down to his shoulders, and jerked it a second time). Nicu's all-time best official lifts are 200.5 in the snatch and 237.5 in the clean and jerk. But those lifts had been done in 1986; during the 1990 time period when I saw him, he was usually hitting around 190/220 in meets. Therefore, 185 and 210 were working pretty close to his top results at the time. In the supplemental lifts, I saw multiple sets of three in the back squats with 250-260, and RDL sets of three usually performed with 250-260. The squats and RDLs with 260 were, as far as the eye could tell, practically effortless. He did not squat with any of the massive weights that many Americans think the top European lifters handle on a daily basis. Also, the jerk was his weak spot and, because of this, he almost always lowered the weight to his shoulders and performed two reps of the jerk for every clean.

But despite the amazing work capacity and kilograms Nicu was capable of handling, the most phenomenal aspect of his training was definitely his technique. When

I first became an Olympic weightlifter, a great coach told me that one of the elements of having perfect technique meant you could "make 50 kilos look exactly the same as 150 kilos." Vlad was the best example of this rule that I have ever seen in my career. Every movement of his body from his back position to his foot placement to his acceleration in the second pull was identical, regardless of the weight on the bar. When he performed snatches and cleans, he would usually power snatch or power clean the light weights, catching them in a high receiving position. And, as the weight got progressively heavier, he would simply catch the bar gradually lower and lower until he was hitting his top weights and catching them near rock-bottom. Nicu jumped his feet forcefully off the platform when he was extending the second pull and going under the bar, producing a loud slap! when his feet hit the platform as he turned his wrists over and caught the weight. Not every great lifter has utilized the same "feet jumping" technique as Vlad, obviously. There are some great lifters who simply lift their feet just high enough to slide them out and re-position them as they receive the bar. But Vlad's technique involved violent jumping of the feet and many lifters, including myself, formed their own technique from emulating him. Everything about his movements was a textbook combination of speed, tightness, precision, and strength. Any weightlifter who wants to be successful would be wise to study the technique of Nicu Vlad, as we all did during our summer of watching him train.

A quick 185 snatch, then some RDLs...

One afternoon, many of the junior squad lifters were in the OTC game room playing pool and PacMan when Wes Barnett stuck his head in the door and told everybody, "Vlad's going heavy in his workout." We all ran out of the game room, across the hockey field, and down the hill to the gym so we could see some big weights. Nicu was warming up in the snatch at the time, and we all quietly took seats around the gym to watch the big show. After his normal warm up, snatching 70, 90, 110, 130, 140, 150, and 160 with ease, he put 170 on the bar. We were all shocked to see him miss the 170, but then he repeated the weight a few minutes later and made it easily. He jumped to 175 and missed the weight behind him twice, and then jumped to 180 and missed that weight twice as well. Most of us were wondering what in the hell was going on, as he was clearly in good shape and strong enough to make these weights. I will never forget what he did next.

He loaded 185 on the bar. This time, as he stood in front of the bar preparing for the lift, he stood motionless, tilted his head back and closed his eyes in the famous Vlad-concentration pose we had all seen him strike on the platform at the Olympics and world championships. He had not done this before any of the other lifts of his workout, and the gym went completely silent. After ten seconds, he reached down, grabbed the bar, and nailed the easiest, strongest snatch of the day.

I learned a lot about mental discipline as I watched this workout. After his missed snatch attempts, Nicu had no reaction whatsoever. He did not get visibly upset or discouraged in any way. His face remained stoic and he simply progressed to the next weight, confident that he would make any technical corrections that were needed. When he got to 185, which I later learned was the weight he had planned to hit that day, he just applied an extra level of concentration and focus. It was a big weight, he was having a bad workout, and he needed to tap into his extra reservoir of inner strength, mojo, or whatever you want to call it. Because he was a world champion, his mojo did not involve jumping around like a crackhead, punching himself in the face, or kicking the bar. His fire burned inside, and it burned hot. And after he made the 185, he simply went on with the rest of his workout. No celebration, actions of deep relief, or pissing and moaning because he hadn't had a perfect workout. It was all just a day at the office for Nicu Vlad.

Then he started performing an exercise we saw him do regularly. It looked a lot like a stiff-legged deadlift, only he bent his knees slightly and displaced his hips backwards as he lowered the bar. He would regularly do this exercise with 250 kilos or more, and he even did a personal record set of 300x3 at the end of the camp. Somebody in the gym asked Nicu and Dragomir what the exercise was called. They said that they did not have a special name for it, and so one of the American lifters suggested that it could be called a "Romanian Deadlift" or RDL. Now, here we are eighteen years later, and this exercise has become a common staple in workout routines all across this country. I've always considered it a privilege that I was present when the RDL was officially named.

The Nicu Vlad Charm School...

Vlad had a fairly quiet, reserved personality, probably due mostly to the fact that his English at the time was relatively limited. With the English that he was able to speak, he was always happy to engage in conversation and joke around. I recall one night in the OTC dorm when a tall swimmer was walking down the hall and accidentally bumped into Nicu, knocking him back a step. The swimmer apparently thought he was a tough guy, because he just glanced around and kept walking without excusing himself. Wes Barnett jokingly told Nicu to go give the guy a beating. Nicu looked at Wes and shook his head saying, "What?" because he didn't understand. Wes pointed at the swimmer and punched his fist into his palm five or six times. Nicu understood, but he stopped Wes and said, "No." Then he punched his own fist into his palm one time, looked at Wes and said, "Just one." He was telling us that he could knock the guy out with one shot!

Nicu also gave out a piece of advice that I now realize is probably the greatest lesson I've ever learned in weightlifting and life in general. This particular junior squad camp had several young athletes who would later go on to become great American lifters in the 1990s. Names like Barnett, Gough, McRae, Patao, and my dorm roommate Pete

Kelley were all there. These individuals were hard working, driven, competitive animals who were hungry to move up in the national rankings. However, there were also several young athletes who had made the junior squad and earned their way to the camp, but showed some of the worst attitudes I have seen in my years as an athlete. These were spoiled brats who whined constantly about the gym being too small, the bars not spinning well enough, the dorms being too hot, the taste of the dining hall food, and every other free benefit that had been given to them. They did not train hard, complained incessantly, back-talked the coaches and OTC staff, and threw temper tantrums in the gym when they missed lifts. Not surprisingly, almost all of them quit the sport within the next few years.

Nicu and Dragomir used to watch these kids silently and shake their heads in disgust. It was obvious what they were thinking. Then, USA Weightlifting magazine decided to do an interview with Vlad, so Dragomir acted as his interpreter to answer their questions. At one point, the reporter asked Nicu what he thought about training with our top young junior lifters. Although I'm not quoting him word-for-word, I remember his answer clearly and it was this: "In Romania, I train on a bar that is bent. My gym has bad lighting and very little heat in the winters. Here in America, you have everything you need to train. It's not in the bar or the gym or the platform… it's in you."

The message, which I consider almost a biblical principle, is that the strength you possess in your heart will be the deciding element in your weightlifting career. Adversity is the name of the game in this sport, and the only factor that can propel an athlete to success is sheer force of will. Physical talent is not enough. There are armies of physically talented athletes out there. The ones like Nicu Vlad, who refuse to allow anything to defeat them, will be the last ones standing. This attitude drove Nicu forward to victory at the World Championship that same year, and then eventually to the 1996 Olympics in Atlanta, where, at the age of thirty-three, he snatched 197.5 in the 108 class, winning the third Olympic medal of his illustrious career.

I could write an entire book about all the other things I saw, heard, and learned during those weeks. Vlad told us that Yuri Zacharevich from the Soviet Union had rack jerked 300 kilos in training. Vlad told us that Naim Suleymanoglu owned eight houses in Turkey. Vlad told us that we were all idiots for spending our recovery time having chicken fights in the OTC pool instead of resting for our next workout. During his trip, somebody printed up some "Nicu Vlad Summer US Tour 1990" tank tops and sold them. I bought one and wore it as religiously as the stoners at my high school wore their Megadeth t-shirts. It was an exciting summer that marked the beginning of some great US lifting careers. I was lucky to be there. We all were.

ARE YOU COACHABLE?
MICHAEL RUTHERFORD

Over the past three issues of the Performance Menu we have examined critical components to the advancement of an athlete's performance development. Step one is a belief in the benefit of the training process. The next step is to evaluate the current status of the athlete and determine the best path for development. This is traditionally accomplished by a battery of assessments and is followed up with a specific goal setting session. The coach and the athlete mutually agree upon the goals to be accomplished. Finally the tools for the job are important in the success. You can have great knowledge of what is to be accomplished but your outputs can stall or be muted with inappropriate program design and inadequate tools.

With the table set, so to speak, it's now time to go to work. The final question becomes, Is the athlete committed to the plan? In short, is the athlete coachable?

The coach is obviously invested at this point, but there is a large psychological, physical and financial investment required by the athlete. This final installment will focus on the athlete's coachability. This writing could easily fit next to step one. Collectively, the contract between parties could be cut off prior to participating in a lengthy evaluation process.

I am particularly passionate regarding this commitment component. I am (was) as an athlete blessed with few natural athletic gifts. Fortunately, I didn't realize it for much of my earlier years in athletics. I somehow out of fear of failure developed a lot of "want to". The minutia that went along with the journey thrilled me. I was determined to get as many of the details correct. In part, this is why I fly heels first into talented athletes/clients who fail to embrace the commitment to the course.

THE OTHER 163

I see the largest majority of athletes/clients only five hours per week. Some I see even less but never fewer than twice. So if at best I see some clients five hours that means that during the other one hundred and sixty-three hours they are solely responsible for execution of the other components of training.

The greatest coaching, elite programming, Eleiko barbells and plates cannot overcome sloppy training practices outside of the training hall. I constantly remind my clients of this fact. I ask for and demand accountability for these other 163 hours in the week.

For some situations there should be accountability checks. This is easily accomplished with the training journal. Certain on-line tools also exist for quick access to data. Athletes will respect what coaches inspect. How many athletes/clients have fallen short of their potential due to poor management of the other 163? I contend that more fail here than with the time in the training hall.

Toughness

Related to THE OTHER 163, is the athlete's mental toughness and tenacity. The word toughness gets tossed around all too often and is liberally applied to certain individuals and situations. Some people like to wear a tough exterior in hopes that everyone else will think of them as cool or tough. This is not tough in my view. Real toughness is not revealed by a tattoo or an exterior. Toughness is revealed by behaviors, choices and acts.

Toughness is choosing the more difficult or less popular path. Toughness is having demonstrated pigheaded determination and discipline even though your decision might not be popular or what the crowd is doing. Athletes demonstrate toughness by doing as their coach has specified. The committed athlete makes the correct choices when they are alone and nobody is there to witness the behavior, choice or act. Now who's really tough?

A Probationary Training Period

In my own practice, I employ a probationary period. There is no promise beyond three training sessions. At the conclusion of these three sessions we can decide if there is a good fit. Sometimes it's not going to be prudent to continue. I've fired myself more times than I care to count. I've trained my senses to sniff out potential problems. I would encourage all coaches to do the same. Your ability to maintain a portfolio of coachable athletes will make you a happier trainer. What will benefit you more? The coachable athlete/client who shares their success or the unaccountable career trend hopper who whines around the community?

While my trained intuition has rarely failed me, in certain cases I have asked the client to complete an inventory of questions. The motive is to help them determine if they are committed to the course of action. I cannot always drop the hammer I prefer mitigation. Coaches could consider such an inventory until they too have developed their intuition about a particular borderline client.

1. I am willing to make the coaching process an investment in myself. I view it as a long-term approach to creating changes in my life. I am not looking for a quick fix.
2. I am ready to do the work necessary to get me where I want to be, and I will let the coach do the coaching.
3. I am willing to change any self-defeating behaviors that are creating a barrier to my success.
4. I accept responsibility for my actions and will not expect the coach to "fix" me, because I know I'm the only one who can make it happen.
5. I have adequate funds to pay for coaching and will not regret the investment. I view coaching as a worthwhile investment in me, not an expense, and I will not allow finances to be a barrier to coaching.
6. I am willing and able to be completely truthful with my coach, and I'm ready to hear the truth from my coach even if it is uncomfortable at first.
7. Coaching is the appropriate process for the changes I want to make.
8. I am able to commit the time needed to make and keep scheduled coaching sessions and to do the fieldwork that my coach asks of me.
9. I'm open to trying new things when my coach asks me, even if they aren't completely comfortable or I'm not convinced they will make a difference.
10. This is the right time in my life for me to accept coaching.

Now score yourself: If you answered "no" to two or more questions, you will need to make some adjustments, either in your lifestyle or in your expectations of coaching, before coaching will be fully effective.

Having a coachable client makes the processes much easier for the coach and allows for the athlete to realize all of their training objectives.

THERE IS NO EVIL TWIN
MATT FOREMAN

Some people lift weights, and some people are weightlifters.

This is one of those "there are two types of people in this world" concepts. In the movie The Good, The Bad, and The Ugly, Clint Eastwood wanted a man to dig a hole for him. So he tossed the man a shovel, pointed a gun at him, and said, "There are two kinds of people in this world... those with loaded guns, and those who dig. You dig." Half of the high school graduation ceremonies in this country each year include some kind of keynote speaker who tries to motivate graduates by saying, "There are two kinds of people in this world... those who watch things happen, and those who make things happen." We love to break society down into categories, and Olympic Weightlifting is a terrific area to draw a big thick line that divides two simple groups: those who lift weights and those who are weightlifters.

Anybody who is a "weightlifter" already knows that they're a weightlifter. And they know the difference between themselves and people who "lift weights" as clearly as we all know the difference between a rattlesnake and a hummingbird. But people who "lift weights" might be a little fuzzy about the qualities that divide the two groups and, consequently, might be confused about which group they belong in. So we need some clarification about the difference between the two groups because it's important for everyone to go through life with a definite understanding of what they are and where they belong. After all, we don't want the Vienna Boys Choir walking into a bar where the Hells Angels drink, do we?

One of the best ways to analyze each animal is to start by observing its behavior. Therefore, here are some simple habits to watch for when you're trying to distinguish weightlifters from people who lift weights. And, of course, you can make up your mind which group you personally belong in after you understand their identifying qualities.

Interest in Weightlifting

People who lift weights think that weightlifting is a fascinating sport. They have seen weightlifting on the internet, read several articles about training and competition, and probably even decided to try it themselves. If they are lucky, these people happen to live in an area where there is a weightlifting gym that has bumper plates, platforms, and a coach who knows how to teach the lifts properly. Once they have given weightlifting a shot and learned a little about it, their enthusiasm grows and they probably start to study the technique of lifters like Pyrros Dimas and Hossein Rezazedeh. They get a kick out of weightlifting, and it becomes a real source of enthusiasm.

Weightlifters believe that weightlifting is the greatest sport in the world and will probably dismiss anyone who disagrees with them as being retarded. They have watched every weightlifting video available on the internet fifty times, the home page on their computer is a weightlifting website, and their screen saver is a picture of an athlete catching a snatch overhead. They probably own a library of DVDs and, if they are truly old-school, VHS tapes of every state, national, and world championship they have ever been able to get their hands on; and they can quote several lines from the Bulgarian documentary "School of Champions" whenever they want to. They have read so much literature on weightlifting that they probably even understand a few weightlifting-related words in Russian. They know how many times per week the Soviet lifters of the 70s and 80s used to train. They know the world records from before 1993 when the weight classes were changed. If they are lucky, these people happen to live in an area where there is a weightlifting gym that has bumper plates, platforms, and a coach who knows how to teach the lifts properly. But if they do not live in an area like this, they will quit their jobs, load all of their possessions in their car, and move to a town like St. Joseph, Missouri or Auburn, Washington where there is a gym with a group of weightlifters who are as committed to the sport as they are. They study the technique of lifters like Pyrros Dimas and Hossein Rezazedeh, David Rigert, Vasily Alexeev, Naim Suleymanoglu, Ronny Weller, Yuri Zacharevich, Rolf Milser, Norb Schemansky, Tommy Kono, and John Davis. They also name their pets after these lifters. Their enthusiasm for the sport becomes less of "enthusiasm" and more "life-consuming hunger." They cannot imagine their lives without weightlifting, nor would they want to.

Training

People who lift weights will set up a workout routine that incorporates the Olympic Lifts. They will put this routine down on paper and stick to it as closely as they can. They will find time in their weekly schedule when they can get to the gym and work out. Even during times when life is busy, they will make sure they get to the gym a couple of times every week. When they work out, they will concentrate on technique and try to perform the lifts as correctly as possible. They will also try to enhance their recovery from each workout through good nutrition, protein supplementation, and stretching. If they have time periods when their lifts are stagnant, they will understand that they have reached a plateau. When they reach plateaus, they will continue to work hard and remain confident that they will eventually start to make progress again.

Weightlifters will find a coach who knows more about weightlifting than they do and ask that coach to write them a workout program. The program exists for one reason: to snatch and clean and jerk bigger weights. They will put this routine down on paper, but they will rarely have to look at the paper because they have the whole program memorized. Their weekly schedule revolves around their workouts, not the other way around. Jobs, school, family, and relationships... these are things that are incorporated into training. If any of these things interfere with training, they have to be modified. If they cannot be modified, they have to be eliminated. It does not matter if life is busy, the car breaks down, finals week is coming up, or it's Christmas Day. Nothing interferes with training. When they work out, they will concentrate on technique and continue to perform the lifts until they are done correctly... no matter how long it takes. Recovery from each workout becomes their lifestyle. On the way home from the gym, they will stop by the gas station to buy a ninety-nine cent bag of ice. When they get home, they will turn on the TV and put the ice on whichever body part hurts the most that day. If they have time periods when their lifts are stagnant, they will refuse to accept it. They reject the very idea of plateaus and their whole attitude about life will start to turn sour until they find a way to start making progress again.

Job/School

People who lift weights will put their workouts as one of their top priorities in life. They will try to find ways to set up their jobs and school schedules to accommodate their workouts. If the gym they train at has business hours that are incompatible with their job hours, they will buy their own weights and build a platform in their garage. They will pre-plan their meals and food consumption for each workday. Often, they will have to bring individualized Tupperware bowls to work in a big cooler and then find time in their workdays to get their small meals of chicken breasts, tuna, and fruit. They will stay committed to their workouts, but they will also stay focused on their education and careers.

Weightlifters will view weightlifting as their occupation. And when people tell them that weightlifting doesn't pay any money, they will tell them to stick it. Weightlifters will select their jobs based on their weightlifting. If a job is too physical or requires too much time on the feet every day, the weightlifter will quit and try to find something else.

The idea of job hours conflicting with training is out of the question. The main reason the weightlifter has a job in the first place is to make enough money to travel to the next national championship. The weightlifter will figure out what time they have to train every day, and then tell their potential employers that they are not available to work during those times. Like the people who lift weights, they sometimes have to buy their own weights and build a platform in their garage. If they have to max out a credit card to buy their equipment, so be it. Their college years will be some of their biggest weightlifting years, and it will be easier to train during this time because college schedules can be adjusted to be more compatible with training. Once graduation has passed and the weightlifter is looking for a way to make a steady living, time management skills will be critical and some sacrifices might have to be made.

Relationships

Advance Warning: This one can get a little sticky

People who lift weights have relationships like most normal human beings. They meet people at parties, go on dates, spend money on clothes and hair products that will make them more attractive to the people they're dating, try to stay thin and sexy (that's for women and metrosexual men), buy gifts for each other, do selfless things to make their partners feel valued and cherished, fall in love, take fun vacations together, argue sometimes, save up money to buy engagement rings (that's for men), get engaged at some special place where the feelings of romance and happiness are like a thick goo that covers everything, get married, procreate, buy gas grills, drive mini-vans, and enjoy life while they continue their love for lifting weights.

Weightlifters have relationships that are slightly different from most normal human beings. They meet people at parties (hopefully before they're too drunk), go on dates at places that serve large pieces of meat, spend money on protein powder and jeans that will fit their thighs, try to get muscular because they believe that being muscular and being sexy are the same thing, buy gifts for each other if there is enough money left over after paying for the plane ticket to the American Open, act selfishly because you have to be selfish to be a good weightlifter, occasionally allow their partners to take fun "weightlifting meet vacations" with them to swinging places like Merrillville, Indiana, argue whenever the non-weightlifting member of the relationship wants the weightlifter to do virtually anything that conflicts with training, buy engagement rings that come with a free set of steak knives (that's still for men), get engaged at the place that serves the large pieces of meat, get married, procreate, quickly decide whether or not the child deserves love based on if they can hit a good bottom position with a broomstick, buy gas grills, drive piece-of-crap cars, and do their best to work out the relationship by getting the non-weightlifting partner to stop complaining all the time.

You were warned

Pain/Injuries

- People who lift weights will reduce/modify their workouts when they experience pain.
- Weightlifters simply accept that pain is part of the game.

Competition

- People who lift weights will compete in weightlifting meets because it's fun.
- Weightlifters will compete in weightlifting meets because it seems like that is what they were born to do.

Frustration

- People who lift weights try to look on the bright side when training is frustrating.
- Weightlifters break things in their homes when training is frustrating.

Hands

- People who lift weights have normal hands.
- Weightlifters have discolored thumbs and calluses that look like little sand dunes.

On and on this story goes...

At the end of the day, weightlifting is one of history's most sacred Olympic sports. Like many sports, it also includes a unique lifestyle that can only be experienced when a person makes the decision to completely commit their life to it. Many full-blooded weightlifters decide to extend their commitment and passion to the sport after their competitive days are over through coaching, directing meets, writing books, working as an official, etc.. The same intensity they brought to the barbell during their younger years becomes channeled into their service to the sport. In prison terms, these are "lifers." They are in it to the end because at some point in their lives, weightlifting became buried in their soul. They all have times when they take their licks, certainly. Many of them have even had moments when they have hated weightlifting. The thought of quitting and walking away from it all... that thought has popped up. But they always come back because they are fanatics, and that's what fanatics do.

And obviously, this fanatical approach is not for everybody. It does not have to be for everybody. There is no law written in any religious text that says a person cannot simply dabble in weightlifting for recreation and giggles. The sport has benefits for everyone. If the individual simply wants to use the snatch and clean and jerk to get a little stronger and more coordinated, great! That is positive involvement in the sport. Even if competitive weightlifting is not a goal and the athlete just enjoys lifting a barbell overhead, then weightlifting has added something fulfilling to their experience. Therefore, the question still stands; are you a weightlifter or a person who lifts weights? Which group do you belong to and, more importantly, which group is the superior one? Who is the perfect child, and who is the evil twin? Who is Cain and who is Abel? You can answer for yourself, but make sure you understand that it does not matter which group you line up with. Anyone who has chosen to make this sport a part of their life, in any capacity, has done something special. In the eyes of the almighty Lord Snatchikus, we are all members of the same tribe. If training with a barbell has done anything to make your life better, then the universe is unfolding exactly as it should.

OLYMPIC LIFTING IN SUNNYVALE: 1960s VERSION
KEN O'NEILL

Catalyst Athletics in Sunnyvale, California. And pretty close to where Bayshore Freeway and Lawrence Expressway meet. Now, that's something real new for Sunnyvale. Or so you'd think.

Not too far from Catalyst Athletics there was once a garage gym, just off the Bloody Bayshore and Lawrence Station Road. Known as Bob's Garage, three of us built it up at the corner of Santa Ynez and Chico. For the early 60s, Bob's Garage was close to state-of-the-art. And all homemade.

The three of us knew each other from high school. We began serious training together as a result of the Sunnyvale Health Studio, one of those chrome plated gyms with M-W-F womens' days, T-Th-Sat mens' days, closed Sundays. All three of outgrew that place pretty quickly. They didn't take kindly to banging out power cleans, rebounded deadlifts, and missed snatches hitting the wooden floor of what had for years been an old-timer grocery store. We moved on, forming our own garage gym.

The sixties were likely the last stand for garage gyms producing real athletes. That was the era during which coaches feared athletes becoming 'muscle bound', the era before gyms grew in number and popularity. Our best choice was to start our own training quarters.

Bob Kemper, Ken Sisler and I all graduated from Sunnyvale High School by 1962. Within less than two years they'd moved all their weights into the garage of the home of Bob's family, all but taking over that garage. Soon outgrowing a scant quarter ton of old time standard barbells and weights — those old ones with the 1-inch diameter bars and plates — we added a York 310 lb Olympic set, along with all the 10, 25, and 50 pound plates we could find. Junk yards yielded flywheels as additional plates, while Markovich and Fox steel yard in Santa Clara became a source of hardened steel one inch diameter seven and eight foot long bars. A power rack custom fashioned from scrap 4x4" construction timber gave us a cutting edge in that early era of racks.

Back in the fifties and sixties there just weren't many gyms, and hardcore training was limited to the Sports Palace in San Francisco and YMCAs throughout the Bay Area. Our little gym in Sunnyvale first drew friends from high school and college for occasional workouts, and more often pure curiosity about what we were up to. Our Saturday workouts became legendary 6-8 hour sessions, while the Sunday 4 hours of squatting were of less public interest. We overtrained for sure, following the rules of those days. Long workouts sipping gallons of milk and our radio blasting KYA top 40 AM rock.

It was only in the early 1980s that the Amateur Athletic Union (AAU) divested itself of Olympic lifting, powerlifting, and bodybuilding. Before that time, the AAU sanctioned all amateur lifting and physique contests. What's more, lifting events were combined with physique championships — most sponsored by YMCAs throughout the Bay Area and California. By 1963, maybe early 64, we were beginning to compete in those events. Of the three of us, Kemper was by far the most talented. By age 20 he sported more than 19" cold upper arms, was pressing a pair of 110 pound dumbbells overhead for sets of 10 after a day of body surfing at Santa Cruz, and was squatting well over 500 lbs. At 5'11" Bob lifted in the 198 lb class for some years, later moving up to the 242 lb class. At the 1971 Pan American Games, occasion of the last official competition in the Olympic press, Bob set that lift's final record at 418 lbs.

During the mid-60s, Bob's Garage became a magnet for Irongame enthusiasts. In that period, the lines weren't draw really tight between Olympic lifters, powerlifters, and bodybuilders — nor wrist wrestlers, odd lifts, strongmen, pro wrestlers, and amateur athletes. We all trained hard together and tried all sorts of lifting. After all, we were a generation in the wake of those doing one arm snatches and cleans with 7-foot Olympic bars, bent presses reaching 300 lbs, dips for reps with 400 lbs over bodyweight, etc. A lot of those guys were drug-free naturals. Steroids were just coming in, and most muscle heads thought they were a new vitamin—and most wouldn't take them. Up until his death in 1964, Ray van Cleef ran Gateway to Health Gym on West San Carlos near the old Sears store — Ray contributed to Strength & Health, and his gym was a stopping-off point for all sorts of athletes. After Ray's death and with the then legendary rise of Kemper, Bob's Garage became a visiting point.

I dropped out of competition by sometime in 1966. By then the playing field was no longer even. Dianobol had become rapidly and widely used. Records shot through the ceiling. What's more, it was no longer confused with vitamin supplements: the dangers of oral steroid usage were becoming well known as casualties already were mounting. Given that situation, there was no point in competing. By 1967 I'd married, moving myself and my share of Bob's Garage to my digs in Palo Alto. After several years of graduate school in Berkeley and a research fellowship in Japan, I returned to the South Bay in 1973. By then Bob's Garage was a memory. Kemper had moved on to the San Jose YMCA, joining the living legends preparing there for upcoming Olympic victories.

Congratulations to Catalyst Athletics — your website photos evidence a dream come true, or perhaps a far more matured version of what we set out to be and do as Bob's Garage. We of that time nearly 50 years ago were informed by visions of natural strength, health, and athleticism: to learn of a contemporary, far more sophisticated version of that vision brings gratitude and joy to this one-third of the Bob's Gym gang. As I approach my 65th birthday, I've now trained for 50 years—I'll cease only when nailed into a box! May the joy of the Irongame be a steadfast lifetime passion for you all.

PLANDOMIZATION
GREG EVERETT

Periodization has become a bad word in CrossFit Land. My optimistic view on this phenomenon is that it's due simply to widespread misunderstanding of what exactly periodization is, how variable its implementation can be, and not only its value when used correctly, but its necessity in some form for anyone but the complete beginner. The cynic in me, on the other hand, believes this vehement aversion to periodization of any nature is more a product of frequent bad-mouthing by individuals in positions of authority who fail to grasp the fundamentals and are much more willing to disparage periodization and its proponents and claim a degree of authority so extravagant it exceeds the intellectual capacity of the totality of the world's coaches and athletes, rather than admit a lack of understanding and spend some time learning from others.

Having said this, I feel a need to clarify that I do believe much periodization is constructed poorly and falls short of its intended goals. This, however, demonstrates an individual's ineptitude or inexperience, not a fundamental flaw in the concept itself.

Part of the problem is likely due to the association of specific models with periodization itself; that is, too many people believe periodization to be a particular structure, likely one they've seen in some internet article (or one of those silly digital journals).

Periodization is simply planning. It's creating a structure to guide one's training during a given period of time. It doesn't necessarily mean a progression from higher volume and lower intensity to lower volume and higher intensity, although this basic trend does have a fair degree of utility. In another sense, periodization is the segmentation of training into blocks of time that allow some degree of emphasis on certain traits over others. The bottom line, the term periodization should be considered synonymous with planning.

Ends & Means

Let me go ahead and distill this entire article to its essence: If you have no plan with regard to your training, you're an idiot. Abrasive, I know, but this point needs to sink in.

The idea that you can make maximal progress without a plan in any pursuit, whether it's athletics, business, or space travel, is absurd. Can you make progress without a plan? Sure. You can pretty much guarantee some degree of improvement over a long enough period of time with consistent hard work. But being satisfied with minimal progress when greater progress is entirely achievable is just stupid.

Does this mean everyone needs to know exactly what they'll be doing every day for the next twelve months? Of course not. Planning comes in many different forms and degrees of precision, and those characteristics will vary according to individual needs.

We can plan everything from a single workout, to a short series of workouts in a week, to an entire year of training. How detailed each of these plans is will change according to individual need, but planning on all of these levels should exist in some manner. Without it, we're just crossing our fingers.

Generalization Specifically

So we have this thing called CrossFit. Its intention is to create fitness, which has been defined by Greg Glassman as increased work capacity across broad time and modal domains. That's fancy-talk for being able to do more shit in less time.

CrossFit is a somewhat nebulous program involving "constantly varied, if not randomized, functional movement performed at high intensity." This notion of randomness has become an eclipsing focus of many CrossFit athletes and trainers. Quite possibly this is because approaching training randomly effectively masks a lack of programming ability and gives one a false sense of programming expertise. Anyone can throw a list of exercises and numbers on a whiteboard; far fewer can create workouts that, over a given period of time, ensure an athlete accomplishes his or her goals.

An entirely random approach to training, in my humble, lowly, uneducated opinion, is a mistake. Being prepared for any random task is not the same thing as preparing randomly for any task. The importance of this point cannot be overstated.

Being prepared for anything means balancing and improving equally, on average over time, the range of athletic traits. The list created by Jim Cawley of Dynamax is a nice guide: Strength, power, speed, endurance, stamina, flexibility, balance, coordination, agility and accuracy.

This balancing of traits is done by improving one's weaknesses without sacrificing one's strengths unnecessarily until every trait is within a reasonable range of equality, at which time elements can be trained in a more balanced fashion (although emphasis of certain elements during certain times will continue to allow greater progress even in a reasonably balanced athlete). How does one improve one's lacking elements of fitness? By emphasizing those elements in training for given periods of time—not necessarily continuously—until they're no longer weaknesses. Sound like anything we've talked about thus far?

People & Places

We have a few basic kinds of people to consider with regard to all this planning nonsense.

First are individuals who must be as balanced as possible—that is, prepared for any contingency—at all times. This includes military personnel, law enforcement officers, firefighters, EMS personnel and the like whose lives and careers depend on being physically capable of managing extreme physical demands without prior notice. A cop doesn't have the luxury, for example, of training for a particularly brutal arrest and control situation a given date.

Competitive athletes, on the other hand, do have competition schedules and know when and where they'll need their particular set of physical traits. Occasionally athletes like fighters will take on last-minute events other than ones for which they've been preparing, but this is comparatively uncommon, and for these athletes, whether or not to take a fight is ultimately a choice, not a requirement.

Finally we have the vast majority of the exercising population—individuals who seek fitness for its own sake, for health, for improvement of their chosen recreational activities, and even for the enjoyment of training itself. These individuals have no schedule at all, and no need to be prepared in perfect balance at any given moment (an exception might be an individual planning to do something goofy like hike up a big ass mountain during a family vacation).

The optimist in me believes it should be strikingly obvious that the training needs of these three groups are not the same; the cynic knows that too many of each group have been convinced that they should all be preparing the same way.

Everyone from each of these groups has strengths and weaknesses. Those weaknesses need to be addressed if that individual is to achieve the level of fitness being sought. Again, these things are addressed by emphasizing particular elements—whether specific exercises or entire modalities—in order to bring them up to speed with the remainder of an individual's abilities.

This need to emphasize certain elements doesn't change among individuals, irrespective of career, sport, or hairstyle; what changes is the degree to which one can emphasize a given element over others. In other words, the less the demand for constant readiness, the more we can temporarily and slightly compromise certain abilities for the sake of improving those needing the most improvement.

Compromise is for Pussies! (and Married Men)

So why should we compromise any element of fitness at anytime? Because in order to genuinely emphasize one element, we need to create slack elsewhere. There is a very real limit to how much the human body can handle simultaneously, and attempting to perform at 100% across the board at all times is a guaranteed recipe for stagnation if not utter disaster.

Interestingly enough, this notion is often dismissed because emphasis and compromise are mistakenly interpreted as specialization and sacrifice. Again, it's critical to understand that it's entirely possible to adjust the degree of emphasis and compromise to be appropriate for any individual in any case.

The fact is that emphasis means greater progress. This cannot be denied without delusion. We can demonstrate this fact by looking to athletic specialists. The strongest athletes in the world, for example, are those who train exclusively for strength and forsake all other elements of fitness that fail to contribute to being stronger in an athlete's event(s). This fact is known to anyone who considers it for a moment, but is often forgotten when entering into passionate discussions regarding fitness.

This rule of emphasis producing greater results can be applied even when fitness is our goal—again, we just modulate the degree of emphasis to better preserve the de-emphasized elements.

Perfect examples of this are Michael Rutherford's Max Effort Black Box and Jeff Martin's Strength Bias programs. Each seeks to maintain a rather high level of fitness while emphasizing strength development, and both have been very successful with accomplishing this goal. Neither sacrifices fitness, and, arguably, actually both improve it by increasing the individual's strength, which appears overwhelmingly to be the trait most lacking in CrossFitters. The athlete's performance on longer-duration metabolic workouts may suffer somewhat, but ultimately, such workouts are less builders of fitness than tests of it, and to a large degree, tests of mental fortitude more than physical ability.

The degree of emphasis in a program is commensurate to the degree of comprise. In other words, with more compromise, we can achieve greater improvement in the trait being emphasized (this is not to say that we necessarily need to emphasize/compromise to a great degree in all cases). This rule is important to keep in mind when creating programs to ensure one doesn't mistakenly expect to be able to emphasize to an extent beyond what is allowed by the associated compromise.

Everybody's Doing It

The funny thing (maybe not funny—more exasperating, I suppose) is that nearly every

CrossFitter does in fact plan and emphasize certain elements to some extent, knowingly or not (the only ones who don't are the same folks who flail around helplessly in the rest of their lives as well). Every CrossFitter knows what he or she sucks at most—and, thankfully, sucking at exercise-related things is discouraged in the CrossFit community (although sucking seems to be quite popular…).

I can't do a muscle-up yet and I feel like a tool! I'm going to drop in more ring dips and false-grip ring pull-ups so I can get one. That sounds suspiciously like emphasis and planning.

So it's being done already—the problem is that it's typically not being done well (it's hard to do something well when you either don't know you're doing it or refuse to admit you're doing it). If more people would acknowledge the need to focus on improving their weaknesses, and learn better ways of training to specifically improve them, we'd find not more specialized athletes, but more balanced CrossFitters.

I am a Specialist. At Everything.

Planning is really not that complicated: Determine a goal and decide on a method of achieving it. The key with goal-setting is being reasonable: don't be the guy who makes a goal of adding 50 kg to his back squat in four weeks. It's far more productive to continually make more modest goals, and to continually achieve them on a more frequent basis. This regular accomplishment of goals also keeps the athlete motivated and training hard and consistently, rather than frustrated and training half-heartedly and sporadically.

The generalist will need to have more conservative long-term goals than the specialist, but often short-term goals for generalists can be more ambitious than their specialist counterparts' because those specialists will be far more advanced in their development. In any case, goals need to be limited in number during any given period—the classic rookie mistake is trying to do everything at the same time to the same degree (Sound like anyone you know?).

This is where creating periods of time to focus on different goals comes into play. If we have a CrossFitter who wants to snatch bodyweight, but also wants to be able to add three more rounds to his Cindy, we have two goals that are not remarkably complementary. This athlete is going to get a lot more accomplished if he or she spends some time improving his or her snatch technique and snatch-related strength while preserving metabolic conditioning as well as possible, and then spending some time improving Cindy-specific stamina while preserving his or her new-found snatching ability, than trying to do both together.

This reality is often dismissed with anecdotes of CrossFitters who added 7,000 lbs to their deadlifts while losing 350 lbs of pure fat and dropping 5 minutes off their Fran times—all while simply following the crossfit.com WOD. This argument, of course, fails to consider the remarkable capacity for adaption of untrained or deconditioned individuals, and the comparatively limited capacity of individuals with many years of smart training under their belts. If an individual is untrained enough, I can improve his deadlift with nothing more than vigorous nose-picking. The point is, what works for beginners (which is anything at all) doesn't work for more advanced athletes. The more advanced an athlete is, the closer he or she is to his ultimate capacity, and the more necessary legitimate planning becomes. Again, for demonstration of this, look to athletic specialists.

Plandomization

Part of CrossFit's effectiveness is the constant variation of the metabolic workouts in terms of exercises, reps, rounds, etc. (as an aside, its biggest weakness is the constant variation and random implementation of strength work).

So how do we reconcile this notion of constant variation with planning for specific goals? Simple: we plan the fundamental structure of our training—the training that is helping us accomplish our current primary goal—and fill in the spaces with more randomized—but smart—training that takes into consideration our secondary goals.

Most often what this will look like (or should look like, considering the current state of CrossFitters at large) is a structured strength program accompanied by CrossFit-style metabolic workouts. These workouts will be varied continually, but they should not be randomly created. At minimum, these workouts should be constructed in a manner than doesn't interfere with the strength work; ideally, they should be constructed with an effort to work toward accomplishing a secondary goal.

A secondary goal needs to be kept just that—it's easy to get carried away and attempt to achieve too much at once, which nearly always results in failure across the board. Secondary-goal-oriented programming would be the emphasis of exercises or elements that have proven to be weaknesses for the athlete in question within actual CrossFit workouts. This might look like increased frequency of pull-ups in metCons for individuals whose pull-ups suck, or an increase in box jump height for an athlete who realizes he or she has been sandbagging with little girl boxes and needs to actually put effort into jumping. It may be spending a few more minutes before and after every workout on flexibility and mobility, or taking a little ego hit and performing dumbbell cleans instead of power cleans in order to shore up bottom-position weakness.

In other words, it doesn't need to involve any kind of extravagant planning—simply being cognizant of minor weaknesses and ensuring such exercises or elements don't continue to be neglected. As those elements improve sufficiently, we move on to the next crop of weaknesses.

This is exactly how I approach the CrossFit programming at Catalyst Athletics. I can tell you exactly what strength work our CrossFitters will be doing six Tuesdays from now, but I can't tell you what metCon they'll be doing that day yet. I plan seven-week strength cycles, but I plan each week's metCons the week prior. When creating these metCons, I consider the strength workout on the same day and the rest of the week, the other metCons that week, and the metCons from prior weeks, along with the weaknesses and strengths I see in our clients. Based on this information, I have goals for them, both short- and long-term, and I create workouts and workout series to accomplish these goals. In other words, while the metCons are constantly varied, they're by no means random.

Work on It

This article is more of an attempt to motivate smarter programming by CrossFit athletes and trainers than to provide actual guidance for such programming. Guidance of that nature requires far more information than can be contained in an article like this—it requires active pursuit of pertinent information, experimentation, and discussion with other professionals.

If you believe you know all there is to know about programming, you haven't done your homework. There is always more information out there, and there will always be someone who knows something you don't. Learn to be unsatisfied with your current abilities.

NORCAL ON RAMP PART 1
NICKI VIOLETTI

The way in which new clients are introduced to your Crossfit program can be the deciding factor in whether you retain them for life (and they refer friends, family and co-workers) or they come for one dose and vanish. Perhaps the most common way affiliates bring in new clients is the "come and try it" approach, often associated with a free session or free week of sessions. With virtually no barrier to entry this can be effective for getting folks in the door. However, the absence of a dedicated entry point for new clients will ultimately hamper your ability to provide high quality coaching as well as your rate of growth as a business.

The following questions are worth some consideration:

What experience do you want each new client to have that comes to your gym? What do you want them to tell their friends and family after the first day? How will a new client progress through your program? Where will they start and where will they end up?

From a coaching perspective, what ideally would be the fundamental skill sets each client would have when they join your classes? Perhaps a decent squat, with the awareness of how to extend the spine? It might also be nice if they knew the difference between active and passive shoulders and had been shown the desired overhead position for the push press. And oh the fabulous deadlift…how many new folks struggle to get in the setup position with a properly extended back? How many are able to lift a 55# barbell without either first elevating the hips or chest prematurely, or flexing the spine?

As a coach and owner of a CrossFit training facility I'm going to make a case for having dedicated points of entry and the utilization of an On Ramp program or similar beginner's workshop

The Early Days

In the early days of CrossFit NorCal we had the "come one, come all" approach to growing our clientele, much like many new affiliates today. We encouraged our existing clients to bring friends to classes and even lured them with specials like "train free for a week." This approach made it relatively easy to grow our business, but quickly became a logistical nightmare. The programming always defaulted to accommodate the new person. Our existing clients didn't get the attention they deserved and as a consequence did not progress as quickly.

This lack of a dedicated point of entry for new clients is especially problematic if you are the sole owner/coach. Here's a common scenario: You have 4-5 clients in a class who are ready to learn muscle up technique. You begin teaching the progression when in walk 2 brand new people, 10 minutes late, wanting to try your free class. They need to sign a waiver and have a conversation with you about their old injuries, etc and then you need to teach them to squat, because there will be squats in the WOD. Meanwhile your existing clients are left in the lurch. Giving free lessons on the squat while your paying clientele is waiting for you to finish, is not, in my opinion, providing the best quality coaching to all parties involved.

A typical way this problem is "solved" is to have a second coach handle your new walk-ins. It seems like a solution, but it's not a viable one. You are a professional who is running a business, and as such you should be paid well for your time. Each service that is provided can and should command a price.

I distinctly remember a turning point for us at CF NorCal late in 2005. There were about 12 athletes in the gym. Robb was coaching a class of 8 athletes and both myself, and Greg Everett each had 2 new people off to the side introducing the squat, etc. I did some quick math in my head to realize that the gross revenue for that hour was about $12. Three professionals pouring their energy and expertise into 12 clients to earn what amounted to $4 a piece. Not a good business model! (This was back when we were charging FAR too little for unlimited training, we had family members and folks on trade and students with obscene discounts, etc. Folks would come every single day, with an effective per class fee of around $3! We've truly learned the hard way!)

Dedicated Points of Entry

If you are an affiliate owner who wants to run a business that sustains your livelihood, as opposed to it being a hobby or second job, you have three primary aims:

- Demonstrate that you are a professional and can get results
- Demonstrate that you are interested in each individual's success
- Have FUN while doing both of the above!

The way to thoroughly demonstrate your abilities as a coach and establish interest in your client's success is to have dedicated points of entry for new clients joining your facility. These points of entry are paths for them to progress into your ongoing classes. (As an aside, the "get them to puke then convert them" approach only works on a tiny sub-fraction of the general population.)

At CFNC we have 2 points of entry for new clients: Private training or the On Ramp class.

- Healthy, orthopedically sound individuals can begin with our 12 session On Ramp class.
- New clients with orthopedic issues are typically private training candidates.

The beauty of having 2 entry points is that you are able to thoroughly bracket your population. The price point of the On Ramp removes the otherwise steep barrier to entry of requiring private training sessions prior to group training. Offering private training allows you to fill otherwise dead hours with paying clientele. Don't overlook the fact that EVERY community has plenty of people willing and able to pay for 1-on-1 coaching.

Building Relationships and Mitigating the Fear Factor

Dedicated points of entry also allow for the development of rapport and relationships, both crucial to growing a service business. Whether in private training sessions or a beginner's class, the coaches and clients get to know each other quite well. It is a safe and less-intimidating setting.

A new client recently shared with me that on her first day she was so nervous that she almost turned her car around and returned home. She was in the middle of her series of private training sessions with one of our trainers and gushingly told me how much she loves our program and how grateful she was that we were in town. After finishing her 12 sessions of private training she is now in our CF Elements classes. She is learning to snatch, she is kicking up into handstands against the wall and she is climbing ropes. She is also a well-recognized professional in our community.

My point is that without a dedicated entry point this woman's experience would not have been the same and we likely would have lost her business after the first day. This woman was scared to death. Had our primary focus been that of proving the toughness of our workouts she would not have come back.

The On Ramp

The NorCal On Ramp is our evolving template for progressing new clients into our group classes. We've been utilizing this program template since June of 2008 with great success.

The On Ramp provides new clients a solid steeping in the movements and upon completion allows them to seamlessly transition into the fast paced group classes. Each session includes a warm-up, skill instruction/review, workout, and stretching/cool down with different topics discussed during each cool down session: nutrition, food logs, etc. We limit enrollment to 10 people with 2 coaches.

On Day 1 we are careful to explain the goals of the class and what clients can expect. We explain that we value and emphasize mechanics and technical mastery and that the primary goal is to provide consistent exposure to the movements and adequately prepare each of them for success in the group class environment.

Upon completion of the On Ramp, the new client feels less intimidated upon entering our existing group classes, and the continuity of the existing class is preserved, as we don't have to slow things down to walk a newbie through the movements.

The Magic of 12 Sessions

The 12-session time frame is key for a couple of reasons. First, almost anyone is willing to try something new for a month, and a month allows for adequate exposure to the movements. We've found that just one exposure to the deadlift, one exposure to the kip, and one exposure to the press, is not sufficient for the raw beginner. A full month of training gives folks a true sense of the power of the CF methodology and it allows us to follow the Mechanics, Consistency, Intensity mantra of CrossFit.

Second, the 12-session time frame also allows for the client to experience transformation on multiple levels: They FEEL better, they LOOK better, and they PERFORM better!

On Day 12 we repeat the same workout that they completed on Day1 and folks consistently shave 3-4 minutes off of their original time. Needless to say they are STOKED! We have found that after the 12th session, when folks see the improvements they have made in just a month, they are ready to sign up for more. It virtually eliminates the need for any sales pitch.

Changes and Adaptations

Our first On Ramp was held in June of 2008. We had 7 people signed up ranging from

21-48 years old. The day 1 workout was the following:

- 200M Run
- 21-15-9
- squat
- bodyrow
- pushup
- 200M Run

Our first crew (who in all estimations was a fairly young/active group) was pretty busted up from this. They were wickedly sore from the pushups and wickedly sore from the squats. Most middle-aged women (your bread and butter clients) don't want to be so sore they can't hold their child or wash their hair.

After that first class we changed the numbers to 15-12-9 and this volume seems much more appropriate. We still get folks who fail on pushups and squats with this rep scheme, and if so, we will cut that individual's numbers mid workout. We will also scale movements if necessary and pushups might be against the pommel horse or GHD if someone is unable to do one from the knees.

A younger male or female who is in relatively good shape will obviously be able to go faster and push harder. We encourage these athletes by showing them our gym records for the workout and challenging them to beat it. Again, our goal here is to progress people according to their needs, not prove that our workouts are tough. Remember, we want to RETAIN these people. We don't want to kill them off day one and have them never come back.

What about Fire Breathers?

I frequently get asked whether we ever allow a younger, fitter individual bypass the On Ramp and just join the group classes. The answer is no. Throwing an uninitiated individual (regardless of age or fitness level) into your class of fire-breathers is not taking interest in the progress of that potential client, nor that of your current clients.

We have uncovered movement deficiencies in the youngest and fittest of our new clients. Everyone benefits from spending some dedicated time working the technique of the movements. In my opinion, rushing someone into a class environment where the competition is much greater only serves to put pressure on that individual to go fast, when instead technical mastery needs to be the focus. Remember, there is plenty of time for these folks to "get some" after some steeping in mechanics! That said, we definitely push the younger, fitter, and cockier ones harder. Typical times for completing the Day 1 WOD range from 5-15minutes. We have the records on the board for the top 5 male and female times and we use this to push the more hard charging types: "the Day 1 male record on this is 4:35 let's see if you can beat it!" And while it's absolutely not our goal, we have still had a couple of young guys head to the bathroom to puke after the Day 1 WOD.

Typical Day 1/Day 12 Times

Everyone sees improvement from Day 1 to Day 12, typically in the 2-3 minute range, but sometimes shaving as many as 5 minutes off the original time. Here is a picture of the whiteboard of a recent class showing their Day 1 and Day 12 times.

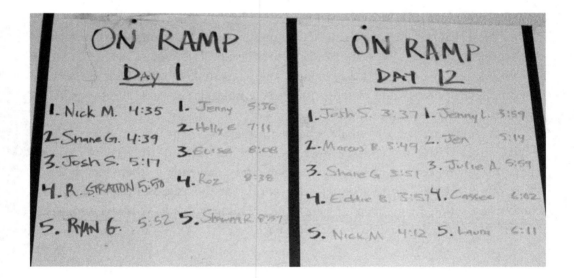

NORCAL ON RAMP PART 2: CURRICULUM
NICKI VIOLETTI

The following is the curriculum for the NorCal Strength & Conditioning / CrossFit NorCal On-Ramp program introduced in the last issue.

Welcome and Introduction

"The emphasis of the On-Ramp is on skill development and exposure to our basic movements. It is designed to prepare you to enter our ongoing group classes. We are going to be hammering technique—both to ensure your safety—and success at the next level."

- We will introduce you to technique and mechanics first, then intensity.
- We will be showing you movements that begin with the relatively non technical and progressively more technical.
- It's important that you are here for each of the 12 sessions as these movements build on one another.
- There will be a workout at the end of each day which will get progressively more challenging as the course progresses.
- The difficulty of these workouts is ultimately in your hands…the degree that you push yourself will determine how much suffering goes on. The class is called "On Ramp" for a specific reason…we want to ramp you up to the level of intensity and output that is inherent in our group classes.
- Shifts in body composition are one of the most motivating ways to measure success. We highly encourage you to take "Before" pictures at the beginning of the On-Ramp class.

DAY	SKILL REVIEW	NEW SKILLS	WOD
1		DROM SQUAT BODY ROW PUSH UP	200M RUN 15-12-9 SQUAT/PUSHUP/BODYROW 200M RUN
2	SQUAT	DEADLIFT STANDING PRESS AND PUSH PRESS WITH PVC	10! MED BALL DEADLIFT PUSH PRESS WITH PVC
3	DEAD LIFT	ROWER THRUSTER	ROW 200 M 10 THRUSTERS *TIME EACH INTERVAL (ONE PERSON RESTS WHILE PARTNER GOES) 3 TIMES EACH (APPROX 3 MIN REST)*
4	DEAD LIFT	KIPPING JUMPING PULL- UPS WALKING LUNG- ES	RUN 200M LUNGE 30 FT 10 JUMPING PULL-UPS 3 ROUNDS
5	STANDING PRESS WITH PVC	SHOULDER MO- BILITY CIRCUIT STANDING PRESS OUT OF RACK KNEE TO ELBOW PROGRESSION	3 ROUNDS OF: 300 M ROW 5 KTE 10 DUMB BELL PUSH PRESS ONE GROUPS WILL REST WHILE 2ND GROUP GOES FOR EACH ROUND
6	Standing press out of rack	Wall Ball Foot clamp on rope	5 rounds for time: 7 wall ball 7 pushup 7 body rows OR 5 rounds for time 10 wall ball 5 pushup

DAY	SKILL REVIEW	NEW SKILLS	WOD
7	DEAD LIFT, START WITH PVC SERIES WALKING LUNGES	KIPPING PULL-UP	CHIPPER: 2 HEATS WITH STAGGER START RUN 400M 15 LUNGES ON EACH LEG 15 BODY ROWS 15 THRUSTERS 15 KTE ROW 400M
8	STANDING PRESS OUT OF THE RACK	BURGENER WU DUMB BALL CLEANS SIT-UPS	10! DUMB BALL HANG POWER CLEAN/SIT UP
9	KIPPING BURGENER WU PUSH UPS	PARTNER BALL DRILLS BACK SQUAT	3 ROUNDS FOR TIME: 400M RUN 15 PUSH UPS
10	ROPE CLIMB BURGENER WU LUNGE	BACK SQUAT DUMB BELL SNATCH RUSSIAN LUNGE	ROUNDS IN 10 MINUTES 10 DUMB BELL SNATCH RUSSIAN LUNGE 25 FT
11	FOOT CLAMP ON ROPE	BACK SQUAT ROPE LOWERS KETTLEBELL SWINGS	200M RUN 20-15-10 KB SWINGS 2 ROPE LOWERS
12	DEAD LIFT KIP/PULL-UP		REPEAT DAY 1 WOD: 200M RUN 15-12-9 SQUAT/PUSHUP/BODY ROW 200M RUN

Day 1

TRAINER A	TRAINER B
WELCOME, INTRO AND WU	VERBAL EXPLANATION OF SQUAT, BODY ROW AND PUSH-UP (TRAINER A DOES DEMO)
PRE-WOD EXPLANATION AND TIMING	RECORDS NAMES/TIMES DURING WOD
COOL DOWN DISCUSSION	STRETCHING

General Welcome and Introductions

WU: 200 Walk/Jog for warm-up, and arm circles and kicks.

Introduce: Squat …Explain movement and demo. Group practice—assess and give feedback. Emphasize:

- Feet under shoulders,
- Weight in heels, first movement is hips back
- Low back curve maintained
- Posture: chest up, eyes forward, neutral neck
- Depth below parallel
- Arms can be out in front to counterbalance
- Full hip extension

If good to go:

Skill practice: Drill team style--We say down… clients squat. Take them up to 10, correcting and adjusting people's form as needed

Introduce: Body Row…Explain progression of strength and skill to achieve a pull-up. It all starts with good movement in a body row. Trainer demos the following: Bodyrow – basic & advanced, Eccentric pullup, Kipped pullup

Have clients practice a few body rows and give feedback. Emphasize:

- Squeeze shoulder blades together
- This is not an arm curl
- Torso is rigid, no bouncing out of the bottom
- Dramatic anterior and posterior scapular movement

- Controlled eccentric recovery—not a rapid drop.

Everybody will do body rows in workout to help strengthen the connective tissue (even if a client can already do pull-ups).

Introduce: Pushup…Demo perfect push-up, and push-up progression alternatives. Emphasize:

- Head/neck alignment: cue eyes looking slightly forward.
- Low back in neutral position: cue pull low back up, tight through core.
- Full depth and extension: cue chest and thighs must touch, and full lock out of elbows.

Have clients practice full push-ups—assess to determine appropriate scaling.

> WOD
> 200M run
> 15-12-9
> squat/pushup/body row
> 200M run

Stretching sequence: hip flexors, and hamstrings on the box, straddle, shoulders, ankles & Achilles

Cool down discussion: Nutrition….BREAKFAST…quality protein and fat. That is HW….good breakfast each day this week. TAKE BEFORE PICTURES.

Day 2

TRAINER A	TRAINER B
WU, SQUAT REVIEW, SHOULDER DISLOCATE INTRODUCTION	VERBAL EXPLAIN/INTRODUCE DL, MED BALL DL, STANDING PRESS WITH PVC, PUSH PRESS (TRAINER A DEMOS
PRE-WOD EXPLANATION AND TIMING	RECORDS NAMES/TIMES DURING WOD
COOL DOWN DISCUSSION	STRETCHING

Inquire about soreness. Talk about connective tissue—and upper body soreness from body rows.

WU: 200 jog and DROM (arms circles and kicks all 3 directions).

Review: squat (just a quick 10-15 squats…enough to check on form).

Introduce: shoulder dislocates with PVC.

- Cue active shoulders, long arms (no bent elbows), open chest

Introduce: deadlift with PVC – emphasize start position/set up and then practice technique with PVC.

- Talk through set up and only have client lift on trainers OK.
- Cue weight on heels, good lumbar curve, long arms Practice using 35# and 55 # bar – rotate everyone through – emphasize start position/set up.

Introduce: Med ball dead lift—and discuss lifting odd shaped objects

Introduce: standing press start position – get everyone set up with PVC

- Cue active shoulders in overhead position.
- Introduce: push press with PVC.
- Emphasize 'dip and drive'…quick pop to full extension with active shoulders
- Pushing up, not forward (head and chin slightly forward in finish position)

WOD

10-9-8-7-6-5-4-3-2-1 reps:
-Med ball deadlift
-Push press with PVC (If client is strong and mobile, load with dumbbells appropriately)

Stretching Sequence: Hamstrings on box, glute stretch on mat, shoulders on wall.

Cool Down discussion: Omega-3s…Fish oil stimulates blood circulation,

- lowers blood triglyceride levels
- reduces the risk of heart attack
- reduces the risk of dangerous abnormal heart rhythms
- reduces the risk of strokes

- lows the buildup of atherosclerotic plaques
- lowers blood pressure
- reduces stiffness and joint tenderness

Day 3

TRAINER A	TRAINER B
INTRODUCE ROWER (TRAINER B DEMOS) DROM	REVIEW DL, VERBALLY EXPLAIN THRUSTERS (TRAINER A DEMOS)
PRE-WOD EXPLANATION AND TIMING	RECORDS NAMES/TIMES DURING WOD
COOL DOWN DISCUSSION	STRETCHING

DROM: Inquire about breakfasts....during warm-up

Introduce: Rowing Technique...Trainer demo how to get in, generally row...and how to safely exit.

- Tall chest/shoulders and extending legs prior to pulling with arms, then returning arms prior to bending knees/returning seat

Have clients row a 500 to practice—trainers evaluate and give feedback.

Review: Deadlift--quickly demo to review, then clients can practice with 35# and 55# bars.

- Be critical on set up—and review with PVC if necessary.

Introduce: Thrusters. Explain and demo (combo of squat into a push press)

- Emphasize full depth and full extension, with active shoulders (head pushes through)
- Cue high elbows, drive through heels, full extension of hips for power

WOD:

3 rounds:
Row 200M
10 thrusters

Time each interval (one person rests while partner goes) 3 times each (approx 3 min rest)

Stretching Sequence: Hip flexors and quads on corner of mat, hamstrings with a strap, straddles.

Cool Down Discussion: Gluten Free…what that means and why? Review HW of eating a quality breakfast…no grains…just protein and fat.

TAKE PICTURES TO POST ON LINE!

Day 4

TRAINER A	TRAINER B
WARM-UP ON ROWER, DROM	VERBALLY INTRODUCE KIP (TRAINER A DEMOS)
REVIEW DL	VERBALLY INTRODUCE JUMPING PULL-UPS AND LUNGES
PRE-WOD EXPLANATION, TIMING OF WOD	RECORD NAMES AND TIMES DURING WOD
COOL DOWN DISCUSSION	STRETCHING

WU: 500 Row (review technique if necessary), DROM

Introduce: Kip

- On ground first—superman/back extension position with PVC in hand to help get body in correct extended position.
- On bar—push head through then pull-back—movement generated from chest and shoulders, not in legs or hips.

Review: Deadlift…modify and add weight. 55# and 65-75#

Introduce: Jumping Pull-up

- Using rings, or boxes on the bar—set up each client in an area.
- Emphasize full extension of arms at bottom of movement and pulling to arm-pits at top of movement.
- Use legs…not just a pull of the arms.

Introduce: Walking lunges

- Long steps, with knee staying above heel---not traveling over toe.
- For balance—step slightly to the right or left of center and turn toe slightly out.
- Full depth—knee should nearly contact ground each step, and then come to a full stand as moving to next forward step.

WOD

> Run 200m
> Lunge 30 ft
> 10 jumping pull-ups
> 3 rounds

Stretching Sequence: Hamstrings on the box, hanging from the rings, ITB band (drop leg across body—while lying flat), shoulders.

Cool Down Discussion: Food logs...grocery shopping email. Also—discuss the impact of gluten.

Day 5

TRAINER A	TRAINER B
WARM-UP ON ROWER, DROM, INTRODUCE SHOULDER MOBILITY CIRCUIT, AND THEN REVIEW STANDING PRESS WITH PVC	VERBALLY INTRODUCE STANDING PRESS OUT OF RACK (TRAINER A DEMOS)
VERBALLY INTRODUCE KTE 9TRAINER B DEMONSTRATES)	PRE-WOD EXPLANATION, TIMING OF WOD
RECORD NAMES AND TIMES DURING WOD	
STRETCHING	COOL DOWN DISCUSSION

WU: 500 Row, DROM

Introduce: Shoulder mobility circuit

- 5 over head pass through with PVC with active shoulders
- 5 overhead squats with PVC
- 5 kips on bar

Review: Standing press with PVC.

Emphasize:

- Shoulder blades pulled together in the back
- Pull head back slightly
- Full extension of arms with active shoulders.

Introduce: Standing press-- taking a bar out of the rack. Emphasize:

- Body becomes rack by allowing bar to lay across deltoids and collar bone
- Split leg (versus feet side by side) stance under the bar on the rack
- High Elbows (wrist/forearm flexibility may be an issue)
- Step out of rack, readjust grip, feet in hip width stance.
- Drop elbows and pull shoulder blades together to prepare for press.

With 15# trainer bar, have each client practice taking bar out of the rack, do 5 standing press, and return bar to rack.

Introduce: Knee to elbow (KTE)...demo progression: full shin to bar, knee to elbow, knee to chest and knee to waist. Emphasize:

- Solid grip
- Keeping long arms and not bending elbows in process.
- Pulling down on bar (similar to kipping motion)
- Keeping head in neutral position and not throwing it back at top of movement.

Have clients experiment with the different progressions of this skill.

WOD:

> 3 rounds of:
> 300 M Row
> 5 KTE
> 10 dumb bell push press

One groups will rest while 2nd group goes for each round

Stretching Sequence: Hip flexors on mat, Glutes on mat, straddle, Achilles, try bridging

Cool Down Discussion: What are we eating for breakfast? How many folks have eating only protein and good fat since we started 10 days ago? Talk about Work to Rest Ratio.

Day 6

TRAINER A	TRAINER B
WARM-UP WITH A 400 M RUN, DROM, SHOULDER MOBILITY CIRCUIT	VERBALLY INTRODUCE ROPE LOWER AND FOOT PIN (TRAINER A DEMO)
REVIEW STANDING PRESS OUT OF RACK (TRAINER B DEMOS)	INTRODUCE WALL BALL (TRAINER A DEMO)
PRE-WOD EXPLANATION, TIMING OF WOD	RECORD DAMES AND TIMES DURING WOD
STRETCHING	COOL DOWN DISCUSSION

WU: 400 run/walk, DROM and Shoulder mobility circuit

Review: Standing press out of the rack, with some load—25#-35#
- Cue safe bar removal from rack—and safe return
- Active shoulders—and solid core (no ribs pushing forward)

Introduce: Wall ball…demo and explain. Emphasize:

- Full depth to "fanny target".
- Use power from hip extension to generate force through arms to ball
- Accuracy and rhythm are key to efficiency.

Introduce: Rope lower/foot pin. Explain safety reason for foot pin (climb up and become fatigue—foot pin can save your arms—and you can safely return to ground).

Emphasize:

- Rope on outside of foot and inside of knee
- Capture rope between sole of top shoe and laces of bottom shoe
- If feet are side by side—foot clamp is less solid.
- To recover, slide top foot to the side—and this allows you to control tension and speed of decent. Have clients practice on rope several times. Trainer can help by holding rope in place to generate correct foot clamp.

WOD:

> 5 rounds for time
> 7 wallball
> 7 pushup
> 7 body rows
>
> OR
>
> 5 rounds for time
> 10 wall ball
> 5 pushup

Stretching sequence: Lying on mat series (hamstrings, ITB band, glutes), stretch wrists and shoulders, review bridging.

Cool Down Discussion: How to eat out? Restaurants that have good choices, and restaurants that will modify…and how to modify.

Day 7

TRAINER A	TRAINER B
500 ROW, DROM, SHOULDER MOBILITY CIRCUIT	VERBALLY INTRODUCE KIPPING PULL-UP AND POP-OFFS (TRAINER A DEMO)
REVIEW DL	REVIEW ALL WOD SKILLS
PRE-WOD EXPLANATION, TIMING OF WOD	RECORDS NAMES/TIMES DURING WOD
STRETCHING	COOL DOWN DISCUSSION

WU: Row 500-1000, DROM circuit and shoulder mobility

Review: Dead lift. Start with PVC lifting series then move to the bars. Should be lifting between 35# and 75#. Be super critical on form—and go back to lighter weight.

Introduce: Kipping pull up. Demo 'pop-offs' and describe how to generate force from shoulder joint. Demo knee drive and hip extension and describe how that adds the 2nd piece of momentum needed to do kipping pull-up. Have clients practice kipping and negative pull-ups as appropriate.

Emphasize:

- Long legs during kipping.
- Put force on bar by trying to pull shoulders as high as possible in back part of kip.
- If time permits—demo and practice hip opening exercises on mat to encourage hip extension for power.

Review: Walking Lunges

- Long steps, with knee staying above heel---not traveling over toe.
- For balance—step slightly to the right or left of center and turn toe slightly out.
- Full depth—knee should nearly contact ground each step, and then come to a full stand as moving to next forward step.

WOD:

> *Chipper: 2 heats/stagger start if needed*
> Run 400m
> 15 Walking lunges
> 15 body rows
> 15 thrusters
> 15 KTE
> Row 400m

Stretching sequence: Hip flexor and quad sequence on mat, shoulders, and hanging from the rings

Cool Down Discussion: Two weeks into this—time to make adjustments to lunch. Keep breakfast the same (quality protein and fat)…transfer those skills to lunch!

Day 8

TRAINER A	TRAINER B
400 RUN, DROM, SHOULDER MOBILITY CIRCUIT	INTRODUCE SOME FORM OF BURGENER WARM UP (CAN BE SIMPLIFIED)
REVIEW STANDING PRESS OUT OF RACK	INTRODUCE DUMBBELL CLEANS (TRAINER A DEMO)
DEMO/INTRODUCE SIT-UP, PRE-WOD EXPLANATION, TIMING OF WOD	RECORD NAMES AND TIMES DURNING WOD
STRETCHING	COOL DOWN DISCUSSION

WU: 400 run/walk, DROM

Review: Standing press out of the rack. 3 sets of 5 at appropriate weight (25#-45#).

Introduce: Dumbbell hang power cleans. Demo each step and have clients perform each step before moving to the next. Take clients through each step without weight, then add weight…connect movement to Burgener Warm-up with PVC.

- Begin with just jumping up and landing—encourage loose arms, and letting shoulders shrug naturally.
- Go through motion without any weight—then add dumbbells.
- Look for full hip extension, and big shrug.
- NO bicep curls!

Introduce: Sit up on the mat. Emphasize:

- Hooking ankles to increase use of hip flexors and hamstrings
- Drive arms up for momentum and to increase turn-over.
- Head must touchdown in the back of each sit up and chest must touch knees in the front.

WOD:

10! Dumbbell clean/sit up

Stretching Sequence: On stomach—press up to stretch abs after sit ups, hamstrings on the box, hip flexors on the box, shoulders against wall, and Achilles.

Cool Down Discussion: Struggles and making both breakfast and lunch quality meals….talk about meal ideas and ways to make quality food portable.

Day 9

TRAINER A	TRAINER B
500-100 ROW, DROM, SHOULDER MOBILITY CIRCUIT	INTRODUCE PARTNER BALL DRILLS
INTRODUCE BACK SQUAT (TRAINER B DEMO)	REVIEW KIPPING AND KIPPING PULL UPS
PRE-WOD EXPLANATION, TIMING OF WOD	RECORD NAMES AND TIMES DURING WOD
STRETCHING	COOL DOWN DISCUSSION

WU: Row 500-1000, DROM, Shoulder mobility circuit

Introduce: Partner medicine ball drills. Soccer throw-in, shot put, trunk rotation, knee to step through.

Introduce: Back squat. Discuss the difference between a CrossFit squat (hips back) and an Olympic lifting squat (hips sit between feet).

- Safely removing and returning bar from/to rack
- Tall chest
- Weight pushing through heels
- Lock breath in for stability
- Depth = hips below knees
- Safely dumping the bar

Review: Kipping and kipping pull-ups

WOD:

> 3 rounds for time:
> 400M Run
> 15 Push-ups

Stretching Sequence: Hamstring/ITB series with strap, shoulders on the wall, wrists, bridging

Cool Down Discussion: Options for after the 'On-ramp' class.

PASS OUT REFERRAL POST CARDS

Day 10

TRAINER A	TRAINER B
400 RUN, DROM, SHOULDER MOBILITY CIRCUIT, AND SIMPLIFIED BURGENER WU	PREVIEW PULL-UP AND INTRODUCE HIP OVER TECHNIQUE ON MATS
REVIEW BACK SQUAT	INTRODUCE DUMBBELL SNATCH
PRE-WOD EXPLANATION, TIMING OF WOD	INTRODUCE DUMBBELL SNATCH
STRETCHING	COOL DOWN DISCUSSION

WU: Run/walk 400

Review: Pull-up or rope climb techniques. For those clients that are ready--take them through hip extension series on the mats---to help encourage hip opening during pull-up.

Review: Back squat

Introduce: Dumbbell snatch. Demo and explain. A snatch uses some similar mechanics as a clean (hip extension and shoulder shrug), but the weight is moving from the floor to over head...versus a clean that is just lifting to shoulder height. Have clients practice without weights—and then add dumbbells.

- Progression of movement.....core to extremity.
- Full hip extension
- Keep weight close to body
- Lock shoulder out on the top (ACTIVE!)

Introduce/Review: Russian lunge. Review the regular lunge, and introduce the Russian lunge. Demo the torso twist toward the front leg—holding weight at chest level.

WOD:

> Rounds in 10 minutes:
> 10 dumb bell snatch R
> Russian lunge 25 ft
> 10 dumb bell snatch L
> Russian lunge 25 ft

Stretching Sequence: Hamstring series and glute/hips on box, Achilles stretch, shoulders. Cool Down Discussion: Making dinner happen....we've done breakfast, we've progressed to lunch...now how to make it work happen.

Day 11

TRAINER A	TRAINER B
500-1000 M ROW, DROM, SHOULDER MOBILITY CIRCUIT	REVIEW ROPE CLIMB/LOWER/FOOT CLAMP
REVIEW BACK SQUAT	INTRODUCE SWINGS
PRE-WOD EXPLANATION, TIMING OF WOD	RECORD NAMES AND TIMES DURING WOD AND LEAD CLIENTS IN THE FINISHER
STRETCHING	COOL DOWN DISCUSSION

WU: Row 500-1000, DROM, Shoulder mobility circuit

Review: Rope climb and foot clamp. Practice rope lower and climb—even if clients have a rope climb.

Review: Back squat

Introduce: Kettle bell swings. Demo and explain. Practice without a kettle bell—just using hands as the weight. Emphasize:

- Hips back as first movement
- Keep torso as upright as possible (don't let weight pull chest down)
- Keep arms long, use hip extension to generate force versus pulling with elbows.

Have clients practice with light kettle bell—and ease them from swinging just to shoulder height—then to forehead height, then all way straight overhead.

WOD:

Team workout: Teams of 3 at least 3 rounds:

> 30 kb swings
> 6 rope lowers
> OR
> 200M run
> 20-15-10
> kb swings
> 2 rope lowers

Finisher: ½ round of Tabata sit-ups, and ½ round of back extensions on mat.

Stretching Sequence: Hip flexor and glute series on the mat, hanging off the rings, shoulders on the wall

Cool Down Discussion: Making food work when you have a family or spouse that doesn't eat the same….possible recipes…

Day 12

TRAINER A	TRAINER B
500-1000 ROW, DROM, SHOULDER MOBILITY CIRCUIT	REVIEW PULL-UPS, KIPPING PULL-UPS
REVIEW DL	PRE WOD EXLANATION, TIMING OF WOD
RECORD NAMES AND TIMES DURING WOD	COOL DOWN DISCUSSION
STRETCHING	AFTER PHOTOS

WU: Row 500-1000, shoulder mobility circuit.

Review: Dead Lift, with appropriately loaded weight

Review: Kipping and Pull-ups

WOD:

> 200M run
> 15-12-9
> squat/pushup/body row
> 200M run

Compare times from first day!

Stretching Sequence: Hip flexor series on the mat, glute stretch, straddle and shoulders. Cool Down Discussion: Signing up for group classes. Final thoughts on food.

THE DISORDERED EATING CHRONICLES: FEED ME
RACHEL IZZO

Girls are crazy; everyone knows that. Between that special time of the month when we'd kill for a piece of chocolate, to our crazy obsessions over our bodies and appearance, it's definitely safe to say that we're all crazy to some extent. And this is especially true with regards to food and body image. When it comes to bodily obsessions and perfection, women most definitely take the cake.

I have had far too much personal experience with the intricate relationship of food, body image, and athletics, and have come to realize how prominent and important it is in society today. Not many people like to acknowledge how prevalent disordered eating and skewed body image is among young women, but talk to most any female and they will have had some sort of issue at one time in their life. Talk to a few more, and a few of them will have struggled for years to overcome an impossible obstacle.

I am one of those women who have been plagued by food, exercise, and body image issues for as long as I can remember. Leaving the comfort zone of my over-active, over-exercising, under-eating, CrossFit-centered world and diving full force into lifting, which caused me to work out less and eat more, was one of the hardest things I have ever had to do. Not all people with disorders think the way I do, nor do they have the same specific issues that I do. But in the following pages, I will use my personal experiences to hopefully shed some light on what goes through the mind of an athlete (specifically an Olympic weightlifter) plagued with these issues, how to train with an eating disorder, and how coaches can help their athletes cope with their illness and to support them through their training and recovery.

IDENTIFYING THE PROBLEM

My background

It's healthy and normal to be concerned about exercise and diet; most of America isn't concerned (hence the obesity problems that are all too common nowadays), and I am usually complimented on my diligent exercise and eating regimen. However, there is a point where diligence and commitment morph into full-blown obsession, compulsion, and self-destruction. But what is that breaking point? How and why is it reached?

I am a perfectionist, not just athletically, but academically as well. Being competitive in the classroom fueled my competitive nature in athletics, which was especially evident when I found CrossFit in 2004, at the innocent age of 14. For some unknown reason, my intense perfectionism, my athletic drive, and my new-found obsession with food (thanks to a week of calorie tracking in health class) planted a seed in my mind that would ultimately be my downfall. Athletics became a tool for burning calories, a competition with my body on how much I could work out; eating became a game, a challenge to myself, seeing how little food I could eat but still be able to function. Such was most of my high school experience. And then came the wonders of the Zone Diet. Suddenly I never had to worry about counting calories; I could count blocks instead! No, I wasn't measuring my teaspoons of olive oil or my 3 cups of broccoli or 4 oz of chicken to count calories! It was all about the blocks! But of course I was just fooling myself; I still counted every calorie, and completely panicked when I didn't know exactly what I was consuming.

So how does this have anything to do with strength athletes? Well, shortly after my discovery of the Zone Diet, I became a full time Olympic weightlifter. No longer could I run 6 miles if I felt guilty about eating a piece of cake; no longer did I feel that same rush after a hardcore CrossFit workout, or feel like I 'deserved' to eat. Working out could no longer be a tool for me to burn calories; I was completely out of my comfort zone. Not to mention I needed way more calories than I had ever consumed before. As a general rule of thumb for protein requirements, lifters need about 1 g per pound of bodyweight. Way more protein (and … calories) than I could ever fathom eating. And the panicking mechanisms have began to churn …

A lifter with disordered thinking is of special concern because of the nature of the sport. Bodyweight is important; performance is quantifiable, and actually matters; women especially want to look good, because singlets are honestly not incredibly flattering. And not to mention the mental aspect of the sport; lifting is incredibly taxing on the mind, and is especially hard on someone who is an extreme perfectionist (like me, and many other women with eating disorders), because no one makes all of their lifts, no one has perfect lifting days. And that can be life or death for someone with an eating disorder, which is exactly what happened to me.

What to look for

It took a while for me to realize that I had a serious problem and needed help. With lifting, it can be especially difficult, but here are a few things to ask yourself.

What is my relationship with food?

If food is your friend, you enjoy it, you know what you need, you are able to let loose and have fun once in a while without feeling guilty … that is good. But if you find yourself obsessing about ratios, blocks, calories; if you find the need to somehow purge after you eat something bad (whether it's by vomiting or through exercise); if food is the enemy … then you have a problem.

The Zone Diet is especially troublesome in my eyes. It is not common in the weightlifting world, but is extremely common among CrossFitters. At first, I believed it was the best thing for me. And initially, it was – for the first time in years I was eating semi-normally. No more starving myself. No more purging through exercise. No more chronic injuries (from lack of protein perhaps? Most likely…). But counting blocks just became a substitute for counting calories; the incessant weighing and measuring only fueled the evil voice inside my head. I couldn't adequately function if I didn't know how many blocks I was eating, which is far from healthy.

Why and how do I eat?

Why do we eat? We need food for fuel. Food fuels are daily activities and our exercise. We need it to survive, to function, and to excel at our sport. Humans are social animals; food is a part of our every day life and should be enjoyed. Sure, food shouldn't be used as a coping mechanism or for emotional eating, but there are many social benefits that come along with eating. People with eating disorders lose joy in food. Food is evil, not good; it becomes a challenge, a feat, to eat as little as possible, to eat as perfectly as possible. Food is no longer seen as a necessary aspect of life.

This is a problem; if what we use as fuel is now our enemy, how can we expect to function? We can't. There were some days I was so starving I could barely concentrate in school; food and hunger was on my mind 24/7. I had chronic injuries in gymnastics and lacrosse; my body was suffering.

Perfection is also key here. I do not starve myself as I did in high school, but the new enemy is perfection. 100% paleo? Low carb? This many grams of carbs per day? It all becomes a challenge, a challenge I can never fully live up to. Because who can honestly eat 100% paleo? Sure, if I really wanted to, I'd go for the bland deli turkey with lettuce at the salad bar instead of the barbecued pulled pork (which is delicious, by the way), which probably has a bit of sugar (although our college cafeteria is fantastic and uses very few extremely processed ingredients). And maybe I should go for the bland turkey every day.

But honestly, who wants to do that? I'd rather enjoy the barbecued pork that isn't 100% paleo than stuff some bland turkey in my mouth. But the Eating Disorder Voice inside my head always yells, "No, that's bad! What you ate is BAAAAD." Same with the low-carb approach. Fruit = bad, because it has sugar. Sweet potatoes? Avoid them like the plague. The normal side of my brain thinks, "What the hell are you saying? Fruit is bad? Sweet potatoes are evil? You can't eat fruit because it has too much sugar, or you'll be eating more than 30 g of carbs a day? What?" But this is what happens when that Little Voice becomes a Big Voice.

How we eat is just as important as why we eat. Do we eat when we're hungry? Do we eat with other people, in a social environment, like in a cafeteria, or with our family? If we go to a social function, are we ok with letting loose and eating less-than-perfect foods? Or do we eat alone, quietly, by ourselves? Are we embarrassed by what and how much we eat? Are we afraid of being judged?

One of the tricks I taught myself was to ignore my hunger. There are times I am so hungry I can almost hear my stomach shout "FEED MEEEE!" But no, I can't eat because I am still a part of the Eat Less challenge that my mind has set up for me. When I do eat, I eat more than the average female because I am a lifter. I am embarrassed to eat in front of others because of this. I avoid social functions because I know the food won't be ideal. I'm in college, and I miss out socially because I'm afraid of food ... and that is a problem.

How do I view myself?

Body image is such a difficult issue, especially for women. Most women go through periods of low self-esteem and negative views of their body; but the problems occur when these negative images overpower the positive ones and last for an extended period of time.

I would spend hours upon hours looking at myself in the mirror and finding ten million things wrong with myself. The list of Bad Things About My Body would've been pages long. I obsessed over every piece of clothing I'd wear, worrying 'Does this make me look fat?' My view of myself was intricately tied to my eating and performance in the gym. If I ate something bad, I immediately looked at myself in the mirror and truly believed that I looked fat. I had a bad day at the gym? The negative self-talk, all the reasons why I'm a failure or why I'm fat, was endless. Not good.

What is my relationship with exercise?

For me, food and exercise are completely inseparable. Food does not exist without exercise, and vice versa. This has been an enormous problem for me, especially since starting lifting, because if I don't feel like I worked out "hard" enough, or if it was a light week, I feel the need to eat less.

Exercise has always been a means of burning calories. If I don't workout for X amount of hours or don't do Y amount of exercises, I don't deserve to eat. Shoot, I ate WAY too much dessert; I'll have to do Murph tomorrow. Exercise became a form of punishment, a way of purging food. Even now, when I'm training for something more than just for fun, I still have this relationship with exercise and food which is an enormous burden and struggle that I deal with every day in my training.

Final thoughts

If you can relate to any of these issues, please get help. No one likes to ask for help, no one likes to admit they have a problem. But these aren't issues that can be easily dealt with alone. Sure I'd like to say I've conquered these demons, that I am completely in control of my training and my mental state; but I am not even close. And there is no way in hell I can do it alone. Especially if you are a serious athlete, it is absolutely vital to get on track, because your training will suffer; mine has tremendously.

Reach out to someone you can trust: a fellow athlete, a coach, teacher, boyfriend, family member. The people in your life that care the most will stick by your side no matter how tough it gets … and it will get tough.

BANANAS, CHOCOLATE AND A BIG RUSSIAN BEAR
MATT FOREMAN

Academy Award-winning actor Tom Hanks was giving an interview once and he was describing a job he had early in his career, before he was a big name, where he had worked with a group of actors and directors who were much more experienced and skilled than he was. It was a tough situation, as he described it, because he was working in a talent pool that was way over his head. However, instead of whining and complaining when he remembered it all, he spoke of the whole thing as a valuable time that made him much better as an actor and a professional. One of the quotes he used during this interview was, "You never learn anything unless you get your butt kicked first." This line always stuck with me and I've come to believe that Hanks was right, in a lot of ways. In application to weightlifting and professional life, I think one of the best moves you can ever make is to surround yourself with people who are better than you. You're forced to work twice as hard and learn twice as fast if you want to move up and become an equal to these people, instead of staying at the bottom of the totem pole and accepting your role as the wanna-be. Obviously, being around people who are better than you is going to put you in a position where you feel defeat and inferiority at times. But that defeat should sharpen your hunger and, hopefully, the end result will be that you found a way to step up your game and compete on an even level with the top players. These ideas are exactly what I think about when I remember a moment in 2000 when I got a chance to compete against the best weightlifter on the planet.

Andrei Chemerkin won the Olympic gold medal in the 1996 Atlanta games. A massive twenty four year-old Russian superheavyweight, Andrei pulled out one of the greatest clutch lifts in weightlifting memory when he crushed a 260 kilo clean and jerk (a weight he had never made before) on his last attempt to defeat Germany's Ronny

Weller and take the gold medal. It was an amazing moment that concluded one of the greatest superheavyweight competitions in Olympic history. After it was over, Andrei went on to establish himself as an almost unbeatable figure during the next four years. He followed up his Olympic victory with the 1997 World Championship, where he duplicated his Olympic final-attempt heroics by clean and jerking 262.5 kilos to once again beat Ronny Weller. Two more world championship titles in 1998 and 1999 gave

Chemerkin an aura of invincibility. Not only was he the strongest weightlifter walking God's green earth, he was also the consummate pressure performer. The big man proved several times that he possessed one of the most important qualities an athlete can have: the ability to put up his greatest performances when his back was against the wall and he only had one shot left. Many people, myself included, began to regard Andrei in the same fashion as Alexeev during his prime. He was the king, plain and simple.

Knowing this, I knew it would be one of the highlights of my career when I found out that I was going to compete against Chemerkin at the 2000 World University Championships in Montreal. I qualified to compete for the US team in the superheavyweight class, and it had been widely advertised that Andrei was going to lift at this meet. I never knew exactly why he chose to travel all the way to Canada for this competition. The meet was held in June, only a few months before the Sydney Olympics, where he was obviously going to be attempting to defend his title. Although there were several outstanding international athletes at this university worlds, no superheavyweights were in attendance that had any chance to compete with the big man. But regardless of any reasons or details, the strongest weightlifter in the universe was planning to show up at this meet and I was going to lift on the same platform. I saw some amazing things on this trip and I learned some of the best lessons of my life. Here's how it went...

Montreal...

When I arrived in Montreal for the competition, the buzz was working overtime. Everyone was talking about Andrei Chemerkin. How much was he going to lift? Was he going to attempt a world record? Why was he competing in this meet? Was he even a university student? I joked to somebody that his college verification paperwork would probably be a cocktail napkin with the words "Andrei goes to school. Signed, Andrei" written on it in pencil. Although there was an entire world championship competition happening that weekend and, interestingly, a world record had been set in one of the lighter women's weight classes, the big Russian grizzly was the main event. After I flew into the airport and traveled to the hotel to check into my room, I turned around in the hotel lobby and saw him walking past me.

It's important to understand that this is one enormous piece of manflesh we're talking about. Andrei was walking near me and he paused for a few minutes to speak to somebody else, and I got a good look at him. His height wasn't overwhelming. I'm six feet tall and I was looking eye-to-eye with him. But the height wasn't what made the impression. This man's head looked like a cannonball. And believe me, that cannonball was sitting on top of a gargantuan pile of muscle. Andrei weighed around 175 kilos at the time (385 pounds, and we'll talk more about his bodyweight later). He was wearing sweatpants, a t-shirt, and a flannel jacket that looked like it could have functioned as a pup tent for a troop of Boy Scouts. I noticed that he had a pack of bananas jammed into his pocket as he walked away. I don't mean that he had two or three bananas, either. Think about when you go to the grocery store and you see the bananas in the produce section, with eight or nine of them attached in a bunch. Just pick up one of these bunches, without picking any of the bananas off, and ram it into your pocket. That's what I'm talking about.

A couple of days later, our competition was getting ready to start and the superheavyweights were in the warm-up room preparing to walk out on the platform for introductions. Our names were called and we were put in a line before the competition director walked us out to the platform. That's when I turned around and saw that it was happening the way I hoped it would... Andrei and I were right next to each other in the introduction line. Although I knew he didn't speak much English, I extended my hand to him and said, "Good luck today, brother." He smiled and shook my hand. Actually, I should say he swallowed my hand with his catcher's mitt of a paw. It was like shaking hands with the abominable snowman. When we walked out to the platform, the crowd went crazy. The announcer went down the line and introduced each athlete one-by-one, and the whole time I kept thinking to myself, "God, I hope somebody gets a picture of me standing next to him."

Side story: After the competition was over, I left Montreal to go home and I was convinced that nobody had taken a picture of us in the introduction line. It was a bummer because Andrei was a living legend and a picture of the two of us together would be a nice addition to my weightlifting scrapbook. I got home, a few weeks passed, and I got an envelope in the mail. Inside the envelope were two or three pictures from the competition, including a nice shot of Andrei and me standing side by side during the introductions. It was a total surprise to me when I got the pictures in the mail, and there was a note inside saying, "I was at this meet watching and I took these. I hope you like them!" The good Samaritan, who I didn't even know at the time, was a seventeen year-old lifter named Carissa Gordon. That's a true story.

Back to the meet...

I had a mediocre day on the platform and placed sixth in the superheavyweight class. Andrei won, obviously, with "light lifts" of 190 in the snatch and 230 in the clean and jerk. No world record attempts, but there was plenty to see and learn as I watched his every move during the competition. First of all, his "stretching routine" was quite a sight. After he put on his shoes, which he had to do by posting his foot against a chair and then leaning forward because his gut was too massive for him to reach his feet, he stood up. Then he hopped off the ground three or four times. And when I say "hopped," I mean he moved his girth up and down by bending and extending his knees. I'm not sure if his feet actually separated from the floor. Then he extended his arms out to his sides and shook his hands like he was trying to get water off them. Then he walked over to a bar loaded to seventy kilos and did his first set of snatches. So much for a thorough dynamic stretch routine prior to working out!

Aside from jokes about his mass and his stretching, it was easy to see why he was a great weightlifter as he progressed through his snatches. His technique was impeccable and every single lift looked exactly the same. Same positions, same speed, same apparent level of effort from seventy kilos all the way up to 170. His competition attempts were 180, 185, 190 and they looked exactly the same as the first set I had seen him do in the warm-up room. The strength of this man was mind-bending. Nothing changed about his attitude, his facial expression, or his state of calm. After the snatches were over, the C&J warm-ups started. This is where I got to see what so many people had talked about for the previous two years.

I'm referring to Chemerkin's clean and jerk technique. Beginning around 1997, Andrei had caused a lot of controversy in the weightlifting world because of a change in the way he performed the C&J. The basic explanation of it is that he no longer caught his cleans on his shoulders. He would go through the pulling movement of the clean and then, during the turnover phase, he would simply turn his wrists over and hold the bar about three inches off his shoulders. Imagine what it would look like if an athlete was holding a clean on their shoulders and then began to press the bar overhead. The position of the bar when it rose to the level of the Adam's apple, that's where Andrei held the bar in the cleans. He would stand up from the squat, go through the normal dip/drive of the jerk, and jerk the bar overhead for a completed lift. At no time during the lift had the bar touched his body, except for the hip drive during the pull. This was freaky to look at and it obviously contradicted a number of rules for proper weightlifting technique. Most people attributed the change in his technique to increased bodyweight. When Andrei won the 1996 Olympics, he weighed 165 kilos and his physique was relatively proportional. However, he began to add several kilos in the following years and, by the 1999 World Championship, he weighed 181 kilos (just under 400 pounds). Much of this additional mass had developed in his upper body. Because of the huge increase in the size of his shoulders and arms, he simply lost the flexibility to hold a clean on his shoulders.

Sounds like a problem, right? Most coaches would tell athletes in this position to lose some weight or do some stretching to fix the flexibility problem in their upper body. I mean, you have to be able to hold the bar on your shoulders to do a clean and jerk, correct? That's where the dilemma started with Chemerkin. This man, believe it or not, could clean and jerk around 250 kilos using this technique. It may sound unbelievable, but I stood next to the competition platform in Montreal that day when Andrei made his last C&J of 230 kilos, and I can positively verify that the bar never touched his shoulders. Not even in the jerk dip! He literally held the bar around the level of his chin through the entire lift. Right or wrong, it was a feat of strength from another universe. Moreover, he had been lifting like that since 1998 and he had continued to win world championships. Despite the fact that his technique violated almost every rule of weightlifting (and physics), the man could still beat anybody on the planet. How could anybody tell him to fix anything?

Time for some kibtzing

In my humble opinion, Andrei fell victim to complacency during this process. He was the best lifter in the world and, for three years, nobody could touch him even if he was lifting with an atrocious technical error. Randall Strossen once approached him in the training hall of a world championship and asked him why he was clean and jerking this way. Chemerkin just smiled, pounded his shoulder with his fist and said, "Strong!" I believe the man saw himself as untouchable, regardless of any mistakes he was making. After his Atlanta victory, he did an interview with World Weightlifting magazine. In response to the question "What do you think of your future chances?" Andrei's response was, "I believe that at the next Olympic Games I will have an easier job than in Atlanta." He actually thought that his competition was going to get softer! However, we all know how this ride ended. A few months after Montreal, Andrei competed in the 2000 Sydney Olympics and got annihilated. Hossein Rezazedeh began his historic reign by winning the gold with a phenomenal 472.5 total. Ronny Weller, Chemerkin's former bridesmaid, won the silver with 467.5, and Armenian Ashot Danielyan won the bronze, leaving Chemerkin in fourth place. The untouchable champion had been shut out of the medals, completely. Eventually, Danielyan's drug test returned positive and he was forced to relinquish his bronze medal to Chemerkin. But regardless, it was a brutal thrashing for a man who many had thought was unbeatable.

So, what can we learn from this?

On the day of the Montreal competition, the sports page of the local newspaper featured an extensive interview with Chemerkin. The headline of the article was a quote from the champion that read, "THE DREAM OF EVERYONE IS TO DEFEAT ME."

After the competition, a teammate of mine approached Andrei and gave him a USA weightlifting pin as a gesture of sportsmanship. Andrei took the pin, glanced at it, and then handed it to somebody else without even acknowledging my teammate.

The man was not modest or humble, or even gracious to his fellow competitors. These are qualities that are, for better or for worse, very common in great champions like Chemerkin. I've heard many stories about Vasily Alexeev that make Chemerkin sound like a contender for Miss Congeniality. Having a healthy dose of ego is an essential ingredient to being great at something. However, there is a caveat to it.

I believe Chemerkin became comfortable with the idea that nobody could beat him. Comfort is the enemy of progress. From my perspective, and this is just one man's opinion, that comfort level laid the foundation for some laziness. Now, can we call a man "lazy" if he is winning world championships? The answer to that question is YES because laziness begins as soon as the individual stops paying attention to all the little details. Some writers have referred to this concept as "believing your own headlines." Andrei's bodyweight increase, from 363 pounds when he won the gold medal in Atlanta to 400 pounds three years later, clearly did not work to his benefit. Basic understanding of physiology tells us that giant increases in bodymass can potentially restrict flexibility, which is especially problematic in a sport that is as dependent on flexibility as weightlifting is. Andrei's upper-body flexibility went in the toilet and he continued to win world championships anyway, with snatches around 200 kilos and jerks around 260 kilos. But he did not make the training adjustments he needed to make to improve his total, and a hungry young Iranian lion was training Clubber Lang-style for the moment when he would have the chance to steal Chemerkin's claim to being the strongest weightlifter in the world. Andrei told a Montreal reporter that the dream of everyone was to defeat him. Those dreams became his worst nightmares before the summer of 2000 ended.

There are two final thoughts to this story. First of all, who am I to critique an Olympic gold medalist and three-time world champion? The man accomplished things that I never did, no doubt about it. This article, in a way, is the mother of all armchair quarterback articles. True, true... But despite these facts, I believe that there are lessons to be learned in everything and I sure as hell believe that the rise and fall of this particular weightlifter has some useful ones.

Second, competing against this colossus was, as I thought it would be, one of the highlights of my career. Although I knew that I had no chance to beat him, it was still a privilege to share the stage with one of the strongest men who has ever touched a barbell. Despite the fact that I think his career could have ended differently if he had taken more careful precautions with the flexibility problems he developed, there is still no doubt about the greatness of his career. Most athletes would sacrifice a limb to have one single moment when they can be identified as the best in the world. Andrei Chemerkin got to spend four years of his life in that moment. His performances were amazing. But, as Tom Hanks said, getting your butt kicked can make you better. Chemerkin kicked a lot of butts from 1997-1999. At the 1999 World Championship, he kicked Hossein Rezazedeh's butt. Then he went to the 2000 Olympics, the one he had predicted in the interview to be "easier than Atlanta." Apparently, Reza didn't get the memo. I guess weightlifting is like a box of chocolates. You never know what you're gonna get.

TEACHING THE OLYMPIC LIFTS IN THE CROSSFIT GROUP SETTING
GREG EVERETT

Sometimes your clients are confused. It's true. Some want to squat to big padded balls instead of just learning where their asses are and squatting like grown-ups all the way to the bottom. Some want to do low-bar back squats. And some aren't very interested in learning the snatch and clean & jerk. Fortunately, as a trainer or coach, it's your responsibility to train your clients according to what they need rather than what they want—if they knew what they needed, they wouldn't be your clients.

This is not to say that as a trainer you get to determine your clients' goals—it means simply that the reason someone is paying you is to determine how best to achieve those goals and to lead them through the process. This often means their doing certain things they may not want to do initially.

When it comes to complex lifts like the snatch and clean & jerk, this lack of interest can make learning a difficult and comparatively unsuccessful endeavor. At least part of the issue is that many in CrossFit—both on the client and trainer levels—don't understand the extent of the lifts' complexity, and consequently fail to put in adequate time and effort to learning both the lifts execution and methods of teaching them. This magnifies the silliness described previously and leads to behavior such as celebrating lift performances like those seen during the snatch event of the last CrossFit Games.

In addition to this, teaching the Olympic lifts in a group setting in which they're not only not the primary focus of training, but in which individuals are typically all at different levels of experience, skill, motivation, strength, flexibility and similar factors, becomes far more complicated and frustrating.

In order to address both basic problems described above, we can create a system of teaching the lifts that accommodates different levels of ability, reduces time dedicated to the lifts within any given training session—which allows a breadth of training as well as minimizes the possible effects of clients' disinterest in the lifts and consequent lack of focus and effort—yet not only remains effective, but is arguably more effective than more focused teaching approaches.

Building the Foundation

The finer details of the teaching system employed by each gym will vary just as all other details of training with vary among CrossFit gyms. There are numerous possible approaches to teaching the lifts in such a setting, and which is used and most effective will vary depending on factors such as how exactly the group training program is administered and the relative emphases on various training components. For example, a gym with a relatively small and consistent clientele is able to do things differently than on with a large and less consistent clientele. Similarly, a gym that emphasizes strength work will have better options than one that uses the common Jazzercise approach of random and extended metabolic workouts with equally random and infrequent strength work. That's another article altogether, but suffice to say if your gym falls into the latter category, you have some fundamental restructuring to do before really worrying about getting this jiggy with the Olympic lifts specifically.

Get Perspective

The first step in develop such a teaching system is learning to consider training in the long term. The failure to do this is a common problem in CrossFit gyms, resulting in random or arbitrary programming that is unable to address long term progress. Your clients will not be training for only a day or a week—why would you approach their training plan in such a term?

Know What You're Doing

This is a fairly important one. If you don't understand the Olympic lifts and how they should be executed, you have no business teaching them to your clients. A Level 1 certification and some CrossFit Journal videos are not an adequate background. There's nothing wrong with such a background—what's wrong is believing or insisting that it prepares you to teach and coach the lifts. Have the integrity as a professional trainer to recognize this and do your homework. Learn more and get better by working privately with qualified weightlifting coaches and attending seminars. (I know of a decent book that might be helpful too.)

Until that point, bring in an outside coach to work with your clients occasionally in a seminar or occasional class format; if this isn't possible stick with the exercises you know how to teach. Anything else is a disservice to your clients, who are likely paying you handsomely for your presumed expertise. They will respect and appreciate you far more for admitting your lack of expertise in a particular special area, than for teaching them poorly. You don't have to be the greatest weightlifting coach in the world—you do need to have a solid grasp of the fundamentals to avoid teaching your clients so many of the ridiculous things they find out later they have to change.

Have a Plan

This ties in with gaining perspective. Figure out what you're doing before you start doing it. This saves everyone time and frustration, and allows far more effective teaching. Having a plan doesn't necessarily mean that even the most minute details are in print three months prior to starting—it means having a level of detail sufficient to guide you to your intended goals. This plan can be flexible, and must be to some extent considering the setting about which we're talking, but at no time should the approach be arbitrary or based on what you happen to feel like doing at the moment.

Shaping the System

Whatever system is finally established, it must take into account a few key elements:

1. Different skill levels among clients in a class
2. Regular influx of new clients
3. Inconsistent training schedules of clients
4. Available time in training sessions for this component
5. Attention span of clients
6. The role of the lifts in the overall program

Different Skill Levels

Unless a gym brings on new clients in a structured group format like an On-Ramp program, and subsequently keeps these clients locked into given class times for the duration of their membership, there is bound to be a broad spectrum of skill and experience among clients in a class (even with such a rigid approach, different clients learn more quickly and perform better than others). With an system for teaching the lifts, we need to be able to accommodate all of these clients, not just teach to a certain level because it's simplest for us. This is easily the most difficult aspect of the process.

The ideal way to address this problem would be to separate clients into different classes based on demonstrated ability. Such stratification is immensely helpful with respect to all aspects of training, but is often very impractical. It means limiting, often greatly, the number of possible classes for each client, while simultaneously increasing the burden of the trainers. There are few gyms that are able to make such a structure work. However, few if any gyms should be unable to separate the absolute beginners from the rest of the clientele—this again can be accomplished by using a system of entry to the program like the On-Ramp classes. This alone makes the task of teaching the lifts far easier and more effective by simply removing the least skilled clients from the equation. They don't factor in until they've achieved a basic level of proficiency with fundamental exercises.

The next best option would be multiple trainers working with the clients in a given class so those clients can be grouped together according to skill level and lead through different training during a single class. While somewhat more practical than separating actual classes, this is still difficult and expensive.

Instead, we need to find a way to have clients function independently enough that a single trainer can run a class without sacrificing the effectiveness of their training or the trainer's ability to provide the necessary instruction. This can really only be accomplished with a genuine plan and structure as discussed previously. In general terms, this means simply determining how much skill variation exists among the clients of a given gym, deciding how many levels of instruction are required to accommodate all of those clients, and then what exactly each skill level will be working on during a given training session. The details of this will be filled out later in the article.

Influx of New Clients

The regular influx of new clients to a CrossFit gym is the source of numerous problems with regard to class structuring and instruction. How this affects the instruction of the Olympic lifts specifically will vary depending on how a gym channels these new clients. A facility that simply jumps new clients into existing classes will have a far more difficult time than one that takes new clients through some sort of introductory class series to establish fundamental exercise proficiency, a base level of work capacity, and a general understanding of how to function as a client within a group training environment. Again, the ideal way of addressing this problem is to use some type of introductory system like an On-Ramp program that separates rank beginners from the rest of the crowd.

Inconsistent Training Schedules

Often one of the most frustrating and limiting aspects of CrossFit style group training is the inconsistent training schedules of the clients. That is, some may come three days each week, and some six; some may come on the same days and times each week, while others show up randomly. This of course makes programming a far more difficult task, and unavoidably reduces the effectiveness of the program for individual clients.

While we can't control clients' attendance, we can prioritize clients and channel our time and efforts accordingly. Our commitment as trainers and coaches should reflect the commitment of our clients—those clients who go out of their way to attend frequently and regularly and train with focus and dedication deserve more attention and effort than those who attend inconsistently and appear to be interested in little more than post-spastic-workout euphoria.

This means programming with your priority clients in mind. This can be done literally—considering the schedules and needs of actual priority clients—or using a theoretical model of your ideal client (as long as it's reasonable). For example, we may program with a consistent 5-day weekly client in mind and simply be flexible for clients who don't fit into this category.

Available Time

How much time in each training session is available for Olympic lift instruction will obviously shape to a large degree what we do. Ideally the instruction and practice of the lifts is taken into consideration when designing the overall structure of the gym's program rather than it being an afterthought. If it is, this will be far less of an issue because adequate time will always be available. If it's not, we will have to work around silliness like medicine ball cleans and sumo deadlift high-pulls in obscene quantities. This just means less time to dedicate to the important things in life like skill and strength.

Client Attention Spans

CrossFitters tend to have comparatively limited attention spans—this characteristic is part of the attraction to a training system that prides itself on constant variation, extremely brief workouts and goals that are by design entirely non-specific. This needs to be taken into account when designing a system of teaching involved and complex movements, particularly when so many clients will have been convinced that the Olympic lifts are not actually technically complex and can be taught adequately in three minutes with a medicine ball.

Part of solving this problem is educating and re-educating your clients regarding the lifts and their role in their training. If your gym's program, from the beginning of each client's exposure, emphasizes the importance of technical proficiency, strength and Olympic lifts, structured programming, and long term planning, you can expect little if any resistance. If instead your program evolves into this from the Jazzercise type of random metabolic conditioning workouts with infrequent and equally random strength training, clients may have difficulty with the transition simply because they're not accustomed to the new format.

As the trainer, it's your responsibility to stand by your decision. Don't feel obligated to explain why the change is being made unless asked. Sputtering on about training theory to clients to aren't interested simply makes you appear unsure about what you're doing and why you're doing it. It's easy to be confident regarding your programming if you develop it logically; if you're not confident in your gym's program, you have some serious re-evaluation and restructuring to do.

This will in part, along with the role of the lifts discussed next, determine how involved and technical the instruction of the lifts is. That is, shorter attention spans mean more focus on drills to teach the body how to lift and less focus on actual technical education regarding the finer details and reasons why.

Role of the Lifts

A final consideration when developing your training system is what role the Olympic lifts play in the overall training program. That is how much emphasis is placed on them relative to other lifts and other types of training, and how will they be used—independently as real lifts, within metabolic workouts, or both. Additionally, this will be part of the determination of how technical teaching is. The greater the role the lifts play in the program, the more technical their instruction will need to be in order to improve clients' execution.

The Lifts within the Training Program

All this talk of mixed skill levels and the importance of technical proficiency begs the question: How do we use the Olympic lifts within metabolic conditioning workouts in a group? The easiest answer is not to. The reality is that the overwhelming majority of CrossFit clients will never reach a level of technical proficiency that makes the lifts' use within metabolic workouts a great idea, simply because the proportion of their training time dedicated to the lifts is minimal.

There are better options for conditioning that won't hinder further development of lift technique while still providing a large metabolic dent—arguably more of one, in fact. Additionally, dumbbell, sandbag, and other implement variations of the Olympic lifts can be used to provide most of the metabolic effects desired from the lifts—these lifts require far less instruction and practice to be effective and are distinct enough to not interfere with technique for the barbell lifts. (It should be noted that these exercises do not include the medicine ball clean, because it is hopelessly lame and has no place in anyone's training.)

Within a CrossFit gym with clients who have established reasonable technical proficiency with the barbell Olympic lifts, these lifts can be used within conditioning workouts if desired. The solution to mixed skill levels within a class is to simply scale the workouts with respect to exercise variation—for example, the top-tier clients may snatch; a middle-tier may 1-arm dumbbell snatch; and a bottom-tier may do jumping dumbbell squats and/or overhead squats. This allows the more advanced athletes to train more effectively, and allows the more novice athletes to train more appropriately without separating them entirely—this helps foster a team atmosphere by keeping everyone performing a similar workout in essence, but doesn't compromise individual clients' training.

To Be Continued

In the next issue, we'll finalize this process with the steps of designing the program itself, as well as a sample program to get you started.

TEACHING THE OLYMPIC LIFTS
IN THE CROSSFIT GROUP SETTING PART 2
GREG EVERETT

Before we continue on this particular adventure, I want to provide some clarification on a few items from the first part of the article. It has been pointed out to me that some of my remarks offended certain individuals, and because this was not my intention, I'm going to take a moment to apologize for any offense that was taken, and to provide my rationale for those remarks. While I may make jokes of certain things, my opinions on them are never without reason.

These reasons are not ones pulled from the ether—they are based on the sum of my training experiences, both in and out of CrossFit. My experience with CrossFit itself dates back to some time in early 2004 when I started working with CrossFit coach extraordinaire, Robb Wolf, and shortly thereafter became a partner in CrossFit NorCal, the fourth affiliate. I had been a credentialed trainer for six years prior to this, but very quickly saw CrossFit as not only an amazing training system, but a community that was beginning to attract the kind of coaches and athletes with whom I wanted to interact, learn and improve. This included people like Robb, Greg Glassman, Michael Rutherford (CF Kansas City), Mike Burgener, Jeff and Mikki Martin (Brand X Martial Arts), and Josh Everett (strength coach, UCR—and not my brother). To this day, these people are some of the greatest contributors to my education as a trainer and athlete, and are good friends— one of the greatest aspects of CrossFit.

Since my start with NorCal, I've had a lot of time to experiment with and evaluate various CrossFit-related protocols with my own clients (I've never counted, but I'm guessing I've worked with at least 10-20 over the years), as well as to discuss such things with other trainers in and out of the CrossFit community. It is on this collective experience that I base my opinions—not whim, fashion or convention.

The Low-Bar Back Squat

Let's take care of this one first since it's such a popular topic. Most readers of the PM are likely already familiar with my opinion regarding the low-bar back squat, and particularly its use by weightlifters.

Generally I confine my opinion regarding the LBBS to weightlifting, but let me turn over another stone and explain my aversion to it for the generalist. First, if you are a generalist, do it… sometimes. Don't replace the back squat with it completely. I say this not because I like the LBBS for the generalist, but because as a generalist, the more exposure you have to more exercises, the better off you'll be. In my opinion, its use should be infrequent and more as a tool for achieving occasional variety than as a staple exercise. I see it the same way I see the box squat—it has a purpose, it can be legit in the right circumstances, but it's not an exercise on which to build a training foundation.

The reasons for this can be found partly in the aforementioned article, but obviously there's more to it since we're not talking about weightlifters here. In short, the squat is the only potential full knee and hip range of motion strength exercise—the bottom position of the LBBS limits the range of motion of the knee and prevents an opportunity for the quad to open the knee joint in its most mechanically disadvantaged angles. We can combine the LBBS with the front squat, of course, to accommodate this desire for complete knee flexion and greater quad reliance, but two problems arise. First, it's a different lift—in a sense more of a core exercise than a leg and hip exercise. Second, individuals whose only other squat is the LBBS invariably perform the front squat poorly. This is due in part to having trouble reconciling the movement pattern of the LBBS with that of the front squat; the former involving an active backward drive of the hips, and the latter requiring simultaneous knee and hip flexion with as direct of a downward path for the hips as possible. This results in front squats with the hips swinging back on the way up and down, which pulls in more posterior chain and reduces the work for the quads, changing the effect of the exercise (and ultimately limiting loading).

The technical causes of this problem can of course be corrected through coaching and practice, but the strength-related causes are more difficult to correct. For an individual who emphasizes the posterior chain through squatting and pulling exercises, the requisite quad strength will simply not exist to maintain the upright posture and hip path that we're after in the front squat. This leads to the poor performance described above, which simply reinforces the current strength disparity around the knee.

Contributing to this problem is the deadlifting and Olympic lift pulling postures typically employed by generalists who use the low-bar back squat. These pulling postures are also designed to emphasize posterior chain contribution and limit knee involvement.

This prevalence of posterior-chain emphasis strength work fails to balance the quad-dominance it is often claimed to be correcting, and simply swings the pendulum to the other side, creating the kind posterior-chain dominance that prevents desirable front squat and Olympic lift mechanics. This limits an individual's athletic development by retarding progress in the lifts and placing too much emphasis on certain elements, positions and movements. For the generalist, attempting to improve in all respects, this should be quite clearly a problem.

Squatting to Balls

The use of medicine balls as depth gauges for squats is not one I endorse, and one I have admittedly ridiculed—not with intentions of insulting anyone in particular, more to make a point that happens to involve what some find funny. There are times very early in the learning stages for some clients during which achieving adequate depth in a squat is difficult, and during which the client's sense of his or her depth is not accurate. In such cases, one method of encouraging better depth, teaching a sense of position, and better engaging the glutes and hamstrings is to have such clients squat to an object of appropriate height.

This practice is not one I object to, because it can be quite effective. That said, a medicine ball is not, in my opinion, an appropriate object for this. If a client is having difficulty of a degree and nature that necessitates this method of teaching and practice, a ball is not only generally too low of a target, but more importantly, is not a stable and reliable platform to support that client should he or she crash at the bottom. If you have a client who is unstable, weak and in such little control over his or her body that they need to be squatting to a target, the last thing you want is that target being one that allows a fall and actually magnifies the potential for damage.

Medicine balls roll, compress, and otherwise provide an unreliable target; more importantly, their height is not adjustable, and no one can tell me with a straight face that people of all statures and abilities should be squatting to an identical depth. Boxes provide a stable, consistent and reliable target and platform for support if needed, and their height can be easily adjusted appropriately for an individual by stacking plates or similar items on top or underneath.

Finally, if as a trainer you decide to use a box in the early stages of teaching an individual to squat, it should be confined to that stage—it is a temporary tool to achieve a specific set of goals. To continue using anything once an athlete is able to squat to proper depth—especially a ball that rolls, allows an individual to bounce, and is very unlikely the proper height—is a disservice to your clients, who need to eventually develop a reliable sense of position on their own. The concepts of "elite" and "unaware of ass location" cannot describe the same individual. (And of course, as was alluded to in the remarks contained in the first part of this article, actually squatting all the way down makes this much less of an issue—it's pretty difficult to not recognize when your hamstrings are pressed against your calves.)

Sumo Deadlift High-Pull

I lumped this exercise in with medicine ball cleans as "silliness" I ostensibly wouldn't allow with my own clients. This is a minor objection, but my view is simply this: Why not just perform a deadlift high-pull? What advantage does a sumo stance provide for this exercise other than making it easier, and why would we want to make it easier? If, for conditioning, we're interested in moving large loads long distances quickly, why would we shorten the distance we can possibly move the weight, and particularly in a manner that reduces the work of the legs and hips but maintains the work of the shoulders and arms?

I actually use kettlebell deadlift high-pulls in our On-Ramp program, but following those few exposures, it rarely comes up again. Once out of the beginning stages of learning, our clients no longer need such an exercise—they can deadlift, clean, snatch and the like with various implements. I'm not completely averse to ever doing high-pulls, as I do feel they have their place in certain situations, but the reality is that in large and frequent doses, they encourage habits that interfere with clean and snatch technique, which is already difficult enough to teach to generalists. The SDHP is absolutely not an acceptable substitute for the clean, and it should not be considered a part of a teaching progression for the clean. It is strictly a metabolic workout exercise, and, in my opinion, is not one of the better options available.

Level 1 Certifications and the Olympic Lifts

I'm actually not sure if my remarks on this topic were among those not taken well by certain individuals, but in the interest of thoroughness, I'll address it anyway. First, I'm not interested in critiquing the curriculum of CF certifications. It's not my business, and I'm happy to leave the decisions to those who make a living running them—I'm going to assume they have good reason for doing what they do how they do it, and that their guiding intention is creating what they feel are the best fitness trainers possible. My point was actually quite simple, and disagreement with it would absolutely baffle me—the Level 1 certification does not prepare trainers to teach the snatch and clean & jerk, and to insist otherwise is completely irresponsible.

CrossFit trainers who want to become competent in teaching the Olympic lifts need—at the very least—to attend one of Coach Burgener's weightlifting certifications. The reality is that no two-day seminar, even on a single topic with an incredible coach like Burgener, can provide as much instruction, practice and experience as is needed to become genuinely competent in instructing the lifts. It should be considered one part of an ongoing process. In fact, I strongly encourage trainers to attend Burgener's cert more than once if possible—the second time through will be even more enlightening with the experience accumulated since the first. This being said, it should be fairly obvious that a two-day seminar that barely touches on the Olympic lifts certainly cannot create great weightlifting coaches. This just means, as one of our weightlifters, Steve, likes to say, staying in your lane—teach what you know, and continue to learn more.

Not being an expert in the Olympic lifts does not make you a bad trainer—posing as an expert to the detriment of your clients does. The experience level of new CrossFit trainers generally parallels that of their clients; that is, trainers will be able to continually improve their experience and abilities at a pace that keeps up with the needs of their clients. It's unnecessary to reach beyond one's scope of experience, then; clients will be better served by instruction and practice of the fundamentals before venturing into more advanced movements.

The Complexity of the Olympic Lifts

Related to the previous was my comment of the general under-recognition by CrossFitters of the technical complexity of the snatch and clean & jerk. This actually can be attributed to a number of sources; let me just say that it's not a surprise when the lifts are given little attention, both within training and in terms of instruction—such a perspective can be expected to develop. Again, trainers are encouraged to spend time with weightlifting coaches and weightlifters—training, watching, talking. Exposure to the weightlifting community directly is the best (and arguably only) way to develop a sincere appreciation for the level of skill required for technical proficiency in the lifts.

This should not be misunderstood as an expectation of generalists to become expert weightlifters—by definition of the term generalist, that would be impossible. It is an expectation, however, that generalists place appropriate emphasis on developing snatch and clean & jerk technique. It should be obvious that the elements of an individual's training that require the most skill require the most practice: the Olympic lifts and the handful of basic gymnastics movements are these elements. Once an individual can perform a thruster, how much practice does he or she really need with it? The only necessary exposures to the movement after it's learned are those in which it's used for training purposes. The snatch and clean & jerk, on the other hand, cannot be mastered in a similar manner and timeframe. Weightlifters perform the competition lifts and variations thereof generally 4-6 days each week, sometimes multiple times each day, for years on end, and continue emphasizing technique improvement. There is not a single CrossFitter, present, past or future, who would not benefit from more coaching and practice in the lifts.

At least once I've heard it said that the Olympic lifts don't even compare in complexity to gymnastics movements. I'll be the first to agree, if we're talking about the entire collection of competitive and training movements. Within the realm of CrossFit, however, gymnastics movements are restricted to a handful of extremely basic ones that certainly don't rival the complexity of the snatch and clean & jerk.

The CrossFit Games Snatch Event

This one may have stung a bit for a number of people, and for that I apologize, but my assessment is not one arising from anything but what I feel are reasonable expectations of a community that strives for and claims the status of elite. The snatch is a competitive exercise that conforms accordingly to a number of technical rules. These rules are not exclusively for the sake of competition, however—there are elements of execution that are important for the sake of athletic development. Two extremely basic ones are that no part of the body other than the feet can contact the ground, and that the bar must be received and held overhead with fully extended elbows. Both of these were violated repeatedly by many competitors, often dramatically. In fact, it seemed at times, the greater the violation, the more people were impressed.

Having said all this, part of the problem could have been resolved by simply not calling the event a snatch—call it a ground to overhead anyhow, and I have no serious complaints. However, if the precision of the exercise is removed, so is much of the point. If the goal is to simply move weight with no concern for how, there are better ways to do it, which move more weight. The only reason I can imagine to hold a snatch event is to distinguish athletes further along in their development to those less experienced—those who have put in the time and effort to develop greater skill than the next athlete. Once you remove the technical requirements, it's simply another strength event—so why not squat, press, etc. instead?

Jazzercise

If you as a gym owner or programmer have no plan, no long-term perspective, no underlying structure and only infrequent and random strength work, you're failing to tap into CrossFit's true potential and are doing your clients a disservice. If this hurts your feelings, quit being satisfied with the easy approach, do your homework, and strive to continue improving the service you provide.

Finally—The Medicine Ball Clean

Of all my potentially offensive remarks, this one may have been the most offensive because of its role in the Level 1 curriculum and its use by many CrossFit gyms. My objection to this, despite the opinions of certain individuals, is actually for very specific reasons.

There are a few relatively minor issues that still manage to chap my ass. One is the head position the athlete is forced to assume with the ball in the "rack" position—tilted way back to make room for the ball. More important is the rack position itself—there is no rack. The ball is supported entirely in the arms, which is understandable to some extent, but the ball is racked with the elbows straight down—not exactly a great habit to be developing for future grown-up cleans. Related to this is the elbow movement of the pull under the ball, which is taught as back and around rather than initiating the pull with the up and out elbow direction that is necessary to pull under a heavy clean. Again, these are comparatively minor problems, but problems nonetheless, and when the ostensible goal is to teach a complex movement as quickly as easily as possible (presumably accurately, as well), it makes little sense to create habits that must be unlearned later.

Next is the instruction to shrug the ball up at the top of the leg and hip extension. Not only should the shrug not be occurring at this point, the manner of teaching encourages hesitation at the top of the extension, which is not a problem when one is cleaning a 20 lb padded ball, but will quite effectively prevent a successful clean with significant weights. The athlete needs to be taught to change directions following leg and hip extension as quickly as possible, and needs to understand that the shrug occurs as he or she is moving down under the implement—it does not elevate the implement. Using an odd-object for an individual's initial exposure to the clean teaches poor body position and stiff arms directed away from the body.

The progression is simply backward. An individual who can clean a barbell can clean anything; an individual who has only cleaned a medicine ball can clean things that look and feel like medicine balls, and only do that in the manner in which one can clean a medicine ball. The transferability is bordering on non-existent. It makes no sense at all to teach a medicine ball clean when one can in the matter of minutes teach a dumbbell clean, which can be taught and executed in a manner that closely resembles a barbell clean, will not interfere with later learning of the barbell clean, will provide quality training effects, and actually has the potential for some legitimate loading.

Finally, if, as CrossFit trainers and athletes, we're so elite, why can't we even teach or perform a barbell clean correctly?

I Hate to Do It, But...

I'm going to anyway. Because this unplanned detour became quite extensive, I'm going to postpone finalizing the article with the actual teaching progressions until next month. Until then, use your medicine balls for real exercises, go to one of Burgener's certs, watch some videos of weightlifters, and kick the medicine balls out from under your clients.

ADVANCED OPTIONS WITH THE MAX EFFORT BLACK BOX
MICHAEL RUTHERFORD

"I guess I'm an awfully good sponge. I absorb ideas from every course I can, and put them to practical use. Then I improve them until they become of some value. The ideas which I use are mostly the ideas of other people who don't develop them themselves."

— Thomas Edison when complemented on his creative genius.

Since 2004 when I first proposed the overlaying of Effort lifting with CrossFit / GPP (Max Effort Black Box aka MEBB), I've worked on numerous template designs. I've listened to athletes and coaches from various walks of life and different sports. The questions have come from those who just love CrossFit and want to do it better to the high school and College coach who want to employ CrossFit but also need more strength.

Several CrossFit Games participants have confessed to using the templates. Testimonials from multiple individuals are littered throughout my blog and on my testimonials page.

To Date here's what we know for certain occurs to the athletic fitness profile of MEBB users:

- Enhanced athletic fitness
- Improved CrossFit Performance
- Improved athletic movement
- Better Training Variety
- Enhanced Power/Explosivenes
- Reduction in orthopedic stress
- Long Term Improvement—No Theoretical Limit
- Increases in lean body mass (LBM)
- Flex use of components

Never quite satisfied with the status quo, I've been working with an advanced template. I've had this out in BETA in different variations since Spring 2009. I want to share elements of this program with you today.

Adding Speed & Volume Tiers

One thing I've fought constantly with any of the MEBB templates was the overachieving, hyperactive "What Else can I do?" personality. If I didn't hand out additional assignments, they would go off the rails and just do something random. This got me to thinking that I needed to consider another way to harness that energy in a productive way.

As a result, in addition to the Effort tier, I have added a Speed tier and a Volume Tier. Adding speed and volume are elements from a concurrent / Westside Template.

Speed Tiers

These are sub-maximal loads (50% of 1RM) executed at maximal velocities. Examples of this would be 10 sets of 2 reps with 50% of the 1 RM squat with 1:00 of rest. Another would be a Hurdle hop or high box jump. Westside barbell founder Louis Simmons has train a number of sprinters with the Concurrent method and speed tier work is an important element in their training plan.

Effort Tier work (Strength –Speed) displaces the Force / Velocity Curve by working on the Force component. The Speed (Speed-Strength) helps to further displace the Curve by working on the Velocity at which the force is applied. (Kraemer and Fleck OPTIMIZING STRENGTH TRAINING 2007)

Volume Tiers

Volume Tiers add dimension to muscle fiber, thickens connective tissue and increases capillary density. Volume Tiers are high-repetition sets reaching close to if not to muscle failure. Think bodybuilders. For the upper body, an athlete could perform 3 sets of 20 reps of suspended push-ups. Bilateral Lower Body Tiers are balanced with unilateral lunge patterns in the Volume Tier. Total body volume work is best accomplished with complexes using barbells or dumbbells.

Effort / Speed / Volume

The advanced template concurrently trains Power, Speed and Muscle density components. The order is Effort Tier, Speed Tier and finally the Volume Tier. A daily session might look like this.

1. Warm Up Moves

2. Hang Power Snatch 3 x 3, 3 x 1
3. Squats 8 x 2 @50% of 1RM
4. Suspended Push ups 3 x RM
5. Glute Ham Raise 3 x 15
6. Post Stretch / Foam Roller

Weekly Template 3/1 2/1

To date our best feedback points to a 3 on with 1 day rest followed by 2 on with 1 Day Rest. We rotate 2 or 3 effort/speed/volume tier days with 2 or 3 CrossFit couplets or triplets. The process for managing all this occurs with a MS Excel designed training tracker.

I must note that selecting ideal CrossFit couplets or triplets takes a keen understanding of the athlete's unique skill set. It's not a perfect science, but let's be frank, nothing in applied exercise science is or has been perfect.

During my Intelligent Exercise Design seminars, we will be tackling the MEBB package from the original construct to this advanced topic. I look forward to discussing the merits of this process in the very near future.

SPEED TRAINING FOR THE NON TRACK ATHLETE
SCOTT KUSTES

If you play sports (you do play sports, right?), you can probably improve your game by being faster. In fact, I can't think of a single sport that doesn't benefit from increased straight-line speed. In baseball, it's base-running. Ball carriers in football want "breakaway speed," while linebackers need "closing speed". A basketball court may only be 92' long, but it involves constant acceleration out of quick cuts.

You could argue that boxers and MMA fighters don't need a great deal of acceleration and speed and I couldn't argue back, so let's just let that one die. But even marathon runners train for speed.

As such, I've been thinking about how to incorporate additional speed training into the program of a non-track athlete's GPP phase. Of course, you won't become a competitive track and field athlete without some specialization, but that doesn't mean you won't benefit from throwing some real speed training into your workouts.

What Is Speed?

To make it simple, speed is power. A fast athlete is a powerful athlete. You'll rarely find someone that's fast in a straight line that can't also hold their own in other athletic endeavors. Sport-specific skills aside, speed has direct carry-over to most anything you could want to do athletically.

When you look at a sprinter, whether it's Tyson Gay or a 40-year old Master's competitor, what you're seeing is "mass-specific force"—the ability to produce force relative to body mass—combined with "rate of force production"—how fast that force can be produced.

Those two things come together to produce stride length, which is effectively how far you're launching your body with each step. Multiply stride length by stride rate and the answer is how fast you can cover a given distance.

How To Increase Speed

So given what we know about speed, we can either increase stride length or increase stride rate to cover ground more quickly. So do you want to go farther which each step or take more steps? Ideally, both, but if you had to pick one to focus on, which would it be? If you guessed that you should want to cover more distance per step, you're exactly right. If you guessed otherwise, sorry.

Now, they're actually interdependent variables, but considering that elite sprinters are turning over about 4.5-5 times per second and the rest of us are probably somewhere around (just a guess) 4-ish, there's far more to be gained from increasing stride length. If we look at the current sprinting god, Usain Bolt, and compare him to other elite sprinters, we find that he's covering 100m in about 40 strides. It's taking the other incredibly fast guys 44-48 strides. Bolt goes farther with each stride, even though all of them are in the same ballpark regarding stride frequency.

In fact, I'd bet that my stride rate is fairly close to Bolt's. But I don't cover 2.5m per stride, and there's the major difference. He might take an extra half-stride per second, but he probably covers an extra 3/4 of a meter on each stride. Stride length is essentially your power output per step, exactly what we want to improve.

How Not To "Increase" Speed

One thing you absolutely do not want to do in trying to increase your stride length is to reach your foot further out in front of you trying to get that extra foot on your stride. There are two big reasons for this. The first one is your hamstrings. They don't appreciate you altering your stride like that and you will be much more prone to injuries. If you want something that will really slow you down quickly, pull a hammy.

The second reason is that, while you may feel like you're going faster, you're not. The farther in front of your body your foot lands, the more braking action you have. You'll also spend more time on the ground and less time projecting your body through the air. Your foot should strike almost directly below your center of mass, about 6-12" in front.

Increasing Strength Output

Let's jump into the important stuff now—where to focus your time to improve your power output. Since power is a combination of how much force you can output and how quickly you can generate that force, additional strength is of obvious benefit.

Now, I'm no expert on building strength. But I can tell you one thing. You want to increase strength without increasing mass. Remember that we're looking for "mass-specific force".

That means you want to use high weights and low reps. You want to focus strength development through the posterior chain since the hamstrings and glutes are the major drivers in sprinting. Beyond those two facts, I really don't care what you do to get there.

You can use Starting Strength, Jim Wendler's 5/3/1, one of the many flavors of 5x5, or whatever other program you find focusing on the major compound lifts: the squat and the deadlift. Just pick one and get stronger.

How strong do you need to be? Being able to squat and deadlift 1.5 times your bodyweight is probably a good starting goal. Additional strength will definitely help, but if you can't pull off these relatively low numbers, you're leaving a lot of potential on the table.

Don't forget to add in some complex upper body work with the bench press, overhead press, pull-ups, and dips. Supplementary exercises that aid the posterior chain can also be added like Romanian deadlifts and Good Mornings.

Increasing Rate Of Force Development

Having more strength relative to your mass is important, but it's not that simple. If it were, powerlifters would dominate on the track. But that's certainly not the case. Mass-specific force is just a measure of strength. To generate power, we need to convert that strength quickly into propulsive force. But even more so than strength, the central nervous system is the limiting factor for, well, pretty much everyone. Therefore, we need to train the nervous system to fire more muscle and to fire it faster.

Plyometrics

Believe it or not, though you may run horizontally, when your leg touches down, you push off with a vertical ground force, not horizontal. Given that, it makes sense to train the body to fire vertically, quickly and forcefully. Enter plyometrics. There are any number of good plyometric programs out there and at least as many bad ones.

A program that I've used successfully can be found online at: http://www.tflinks.com/articles/training/a001.html?2. I like this program because it has a gradual build-up from low to high intensity.

A word of caution: Do not overdo it on the plyometrics. These are incredibly ballistic exercises and will injure you. I know you think you're prepared and are in great shape and can handle it. So did I before I damaged a hamstring tendon last year, leading to two months of sub-par training. Start slow, do less than you think you can do, and build up over a 4-6 week period.

In fact, if you use the program I linked to above, start at the lowest intensity for three weeks, then move up a level for another three weeks, and so forth. You might laugh at the ease of these early workouts. They might not feel taxing. Do them anyway. That's my caution. If you damage yourself, don't blame me.

Loading: You will be doing plyometrics no more than once per week. This one session will encompass 80-120 high-quality jumps per session. And that's it. Go home and rest.

Olympic Lifts

No discussion of force development would be complete without touching on the Olympic lifts: the clean and jerk and the snatch. I don't think that the snatch is really necessary for a non-Olympic lifter. Heavy, low-rep clean and jerk, on the other hand, is a good addition to your workouts. You can probably even limit yourself to the hang power clean for maximum "bang for the buck".

A discussion of programming is beyond the scope of this article. Greg Everett would be the man to ask that question to and his Catalyst Athletics Workout of the Day seems as good as any for ideas on programming the lifts.

And Of Course, Sprinting

No disrespect to Olympic lifters and powerlifters, but all theory aside, the best way to get good at running fast in a straight line is by... running fast in a straight line. The lifts are excellent, but they are supplements to speed training. Specificity of training says that you'll get more out of sprinting. Remember that the limiting factor for most athletes is the rate at which the nervous system will fire. By sprinting, you're teaching the body to fire those muscles quicker and optimizing fast-twitch expression.

Think of sprinting as the ultimate plyometric exercise. As the foot lands on the forefoot, the heel is pressed down, loading the Achilles tendon and calf muscles in just a few hundredths of a second. The quads are loaded during heel recovery and the hamstrings are loaded during the forward leg swing. Once you get to top speed, it becomes a very efficient motion using muscle and connective tissue elasticity to maintain speed. Effort is still required, but not the same amount as during acceleration.

A Couple Final Points Of Training Advice

Mind Your Ankles

I attended a USA Track and Field Coaching Certification back in June and came back with some ideas for improving my own training. One of the big ones was ankle strength. As we know from the used-way-too-often, but very true, cliché, "A chain is only as strong as its weakest link." The ankle is the smallest and weakest joint in the leg. When running properly, you are generating forces of about 4 times your bodyweight, all with one leg. It's a good idea to make sure all of that force is going into the ground, not being lost to sloppy joints.

Some of these college coaches had used ankle strengthening exercises with their athletes to improve their running and attributed at least part of the year-over-year improvement to these exercises. I incorporated some simple ankle strengthening as well and feel that it has helped. Here are a few ideas, but the Internet is full of ways to get your ankles stronger. Yes, there is a place for isolated training.

- Walking in sand
- Standing on one foot
- Standing on the toe's of one foot

Unilateral Exercises

I have also come to the conclusion that since 100% of the time when you're running, you are doing so on one leg, there is a benefit to doing single leg exercises, both loaded and unloaded. The list of choices is long; to name a few:

- Pistols
- Split Squats
- One-leg Deadlift/Romanian Deadlift
- Step-up

Everett and others in the lifting world probably have some additional ideas.

The Key For The Generalist: Carry-Over

So why should you care if you can cut a 12.25-second 100m or 56-second 400m? What is that really going to do for you? Think about the guys and gals that pick up a program like CrossFit after a long time training in the powerlifts or Olympic lifts. After a short adaptation period, they typically have no problem blowing through workouts with high reps, but light weights, like Fran, Grace, and Diane. Why? Because the weights are such a small percentage of their maxes.

Aerobic Capacity

Similarly, a 50-second 400m runner should be able to cut a 5:00 mile with only a little additional training. You're talking about sustaining 67% of his top speed. Compare that to a 55-second 400m runner; he's running at over 73% of top speed to pull that off. A guy with a 60-second 400? He's putting out nearly 80% to pull off the same 5:00 mile (a pace that is probably virtually impossible).

That doesn't necessarily mean the faster short-distance runner will be faster over the longer distance. But he has a greater potential to do so because he has a greater speed reserve.

Take me for example. Two years ago, my best mile was a 6:47 (a very painful mile, I recall) and if I remember correctly, my 400m time then was around a 1:03. This year, I finished the season with a 52.5 400m and recently tested my mile at 5:50 simply by maintaining a set pace. Perhaps I could go a bit faster with someone to push me around the last couple laps, but regardless, in the last two years, I've brought my mile down nearly one minute. How did I do that?

It wasn't by training for the mile, that's for sure. I've done absolutely no training for running a mile. In fact, in my training, I don't recall any days where I ran more than 500m in a single run. But my general speed is high enough that a 5:50 is only 60% of my 400m pace, down from 62% for that 6:47. You see, increasing my speed and glycolytic ability directly affects my aerobic ability, though I'm actually maintaining a lower percentage of my max than I was two years ago.

Adding just a little training for the mile could probably push me to around 5:30. While it's no record-setting pace (and likely not even competitive in Master's Track and Field), it's a time few people that slog miles and miles can do, even with tons of training.

Balance

In the past year, I've also seen an improvement in balance-related activities. For instance, I can now bang out 10 straight pistols on each leg with no problem. Until recently, I hadn't done pistols in probably six months and had trouble getting more than 3 or 4. My first time attempting them a few weeks back, I hit 10 with ease.

When I go trail riding, my control of the bike is vastly improved, though I just hit the trails for the first time in a year recently. I can control the bike around low speed, uphill turns much better and can power through parts of trails that used to have me walking the bike.

Vertical Jump

I've seen an improvement in my vertical jump of 1.5-2", up from 28" about 18 months ago. I can only attribute the improvement to my sprinting and long jumping training since I've done no focused jump training.

Lactic Buffering and Anaerobic Recovery

Going back to that trail riding, I notice that I'm able to sustain power output on longer, steeper hill climbs with relative ease. The acidosis build-up used to have me stopping 2/3 of the way up some of these hills that I can now push through. My legs still scream at me, but my muscles don't give out. Similarly, I can recover from repeated bouts of hill climbs very quickly.

For people that think specialized training has no carry-over to activities outside of that specialization, they're flatly wrong. There are certain skills that transfer very well to other domains:

- The ability to control one's own body (gymnastics)
- The ability to control external objects (Olympic lifting, powerlifting, strongman)
- The ability to propel yourself quickly (sprinting and swimming)

You won't see a 1-to-1 carry-over, but improving your power output in any of these realms will definitely improve your power output in other realms.

The Two Major Components Of Your Sprinting

Now it's time to get into what you really care about: how do I get faster? When you get down to it, every time you sprint, there are two broad components: maximum velocity and speed-endurance.

Maximum Velocity is just what it sounds like. What is the highest speed that you can hit, even if only for a millisecond? Go back and reread all of my rambling prior to this. Increasing maximum velocity (raw power output) is what I've been discussing.

Speed-Endurance is also pretty much just what it sounds like. It's the ability to maintain a very high percentage of your maximum velocity. This is further sub-divided in the Track and Field world into terms like Alactic Short Speed Endurance, Glycolytic Short Speed Endurance, Special Endurance 1, and Special Endurance 2. But forget all of that... it's not important for what we're doing.

We're basically dealing with energy systems here, primarily the phosphagen and glycolytic systems when dealing with sprints, which is considered to be anything up to 400m. Realistically, however, even a 100m race has a speed-endurance component. In fact, once you get beyond about 40-50m, you're into speed-endurance, a fact that will come into play in programming.

Three Sample Templates

I assume you're not aiming to become a Track and Field competitor and as such your goal isn't to specialize in the sprints or any other event. Therefore, the goal is to work speed training into your general conditioning program, maintaining a good base of general fitness with a focus on speed.

I've thought through some different theoretical frameworks for incorporating a speed bias into your training. Descriptions of these workouts are below.

8-day cycle (3-on, 1-off)

1. Speed
2. Heavy lifting
3. Short Metcon
4. Rest
5. Plyometrics
6. Heavy lifting
7. Speed-Endurance
8. Rest

9-day cycle (2-on, 1-off)

1. Speed
2. Heavy lifting
3. Rest
4. Plyometrics
5. Short Metcon
6. Rest
7. Speed-Endurance

8. Heavy Lifting
9. Rest

14-day cycle

1. Speed
2. Heavy lifting
3. Short Metcon
4. Rest
5. Plyometrics
6. Short Metcon
7. Rest
8. Speed-Endurance
9. Heavy Lifting
10. Short Metcon
11. Rest
12. Tempo
13. Heavy Lifting
14. Rest

You can plan longer cycles if you'd like, but if you're not actually competing, it's probably just a lot of wasted mental effort. For someone just wanting to add some productive speed training to their workouts, the basics will get you there without over-planning and too much concern about periodization and all that.

My preference is for the 9- or 14-day cycles. More rest means higher quality work. Higher quality work means better gains. It also allows for sprinting days (speed and speed-endurance) to follow rest days. It's really hard to sprint when you're sore from lifting and I've tried to structure the cycles based on my experience of what works well on following days. Your mileage may vary.

The 14-day plan allows for working in more metCons if you really want to focus on that aspect while still adding some speed work, along with additional max effort lifting days.

Warming Up

You wouldn't just rack up your max squat and jump under the bar without working up in a progression to that weight. (Please tell me you wouldn't do that!) Similarly, it's a bad idea to go straight into sprinting without a proper warm-up. Recall that you're generating and absorbing forces equivalent to about 4 times your bodyweight. That's a lot of stress on the muscles and connective tissues.

Along those lines, it's a good idea to warm-up properly before you start hitting these speed workouts. I spend about 15 minutes warming up with these drills before I get into my workout:

- A-skips (forward and backward)
- B-skips
- Ankle hops - bouncing using only the ankles
- Straight leg runs
- Leg swings, forward and side
- Light Bounding
- Power Cariocas - A simple crossover, but driving the front leg down powerfully.
- Deep lunge holds to stretch hip flexors

I do each of these for about 30-40m, in no particular order, with a jog back to the start, then do 6-8 sprints. With the warm-up sprints, I start at about 15m and work out to 60m, increasing intensity and distance. Basically I do something like this: 15m @ 70%, 25m @ 80%, 30m @ 80%, 40m @ 80%, 50m @ 90%, 60m @ 95%. Then I rest 5 or so minutes to let my heart rate come back down and get into the workout.

These Are A Few Of My Favorite Workouts

Finally, here are some simple workouts I use that target the desired attributes of the day. The basics should work for you if you haven't been training speed, so resist the urge to over-complicate your workouts.

Naturally, you can create your own workouts, but keep the principles of the workout type in mind. Make sure you are actually working speed on speed days and not putting speed and speed-endurance together.

To clarify one term, an "on the fly" rep means to enter the work zone after accelerating to speed with a 15m run-in. You do not time the acceleration zone. If "on the fly" is not signified, you're working from a dead start.

I've put together a spreadsheet that will help you figure out your goal times on each of the speed-endurance and tempo workouts that can be found on fitnessspotlight. com. I've focused all of the goal times for speed-endurance and tempo runs on your 400m time as it's easier to maintain timing accuracy when self-timing and it's more appropriate for the generalist.

Speed

Speed workouts are low volume, high-intensity, focusing on running full-out for short distances with full recovery between reps. This allows ATP/CP stores to refill between efforts, keeping the intensity high, and reducing aerobic fatigue. I aim for no more than 10 runs per workout and no more than 50m per run, often far lower on each of these. Rest periods are about 1 minute per 10m, so 4 minutes for a 40m sprint.

- 6 x 40m, on the fly - A 40m sprint with a 15m acceleration zone. Hit top speed at the 0m mark and maintain for 40m.
- 4 x 15m, 2 x 25m, 2 x 35m, 2 x 40m - Just as it sounds, from a 3-point start.
- 8 x 30m hill sprints, alternating uphill and downhill - use a very low-grade hill (3-5%) such that your stride is not altered.

Speed-Endurance

Speed-endurance workouts focus on hitting a desired speed and maintaining it. This is typically done at your pace for a long sprint, such as a 200m or 400m. Rests vary from long but incomplete to very long for full recovery. Yes, you should really rest that long. Speed-endurance work is very taxing and will do wonders for improving your anaerobic capacity.

- 2 x (4 x 200m), rest 4:00/8:00 - 2 sets of 4 x 200m with 4:00 rest between reps, 8:00 rest between sets. Use 100% of your 400m goal time.
- 3 x 500m, rest 15:00 - Use 90% of your 400m PR.
- 2 x 250m, on the fly, rest 25:00 - Use 100% of your 400m goal time.

These are ambitious volumes and intensities, so dial them back as you need in the beginning. You don't have to be exact, but aim to be within a half-second either way. Do not try to blow each one out at 100%. You can run 200m faster than you can run 400m; that doesn't mean you should aim to run a 100% effort 200m on that first workout listed. Again, keep what you are training for the day in mind.

Tempo

Tempo workouts focus on maintaining a set percentage of your best time, typically in the 75-90% range. This allows a build-up of lactate and acidosis, coupled with short rest periods, forcing the body to improve lactate turnover and hydrogen buffering. The other goal is to teach you to run relaxed and maintain form.

- 6-10 x 150m, rest 3:00, 75-90%
- 4-8 x 400m, rest 3:00, 75-90%
- 2 x (500m, 400m, 300m), rest 3:00/6:00, 75-90%

Start at the lower end of the prescribed percentages and reps. You can lengthen the rest periods to 4:00 if necessary. Increase intensity, then increase volume. Do not increase both at the same time.

Focus on Quality

You hopefully noticed that there is a time component to all of the speed-endurance and tempo workouts. This isn't just "go out and run hard". It's "make sure you hit your target times". It's "keep the quality high and end the workout if you can't make your targets". It's goal-oriented. Obviously I can't stop you from slogging through a string of sub-par workouts, but I can tell you that it won't get you to where you're going.

If I had a more sophisticated setup, there would be a time component to speed work too, but I don't, so I base that on feel. If I don't feel like the intensity is there and I'm not getting up near top speed, the workout is over. Trying to train the nervous system to fire powerfully with sub-maximal work is a futile effort.

What Not To Do

I've seen it quite a few times. Someone decides to add "sprint training" to their workouts and the workouts are something along the lines of 10x100m with 1 minute (or perhaps 2-3 minutes) rest. That's not a sprint training workout. That's a conditioning workout and may have a place in your program, but it's not going to make you faster. There will be far too much fatigue to truly sprint. Remember that just because you're moving faster than your 5k pace doesn't mean you're sprinting.

Speed training uses a different mentality than you're probably used to. More is not always better. Less rest between reps is not always better. If you are actually committed to improving your speed, proper rest between reps and maintaining quality of work is the most important factor. Save the metcons for metcon days and treat speed training as you would a heavy lifting day. Don't make your speed training into a running-focused metcon.

Rest means rest. Not jogging around, not doing pushups or pullups. It means walking, standing, sitting, or even laying and waiting. Literally, on my long rest days (like the 2 x 250 with 25:00 rest above), I sit/lay out of the way on the track and watch other people do their thing. Then I get up and go again.

Make It Yours

This is all hypothetical and untested, but I'd love to get some feedback if you give this a shot. My training is 100% Track and Field focused, so I don't work in metCons and I cycle my lifting, speed, acceleration, plyometrics, and speed-endurance work differently depending on where I am in the season. As such, nothing about this is set in stone, but is intended as a starting point for someone that wants to emphasize speed while still maintaining a level of "general fitness" (though I could easily argue that Track and Field would do that).

I kind of look at it like another iteration of the ME Black Box by Coach Rutherford, only with a speed bias. Tweak it, play with it, give feedback.

PERCENTAGE BASED MEBB
MICHAEL RUTHERFORD

One poor assumption I have made with regards to lecturing on the Max Effort Black box deals with the athlete's experience with finding the daily max effort. I'm up there babbling about finding that best effort for 5, 3 or 1 on a particular move and then suddenly it hits me—The majority of my audience is lost. I often times get the same tilted head, glazed over look my Airedales give me when I'm talking to them. It's bad coaching on my part and I regret that. Failure breeds innovation. So now we have another way.

After a month on the road, in front of friends, coaches, and athletes I returned to base to tweak out a thing or two. I broke out some training logs, a calculator and excel spreadsheet and found an alternative route to working through the three weeks rep rotation. This is nothing new to those who follow, practice and study the world of strength and conditioning. It's just a method that I have avoided to keep things a bit less cumbersome and a bit more intuitive.

As a refresher, a particular movement is selected from an inventory of total lower and upper body movements. The first week is an introductory week of 5s, followed by a week of 5 x 3 and finally a week of 5 x 1. The objective each time is to reach a best effort work set on the final set of the day. It's at this point where difficulty arises in determining how to progress and arrive at that final work set. Percentage based MEBB to the rescue. Now Fans and coaches can plug their athletes into a max and have all their Sets calculated out for the three weeks.

You will need one or all of the following. A chart, a calculator or an excel spreadsheet to do the work. I would suggest finding any one of 1000 max charts or formulas available on the Internet.

If you don't have a max for an athlete then just do some conservative projections and have them start. Here you go.

MEBB PERCENTAGE BASED PROGRAMMING

WEEK 1	WEEK 2	WEEK 3
5@55%	3@63%	1@70%
5@63%	3@70%	1@77%
5@70%	3@77%	1@85%
5@77%	3@85%	1@93%
5@85%	3@93%	1@100-101%

I can already anticipate the outcry at the oddball percentages. Yes, you can round up to 65,80,and 95 percentages to make your chart neat and tidy.

You can also make your own chart with MS Excel. Find a business/accounting or math friend to help if you are like me.

1RM	101%	93%	85%	77%	70%	63%	55%	50%
50	51	47	43	39	35	32	28	25

Total body moves for the week of 5s and 3s May require a reset after each set for many. No big deal. Dump it safely and go again.

I hope that this helps with the difficulty on finding a best effort and keeps you on track.

SEVEN DAYS OF HEAVEN:
PLANNING YOUR TRAINING PART 3
MATT FOREMAN

This will be the third and final installment in our three-part series on planning out your training. Two months ago, we examined the challenges of selecting goals and picking out competitions for a given year of training. Last month, we looked at the week-by-week loading progression for a training cycle that would lead up to one of those competitions. This month, we will narrow the subject down just a little more and take a look at how to set up a basic week of training. Seven days, seven days... The possibilities are endless.

Before we get into the meat of the subject, let's face reality. This is part three of a series of articles. And I think we all know the possible disasters that can occur when you get to a "part three" scenario. The Godfather Part III was a lousy movie. Return of the Jedi was the third part of the Star Wars trilogy and look at it, for crying out loud. You had a bunch of muppets running around killing stormtroopers with homemade spears. Awful stuff, truly. Therefore, the goal here is to build up to a flaming climax. We want to make sure that this grand finale doesn't follow the sad tradition of third-part flops. Everybody should walk away from this month's article feeling like they could sit down at their computer and design a training program that will lead to continual progress, consistent strength development, injury-free training and new personal records.

Setting up a weekly training program presents you with some interesting demands because, as with all other elements of training, it will depend on the particular situation of the individual you're working with. What we will attempt to do here is put forward a weekly training plan and also address some ways that it could possibly be adapted or retooled to meet the needs of different athletes. Before we actually take a look at this weekly plan, it benefits us to throw out a few general training ideas that need to be taken into consideration.

Exercise Sequencing

Exercise sequencing, how's that for fancy terminology? It's almost like we have Mike Tyson here with us, creating his own vocabulary as he describes how ludicrous it is for his opponents to think they can depenetrate his impregnable defense. Praise be to Allah.

Exercise sequencing simply describes the order of your exercises in a given workout. If one workout is going to contain four exercises, which ones should be performed first and which ones should go last? For example, let's say an athlete wants to do snatches, back squats, some abdominal/core exercises, and clean pulls in one workout. What order should they follow?

Rule #1

Generally, the exercises that are most dependent on speed should be performed first. The athlete will be freshest and "snappiest" at the beginning of the workout before fatigue has set in from other exercises. Towards the end of a workout, after strenuous work has taken place, the athlete's explosiveness will be somewhat diminished. Trying to perform speed exercises at this point will not be optimal. In the workout example we're discussing here, which of the four exercises is most dependent on speed? The answer is obviously snatches. This means that the snatches should be done first.

Rule #2

Exercises that are closely movement-related should be performed in sequence. This means that if an athlete is going to perform snatches at the beginning of a workout, the exercises that immediately follow the snatches should be the ones that are most similar to the snatches. In this workout example, which exercise is the most movement-related to the snatches? The answer is the clean pulls. Although the snatch and the clean are different exercises, the triple extension of the pulling movement is a common factor between the two. After the athlete has finished doing snatches, the pulling movement will be "warmed up," so to speak. Because of this, the clean pulls are a good choice following the snatches because the pulling from the snatches will transfer into the clean pulls. Also, going back to Rule #1, the clean pulls are probably the second highest speed exercise in the workout. The snatches will be the most dependent on speed, and the clean pulls are second in the ranking order.

Rule #3

All of the barbell exercises should be completed before moving on to supplemental work. Having said this, the squats should be done after the clean pulls. After the squats are finished, the bar can be put away and the athlete can perform auxiliary exercises such as core strengthening, plyometrics, grip training, etc. Personally, I like to finish each workout with hanging leg raises, two or three other core exercises such as crunches or planks, and crush gripper training. I also like to stretch for ten minutes after each workout. Post-workout stretching should be a permanent part of your training program. Therefore, the workout should look like this:

1. Snatch
2. Clean Pulls
3. Squats
4. Core/Abdominal work
5. Stretching

Variations:

These rules are effective guides for planning your workouts. However, it must always be stated that adding some occasional variety and changing things up can pay big dividends. For example, I once decided that I was going to experiment with performing my strength work at the beginning of my workouts, followed by my speed lifts. I deliberately wanted to be fatigued from heavy strength lifts (squats) prior to the speed exercises such as snatches or clean and jerks. The idea here was that when I finally got to a competition and performed snatches and clean and jerks without the pre-fatigue from squats, my explosiveness would be greater. In other words, the bar would feel lighter on meet day. I trained like this for around six weeks and then went to a meet. Did it work? I don't think I noticed a big physical change, either positive or negative. I basically felt the same on meet day as I usually had in other meets. But it was fun to train differently for a while. I once snatched 140 kilos (around 90% of my max) immediately after back squatting 250x5, and I think there was a mental benefit from this because I basically started believing that I could snatch 90% anytime, anywhere, regardless of anything.

OFF DAYS!!!

You might decide that you want to train seven days a week. I wouldn't, but you can if you want to. If you choose to go this route, you won't need to worry about off days because you won't have any (until you enter the hospital).

But for those of you who are trying to decide how many days a week to train and which days you should take off, here are a few thoughts. First of all, you have to ask the question, "How many days a week should I train?" If you talk to ten different coaches about this, you'll probably get ten different answers. I've known elite lifters who train six days a week, and I've known elite lifters who train three days a week. There is no rule set in stone that applies to everybody. When I was doing the best lifting of my career, I trained five days a week. After a few years of this, I changed to four days a week and guess what? I continued to do the best lifting of my career and even made some solid improvements.

As we have said repeatedly in our series, things are dependent on your personal schedule. Your job might completely dictate how many days a week you can train. If you have a job that only allows you to get to the gym three days a week, then you will have to set up a three-day-per-week program. Nothing complicated there. But it you're in the fortunate position of having as much time as you need to train, then the questions really begin. Selecting which days are going to be your off days is a strategic move. Logically, it makes sense that you will want to take your off days when you will need them the most. How can we accurately gauge when that will be?

Sundays

I've taken Sundays off throughout my entire career, and I think most lifters do as well. Some people have religious obligations that prohibit them from training on Sundays. Some people believe that weightlifting is their religion. Regardless, Sunday is generally a good off day because it freshens up the athlete for the coming week. There's a sense of completion that accompanies Sundays. A feeling tends to come over people that tells them their work for the week is done and it's time to relax, mentally unwind, and enjoy the day before the grind starts again on Monday. This is probably why NFL games are televised on Sundays. They practically force America to the couch. One of the best lifters I've ever trained with told me, "If you're a lifter, Sundays are for laying down, eating, and napping." Truer words have never been spoken.

Between D-Day and Armageddon

There should always be a day off between two workouts that are extremely demanding. One way of approaching this is to arrange your most difficult workouts around an off day. For example, you could plan an off day on a Wednesday if you know that you're really going to be hitting it hard on Tuesday and Thursday. If you're planning to take Sundays off, as we mentioned earlier, then it makes sense that Saturday and Monday would be big workouts. The overall thought here is that there has to be a structure to your training week. Off days should not be random. If you have a job situation where you know that you won't be able to train on Saturdays and Sundays, then your Friday and Monday workouts should be the ones where you plan to get the most intense work accomplished.

Finally, an example...

Now, with all those theories and rules lying on the table, let's just quit beating around the bush and put one week of training down on paper. Here it is:

Monday

- Cleans
- Clean Pulls
- Back Squats
- Straight-Legged Deadlifts
- Abs

Tuesday

- Rack Jerks
- Power Cleans
- Standing Military Press
- Abs

Wednesday

- Snatches
- Snatch Pulls
- Abs

Thursday

- Clean and Jerks
- Clean Pulls
- Stop Squats
- Straight-Legged Deadlifts
- Abs

Saturday

- Snatches
- Snatch Pulls
- Front Squats
- Abs

I didn't list stretching in any of these workouts, but it should be included in all of them.

There you go. Now, let's take a look at some reasons for why this week looks the way it does.

1. Thursday and Saturday are big workouts, hence the day off on Friday. Plus, the athlete will be training four days in a row throughout the week (Mon-Thurs), so he/she will be ready for a day off by Friday. Sunday is a day off for the reasons already mentioned.

2. Three squat workouts per week is a good plan for a competitive Olympic lifter. Some coaches actually have their athletes squat four or five times per week, with more moderate weights. I personally have found that doing three squat workouts per week and really hitting those workouts hard will be most effective.

3. Doing rack jerks on a day that follows a squat workout is part of the design. The legs will be fatigued the day after squats. Performing rack jerks when the legs are fatigued simulates how the athlete will feel during a heavy competition clean and jerk, where the legs will be fatigued after standing up with the heavy clean. If the athlete can adapt and learn to use the legs in the jerk effectively on Tuesday after the tough Monday squat workout, there will be a benefit in the full clean and jerk.

4. Following the competition lifts with a pulling exercise is a good way to strengthen the movement. In other words, always do clean pulls after cleans. Always do snatch pulls after snatches, etc.

5. Straight-Legged Deadlifts are designed to strengthen the lower back, stretch the hamstrings, and prevent injury. This exercise does not need to be performed with enormous weights. It is performed with a barbell, but it should be viewed as an auxiliary exercise.

Adaptations

This program is specifically designed for athletes who are completely concentrating on Olympic Weightlifting. If the athlete is planning to incorporate other athletic endeavors into their training, such as running or mountain biking, then the program would need to be restructured. The intensity and workload of this program will not leave much energy left for additional pursuits.

Age issues must be considered. I would not have a thirty year-old athlete train five days a week in this manner. If a thirty year-old wanted to train five days a week, the intensity of the workouts would need to be reduced. I've trained at twenty years old and I've trained at thirty years old. The simple fact is that the body just doesn't recover as quickly as the years pass by.

In this particular training week, the two competition lifts (snatch/clean and jerk) are not trained on the same day. This is simply a basic look at how to build a training week. For a competitive weightlifter, it is important to train the competition lifts together on the same day to simulate actual meet conditions. This training week would need to be organized a bit differently to accommodate that principle.

There are a few other things I would like to add about this program, along with program design in general. First of all, the five-day training week I outlined in this article looks very simple. There aren't any magic exercises in there. In fact, some people might take a look at it and think that it doesn't look like enough work to make big progress. I've shown this training week to several lifters over the years and had them give me the same response, "Wow, this doesn't look very hard."

Okay... When I moved to Washington in 1993 to train with the Calpian Weightlifting Club, I began using the exact same five-day plan I described in this article. It was very different from how I had trained in the past, but I had been stuck at the same weights for over a year and I needed a change. I came to Washington in January and had a best competition total of 265 kilos in the 99 kilo class. After eleven months of training this way every week, I totaled 300 kilos at the same bodyweight. Now, it's important to understand that I was pushing myself extremely hard within this framework, as were all the lifters in our club. Our coach had our daily workout weights planned out throughout our entire program, but we were not hesitant about deviating from the plan and loading up personal records on the bar if the time was right to go for it (remember last month's article?). It was a sensible, organized approach that also encouraged aggressiveness and breaking new ground. All of the information from this article, along with the preceding two articles in this series, give you a solid idea of how I've trained throughout my career and how I've trained other athletes.

And because of our thousand-ways-to-skin-a-cat understanding, it's important to acknowledge that this isn't the only way to train successfully. Can you go from 265 to 300 in one year training differently than how I've discussed? Absolutely. Weightlifting coaches sometimes make the same mistake as some religious leaders; they basically say, "Only I am right, everyone else is wrong." The point that I hope we all understand is that there are certain commonalities that make for smart training, even if the daily routines are dissimilar. Despite individual differences in workout frequency, loading progression and exercise selection, every coach will have to use some good old-fashioned horse sense when it comes to program design. "Horse sense," for those of you who weren't lucky enough to grow up in the boondocks, is a term that refers to sound practical judgment. Sound practical judgment, along with a fantastic work ethic, unrelenting commitment, and high pain tolerance will usually make you a better athlete, coach, spouse, parent, professional, or Jedi Knight. So file down your calluses and get to work, and may the force be with you.

ESTHER GOKHALE: PERFECTING POSTURE
YAEL GRAUER

Esther Gokhale has been called the Michael Pollan of posture, but perhaps a comparison to nutrition pioneer Weston Price would be more accurate. Weston Price was a dentist who conducted ethnographic nutritional studies across diverse cultures, synthesizing dietary principles held in common by cultures that were not ailed by modern diseases. Gokhale looked to native people, ancient Greeks and young children to synthesize what kinesthetic principles led to their ease of movement and back health.

Gokhale, a Harvard and Princeton-trained biochemist (as well as an acupuncturist), suffered from back pain in her 20s. She was awake every two hours, walking around her neighborhood in a vain attempt to relieve the agonizing pain she was in due to an L5/S1 disc herniation. Because she was nursing, pain medications were not an option. Although Gokhale had back surgery for the herniated disc, her sciatic pain returned a couple of years later and the doctors recommended a second surgery. Gokhale, instead, studied at the Aplomb Institute in Paris, took anatomy and anthropology courses at Stanford, and travelled all around the world; observing, interviewing, photographing and filming people in countries where back pain is virtually unknown. Gokhale also looked to babies, ancient statues and photographs from the past to better understand the blueprint of our skeletal structure, the laws of nature that are being ignored and leading to back pain.

Back pain is rampant in this country. It affects around 80% of individuals, and is the second leading symptom of physician visits. It is the leading cause of work-related disability. The direct and indirect treatment cost of back pain is estimated at around 100 billion dollars annually. Many reasons for back pain have been posited, including excessive sitting and standing. But Gokhale's research makes most of these theories fall flat, as she has observed and photographed weavers, basket makers, potters and others who spend their days engaging in activities which require them to sit and stand for many hours. Gokhale asserts that the back problems in modern industrialized society are directly related to poor posture.

Good posture, however, is probably not what you think it is. According to the Gokhale Method, what most people do when attempting to "stand up straight" is not good posture, as putting your chin up and chest out (for example) leads to exaggerated spinal curves. Trying to stand straight (usually with a retroverted pelvis) often leads to a ping pong match between a tense and upright posture and a slumped and relaxed posture. We're going for a relaxed and upright posture, so that it can be maintained. Only with proper (anteverted) pelvic position can your bones stack properly, allowing you to relax your muscles and improving both circulation and the health of tissues around the spine.

Proper posture is standing with your tailbone back and ribcage forward, shoulders slightly behind the body. Your pelvis is tipped forward and sacrum angled back. The lower border of your rib cage is flush with the abdominal contour. There is a soft angle at the groin between the front of the torso and legs (permitting the femoral arteries, veins and nerves to function at full capacity). Whether standing, bending, sleeping, sitting or walking, you are using your muscles and sparing your discs. You breathe into your chest and spine, improving the rib cage, massaging and mildly lengthening the spine and stimulating good circulation. Athletes take note: Proper posture and movement makes you less prone to injuries and joint degeneration, in addition to enlarging your rib cage— leading to greater lung capacity.

The J-Spine

Many lumbar support cushions, cervical pillows, TLSO body casts and even modern clothing and furniture accentuate an excessive curvature in the lower lumbar and cervical spine, flattening the lumbo-sacral curve. This leads to a distorted and compressed spinal column. In her book and classes, Gokhale compares medical textbooks from the past and present. A 1911 diagram of the spine shows a gentle curve, with elongated lumbar and thoracic spinal contours. In contrast, a similar diagram in a 1990 medical book shows increased curvature in both the lumbar and thoracic spine. Numerous factors are likely responsible for the cultural drift-- the influence of the fashion industry, how children are carried and held, modern furniture and a disruption of a kinesthetic tradition between generations included among them.

What Gokhale calls the J-spine is a far cry from S-curve touted by chiropractors or the tucked pelvis recommended by yoga practitioners, but is anthropologically informed and positions one's body weight evenly over the heels. And although it is not commonly accepted amongst chiropractic circles, medical literature indicates that reducing spinal curvature reduces pain and alleviates compression. Patients with more upper lumbar curvature and less lower lumbar curvature have more pain. The converse is also true. Gokhale teaches people how to stand with an anteverted pelvis and with a significant and pronounced angle in the lumbo sacral arch (L5/S1.) The shoulders are positioned posteriorly relative to the torso. The arms are externally rotated, angling to the back of the torso, with externally rotated thumbs facing forward. The chin is angled down, elongating the cervical spine. The feet point out at an angle of 10-15 degrees.

One need only turn to evolutionary biology to understand why the L5/S1 curvature is important. When we evolved from being quadrupedal to bipedal, the L5-S1 disc became wedge shaped. Anteverting the pelvis preserves the wedge-shaped space accommodating the disc. Tucking the pelvis, on the other hand, forces a wedge-shaped disc back into a cylindrical space. This causes the L5/S1 disc to bulge, herniate or sequestrate due to pressure it puts on the anterior part of the disc, wearing out its fibrous exterior.

According to Gokhale's research, a tucked pelvis can also compress the pelvic organs into an unnaturally small space, compromising their shape, orientation and function and possibly contributing to irritable bowel syndrome, constipation, prostate issues in men and fertility issues in women. When the pelvis is tucked, the pubic bone doesn't support the pelvic organs. This leaves all the work to the pubo-coccygeal muscle instead, likely predisposing women for organ prolapse and urinary incontinence. Also, since the hamstring muscle attaches to ischial tuberosities (sitz bones), a retroverted pelvis shortens the hamstring muscles, thereby increasing susceptibility to injury.

In addition to teaching us how to stand, one can also use Gokhale's wisdom (synthesized from village Africans, Tahitians, Cambodian Bodhisattva figures, Greek statues and children) to learn how to sit properly. Gokhale teaches two types of sitting-stretchsitting and stacksitting. Most people alternate between hunching (compressing the discs and leading to spinal degeneration) and swaying (which also compresses the discs but, as an added bonus, compromises circulation as well). Pulling the shoulders too far back stresses the rhomboids, and hunching the shoulders too far forward compromises the brachial plexus. Stretchsitting instead, therefore, is particularly cogent. It is basically a subtle but effective form of therapeutic traction, lengthening the long muscles of the back, and decompressing the discs. The neck, too, is lengthened and aligned, preventing cervical disc and nerve damage. (Stacksitting simply involves sitting with a well-positioned anteverted pelvis.)

Probably my favorite exercise was glidewalking. Most people (myself included) come into the Gokhale Method Foundations course with a gait that underuses the gluteal and leg muscles. Therefore, your back is twisting, swaying or hunching as it jerks with each step. This is quite jarring to the weight-bearing joints in the body—knees, hips, spine. Instead, the butt and legs should contract strongly, propelling the body forward, sparing the back.

Glidewalking strengthens the glutes which supports pelvic anteversion, stretches the psoas during the push-off, strengthening the foot muscles. The swing phase of walking restores healthy joint space between the head of the femur and acetabulum. But my favorite part of the walk is the resting position, especially one version in which the back heel is raised with all muscles relaxed. This occasional rest phase, incidentally, is what gives native women carrying baskets or clay pots on their heads such a graceful, cerebral gait.

Walking was difficult. I have in the past tried to simply put my hands on my quads, hopefully activating the power of reciprocal inhibition. That never quite seemed to do the trick, as my overdeveloped quads still did most of the walking. Gokhale's method uses the psoas and glutes, which is difficult with a tucked pelvis. (Incidentally, it is the gluteus medius, not the gluteus maxiums, that most people underuse.) And I don't think I would've learned how to leave my back heel on the floor without Gokhale practically stepping on the back of my shoes as I walked, grasping my Achilles tendon with her toes.

Walking incorrectly contributes to overused joints and underused muscles. Instead of strong muscles and joints we get weak buttock and leg muscles and worn joints. Glidewalking, on the other hand, propels the body forward smoothly, sparing the joints and strengthening the muscles. Proper posture is not limited to simple everyday activities but also to athletics, of course. Photographs in Gokhale's book and slideshow feature Kenyans and Olympians running with an upright torso and anteverted pelvis—whether leaning forward or not, anteverting the pelvis increases the contribution of the glutes to our stride.

It is also great for bone health. As I learned in college from a little old lady who wouldn't let me carry her groceries for her, weight bearing bones need a healthy level of stress to prevent osteoporosis. Standing with the main weight bearing bones vertically aligned over the heels is a good start. Walking properly is the next step. If weight bearing bones are not stressed they do not remain strong, as calcium leaches from the bones or is inadequately deposited, leading to osteopenia or osteoporosis. Letting the correct bones bear weight provides the healthy stress that keeps bones strong. (Stress on wrong parts due to misalignment, on the other hand), can lead to arthritic changes such as bone spurs (ostophytes). And putting one's weight to far forward to the middle or front of their foot (instead of the heels) stresses the bones and leads to bunions, sesamoid bone fractures and plantar fasciitis.

Knee problems are also a symptom of incorrect posture and movement. Many athletes report that their knees rotate inward while squatting. This is correlated with the pronation of foot and underuse of buttock muscles, making the knee joint more prone to injury. Rotating the knees outward is also no picnic and increases chance of torn ligaments, frayed menisci and arthritic changes in knee. And locking the knees, as I learned in high school marching band, inhibits good circulation (though thankfully none of us passed out).

Unlike books of back exercises and videos on back safety shown at workplaces nationwide, Gokhale teaches participants hip hinging—a particular form of bending from the knees which increases one's reach and improves arm and buttock position, whether you are outwrestling someone much stronger (like Gokhale's son did) or are gathering water chestnuts for seven to nine hours a day Burkina Faso (like the women Gokhale photographed, who incidentally have no complaints of back pain). This particular exercise is far more challenging than one would think, and esther warned us not to try lifting anything until we had perfect form (sound familiar?)

Another mistake in walking is parking the hips forward. This leads to numerous problems. Specifically, it can misalign the head of the femur in the hip socket (acetabulum); tensing muscles that bridge the area, reducing the natural gap between the ball and socket, resulting in bone-to-bone contact which can lead to arthritic changes or worse. Hip misalignment can also occlude femoral arteries, veins and nerves, affecting circulation to and from the legs and feet. My lifelong problem with cold feet and slowly healing leg injuries, explained instantly.

Gokhale also teaches one to protect the "inner corset," or set of muscles around the torso that helps lengthen and stabilize the spine. I always wondered why simple Russian twists (with or without a medicine ball) hurt my back. If the spine is compressed, twisting it can damage it—but activating the inner corset (isolating the internal and external obliques and abdominal transversus muscles from rectus abdominus) protects it—allowing you to lengthen and support your spine without distorting it, periodically stretching your erector spinae muscles.

Gokhale synthesized the information from years of study into an award-winning book, 8 Steps to a Pain-Free back, to teach others how to re-establish their body's structural integrity through healthy posture and movement, regaining pain-free living. Although Gokhale's book is informative (I was particularly drawn to the beautiful photographs from different cultures), some people need gentle hands-on guidance to help with specific postural issues or body types. I was thrilled when Gokhale came to my town. The personal attention from a well-trained eye (who was able to quickly comment on very specific postural issues with pinpoint accuracy) was just what I needed.

The idea of establishing a baseline for health, pain-free posture and movement in just 9 hours, without expensive equipment or continual treatments, seems like a dream come true. Although those with particularly difficult cases might need additional interventions, before/after pictures and our own experiences show that habits can be changed fairly quickly. The three day intensive, comprised of two 1.5 hour lessons a day for three days, included a visual component (with an informative slide show), discussion, lecture and an extensive kinesthetic component, with gentle hands-on guidance.

FUNKY LOCKOUT BLUES: FIXING THE JERK
MATT FOREMAN

When I was in my early twenties, I drove a 1981 Chevy Malibu station wagon. I bought it from my parents when I finished high school and drove it until I graduated from college and got my first full-time job. I loved this car, but it was one of the biggest pieces of crap in the galaxy. Every morning when I left my house to go to class, I would sit in the front seat of my car, put the key in the ignition, and pray to Valhalla that it would start. Sometimes it started, and sometimes it didn't. And if it didn't start, I had to combine some fast thinking and a kaleidoscope of foul language while I tried to get it running so I could make it to class on time. This probably happened seven or eight times a month... for six years. That's frustration, jack.

However, that wasn't the only frustrating pickle I ever had to grapple with. There have been others, obviously. And every one of you reading this article can think of your own predicaments from the past or the present where some common irritation keeps popping up. Your junker car, your annoying spouse, your lack of math skills, your toe fungus, whatever. The reason we're talking about this stuff is because there is probably nothing more frustrating for a weightlifter than not being able to complete the jerk after a successful clean. You've put in all the effort to clean the barbell, it's sitting on your shoulders, people have their cameras ready, the judge's finger is twitching on the white light button, and you crush the hopes of everybody in the room because you just can't find a way to stick it over your ears and complete the entire clean and jerk. All that effort in the clean was for nothing and now your mom is embarrassed because you're a lousy, disgusting jerker. For some athletes, this almost seems like an unconquerable nemesis. That's why this article is about jerking, plain and simple.

You need to know that I feel your pain, brothers and sisters. For the first few years of my weightlifting career, I was in this exact same swamp of failure. I had a fifteen kilo difference between what I could clean and what I could jerk, and I missed more jerks than I made in competition during this time. It was ridiculous. I knew how to perform the jerk, I was strong, my technique was solid, but the weight just wouldn't stay overhead when I was attempting my heaviest lifts. It was enough to make a grown man weep. If there would have been Jerk Prozac available, I would have had it loaded into a Pez dispenser.

This lasted until I was around twenty. And then I learned some things. I made some changes. I fixed a few problems that I had never thought of fixing because I didn't even know they were problems. By the time I was twenty-four, I was a legitimate jerking machine. I don't think I missed three jerks in competition for the next four or five years and I was lifting 30-40 kilos more than I had been in the younger years. So now, believe it or not, I'm going to hand you some of the solutions I discovered on a silver platter. You're about to become a better jerker as you sit where you are. You'd better be ready.

Make sure you're fishing in the right pond

First of all, this article is not going to be a technical analysis of how to perform the jerk. If you want that, then you need to buy Greg Everett's book, ask a coach to teach you, or watch some videos of Wes Barnett. All of those things will explain how to achieve technical magnificence in the jerk. Instead, we're going to look at some practical ideas to improve the jerking prowess of an athlete who already has a solid foundation of knowledge and technique.

One of the easiest steps in the jerking equation is to figure out if you're using the correct style. Are you going to be better at the push jerk, the squat jerk, or the split jerk? Right away, we need to make sure we're clear on the terminology. Split jerking is the most common jerk technique in weightlifting. This is the easily recognizable form where the athlete punches one foot forward and one foot backwards to lock the bar overhead in a sort of stride position. If you go to a weightlifting meet, the vast majority of the lifters you see will use the split jerk. The squat jerk, on the other hand, is a technique where the athlete punches under the bar by jumping the feet slightly out to the sides and descending into a deep squat. The bottom position of this jerk looks like a clean-grip snatch, and it has been popularized by some world-class lifters. Chinese Olympic Champion Zhan Xugang probably has the greatest squat jerk in history, and studying videos of his technique will give you a solid idea of what it's supposed to look like. Finally, the push jerk is a basically just a shallow version of the squat jerk. The feet are jumped into the squat position when punching under the bar, but the athlete does not descend into a full squat. Most push jerkers catch the weight in a position that looks like a half-squat. Some coaches refer to the push jerk as a "power jerk," which is fine. Greek legend Pyrros Dimas is one of the most famous push jerkers in history, although some of his biggest lifts drove him down deep enough into a position that was close to a squat jerk.

There is no rule written in stone that dictates which style of jerk an athlete should use. Whichever style gives the athlete the best results is the correct one for that particular individual. Most weightlifters in the world use the split jerk because it has historically yielded the highest marks. Most (not all) world records in the clean and jerk have been set with split jerks. However, this does not make it the universal rule for everyone. Some athletes are simply more comfortable with push jerking or squat jerking. Pyrros Dimas and his Greek teammate Kakhi Kakhiashvili both won three Olympic gold medals using push jerks. Dimas actually converted to the split jerk briefly in 1993 and the change simply did not work for him.

As a coach, my personal preference would be to teach the athlete how to perform the split jerk with the intention of using it exclusively. However, all weightlifters should also be taught how to perform the push jerk and it can be used as a terrific assistance exercise. If time passes by and the athlete has sustained difficulty with split jerking, it would be wise to give the push jerk a try. If the athlete learns the push jerk and quickly exceeds his/her best split jerk results, the coach may want to consider a full-time conversion. Obviously, this will need to be given attention on an individual case-by-case basis. The squat jerk will probably be a little trickier because of the extreme flexibility and strength it requires. The athletes will basically have to be able to perform a narrow grip overhead squat with the same weight as their top cleans. This requires a very special type of athlete with unique leverage.

Caveat! Caveat!

Although the idea of converting a split jerker into a push or squat jerker is always a viable option, a warning that needs to be mentioned is that the coach shouldn't rush to convert the athlete away from split jerks simply because the athlete is having difficulty. There are ways to fix a sloppy jerk without switching styles. As mentioned above, this article is not a tutorial on how to perform a jerk. However, it will examine some common mistakes and how to fix them. Here are a few of them:

Problem: The athlete is trying to jerk the bar with the upper body instead of using the power of the lower body. This is an easy one to spot. The next time an athlete has a bar on the shoulders and is preparing to jerk, take a look at the athlete's hands. If you can see that the athlete is gripping the bar tightly with the hands, it means he/she has already started to prepare for an arm-initiated movement. White knuckles, straining forearms, and purple fingers don't lie. If athletes attempt to jerk the bar overhead using the strength of the upper body, it will be a disaster. The arms and shoulders are simply not strong enough to lift a maximum clean weight over the head to a locked position. The power to complete the jerk has to come from the lower body.

Solution: Tell the athlete to loosen their hands before attempting the jerk. Some great jerkers even have the fingers slightly opened prior to the dip. Loosening the hands forces the athlete to use the legs. When I was getting started in weightlifting, I once heard a coach say that the drive of the legs should generate enough power to elevate the barbell to the level of the forehead, and that the arms shouldn't even be actively used until the bar is passing the scalp and the split has begun. This is an interesting way to describe the movement and just might be the proper verbal cue to give one of your athletes the correct mental perception of the lift.

Problem: The athlete is driving the bar forward when it comes off the shoulders and the lockout is not directly over the head. This could be caused by a variety of culprits. Therefore, multiple solutions are in order.

Solution: The athlete might be letting the elbows sag down during the dip phase. Watch the jerk from the side and see if the elbows are drooping when the athlete dips with the legs. If the elbows are drooping, then the shoulders are rounding forward as well. Both of these will cause the bar to be driven forward, away from the body, during the drive phase. A useful verbal cue for this problem is "big chest on the dip." When the athlete thinks about spreading the chest and maintaining a strong upright posture during the dip, the elbows are much less likely to sag because the position of the shoulder girdle will force them to stay up.

Solution: The athlete might have tight flexibility in the overhead position. Obviously, stretching is a necessary element to fixing this. However, jerks from behind the neck can be extremely beneficial in this situation. If you are unfamiliar with this exercise, it's exactly what it sounds like. The bar is placed on the back exactly like a back squat, and then the athlete simply performs the jerk. Because the starting position of the barbell is already behind the ears, the athlete has a much better chance of locking it out in the correct position over the head.

Solution: The athlete might be pushing the hips back (instead of straight down) during the dip phase. If the hips start to shift backwards during the dip, the resulting drive will be forward instead of straight up. Telling the athlete to "dip through the heels" is often helpful here. The athlete must mentally imagine the hips dropping straight down between the heels. Likewise, the athlete might also have his/her bodyweight on the front of the foot prior to the dip. This can result in the same forward problem. "Dip through the heels" will obviously communicate to the athlete that the weight should not be on the front of the foot before the jerk is initiated.

Problem: The athlete is having trouble locking out the bar on straight elbows overhead. This is clearly a technical problem and it is also one of the most common rule violations in the sport (pressout). Although there are some technique changes that can be made to fix a poor lockout, it must also be acknowledged that the problem could simply be a structural issue with the athlete's elbows. To state it clearly, some people just have really lousy elbow lockouts. The arms don't completely straighten and the athlete has all kinds of wobbly, bendy issues when the bar is overhead. These people will struggle with the Olympic lifts, period. However, let's make sure we understand that it is still possible to be a successful Olympic lifter even though the elbow lockout is shoddy. It's been done before.

Solution: Poor elbow lockout could be fixed by adjusting the width of the grip. The athlete's hands might need to be widened (or narrowed) to give the straight, snappy lockout we're looking for. This will obviously need to be considered in conjunction with the most beneficial grip for the clean, since the clean and jerk is a two-part movement. Poor lockout could also be caused by improper timing. If the athlete's feet are landing and planting on the platform too early, the elbows might still be fighting for lockout when the lower body has already fixed itself into position. Telling the athlete to synchronize the feet landing with the elbow lockout can give a proper sense of timing.

Some lifters will struggle with jerks their entire career. Stand behind an athlete sometime and look at their shoulders. You'll usually figure out which ones will be the best jerkers simply by seeing their physical structure. If the athlete has narrow, sloping shoulders, then jerking will be tough. The upper body is going to have to work extremely hard just to support the barbell during the dip phase because the shoulders naturally have a downward contour to them. Then, on the other hand, look at the athletes who have a square, wide look to their shoulders where the span from deltoid to deltoid looks like the top of a box. These will be the best jerkers because the barbell has a natural plateau to rest on while the dip and drive are taking place. Look at it this way; what would happen if you sat a fifty pound block of concrete on top of a cardboard toilet paper roll? The toilet paper roll would get crushed because it's just not a strong enough support base. Now, what if you took that same concrete block and sat it on top of a dictionary? That dictionary would have a much better chance to support the block because of its density and size. Likewise, an athlete with a wider, thicker support base for the barbell will probably have a stronger jerk than an athlete with a narrower, thinner base. This is why increased mass in the upper body often leads to greater results in the jerk.

There is nothing nicer than seeing an athlete absolutely stick a perfect jerk after a tough clean. American legend Jeff Michels was thrilling to watch because many of his best jerks were popped into lockout after tough, grinding, screaming cleans. Some people have a natural knack for it. And then there are the unlucky ones, who go to meets and clean massive weights easily only to have the jerk come crashing down on them like a fighter jet being shot down. Those are the ones who have to put in extra work, end of story. However, as a former pathetic jerker who went to jerk rehab and eventually developed into a jerking assassin, I can tell you that the struggle is worth it when you start getting those down signals. Happy jerking, amigos.

GET YOUR HANDS OFF MY BURRITO...
AND OTHER TEAM BUILDING STRATEGIES
MATT FOREMAN

I remember my first teaching job. I was twenty-five, graduated from college, and I got a job working at a private high school. The school only had two hundred students, around thirty teachers, and it was very centered around the idea of "building close relationships" throughout the campus. The school's mission was to educate students and, at the same time, strengthen the bonds between the faculty and the student body. If the whole thing sounds suspiciously close to a bunch of people holding hands around a campfire and singing Kumbaya, that's because it was. It was a lot like the final scene of the movie The Wicker Man, only we weren't burning a giant statue with a human being inside.

Anyway, one week before my first year of school started, the administration took the entire faculty on a two-day "team building exercise." Basically, we all packed up some gear and went out to a camp in the forest where we spent forty-eight hours doing activities that were intended to make us closer friends through working together. We had to get into groups of five and scale our way across a rope bridge, we had to problem-solve little dilemmas that were assigned to us, we had to do that thing where we all lock hands in a tangled bunch and then twist our way out of it without letting go of each other's hands, that type of stuff. Did it make us closer colleagues? I think it made me closer to five or six people that I really liked. But most of it was so irritating that I wanted to light the entire camp on fire by the time we left. Maybe it really was just like The Wicker Man after all?

That little tale is about TEAM BUILDING, which is what this month's article is focused on. Many of you who read the Performance Menu are gym owners, coaches, or personal trainers. Your livelihood is dependent on finding people who are willing to commit to a training relationship with you and pay you money to work with them. You probably also realize that the market is flooded with other trainers, coaches, and gym owners who are trying to do the same thing. What that means is that your services are going to have to be special, in some way. You're going to have to offer some kind of X-Factor that makes people choose you instead of other trainers. And that's where team building comes in.

People want to feel like they're a part of something special. That's why kids join sports teams. That's why kids join gangs. That's why adults get married. That's why people pay for memberships to the National Rifle Association or the American Civil Liberties Union (two groups that really love each other, by the way). That's why big families have reunions and...hell, that's why people have big families. Everybody wants to have an experience where they know that they are a member of a tribe. Therefore, that's why we're going to throw out a few suggestions about how you can make your clients and athletes feel a stronger loyalty to your gym, your team, or you personally. The stronger their loyalty is, the more committed they're going to be. The more committed they are, the longer they're going to stay with you and help grow your business.

Two little asterisks first. A) Some of you are still athletes and you haven't started training people yet, so you'd rather hear about some training-related subject to make your squats go up. Please just hang in there, though. You'll probably coach people someday and this information will come in handy when that day arrives. B) Some of you Son-of-Sam types might be huddled in front of your computer, twitching furiously, and saying, "Bull—t! I don't want to be a part of anything. Everybody needs to leave me alone!" If that's you, then I apologize for wasting your time. Have a glass of milk, put down the ice pick, and relax.

Hail Caesar!

One of the first ideas I have about this deals with leadership. If you are the manager, coach, or owner of your training business, then you have a great deal of responsibility on your shoulders because people want strong leadership. Regardless of the area or setting, people always look to the leader of the group for guidance and examples of behavior. You may not even know it, but your personality is shaping the attitude of your entire clientele. Let's say, for example, that you are the coach/manager of a facility where people want to learn how to lift weights and train. The thing you need to realize is that it is your job to teach those people how to perform the lifts of the workouts, warm up properly, use correct technique, etc. This is obvious. But many coaches and trainers forget that the people they coach are also going to develop their training attitude based on the example they see from the leader.

The leader sets the tone for the entire group personality. If the leader is friendly, enthusiastic, intense, helpful, and disciplined, then the people who work under that leader will adopt those same qualities. Likewise, if the leader is negative, panicky, lazy, or cynical, then those characteristics will start to surface in the athletes and clients. It won't even be a conscious decision on the part of the trainees. They will simply come to the gym every day and mimic the behavior they see from the person who is in charge.

I have seen great examples of both the positive and negative in this area. One of the first coaches I had in my sports career was a man who made everyone around him worse in some way. He knew the fundamentals of how to coach his sport and he had a decent level of experience, but his personality was lousy to deal with. He was one of those coaches who enjoyed doing cruel things to people. He liked to make insults, he was pushy and domineering without being a positive motivator, and he frequently spoke negatively about his athletes behind their backs in a way that ensured they would eventually hear it through somebody else. Not surprisingly, every member of the team he coached (including me) exhibited the same behavior. The team was filled with drama, hostility, and most of the athletes on the team wanted to see other people fail. What was the end result? Usually, his athletes had frustrating careers where they never reached their potential, and then they quit and walked away forever.

So this was an example of a coach who was a terrible leader, but it has also been my good fortune to work with some fantastic examples that went in the other direction. Two years ago, a very good friend of mine retired from a thirty-year career in coaching track and field. It would be a ridiculous understatement to call this coach a dynamic personality. His level of intensity, sense of humor, and commitment to the success of his athletes was unlike anything I've ever seen. He was one of those coaches who could take athletes with mediocre talent and elevate them to championship levels by making those mediocre athletes see themselves as champions. He reached inside them and pulled the greatness out, no matter how deep it was buried. If any of his athletes did anything lazy or disrespectful, he would give them some of the most brutal tongue-lashings I've ever seen. But the athletes would walk away from it feeling like they had let their coach down, not vice versa. They would have tears in their eyes because they knew they had disappointed one of the great influences of their lives, but this coach would always make sure the athlete was not completely crushed. Every butt-chewing ended with a positive message that tomorrow was a new day. What was the end result? This coach's teams won championships for three decades, athletes flocked to his program like the Pied Piper, and grown adults came to his retirement party to thank him for the way he prepared them for life.

Both of these coaches formed their teams through the way they conducted themselves every day. Whether you know it or not, you're the leader and your athletes are watching everything you do. Make sure they see the right things.

Got My MOJO WORKIN!

What's the mojo in your gym? Please do us all a favor and don't act like you don't know what "mojo" is. You know what it is as clearly as you know what you look like naked. However, I'm willing to accept the idea that the actual term "mojo" might be a new one for you, so here's a quick analysis.

The mojo of your gym is the general atmosphere. It's a description of how much "juice" you have in your gym environment. Still confused? Okay, go someplace like a mortuary, a library, or an Arizona Diamondbacks game. Low mojo, baby. Seriously low mojo. Now, go to an Irish pub on St. Patrick's Day. Completely different level of mojo. Get the picture?

Do the athletes in your gym cheer for each other when they're attempting big lifts? For that matter, do the athletes in your gym know what constitutes a "big lift" for the other members of the gym? In other words, are your athletes interested enough in each other that they know what the team's personal records are? They should. Your gym has a have a team concept, and everybody has to feel like they're a part of that team. If you haven't actually established a team name, you should do it. Get them to think they're a foot soldier in your army, and then get them to believe in the concept of DEATH BEFORE DISHONOR.

Every gym has a few lifters who are identified as the "big dogs." These are simply the strongest and most respected athletes in the house. When newbies start training in your gym, it doesn't take them long to figure out who the big dogs are. So think about what it means when that newbie is getting ready to attempt a new personal record snatch and he/she hears one of the big dogs yell out, "Let's go! Pull hard and stick it!" That newbie just got a huge blast of adrenaline, and guess what? You've just had a team-building moment in your gym. That newbie feels like a part of the gang, and you've probably got a new member on your hands.

Camaraderie is everything, as long as it's combined with focus. It's incredibly helpful to have the members of your gym liking each other, wanting to befriend and support each other, etc. However, the leader always has to make sure that everyone's minds are on their work. Conversations and laughs are great, but the intensity must not be made to suffer. If a Chatty Cathy starts training in your gym and people start getting distracted from doing their job correctly, then it is your job to step in and let Chatty Cathy know in a helpful, positive way that she needs to learn to shut her mouth at the appropriate times. Lastly, you might have the occasional prima donna come through your doors. This, as we all know, is the athlete who wants the entire gym to revolve around him/her and expects everybody to bow down. How much do you, the leader of the gym, let this prima donna get away with? Do you let your other athletes see you cater to this prima donna and lavish special treatment that the gym scrubs don't get? If you do these things, then you're going to lose some people. Some of your team members are going to watch you coddle the prima donna and they're going to start to think you're full of bunk. If one of your lower-ranked athletes gets angry and throws a fit after missing a big lift, then you need to handle it and exert a little authority so everybody knows how things work in the gym. But then you have to make sure you give the same business when the prima donna throws the same fit. As soon as your team senses that there are double standards in the gym, they're going to start buying out.

Finish with a BET...

If you ever want a fun, exciting way to get some motors running in your gym, try establishing challenges and bets for your athletes. Here's an example. During the years when I trained in the Calpian gym in Washington, we had a tradition for our Tuesday workouts. On Tuesdays, the entire team did rack jerks. That was the big highlight of the day. As time went on, lots of wagering and challenging started to surround the Tuesday jerks. Sometimes, one lifter would challenge another one head-to-head. Let's have a jerk contest and the loser has to buy the winner a burrito after the workout. Or, lifters of different bodyweights could challenge each other with bodyweight handicaps. Or maybe the challenge could be to see who gets the closest to jerking a personal record that day, and the loser had to unload everybody else's bar afterwards.

You get the idea. Find creative ways to get the competitive vibe running in your gym, and provide some kind of tangible rewards. Before you know it, you've got a situation where personal records are falling left and right...all because of a burrito. This also provides a way for some of the big dogs to occasionally be in a situation where they have to fight like hell to stay ahead of one of the weaker lifters. The point here, and the point to all of this, is that it is the task of the gym leader to develop the entire program. Everything including equipment rules, scheduling, conduct and behavior, inter-squad competition, and good old fashioned family atmosphere is part of the vision of the coach, manager, or whatever title you want to give yourself. Most people feel more comfortable and confident if their leader is a strong alpha personality. If there comes a time in your career when it's your turn to run the show, make sure you find a way to build something special. Don't just tread water.

SO RUNS MY DREAM, BUT WHAT AM I?
MATT FOREMAN

Not long ago, an old friend of mine posted some information on the internet about using barbell exercises to strengthen and rehabilitate an athlete who had a severe problem with scoliosis. The story he posted was under the title "The healing power of the barbell."

That title caught my eye because it made me think about something from my own personal history in the iron game. When I first glanced at the words "the healing power of the barbell," I initially thought about the ways in which a person can be healed. Obviously, most of us think about healing in the context of injury recovery. We strain connective tissue, pull muscles, and tweak our bodies in a variety of different ways when we're fighting for bigger lifts and greater strength. Then our physiology has to heal and repair itself after these traumas. It's part of the game, nothing new to anybody.

However, that title took my brain in another direction. Aside from physical aspect of it, I couldn't stop thinking about the idea of being healed in other ways. We go through times when we're frustrated or discouraged from lack of progress. We also experience defeats, either on the competition platform or in the bigger contest venue known as life. Some people walk through their lives carrying around scars and baggage from early experiences that were almost impossible to deal with in a positive way. And the thing we all have in common is that we all look for ways to heal ourselves after we've gone through hell. Some people pick destructive paths such as substance abuse or criminal activity because it seems like it will erase the pain, at least for a little while. Some people adopt pets. Some people learn to play a musical instrument. Some people submerge themselves in their professions or their relationships, thinking that constant focus on a certain area will eliminate any focus on the other areas that are difficult and depressing. Then, some people simply become bitter and vengeful because they want to build a brick wall around their soul and never give anybody else a chance to cause damage.

How does all of this connect to barbells? Seriously, how does all the Dr. Phil-type discussion lead us to a place where we can get some useful information out of this month's issue of The Performance Menu? Well… let me say a few words about that.

I love the 90s...

Aaahhh, 1998... I was twenty-six years old and at the top of my weightlifting game. My first Olympic weightlifting competition was in 1990. After spending a few years fumbling around in training and getting limited results, I decided to take this weightlifting thing all the way. I packed everything I owned into my 1981 Chevy Malibu station wagon, left my home in sunny Arizona, and drove up to rainy Washington so I could train for the legendary Calpian Weightlifting Club and be coached by John Thrush, the best weightlifting coach in America. The next five years of my life were brutal as I fought the weightlifting wars and attempted to work my way up the national rankings. Frustration? Plenty. Plateaus? Several. Best years of my athletic life? Absolutely, jack.

Things started to pay off around 1997 because I moved up to superheavyweight from the 105 kilo class and my lifts shot up like a rocket. My breakout meet was the 1997 American Open in St. Joseph, Missouri where I snatched 150 and clean and jerked 180 for the first time, weighing under 120 kilos. For the next year and a half, I continued making progress and consistently won medals at all the top national meets in the United States. Times were fun. As H.I. McDonnough once said, they were the salad days.

However, lifting big weights and winning medals were only pieces of the entire puzzle. One of the best parts of being on the national weightlifting circuit was the friendships and bonds you formed with other lifters from around the country. This was always one of the elements of the lifting world that I loved the most. Even though one lifter lived in Florida and another lifter lived in Michigan and they only saw each other three or four times a year at national meets, it still felt like family. Everyone was around the same age, and the connection we all had through the sport we loved was an extremely tight link. I've always considered weightlifting a tribal sport, and being members of the tribe that competed at all the big meets made us brothers, sisters, cousins, and so on.

During these years, I ran with a crowd of lifters that liked to train hard and play hard. We were not choir boys. Maybe we would have been better weightlifters if we had played by the rules and spent all our post-competition time sitting in our hotel rooms and writing out our new weightlifting goals on Embassy Suites stationery, watching a Sandra Bullock movie and treating ourselves to a nice bowl of ice cream. I don't know for sure. What I do know for sure is that we liked going to bars, we liked drinking beer, we liked female companionship, we liked being young and strong, and we liked pushing the limits of safe, socially appropriate behavior. I'm surprised we didn't all grow up to become United States Congressmen.

One of my closest friends during this time was a lifter from Sacramento named Greg Johnson. Greg, like me, was a former football player-turned weightlifter and I think it's safe to say that he and I were sculpted from the same block of cheese. Along with Coach Bill Kutzer and a great pack of fellow weighlifters, Greg built the Team Sacramento Weightlifting Club from the ground up. Throughout the late 90s, Team Sac was consistently an impressive power at the national level. Their men's and women's teams were competitive, and the overall personality of their group was a lot like the Calpians. They had a coach who was a very good man and wanted nothing but the best for his lifters, who he treated like his own kids. They had a gang of athletes who trained hard, and they showed a noticeable enthusiasm and positive team attitude in all the things they did. We competed in all the same meets, we partied together, and we grew very close. Greg even had family in Washington State, so we would often see him a few times a year when he came to our gym to train while visiting. Although we lived in different areas, I considered Greg a brother in iron.

We all went through the salad days together. Down in the Sacramento area, Greg lifted, coached, and directed local meets that were fun and intense. Up in Washington, I did exactly the same thing with my club. The world was our oyster, and then things changed.

Losses...

As Jim Morrisson once said, "The future is uncertain and the end is always near."

On July 24th, 1999, I dislocated my knee during a 187.5 clean and jerk at a local meet in Auburn, Washington. It was less than a year before the 2000 Olympic Trials, which had been the ultimate goal of my career. Hell, it was the ultimate goal of my life. Weightlifting was practically my entire reason for breathing. I don't know if it was healthy or balanced to look at the world this way, but being a lifter was the most important thing in my existence. The Trials were around the corner, I was in the best shape of my life, and it was obvious from my training that much bigger lifts were about to fall. Now, I should mention that our 2000 Olympic Team consisted of only two men (who turned out to be Oscar Chaplin and Shane Hamman), and I knew I wasn't going to be in the mix for the top spots to go to Sydney. I was at 155/185 with the potential to maybe hit around 160/195, which clearly wasn't serious Olympic contention. But it didn't matter to me because from the time I first became a weightlifter, I knew that having the chance to compete in the Trials was a sacred honor that separated you from the pack in our sport, even if you didn't make the Olympic Team. I wanted it so bad, I couldn't stand it.

Then, when I had that 187.5 jerk over my head and I felt the bones in my knee separate, I knew it was all in jeopardy. It was a bad injury. After getting the MRI and speaking with a top surgeon, my options were clear. If I had surgery to repair the damage, I would be looking at almost a year of rehab. Or, I could skip the surgery and try to get back to my top lifts through strengthening the joint and physical therapy. The only choice I had to possibly make the Trials was option #2, clearly, so I skipped the surgery and started training again as soon as I could.

To make a long story short, I didn't get back to my top lifts after the injury and the 2000 Trials passed me by. My discouragement and disappointment were extreme, to say the least. In fact, I had practically decided to get out of Olympic weightlifting by 2001 because I couldn't stand the frustration. I spent the next three years squatting and deadlifting in the gym, only because I couldn't imagine my life without lifting weights. But there was no real focus, no real hope. I resigned myself to the idea that competing in the Olympic Trials was just something I was going to have to let go. This realization was like acid in my mouth, and I didn't handle it well at every given moment.

Then, the universe provided one of those moments when you snap to attention and look at everything just a little bit differently. I had been in the middle of a three-year pity party for myself when I woke up one day and found out that my old friend Greg Johnson, who I had continued to keep in touch with outside of weightlifting, had been killed in a car accident in early 2003.

It's an understatement to say Greg's death was an immensely painful blow to everyone who knew him. The news of his passing hit us like a hammer to the chest. He had a young son, he had recently been given a strength coaching position at Stanford University, and his hard work on the local weightlifting scene in California had nourished the sport in a valuable way. It was difficult for all of us to comprehend how such a bright light in the weightlifting world could be snuffed out so early. I think there are many people out there who still haven't come to terms with Greg's loss. It certainly made me ask some questions about life that I still don't know if I've found an answer for.

And a few months after it happened, his Team Sacramento family showed their typical classy character by announcing that there would be a Greg Johnson Memorial weightlifting meet in Sacramento in August of 2003. Just as Greg would have wanted it, the competition was going to be held on a beach, right next to the water, with loud music blasting and big weights flying. It was a chance for weightlifters to pay their respects to the memory of a good friend, and I made the decision that I was going to fly down and compete as soon as I heard about it. I had been out of competitive lifting for almost three years at the time. I had no plans to put together any kind of impressive total, and it didn't matter at all. What mattered was the having the chance to honor a fallen friend in the most appropriate way I could imagine, by lifting big weights on a platform with his name painted on it.

The 2003 Greg Johnson Memorial

When I arrived in Sacramento the day before the meet, it's fair to say that I was not exactly in the greatest phase of my lifting career. I had maintained some decent strength through the powerlifting movements I had been doing in the gym, but I wasn't ready to snatch or clean and jerk anything impressive. It had been almost a year since I had done a snatch in training. I had no idea what I could expect. And on top of all this, I had just gone through a very painful divorce. It wasn't the rock-bottom time period of my life, but it was a long way from the salad days.

Brett Kelly, Greg's close friend and Team Sac teammate, offered me a room in his house for the weekend. The day before the meet, all the volunteers got together to haul the weights, platform lumber, and meet supplies to the beach and set up for the next day. I wanted to be in on all of it, regardless of how tired it made me for the meet the next day. We all worked until sundown to prepare the competition area, and then we went out to eat burgers, drink beers, and tell Greg stories. When the meet began the next day, there was something in the air. In twenty years of weightlifting, I don't think I've ever seen a competition where there was as much happiness, enthusiasm, mutual support, and weightlifting camaraderie as there was at this meet. To put it simply, everything was perfect. The sun was shining, people were smiling and lifting with everything they had, the music was blasting, and lots of fans had showed up to watch the action. In other words, it was exactly the way Greg would have wanted it.

And the crazy part of the whole experience is that I had an incredible day of lifting. I went three-for-three in the snatch, nailing an easy 142.5 on my last attempt. In the clean and jerk, I made 155, 165, and cleaned 170 for a narrow miss in the jerk. These weights were still well below my personal bests, but they were much better than I had expected. However, more important than the weights I lifted was the way I felt on the platform. I felt the energy of this meet in my bone marrow. I felt the spiritual presence of a lost friend who gave everything he had to make people better weightlifters, and all the smiles and laughs we had shared as we sat on barstools and toasted the prime years of our youth. I felt the disappointment and pain from the last three years of my life melting off me like frost every time I chalked my hands and stepped on the platform. I howled at the sky like an animal after successful lifts. People were screaming, "Do it for Greg!!" as I reached down to grip the bar and I knew, for some reason, that all of my pathetic little problems were no bigger than the molecules of dust that rose from the platform when the bumper plates came crashing down. This moment... this perfect moment was a healing experience for me. The loss of my weightlifting dream and the loss of my marriage evaporated into the air of that beach as I held that barbell over my head. After my last lift, with the applause and appreciation of the weightlifting family still ringing out, I took off my weightlifting shoes, ran off the platform, and dove into the cool water. The waves rippled as I rose to the surface and floated on my back for a few minutes, looking at the blue sky and listening to the meet announcer laughing into the microphone and thanking the crowd for coming out to watch the meet. I can tell you right now, seven years later, that it was one of the happiest moments of my life.

I got out of the water, dried off, and Brett started handing out the awards to the athletes. The biggest award of the day was an enormous trophy that had "The Greg Johnson Memorial Award" engraved on the plate. Team Sacramento had designed the award to be given to the athlete who, as they phrased it, demonstrated spirit and intensity on the platform that would honor Greg Johnson's memory. They gave me this trophy, and it stands on a cabinet in the den of my house. I'm looking at it as I type these very words.

The aftermath...

When I came home from this competition, I had the fire back in my guts. I was encouraged by the lifts I had been able to make at the meet and it occurred to me that I wanted to give my weightlifting career another shot. Four months later, I won the silver medal at the American Open. Four months after that, I placed fourth at the Senior National Championships and qualified to compete in the 2004 US Olympic Trials at the age of 32.

In a twist of poetic justice, I traveled back to good old St. Joseph, Missouri for the Trials. My knee was hurting, training hadn't gone perfect, I had no realistic shot of actually making the Olympic Team, and I didn't give a damn about any of these things. With the help of a departed friend, I had dug myself out of a black pit of self-doubt, and I stood on the Olympic Trials competition platform with my final clean and jerk completed over my head. Somebody in St. Joseph must have known something about my comeback situation because after my lifting session was over and the fans had all left the auditorium, the name "Foreman" stayed illuminated on the scoreboard. I found a chair, sat down next to the platform, and stared at that scoreboard until the custodial crew told me that they were shutting off the lights and locking the building up. Then I went back to the meet hotel, cleaned up, and went to meet some old friends for beers.

I've spent a lot of time since the 2004 Trials thinking about how this whole story unfolded. Greg Johnson's death was a tragedy that nothing can cure. It made my knee injury and personal problems look like a game of tiddlywinks. Many of you who are reading this article have felt your share of dark moments just like these. Certainly, some of you have even walked through hellfire that was much hotter than anything I've spoken of. You might even be feeling the flames of those fires right now. And I don't have any magic words for you that are going to fix anything. Nobody does. All I can offer is the idea that there is a healing out there somewhere, and it probably lies in the thing you love most. After all the years of frustration, my healing came from doing the most obvious thing I could think of... going back to weightlifting. Weightlifting was what I loved most, and my salvation had been right in front of my face the whole time. Maybe we're all part of a bigger plan, and that plan is going to drag us over some rough territory at times. Maybe there is no plan, and everything that happens to us in life is just random activity. Either way, there are a few things I know for sure. Life is a beautiful thing, the world is a fine place, and the best thing we can all do is try to find love and happiness while we've still got the chance. The title of this article is a line from a poem by Alfred, Lord Tennyson. He wrote it after his best friend died in 1833. The last line I'll give you is from Bob Marley: "Everything's gonna be alright."

WHEN THE OLYMPIC LIFTS AREN'T APPROPRIATE
GREG EVERETT

The Olympic lifts are not for everyone. I'm sure that sounds funny considering the source—most people who don't train in our facility assume that all we do is Olympic weightlifting, even with our fitness clients. This is of course is not a logical assumption, but understandable to some degree based on our reputation for being totally awesome.

As it turns out, our fitness clients actually don't do the Lifts extraordinarily frequently. As much as I'd prefer simply instructing and coaching them over anything else, what's appropriate and effective for a given set of clients has nothing to do with my personal proclivities (nor those of any other trainer or gym owner). If it did, our fitness classes would consist of us sitting around watching IronMind lifting videos, eating nachos with triple steak, and drinking cold, crisp, refreshing Arnold Palmers. But alas, I and the other trainers have to actually train people according to their goals and abilities.

We have four basic sets of individuals training at Catalyst. The first is our weightlifting team—this is comprised of competitive lifters and a few who are not yet competitive but will be soon whether they know it or not. The next is strength and conditioning clients who are training for particular sports. The third set is our collection of personal training clients, whose goals cover the spectrum of possibilities. And the final is our fitness class folks.

The first group is pretty simple—they snatch and clean & jerk their faces off along with plenty of other heavy related lifts five days a week; they sit around a lot between sets and talk about food and the distastefulness of endurance sports (by endurance, I mean anything beyond a single 10 second effort).

The S & C folks are easy because they have very clear goals and tend to be more naturally athletic and experienced than many other individuals; likewise, personal training clients are extremely easy because everything can be individualized completely, and generally these folks have well-defined goals, and if not, can develop some with the guidance of their trainers.

The final group is the toughest to work with for a number of reasons, such as undefined or disparate goals, a broad range of experience and ability, and inconsistent training schedules. Generally, these individuals are simply interested in "getting fit" and looking better naked. It then becomes my job as the guy who does all the programming here to determine what exactly fitness is and how best to help such a group achieve it.

Many of you reading this are familiar and may even agree with the CrossFit definition of fitness—personally I was a big fan when CrossFit was using Jim Cawley's 10 traits and aiming for competence and balance among them—strength, power, speed, endurance, stamina, flexibility, coordination, agility, balance and accuracy along with the idea of balancing the capacities of the three metabolic systems—I'm not remarkably excited about the current state of things with regard to definitions and methods.

This is not to say there are not elements of CrossFit that I believe in and implement—there are, and I'm grateful to be familiar with them. However, they are elements from an older and long-forgotten CrossFit, and they comprise only a segment of what we do.

In any case, these individuals perform strength work, conditioning work, dynamic and static mobility and flexibility work, and corrective/preventative work. Their strength work draws from an array of disciplines, but always relies on a foundation of the big basics: barbell squatting, pulling and pressing variations. There are periods in which they will do more obscure strength movements such as unilateral squat variations and the like in order to ensure stability and balance and provide enough variety to prevent boredom and staleness.

Their conditioning work consists of more traditional conditioning modes like running and rowing of various durations and intensities; interval work with various monostructural and mixed-modal efforts; dumbbell, kettlebell, barbell and other implement complexes; circuits with an array of movements and implements; and CrossFit-style mixed-mode circuits (with properly executed, rationally-chosen exercises, to be clear).

Within conditioning workouts, they will often use Olympic lift variants with dumbbells, sandbags or other non-barbell implements. Occasionally they will use a barbell Lift variation such as a power clean within a barbell conditioning complex—but with few reps and in a situation that both demands and allows an actual power clean. And never will they use the full barbell Olympic lifts in a conditioning workout as is seen with some CrossFit workouts.

Attempting to curb my circumlocution, let's get to the point: The Olympic lifts are not appropriate for everyone at every time. As I already said, I'm of the opinion that they're essentially never appropriate within a conditioning workout (with the occasional exception of lifts like power cleans at low rep numbers in a controlled and technically sound barbell complex). Additionally, there are individuals for whom the Lifts will simply never be appropriate. My 95 year-old grandmother, for example, has no business snatching and clean & jerking (and no, not even with a PVC pipe—what on earth would that accomplish, exactly?). An extreme example certainly, but the point remains—there are individuals who will seek the guidance of a trainer who do not need the Olympic lifts, and for whom the performance of which is downright silly and dangerous with no arguable benefit. (Yes, the needs of Olympians and grandparents DO differ in kind, not just degree.)

The reasons for this are pretty straightforward. First, the Lifts require a great deal of flexibility that many individuals do not possess, and in many cases, will never possess even with aggressive and consistent work. Without the requisite flexibility, the Lifts are simply not safe with loads that would be effective, like any other activity performed without adequate flexibility. Along these same lines, many clients will have residual limitations from previous injuries that prevent the safe and effective performance of the Lifts.

A reasonable level of strength is also necessary for the Lifts to be useful. Don't argue with me about how beneficial it is for someone to snatch a length of PVC—it's not. Unless it's a temporary stage in a long term learning process that culminates in snatching legitimate weights with sound technique, it's a waste of time and an indication of confused priorities.

Additionally, the ballistic nature of the Lifts means the joints and supportive structures of the body will experience and need to be able to manage high levels of force. The capability to cope with this kind of stress is not innate, and must be developed over time, like most other physical qualities, which arise as a response to certain stressors. Smart programming introduces these stressors and plans the athlete's exposure to them in a manner that provides progressive increases in volume and magnitude with ample recovery time.

In short, when a client walks into your gym, you better have a plan to prepare him or her to perform EVERY exercise they'll be doing safely and effectively, and you better have good reasons for EVERY exercise and workout you expect him or her to do.

Speaking of rationale for exercises and workouts, how many of our fitness clients need the extraordinarily great levels of hip and knee explosiveness that demands the use of complex exercises like the Olympic lifts and advanced plyometrics? I can tell you exactly how many—zero. This doesn't mean these things are not potentially beneficial for them if implemented properly, but their absence or presence will not be the difference between fit and not fit. This is much different than the situation of certain athletes for whom the absence or presence of properly implemented Olympic lifts can have significant effects on performance and be the difference between winning and losing.

The idea of training every day fitness clients like high-level athletes sounds nice and is exciting for those clients, but the reality is that these people are not high-level athletes, and training people is not a conceptual endeavor—there are very real issues to contend with, and very real possibilities of injury and slowed or absent progress when trying to implement inappropriate programming. High-level athletes have years of frequent, well-planned training under their belts that has prepared them for their present training—for a perfect example of this, consider gymnastics and what the kids at each level do. The idea that you can skip over those years of preparation and casually jump into advanced training is horribly misinformed.

It's not simply an issue of safety either, but also of effectiveness. A good example is strength work and programming. Few fitness clients will ever reach a level that requires complicated strength programming like would be seen with competitive weightlifters or powerlifters. Non-strength specialists will simply not get close enough to their genetic ceilings to require such degrees of jiggification. The same goes for tricks like accommodating resistance and similar methods—an adult male with a 200# max back squat doesn't need to be using bands and chains. In fact, not only are inappropriately advanced programming and methods unnecessary, they can be considerably less effective than simpler approaches for such clients.

The previous did NOT say: Make your clients' training easier. This idea of adequately preparing your clients for future training and using appropriate methods and exercises has nothing to do with the difficulty and demands of their training, or whether or not they're willing to work hard. While it's true that some fitness clients don't want to push themselves as hard as you'd like them to, there are quite a few who are more than willing to put themselves through surprising levels of pain and discomfort for the ostensible end of fitness (the popularity and rapid growth of CrossFit demonstrates this well). In our entire gym, we don't have a single client who doesn't put forth sufficient effort.

However, within any group of individuals who are willing and eager to push themselves to such a degree, you will be hard pressed to find those who are also able to display the kind of discipline and foresight to critically evaluate their needs, create a rational plan based on these and their goals, and to commit to the necessary training even when it doesn't suit their whims at every given moment.

Typically the kind of work that needs to be done for the sake of preparation for things like the Olympic lifts and other more advanced training is simply not that fun. No one really enjoys things like glute activation exercises or goofy rotator cuff work with infant-size dumbbells. Those with adult ADD may grow bored with their current pool of exercises and want to play with everything under the sun for no other reason than variety. I'm not impressed by the individual who is willing to exercise to the point of vomiting or a loss of bladder control—this is not that unusual. What I'm impressed by is the individual who shows up every day at the gym, does what is necessary, doesn't complain, doesn't look for recognition, does what's necessary outside of the gym to support their training and goals, and continues this process consistently for years.

The idea of smart, appropriate progression is not limited to any particular set of people or training method; it applies to all training, and to all learning, for that matter. We can apply the same principles to weightlifting, strength & conditioning for high school athletes, CrossFit, Pilates, and just about anything else.

This is where the discipline becomes critical—there are times in which what you need to do is not what you want to do. This of course is not to say that you shouldn't be doing what you want—that's exactly what you should be doing. But if what you want is something that requires work, there will be requisite steps along the way that aren't wholly enjoyable.

So what does all this tangential bluster mean with respect to the premise of the article? It means:

1. Your fitness clients don't necessarily need to be doing the Olympic lifts.
2. If your fitness clients will be doing the lifts, you need to prepare them for it.
3. If your clients are going to be doing the lifts, make sure they're really doing the lifts rather than just humping a barbell like a three-toed sloth on Ritalin.
4. As a corollary to Number 3, doing the lifts means actually using enough weight to produce some kind of improvement in athleticism.

So let's tackle these points with some semblance of order and organization (to mix it up a bit). But let's do it backwards.

Four: This doesn't mean max weights. In fact, if you're looking to work speed and power, max weights are not appropriate. You'll see the best results in the 70-80% of max range. Take the time to teach your clients proper lift execution and provide them adequate time and exposure to develop technical proficiency before introducing significant weight increases. As I've said about a million times, keep a long term perspective and accept the fact that proficiency is worth the time and energy investment.

Three: This is essentially the same as Four without the first two sentences. Find ways to teach your clients how to lift properly, and continue demanding excellence.

Two: Make sure you take a rational approach to progress. Can your clients squat, deadlift and press with consistently excellent technique and decent loads? If not, why on earth are you teaching them to snatch and clean & jerk? Do your clients have significant flexibility limitations that prevent them from achieving sound positions and performing the correct movements? If so, they're not ready to snatch and clean & jerk—help them get ready.

One: Determine appropriate exercises based on who your clients are and what they need, not what you feel like doing yourself. Do you want Joe and Jane Fitness to be strong, agile, mobile and explosive? Of course. Will they ever be any of those things to the same degree as a lifetime high-level athlete? Of course not. Do they need to train the exact same way as those advanced athletes, and should they? Of course not. Should they be allowed and encouraged to do things like the Olympic lifts if that's what they're interested in doing? Of course! But it's your responsibility as a trainer to help them prepare for it.

So with regard to Number One, what do we do to work on explosiveness when we've decided that the classic barbell Olympic lifts are not appropriate? First, we do all the typical barbell squatting, pulling and pressing variants to continue developing a foundation of strength. Second, we have myriad (yes, it's myriad, not a myriad of) options for explosive movements that neither require the technicality of the Lifts nor the potential for injury with improper execution. Any movement that involves driving against the ground and/or extending the hip aggressively fits into this classification. This includes the dumbbell Oly lift variations (preferably power), kettlebell swings (if done correctly), box jumps (that's box jumps, not ankle hops with foot lifts), squat jumps, broad jumps, jumps from the power position with dumbbells or the like, and quite a few other options if you're creative.

What if your clients want to learn the Lifts for the sake of learning the Lifts, rather than because they think or have been told they need to in order to be "fit"? Then by all means, teach them and encourage them. But again, do it properly—with respect for long term progress, technical proficiency and adequate physical preparation.

Take the time to evaluate the circumstances and your clientele and make sure you know exactly why you're doing what you're doing. They're paying you good money to help them achieve THEIR goals, whether or not they align with your own, to ensure their training is effective, and to keep them safe and healthy.

MOTIVATION
AIMEE ANAYA EVERETT

While I have been wanting to write this article, and my good friend and training partner, Kara Yessie, has been encouraging me to write it, I was avoiding it simply because I didn't want it to seem as if I were pulling out a page in my diary for ya'll to read. But I figure someone other than me may struggle with this little thing that is a pretty important factor in one's training: motivation.

Let's start from the beginning. Well not the true beginning; the beginning of my new beginning. I was lifting pretty well in 2007 until I got hurt, then continued to train hurt, continued to be hurt, when it all came to a tearing halt (literally) at a very disastrous American Open in December 2007. I spent most of 2008 recovering from a gnarly injury, mostly because I wouldn't stop training (big mistake), even though I wasn't on a program and would just do random stuff every day (another big mistake). In 2009, I was almost ready to think about training for real again, and the thought of competition was on my mind, but barely. We had just moved, I was working on my thesis for my MA in Psychology, we were opening a new gym, and I was still hurting 88.737% of the time during training. While I had increased my 2-3 days per week of training to 3-4 days per week, it was purely because I hated being skinny and weak. I really wanted to lift big weights, but I wasn't motivated to do so. I wanted to start competing again, but I wasn't motivated to do so. I wanted to be motivated, but I was too busy pretending to be motivated to actually work on being motivated.

Then, with three people who weren't even lifters, the beginning started.

Jolie

We were hosting a seminar at our gym at the end of January of last year and during the break we were training. I had just finished snatches and had moved on to rack jerks. In those days, I pretty much snatched, jerked and back squatted every time I trained, because those exercises hurt me the least, and well, I was not on a program, and was only doing stuff I liked, while pretending it was really effective. A little gal walked in and was sitting with some other folks watching us train. I jerked 105, and I saw her quickly calculating on her blackberry how much was on the bar; apparently I had caught her attention. A couple days later I received an email that said, "Will you train me?" That was the start of Jolie and I.

From coaching Jolie (in CrossFit and O-lifting), I learned a tremendous amount about having undeniable drive. This girl put 137% in to every training session, she poured herself in to her workouts, and she made me realize that I was falling way short as an athlete. She was the first to show me motivation, and through her, I found what I had lost; the desire. Coaching Jolie helped me become a better athlete. She demonstrated the passion to always push herself past what she thought she was capable of, and she did that for me, because I was asking her to. Jolie never quit during a hellacious metCon, she never stopped when it got heavy, and she rarely stopped when she started missing. She has the most amazing will and guts I have ever seen—she didn't want to let me down, and she refused to fall short of what she desired—and through that, I realized how selfish I had been with my own training. I couldn't remember a time that I had ever given more than 90% effort in my training. I treated my lifting like school; I knew I could cruise through and get As and Bs, so I never put in any more effort than I had to. If I could get a B+, than why work harder to get an A? I know! Bad attitude. But this is exactly what I did in training my whole career. I always stopped short of what was hard for me. After a couple months working with Jolie, I was still pretending to be motivated, if we are being honest, but I was starting to have more desire, and was coming close to having more drive to become motivated. Jolie gave me desire, something I had lost with the injury. She helped me to believe again.

Jocelyn

I went to a certification in March of 2009 and saw a gal with strong legs that made me incredibly jealous. I knew who she was because Coach B had emailed me asking me to touch base with this gal, Jocelyn, who he had worked with a bit in the lifts, and he thought she would appreciate some help in preparing for the CrossFit Regionals. Shortly thereafter, I contacted her and invited her to our open gym on Saturday, and that became the start of Jocelyn and me. Through coaching Jocelyn, I learned how an athlete is supposed to fight. I envied her mental strength, and became resentful of my lack thereof. Jocelyn had been a pitcher for UC Berkeley, and in 2002, toward the end of her senior year, her sister was found brutally murdered. Something that is supposed to bring you to your knees, to shatter all your motivation and will to continue to compete, gave her the anger and fire to be better than she had been before. One week later, Jocelyn was back on the mound, pitching the game of her life. She struck out 15 and allowed one-hit against Arizona, and she led her team to Cal's first NCAA women's National championship in any sport. She went on to play professional softball for six years, and eventually found CrossFit (and now is focusing on her lifting career, thank Budha! She is hooked!). Coaching Jocelyn taught me how to be tough. Unstoppable. She has been an amazing athlete to coach, and an amazing lesson in mental stability. Watching and coaching her really got me serious about thinking about becoming motivated again. Jocelyn gave me fight, something I doubt I ever had. She taught me to approach everything without fear. She is my hero. In a very non-cheesy-superman-as-your-hero-when-you-were-a-kid kind of way.

Tamara

Tamara Holmes is strength. This girl can kick anyone's ass, anytime, anywhere, without training. In mid-2009, I invited her to the gym out of pure selfishness. I saw something in her that I was dying to have, and I wanted to absorb it as quickly as possible. So of course I told her to come in for some training with the girls (Jolie and Jocelyn), and used my wanting to coach her as an excuse, when I really just wanted her to be my training partner. Which is exactly what she became. Coaching Tamara showed me what it is to be a strong girl. This girl can skip training for a month and come in and power snatch 75 kg and power clean 103 kg without even warming up. Tamara has been amazing for my motivation, simply because I don't want her to beat me in the gym. She talks a big game, she doesn't care what people think of her, and she lifts the hell out of some barbells. I knew Tamara had my back when she said, "We are accepting applications to our club of bad bitches. But don't get it twisted, we invented platform swag and can't let just anyone join. Don't even think about applying unless you have a 200kg total. If you don't know what that is, turn around and take your weak ass game back to Curves." Shortly after Tamara started coming to the gym, I stopped pretending that I was motivated and seriously became consistent in working hard to dig deep. Tamara gave me humor, and most importantly, strength.

Coaching them, to help me

In the summer of 2009 I knew I was ready to get on a program, and get on the path to compete again. I was finally feeling fabulous after dealing with injuries and pain for almost two years. Coaching these three amazing gals helped me find the things I was lacking: desire and belief, how to fight and to be without fear, and strength. I had found motivation through coaching these girls; I had given so much to them, and unknowingly, they gave even more to me. I poured my heart into their success and their improvement because all three of them were teaching me valuable lessons, irreplaceable tools, and they had given me something that I had never had—the motivation to actually want to be the best. To want to go beyond what I ever had before. To coach such amazing athletes has made me want to be equally amazing. I have never told them how much each of them meant, in very different ways, in jump starting my weightlifting career, becoming such astounding friends and mentors, and the key to hanging on to motivation for dear life. Through coaching them, I almost felt as if I had fallen short for my own coach. I wondered if I ever gave Coach B what these girls had given me, and for that I was deeply regretful and vowed to give him (and now Matt) everything I had, every single day. I had someone else to be motivated for.

Motivation in other forms

By the end of 2009, I had the motivation, but I needed the direction. I harassed Matt Foreman to do some programming for me since my coach was traveling all over the world and was as busy and popular as Britney Spears. I had a fabulous new training partner, Kara Yessie, who happened to move here, thankfully, right after I had opened Pandora's box [to motivation]. I had three tough chicks to coach (and ultimately learn from), I had a fantastic new program that came with a coach, other than Coach Burgener (who I miss terribly, although I feel he thinks the break from me, and Jack Daniels, is like a much needed vacation), willing to put up with me, I was motivated, I wasn't hurting, and for the first time in my life, I was putting everything I had in to every single training session and I was finally ready to come out and play with the big girls.

Fast-forward to 2010, and the road to Nationals… Aimee the athlete was hitting numbers in training that surpassed her lifetime competition PRs, and far exceeded anything she has ever done in the gym. She was consistently hitting above 95% the 6-7 weeks before Nationals, all her lifts were feeling easier and easier. However, Aimee the person hit a lot of nasty bumps in the road, and had a lot of tears, a lot of heartache, and a lot of punches all coming from different directions. Each punch that came, Aimee the athlete would draw from Jolie's desire, Jocelyn's fight on that pitching mound (When approaching a bar, I often thought… If Joc can deal with THAT, than I can certainly deal with THIS), and Tamara's undeniable strength. She would look over at Kara, and see the support, sing a tune in her head, and approach the bar as if Aimee the person didn't exist. The athlete had hung on to that motivation despite what the person was going through, and she excelled. Four days before Nationals, on June 8th, Aimee the person found out she was very sick and couldn't travel. Aimee the athlete was crushed because she had a chance to make the world team, and was in the best shape in her life. Aimee the athlete felt herself slipping back in to that dark hole of where she had found herself in 2007 post-injury—the place where motivation doesn't exist, where fear grabs hold of you and doesn't let go.

A new, young form

This past weekend I was at School Age Nationals helping in the warm-up room with the cards. I am so glad I was there at that moment, and know now that I was supposed to be right there at exactly that time to bring me out of that hole. A young girl, Megan Poole, was competing as a 63 in the 16-17 year division. She was in the #2 spot fighting for another 63 girl's #1 spot, in order to be the one athlete chosen to go to the Youth Olympics. She ended up not moving in to the #1 spot, but let me tell you why she touched me, why she is going to be better than that #1 girl, and why she reached in to the hole and pulled me out without even knowing it. This girl has the most amazing fight, the most incontestable competitiveness, and is absolutely the most precious thing to have ever touched a barbell.

Both girls opened with 95 kg in the clean & jerk, and both girls missed their first attempt. After her first miss, she walked back to the warm-up room to get ready for her second attempt. I was rooting for her and I didn't even know her. Both girls then missed their second attempts, and Megan came back to her chair with everything written all over her face that I had felt many, many times in training and in competition: the fear, the determination, the doubt, the desire to win, the wanting to gain control, the hard work, the raw emotion, the begging yourself to make the lift. The tears in her eyes got to me because I knew what place she was in at that moment.

Both girls missed their third attempts, and Megan was shattered, and in tears, and broken. But to me, she was a fighter who put more on that platform with her misses than I had ever given with my makes. She left more on that platform than many lifters do in their whole careers. She has an enormous amount of mental power, which she possibly doesn't even know exists—and is exactly what is going to bring her out on top in the end. She is my hero, a true champion to have what she has at such a young age. She has given me the new motivation to come back after missing Nationals, and fight even harder, train more fiercely, attack each lift even more. She will likely never forget that day, and neither will I. She is going to be great, and not even knowing her, I am so proud of her.

How does this help anyone or anything?

I am a person with real issues, but I can also still be an athlete. I have worked really hard to get to this place and I refuse to fall back to not-so-motivated-and-wimpy 90% Aimee. Motivation comes in many different forms, and it has taken me a long time to find it, draw from it, and run with it. Who knew coaching some girls, and getting a new training partner from Canada would be the key to my motivation? Who knew watching a young girl leave her broken heart on the platform would make me realize there are other chances, and to never walk off the platform with a regret- miss or make?

So while this seems like it is indeed a page out of my diary, my intent is to tell you that motivation is there, even when you feel you have none. Any coach is lucky to have an athlete who teaches you as much as you teach them, and I have three! I look back at all the years I have been the athlete, and hope that I have taught Coach Burgener and Matt something they can hold on to. I found it, finally, after years of searching, and I am hanging on and keeping it very close. If you are a coach, or an athlete, find it, keep it, and don't let it go. And when that little guy hops on your shoulder to try to take away your motivation, keep in mind what my coach Matt says: "That fucker doesn't know shit about weightlifting.

THE ROLE OF STRENGTH IN WEIGHTLIFTING
GREG EVERETT

While the premise of this article may at first strike readers as odd, considering that weightlifting, despite considerable elements of skill and speed, is very clearly a strength sport, there exist quite a few perspectives regarding the role of strength in the training of weightlifters; or, more accurately, regarding the appropriate degree of emphasis of what might be considered non-specific strength work.

The spectrum is represented on one end by Bulgarian-style training, involving little other, if anything at all, than the classic lifts and squats; the other end is represented by more of a powerlifting influence, involving a relatively large volume of general strength development with exercises like squatting, deadlift and pressing variations.

With weightlifting, as is the case with all physical training, we are possessed of few irrefutable facts, and constantly inundated with ideas, theories and anecdotes. And as with just about everything involving opinions, arguments and full-scale warfare continue to rage unabated (thanks in large part to the wondrous liberty and absence of consequence provided by the internet).

Also like with most similar endeavors, success is being achieved with a variety of methods, proving that no perfect approach exists—or at least that it has yet to be discovered.

Strength

Strength is a physical quality that is manifested in many different forms, some of which, it turns out, have little or nothing to do with each other in a practical sense. The most pertinent example in this case is the transfer of slow strength to explosiveness, or, more accurately, the lack thereof. Both anecdote and research have demonstrated that the ability to move very heavy weights slowly does not transfer well to the ability to move weights explosively; however, training explosively can improve an athlete's ability to move very heavy weights at any speed .

This is the basis for many weightlifting coaches' aversion to exercises like deadlifts—they want to avoid slow, grinding movements for fear of limiting the athlete's ability to perform a similar movement explosively.

On the other hand, it's often argued that developing and maintaining a greater base of less than perfectly specific strength will provide more potential for classic lift performance. For example, if an athlete is able to clean 70% of his best deadlift, it seems logical that a heavier deadlift will result in a heavier potential clean.

Considering various weightlifters, the truth appears to be far less simplistic. It's not uncommon for weightlifters who never train the deadlift to out-deadlift their deadlifting counterparts. Of course, there are also plenty of examples of successful weightlifters who do employ the deadlift regularly.

Kendrick Farris is currently the best weightlifter in the US (he has cleaned and very nearly jerked the current world record as an 85 kg (187 lb) lifter—218 kg (480 lbs)), and accordingly, is often used for examples of effective training methodology. His coach, Dr. Kyle Pierce of LSU Shreveport, employs a system of classic periodization and a considerable volume of basic strength lifts such as deadlifts. Farris is extraordinarily strong; for example, he recently back squatted 235 kg (518 lbs) for 10 reps.

On the other end of the spectrum is Pat Mendes, who trains with coach John Broz in Las Vegas. At 130 kg (286 lbs), Pat has snatched 200 kg (441 lbs) and cleaned 230 kg (507 lbs)—2.5 kg more in the snatch and just 7.5 kg less in the clean & jerk than Shane Hammon's American record lifts—at the age of 19. Pat trains with Bulgarian-type methods, relying on the snatch, clean & jerk and front and back squats for the overwhelming majority of his training.

Would either be better having trained the other way? It's impossible to know. What we do know is that both ways can work. The Bulgarians have their stripped system of heavy classic lifts; the Chinese have a system of huge variety and a great deal of strength work. Other countries have systems using elements of both. All are producing extraordinary weightlifters.

Us Against The World

The US's performance on the international weightlifting stage has been less than impressive for the last few decades. Opinions vary on the reasons for this, but no one denies the fact that Americans are lagging far behind.

The trite phrase being tossed around the internet is, "American weightlifters just aren't strong enough." Such a statement is as useful and insightful as telling a sprinter he isn't fast enough. The question is how this can be changed, and this is where the arguments begin.

The idea that the US's poor international performance can be attributed to a single reason is silly at best. There are myriad factors contributing to the current state of weightlifting, and to neglect some to focus on a few that seem easier to correct is securing failure.

The more dominant countries in the sport have extensive infrastructure that provides for the recruiting and development of appropriate talent for the sport. They have cultures that recognize and appreciate weightlifting and weightlifters. They have fewer alternate sports to divert weightlifting talent. They have a greater number of lifters. And always looms the fact that drug testing in many of these countries is questionable, and by most accounts, drug use is commonplace.

In the US, weightlifting is an extremely obscure sport. Even if potential athletes happen to be exposed to it, there is little motivation to become involved. Sports like football, baseball, track and field, and gymnastics offer far more potential for financial and social success; additionally, these sports are ubiquitous, and coaches, facilities and related programs are easy to find. In contrast, weightlifters often must go to great lengths to even find a gym in which they can perform the lifts, let alone a qualified coach.

Considering the disparities in the circumstances, it's little surprise the US is not a leader in the sport. To chalk it up simply to inferior training methods is nonsense.

Making the Decision

If it's true, as it appears to be, that no single approach is best and that multiple methods can be effective, how does a weightlifting coach or weightlifter decide how to train? This is a decision that will hinge on multiple factors, but in all cases, it must be made in accordance to the needs of the lifter and his or her response to any given method. The biggest mistake any coach or athlete can make is to remain rigidly committed to a single approach when it becomes apparent that it no longer works or never worked in the first place. Experimentation carries some degree of risk, but it also provides the opportunity for discovery.

In a system that starts lifters at a young age with no previous athletic experience, a more consistent plan among athletes is possible. That is, these athletes can be collectively developed according to common need—the instruction and development of classic lift technique, the development of general and specific strength, and the development of work capacity.

In the US, there is essentially an absence of a system. Weightlifters typically arrive at the sport at later ages following other athletic careers. As a result, there is far more variation in the abilities, capacities and needs of US weightlifters, and consequently no simple prescription can be applied across the board. If a lifter is extremely strong, but technically unsound or inconsistent, it makes little sense to emphasize strength work over classic lift work; if a lifter is technically sound but simply doesn't have enough strength, strength work can be prioritized and classic lift work reduced. This kind of individualization can be difficult to implement with large groups of weightlifters, but fortunately, such groups really don't exist in the US.

The bottom line is that without a huge pool of athletes appropriate for the training, training must be made entirely appropriate for the athletes in order for any reasonable level of success to be achieved.

THE ESSENCE OF TIME
JOE KENN

In sports, when the word "time" is used in a conversation, most discussion will be focused on an individual's 40-yard dash, or how fast they can cover 40 yards in a maximal effort sprint. This is usually discussed in seconds, as in, "My running back ran the 40 in 4.37 seconds."

In the structured programming of competitive athletics, the essence of time is a critical point of the planning process for the majority of strength and conditioning coaches across the nation. There are many ways to view the term "time" and how it applies in many different parameters of the training plan. Below is my opinion on the "manipulation of time" in several areas, as it applies to training.

Time: The Long and Short of It

The development of a highly successful program is going to be gauged on the development of long and short term planning. Coaches should develop a Quadrennial plan for their athletes' high school or college careers. The term Quadrennial Plan comes from Olympic Training programming as it relates to the 4-year training process an athlete goes through preparing for the Olympic Games. The Quadrennial plan works fairly well with high school and college athletes because we generally have them entering their freshmen year and continue to work with them through their senior season. Typically, this is a four-year process. As strength and conditioning coaches (and at this level, we are really general physical preparedness specialists), we can develop an approach that sequentially improves on the general physical fitness attributes necessary to achieve improved athleticism. It's up to an athlete's sport specific coach to improve their specific "on-field" abilities. We train the general; they train the specific.

As we set up the goals of Quadrennial Plan, we must now shorten the time period down to four specific annual plans. As the athlete goes through your program, the goals and expectations of the program should change with the athlete's increased training age.

Once the goals of the annual plans are set, we now move onto the short-term goals of the yearly plan. These short-term goals are usually broken down into multiple four-week time periods. Four-week periods are usually termed mesocycles or blocks, and they will have specific adaptation goals that your athletes will be working hard to achieve.

Long term planning for professional athletes is going to be slightly different. I have studied and discussed this at length and have found coaches tend to look at the longevity of the athlete's career in "years of service." I have spoken to several coaches who break up the long term plan similar to this; rookies to year three, year four through year seven, years eight through ten, and finally ten plus.

This is a basic overview of the essence of time as it relates to programming an athlete's career. As with any programming issues, there are always exceptions. This might include athletes who transfer in, athletes who leave early for the professional ranks, athletes who exceed the norms for their general training age, injuries, etc.

Training Session Duration

If you read enough material you will find that there are several opinions on what the optimal training session duration should be. Should it be no more than 60 minutes? 90 minutes? Do you include the warm-up in this time? The responses are as varied as the coaches.

I think one of the biggest issues of time spent in specific training sessions will be based on your specific situation. For example, college strength and conditioning coaches are working off of an NCAA governed allotment of eight total hours a week of training. In some cases, as with basketball, this may be reduced to six hours because the position coaches can do individual position specific work with their athletes up to two hours per week. In the high school level, your training session duration may be designated by the length of each class period. As you can see, though training has its scientific factors, the coach's ability to be creative in program design is at a high premium.

My goal for a strength training session is 75 minutes. This includes the "warm up," though I prefer to use a term borrowed from Coach Charles Staley: pre-activity preparation. If we have scheduled a running session, our goal time for the session is less than 60 minutes. Our Linear and Lateral Speed Sessions can range from 15 to 45 minutes, depending on the mesocycles. The majority of the time we are in the 30-minute range because we usually follow this session with a transition to the strength training session of the day. Depending on the goals of the training blocks, conditioning sessions can run between 45 to 120 minutes. The latter is usually during the final stages of a football summer program when we are in a block of training in which the conditioning session is organized similar to an actual practice. When we are in this block of training the time demands on the other components of training decrease.

Repetition Speed (as it pertains to strength training)

Speed of movement is another exciting aspect of time that can bring about a tremendous amount of discussion. This is one factor of time that I have really worked hard on defining and differentiating in my own training as it relates to strength movements. Why? So I have a better ability to relate to my athletes the type of training response we are hoping to achieve.

First, my recommendation as it pertains to training athletes is to always perform the concentric portion of a movement with maximal concentric acceleration. This is based off of Fred Hatfield's Compensatory Acceleration method and Vladimir Zatsiorsky's Dynamic Effort Method, made popular by strength coach Louie Simmons. This especially pertains to movements that are not classified in the Olympic Weightlifting category. The goal is to perform the positive aspect of the movement (concentric phase) as explosively or fast as possible.

How fast or explosive the movement is completed is related to the external load of resistance based on training intensity, but the athlete's mental intent must be on being fast. The external load will also determine how fast one must begin to decelerate the bar before completion. In general, the lighter the load, the sooner deceleration of the movement occurs.

When training intensities are lighter, coaches of advanced athletes could implement the principle of accommodating resistance, popularized in the U.S. by Coach Simmons, into the program. In short, accommodating resistance means varying the resistance (implementing chains or bands) to mimic the increased/decreased strength levels of the changing lever angles during the entire movement. In the case of the concentric phase of the movement, the load gets heavier as the athlete completes this phase, allowing for a longer acceleration time.

As far as the eccentric or negative phase of the movement, I recommend what I call a "strong eccentric." This is usually between one to three seconds, but I am not asking my athletes to mentally count this out. I prefer to see the athlete control the external load to help develop eccentric strength as well as the stabilizing muscle groups of the movement. Here are some examples of how to vary speed of movement. Tempo as it relates to repetition [rep] duration is a term popularized by Strength Coach Charles Poliquin. Utilizing a tempo based repetition we will place a specific time for each phase of the movement. I have slightly manipulated Coach Poliquin's model to suit my needs. An example of a specific repetition tempo for our athletes might be [X-2-1-1]. This is a standard tempo we would use with most of our major and secondary assistance movements. The first number "X" coincides with the concentric phase of the rep. As I mentioned earlier, I am a proponent of maximum concentric acceleration so we are looking for an explosive intent. The second number is the eccentric phase which equals 2 counts. This can be measured easily by using a 1-1, 2-2 cadence. The third number relates to midpoint pause/contraction time and the fourth number relates to completion pause before performing the next rep. By adjusting the tempo scheme of the rep, we can elicit different training stimuli.

I also want to add two training tempo manipulations. I utilize Iso Miometric/Iso Dynamic and Sub Max Eccentrics. These two training tempos are from Christian Thibaudeau and are part of my regime training cycles that I learned from Coach Buddy Morris and Coach Tom Myslinski. An Iso Miometric/Dynamic protocol is based on a 6-repetition set in which the midpoint pause/contraction time is manipulated. Repetition one has a 6-count midpoint pause and for each following rep you decrease the midpoint pause 1 count. A Sub Max Eccentric Set is a fixed tempo of a 6-count eccentric phase for each rep. The standard rep count per set is six.

These are excellent alternatives to high repetition hypertrophy training because we have manipulated the all-important aspect of time. Based on the principle or T-U-T, Time Under Tension, we can elicit a hypertrophy effect with fewer reps because we alter the repetition tempo to match the time demand. In the majority of articles I have read on the subject, it is recommended that an individual set must have a T-U-T of at least 40 seconds to elicit a hypertrophy response.

Obviously, this is an overview and one man's perspective on these aspects of Time. My goal was to stimulate the thought process and for you to evaluate how the Essence of Time is an important part of the program design continuum.

Here are some other components of time to dwell on: rest and recovery time. Work: Rest ratios in your speed and conditioning sessions, and improving your density of training. Rest and recovery as well as nutrition may be more important than any other training modality. Are your work to rest intervals properly developed for the energy system(s) you are trying to improve? Or can we improve density of training by manipulating rest times between sets and pairing movements?

There are numerous factors that need to be considered in the process of program design. Time and its many derivatives is just one of those factors that has numerous influences in programming. In the end, be practical and creative and your athletes will succeed.

IT'S NOT A RACE FOR LAST
JOE KENN

This July, my youngest son Peter was going through his first training camp of organized tackle football and I was very excited. With football, as with most other team sports, practices are pretty much all the same; start off with a warm up, move to position fundamentals, follow with some group/team work, and finish up with conditioning. It was during the conditioning portion of my son's football practice that I heard one of the greatest motivational lines I've heard in my 34 years of playing sports and coaching.

On that humid summer evening, Coach Phillips was running his team of twelve year olds through sprint drills. The sight of those boys running sprint after sprint, arms flailing and heads bobbing, was one that made me laugh. I knew some of them were running for the first time all summer. Coach Phillips probably knew it also because when he noticed several boys lagging he yelled, "It's not a race for last! " "It's not a race for last"…as soon as I heard it, I knew it would be a great line to use down the road. I didn't want to forget it so I quickly texted it to myself. So, thank you Coach Phillips. I have officially stolen it.

Now, as I watch conditioning drills for my own team, I keep this quote in the back of my mind. I have yet to use it as motivation for my athletes, but try to think about what it actually means to me. I have an idea of what Coach Phillips was trying to get out of his team, but I am looking for something deeper. I continue to evaluate my team as well as the quote. In doing so, I think of past summers with other teams at different universities for a way to define it. I contemplate how to apply it to my athletes, staff and colleagues.

As I look to define It's not a race for last, let's examine this scenario: a typical interval conditioning session. Whatever distance you are running, you will have athletes that fall into several categories.

The first one is what I call The Rabbits. These athletes are the ones that set the tempo for the rest of the group. They pride themselves on finishing each rep at the front of the pack. They beat designated goal times.

The next group of athletes is The Back of the Pack group. No matter how hard they try, they will never make the designated goal times because goal times are based on average norms. Some of these athletes may be the fastest on your team in short sprints but on distance intervals, they are cooked. Other athletes are just not meant to run. I have a tremendous amount of respect for these athletes. My goal with these athletes is for them to improve and to bring them closer to the third group that I call The Pace.

Pace Athletes are divided into two types. The first type, are those who perform drills with solid effort but finish slightly behind The Rabbits. The second type, are the newly named It's Not a Race for Last group. These athletes do just enough to finish the drill and remain invisible. These athletes cross the goal line just as you say, "Time". They extract just enough energy to "not be called out" but never enough to get them to the next level. They think no one is watching them. Really good coaches have every eye on them because these athletes will get you fired.

The It's Not a Race for Last group or person can occur on any team, staff or organization in any situation. That is because the simple definition of It's Not a Race for Last is COMPLACENCY. Every large group working toward a common goal will have individuals who are just trying to get by. They are satisfied with the current situation wanting no more or less. Some don't see themselves as this type of person. These are the ones who become problem issues. They can't see why they are asked to give more or step out of their comfort zone. These individuals always have an excuse as to why they can't do something or why they were late, absent, or missed a deadline. It's never their fault. When things go bad, they become locker room lawyers. They don't like to be called out in front of their peers for lack of effort and usually try to bring others down with them. In my world, these athletes may have extreme talent but they lack motivation and are easily distracted. In their minds, they are Ballas who are going to the League. As for me, they think I don't know what I am talking about. If you get too many of these athletes on one team you are sure to find failure.

So, how do you correct this problem? Whether through recruiting or interviews, make sure you have a process that allows you to evaluate an athlete's Positive Tangibles. Does he look you in the eye when introductions are made? Does he have a passion in his voice when discussing the possibility of being part of your program? Is there a strong work ethic built into his family makeup? Is being part of a successful venture important to him? Is he willing to evaluate his skills to be the best at his position? Does he have a leadership gene? It's my opinion leadership is an innate ability that cannot be taught. I have been involved in numerous projects designed to teach leadership skills to student athletes only to find out that leaders already know how to lead. You can give individuals the tools to lead but you cannot get them to operate those tools if they don't want to.

How do you change the culture of athletes in your organization? You must be willing to judge each athlete individually. Each athlete will have something slightly different that makes them an It's not a Race for Last athlete. You must be willing to draw out their best qualities. In some cases, it will be easier to assign someone else to work with or supervise them. Having a diverse staff will be to everyone's benefit. A diverse staff with slightly different personality traits blended to match your overall coaching culture will help you bring out the best in every athlete. Sometimes an It's Not a Race for Last athlete for you will be a different athlete for one of your staff. Together, you can figure out what motivates the athlete, building and mending the relationship so that the athlete feels you care for him and have his best interests at heart.

Keep the It's Not a Race for Last athletes engaged in the developmental process. It can be as easy as playing the type of music they like to hear or an incentive program in which they are rewarded. Be open to new ideas and consider numerous ways to motivate them. Good luck and thanks for reading.

REEVALUATING LOWER BODY TRAINING
JOSH HENKIN

Far too often as coaches we read articles that are full of scientific research, but a lot of times bridging that gap to practical application is far more difficult. One of the biggest challenges to coaches is fitting in various types of training with their athletes or clients in just a few sessions a week. How do we combine all the necessary components of proper training, maximal strength, speed, agility, deceleration, acceleration, change of direction, isometric strength, endurance, and sport-specific training?

The truth is that many techniques we use cover more than one aspect at a time. If not, a coach needs to reevaluate their training philosophy. A component of training that has been receiving a lot of attention is the concept of stability training. Joint stability seems to be a cornerstone of any training program. However, what makes up stability training may not be so clear.

The Stability Component

Stability can be as vague of a term as "strength" is. Without overly complicating terms, a definition I like is this: "Joint stability refers to the resistance offered by various musculoskeletal tissues that surround a skeletal joint. Several subsystems ensure the stability of a joint. These are the passive, active and neural subsystems. The opposite of stability is instability." (1)

For a large majority of coaches, such a definition isn't overly helpful. A more practical definition may be, "the effective accommodation of the joints to each specific load demand through an adequately tailored joint compression, as a function of gravity, coordinated muscle and ligament forces, to produce effective joint reaction forces under changing conditions.

Optimal stability is achieved when the balance between performance (the level of stability) and effort is optimized to economize the use of energy. Non-optimal joint stability implicates altered laxity/stiffness values leading to increased joint translations resulting in a new joint position and/or exaggerated/reduced joint compression, with a disturbed performance/effort ratio." (2)

Truthfully, this doesn't seem to help that much either. For most coaches, stability training and slow isometric movements are typically done on the floor. It is almost seen as a "necessary evil" that takes some time from our normal training; drills that we feel obligated to do and try to get over with as fast as possible. While such drills may be necessary, the progression to more dynamic and real world base drills is far more important in performance related endeavors.

Sport-Specific Stability

The truth hurts, but real sport-specific training is beyond most coaches. REAL sport-specific training requires a highly developed knowledge of biomechanics of sporting actions that occur during the sport. The nice part is most athletes are not prepared to perform true sport-specific training because they are not "fit" enough to benefit from the training. However, we do need to understand that our training does need to progress to speeds and challenges that are faced in real world and sport.

One of the easiest ways to achieve stability in more practical ways is to emphasize the role of single leg training. Of course, most coaches already use single leg training in one form or another, but rarely give it the attention it truly deserves. No, you don't have to stop your bilateral lifts, but looking at the role they play in your training is important.

Some coaches are still believers in the idea that squats, deadlifts, and Olympic lift variations will take care of most lower body and stability type of training. Yet, even non-field sports such as Olympic lifting have even used single leg training as a means to improve these very qualities for their competitive lifts. Research also tends to support that utilizing one-legged drills is important for several reasons...

Maximal Muscle Contractions: A 1978 study demonstrated that unilateral leg extension exercise created higher levels of maximal voluntary muscle contraction than bilateral leg extension training. (3) Yes, I know, LEG EXTENSIONS! This can't really be indicative of true functional and sports training. Yet, another training study does support this in a more functional environment.

Higher Ground Reaction Forces: "Ten well-trained male volleyball players performed one-legged and two-legged vertical countermovement jumps. Ground reaction forces, cinematographic data, and electromyographic data were recorded. Jumping height in one-legged jumps was 58.5% of that reached in two-legged jumps. Mean net torques in hip and ankle joints were higher in one-legged jumps. Net power output in the ankle joint was extremely high in one-legged jumps. This high power output was explained by a higher level of activation in both heads of m. gastrocnemius in the one-legged jump. A higher level of activation was also found in m. vastus medialis. These differences between unilateral and bilateral performance of the complex movement jumping were shown to be in agreement with differences reported in literature based on isometric and isokinetic experiments." (4)

Most sporting actions are determined by ground reaction forces. Typically, greater speed and power is developed by creating higher ground reaction forces. The majority of sports have a transition phase of our base of support being applied only by one leg, whether this is in straight ahead running or change of direction. This may mean that more advanced forms of training is spending more time learning how to develop power and strength on one leg.

However, how does this all transition back to the idea of providing body stability? Reducing our body support has a profound impact on how our body recruits different muscles.

Studies have shown in just bridging exercises the body recruits more muscles in a less stable position than more stable. "In general, the ratio of the internal/external abdominal oblique activity was about 1. However, during the unilateral bridging exercise, the ipsilateral internal/external abdominal oblique activity ratio was 2.79 as a consequence of the significant higher relative activity of the internal oblique compared to the external oblique." (5)

Single leg drills tend to work more the adductors, gluteus medius, and gluteus minimus than their bilateral counterparts. This is tremendously important, as much of our pelvic stability is reliant upon the strength of these muscles. If our pelvis is more stable, our ability to exhibit force goes up. In fact, weakness in these muscles can show themselves in problems such as Trendelenburg gait where the SI joint and lumbar spine can be at great risk of injury.

Where to Start?

It may not be that hard to convince people that they should utilize single leg exercises. However, many do not have a definitive system in which they implement these movements. Just as with any training, we need to lay down progressions for proper usage. If we are not aware of the impact of jumping into advanced versions of single leg training, we can easily set-up our athlete or client for injury as forces applied to the body in single leg training aren't just double that of bilateral, but can be exponentially higher.

1. Stable before unstable: A good rule of thumb for just about any form of training, this is especially true in single leg training. Most coaches rush into single leg plyos or stepping versions of lunges without observing if their client can demonstrate control and proficiency in safer environments. A base level exercise for dynamic lunging would be a static position. Watching for proper stride length, knee valgus, and lower leg control is key in being able to provide appropriate more advanced forms of single leg training. In drills such as step-ups, working from a low step in a slow controlled manner is the correct starting point where many coaches work from higher steps that often cause compensation.

Beginner Series:

- Stationary Single Leg Squat
- Stationary Single Leg Squat Lateral
- Stepping Lunge Forwards

Intermediate Series:

- Stepping Lunge Reverse
- Stepping Lunge Lateral
- Elevated Rear Leg Single Leg Squat

Advanced Series:

- Rear Crossover Lunge
- Mixed Patterns
- Suspended

2. Work on Different Loading Patterns: The placement of load is commonly a neglected aspect of programming. Beginning with the load down by the hips either holding a dumbbell or kettlebell places the load through the body without much of a change in center of gravity. We can go through a progression of placing weight on the upper back, front of the body, and overhead. These variations all change the center of gravity and perceived load. More advanced loading patterns can be sandbag shoulder, one-arm weight overhead, mixed loading patterns (one arm up, one arm down), etc.

Beginner Series:

- Down By Side
- Goblet

Intermediate Series

- Front Rack
- Overhead

Advanced Series:

- X Series 1: One down by side, other in front rack
- X Series 2: One in front rack, other overhead

3. Range of Motion (ROM): A simple principle of loading and progression is to alter the range of motion. Whether it is due to mobility and flexibility issues, or confidence and strength, ROM is a vital component of any drill. The eventual goal of any lift should be to obtain optimal ROM. This can vary depending upon one's structure, but identifying what is optimal for that individual should be identified in early stages of training. Increasing ROM can be a means of raising intensity of any drill and decreasing the ROM is can serve as an important means for progressing individuals that show significant signs of instability.

Progressional Series:

- Front Foot Elevated
- Flat on Ground
- Rear Foot Elevated
- Suspended

4. Complexity: An often-overlooked variable is exercise complexity. This can be much hard to quantify, but can be powerful in accomplishing goals of improving stability and performance. Increasing complexity by changing stepping patterns, mixing loading patterns (cross patterns for example), and increasing speed can fit into this category, as the body now relies on different neural loops to guide the performance.

Examples of Complexity:

- Rotational Lunge
- Split Snatch
- Lateral Step Swings
- Suspended Squat Thrusts
- Staggered Cleans

Having a series of specific progressional series for lunging, single leg squatting, single leg deadlifts, step-ups, and single leg explosive lifts is critical. While most coaches are quick to implement single leg bounding and plyometric drills, these preparatory series can do a lot for performance, by allowing coaches to properly utilize more advanced training techniques when necessary.

Notes

1.Panjabi MM. (1992). "The stabilizing system of the spine. Part II. Neutral zone and instability hypothesis."]. J Spinal Disord 5 (4): 390–7.

2. Vleeming A, Albert H B, van der Helm F C T, Lee D, Ostgaard H C, Stuge B, Sturesson B.

3. 'Contralateral Influence on Recruitment of Curarized Muscle Fibers during Maximal Voluntary Extension of the Legs,' Acta Physiologica Scandinavica, vol. 103, pp. 456-462, 1978).

4. A Comparison of One-Legged and Two-Legged Countermovement Jumps,' Medicine and Science in Sports and Exercise, vol. 17(6), pp. 635-639, 1985

5. BMC Musculoskelet Disord. 2006 Sep 20;7:75.Trunk muscle activity in healthy subjects during bridging stabilization exercises.Stevens VK, Bouche KG, Mahieu NN, Coorevits PL, Vanderstraeten GG, Danneels LA.Department of Rehabilitation Sciences and Physiotherapy, Faculty of Medicine and Health Sciences, Ghent University, Belgium. Veerle.Stevens@UGent.be

PULL
MATT FOREMAN

I've learned a lot about the Catalyst Athletics crowd since I've been writing articles for Performance Menu over the last two years. Some of the things I've learned have come from reading the forums on the Catalyst website and checking out what people are talking about, and I've picked up other things through the connections I've been able to make in recent months with people in "the network." When I talk about "the network," I'm referring to people who are Catalyst readers, WOD followers, and lots of other people who like to blend the Olympic Lifts with several different forms of training to gain strength. I'm really enjoying you network folks, and there is one interesting (and refreshing) fact that I've been able to observe. You guys like the deadlift.

It seems like every time I read something from the Weightlifting & Powerlifting forum on the website, there's a thread where people are discussing the deadlift. You people love it, and I can't say I blame you. The deadlift was my first love in the iron game. Well... maybe not my first love. I guess the bench press was actually my first love. But my bench press love wasn't real love. I know that now. My bench press love was like the love you have for a high school girlfriend. It's not true love, but it seems like it at the time because you're getting a lot of cool immediate rewards. And likewise, it wasn't until after I had wasted a lot of time and energy on my bench-press-first-love-not-really-but-it-seemed-like-it that I finally discovered the deadlift. And the love for the deadlift is the love that lasts a lifetime.

Now, everybody and their crippled grandmother has written an article about the deadlift. If you've been around strength sports long enough and done plenty of reading, you've probably heard a lot about technique, training methods, benefits and hazards, etc. of the deadlift. Regardless, I'm going to write a deadlift article anyway because I am absolutely positive that I can give you some information that will benefit you, and I'll bet my medulla oblongata that some of it will be stuff you haven't thought about before. Nobody has been this confident since Johnny Cochran. So whether you're an Olympic lifter, generalist, strength coach, powerlifter, or human being who wants to live a better life, read on and soak up the knowledge.

Why do we love it so?

As most of you know, the deadlift is one of the three competitive lifts in the sport of powerlifting. Several phenomenal world record lifts have been pulled since powerlifting became an organized sport decades ago, from Lamar Gant's 688 pound pull at 132 bodyweight to the heaviest deadlift of all time, Andy Bolton's 1008 pounder. That's right. Human beings have lifted those weights. Some people have called the deadlift "the best overall test of a person's true strength level that can be performed with a barbell." I agree with this. When a person is locking out a heavy deadlift, there are very few things in the world that will give the same feeling of complete physical exertion.

If you follow powerlifting at all, you know that the last twenty years has seen an explosion of supportive gear in the sport. Canvas squat suits and denim bench press shirts have been invented that have allowed powerlifters to add 200-300 pounds on these lifts through the supportive slingshot effect they provide. Many people (myself included) believe that this equipment has gotten totally out of control and blemished the sport. However, nobody has ever been able to find a piece of supportive gear that adds tons of phony pounds to the deadlift. Sure, some lifters wear supportive suits in the deadlift that are fashioned much like the squat suits, but their effect on the lift is generally considered minimal. In fact, many of the top lifters in the world still pull their competitive deadlifts in regular wrestling singlets because the supportive suits don't help that much. This situation has allowed the deadlift to remain relatively pure in terms of comparison of the top numbers from thirty years ago and the top numbers of the world's current best. While the squats and deadlifts from the 70s and 80s have been left in the dust by today's supportive-gear-enhanced lifters, the deadlifts of former icons like Vince Anello and John Kuc still stack up today as some of the finest pulls in history.

One of the things about the deadlift that I personally find interesting is the fact that it seems to be the one major strength lift that people can still perform fairly well in old age. We all know that our strength starts to go downhill as we get older. That's not a news flash. But if you spend enough time in strength sports and do enough reading, you'll notice that some lifts go downhill faster than others as we get older. The Olympic Lifts, unfortunately, are some of the prime culprits in this dilemma. The snatch and the clean and jerk rely on explosive power and flexibility, which are two areas that don't hang around long once the gray hair starts to pop up. Don't get me wrong, there are still thousands of old masters weightlifters in the world who are performing the Olympic Lifts into their fifties and sixties (and older!). But the poundages take a major nose dive and the technique of a sixty year-old lifter is usually much slower than a twenty year-old (no offense meant; anybody who is still snatching at sixty is a god in my eyes). The same thing holds true for squatting and bench pressing, because the knees and the shoulders often don't hold up well to all the pounding and compression as the years pass.

However, the deadlift has some interesting features that seem to make it a more favorable lift for geriatrics. It's probably because it's easier on the knees and shoulders than the aforementioned squats and Olympic Lifts, and the nature of the lift increases postural core strength. I'll give you an example of what I'm talking about. At a recent powerlifting contest in Florida, 64 year-old Bob Gaynor pulled a 680 pound deadlift in the 198 pound weight class. Yeah, seriously... The current all-time world record in the 198 pound class is 859 by Ed Coan. That means Bob's lift is 79% of the biggest lift in history in his weight class, and he's 64. Believe me brothers and sisters, there are no 64 year-old Olympic Lifters who are snatching or clean and jerking 79% of the world record. The current clean and jerk world record in the 208 pound weight class is 510 pounds by Poland's Simon Kolecki. 79% of that record would be 403 pounds. Try to find a 64 year-old who is clean and jerking 403 pounds. You'll have better luck looking for the Loch Ness Monster.

Of course we all know that there aren't a whole lot of Bob Gaynors running around in the world. Bob is a freak of nature, no doubt about it. But if you read Powerlifting USA magazine and look at the meet results section, you will routinely see lifters in their fifties and sixties who are still pulling well over 500 pounds. I just competed in a powerlifting meet last weekend where two men in the 60-64 age group pulled well over 500 and another lifter in the 50-54 group did 589. And speaking of that meet I lifted in last week, I think I might have figured out a training secret that has allowed these old geezers to keep yanking big iron. Wanna know what it is?

Heavy singles?

I decided to try a little experiment at this recent meet. Before I tell you how it worked, let me give you some background. Throughout my lifting career, I have always trained the deadlift by deadlifting heavy... plain and simple. When I did my biggest deadlift (672 pounds) back in 2003, I was deadlifting once a week and basically always performing doubles and singles in the 620-650 range. I didn't do much high-rep training and, because I was only 31 at the time, my body handled it pretty well.

Now, I'm 38 and it's just really damn hard to pull maximum singles and doubles every week. I've found that at this age, heavy deadlifts take a few weeks to fully recover from. My recovery time isn't nearly as good as it used to be, and having a full-time job makes it really tough to have a lot of energy at the end of the day when I hit the gym. So when I decided to compete in a powerlifting meet recently, I made a decision to experiment with my training a little. First, I established a goal for how much I wanted to pull at the meet. Considering where I am in my lifting life right now, I set 570 pounds as the goal. I had knee surgery back in June and I pulled a tough 545 six weeks later, so 570 looked like a weight that would make me happy for now. Then, I decided that I was only going to use sets of five reps with lighter weights in training because my body just won't take the pounding of heavy singles and doubles right now. So I calculated out how much I needed to pull for a set of five reps to give me a projected one-rep max (1RM) of 570. I used the following formula:

weight x number of reps x 0.0333 + weight = 1RM

I wish I could take credit for inventing this mathematical equation, but I can't. I've read it in various places over the years. I most recently read it in Jim Wendler's 5/3/1 book. You multiply a certain weight by how many reps you complete, then multiply that number by 0.0333, then add the original weight to that number, and the result is your projected 1RM. For me, it calculated like this:

490 x 5 x 0.0333 + 490 = 571

This meant that I needed to pull 490 for a set of five reps to put my projected 1RM at approximately 570. And that's what I did. I used a simple progressive overload program for eight weeks and then, three weeks before the meet, I pulled 490x5 and that was the heaviest weight in attempted in training. It was a challenging set, but definitely not the hardest thing I've ever done.

When I came to the meet, I pulled 501 on my first attempt, 551 on my second, and then finished with 567 on my third attempt. The weight was difficult, but probably not even in the top five toughest deadlifts I've ever pulled. I could have done 573 or maybe 578, probably not much more. So the formula was very accurate, and I was able to hit a big lift in competition without wrecking myself in training. I'm already planning to use this method again. My next goal is to get back to a 600 pound pull, and the formula says I'll need to do 515x5 to hit a 600 pound 1RM. We'll see how it goes. Those of you who want to improve in the deadlift might want to give this method a try. It worked for me.

Other musings...

Here are some rapid fire ideas for you:

Question: What is the best assistance exercise for the deadlift?
Answer: The squat

Question: Can you make progress in the deadlift without heavy squatting?
Answer: Yes, but you'll make more progress if you're increasing your squat strength.

Question: What are the most important technique tips for the deadlift?
Answer:
1. Try to keep your back flat
2. Think about pushing down on the floor instead of pulling up on the bar.

Question: Will heavy deadlifting cause back problems?
Answer: If you use good technique and train correctly, there is very low risk of back trouble.

Question: Is it bad to pull with a rounded back?
Answer: In my opinion, yes. There's only one Konstantin Konstantinovs, and you're not him.

Question: Do heavy deadlifts improve your Olympic Lifts?
Answer: Not really. Heavy deadlifts are slow, and weightlifting is a speed sport. Snatch and clean pulls are much more effective tools to improve in the Olympic Lifts. Of course it's worth mentioning that there are some good lifters who occasionally use deadlifts, but the vast majority don't do them.

Question: Is abdominal work important in the training of the deadlift?
Answer: Absolutely. It's important in everything, period.

These days, everybody wants something that will keep them feeling young. Women run to Botox; men run to Viagra. Nobody wants to feel old, so they'll do practically anything to keep feeling young. So let's agree that there are few things in the world that make a person feel older than a sore lower back. How many of us can think back to when we were kids and we watched our dads grunt like rhinos when they stood up out of their recliners? Their fat guts were pulling their lower vertebrae out of whack, and they let the whole house know about it when they had to get on their feet. Then we go to the airport and see the poor old people who are wheeling their luggage across the terminal with permanent curvature in the spine. It's rough to look at.

I don't know everything about the solar system, but I would just bet that most of these people didn't incorporate a sensible lifting program into their lives. I would even guess that many of these same people spent most of their lives telling others that lifting heavy weights was bad for your back. You probably don't hear those comments from Bob Gaynor. Deadlifting is a terrific exercise for increasing strength and having fun in training, and I'll even say that it can make your golden years more golden if find ways to keep training it productively.

We talked about love in the beginning of this article, so think about being in love with somebody and then apply the same principles to your deadlift training. As the years go by, you have to think of creative ways to tolerate each other if you want the relationship to stay alive. The same thing goes for deadlifting. Think outside the box and don't ever give up, and before you know it you'll be seventy years old with strong spinal erectors and smiling like Peppy McHappystein.

THE RITUAL OF COMPETITION
DANIEL CAMARGO

Athletes are a unique breed of people who bring a sense of passion and ego to any activity they participate in. This is not only accepted but also encouraged. There are athletes who may play a sport for recreational purposes, join an athletic club for social reasons or train at a gym for personal enrichment. But for some athletes, there is a deeper calling to sport. I'm speaking of an athlete in the truest sense of the word – a competitor. Competitors have taken their athletic prowess to a new level and opt to challenge themselves in the arena of competition. They believe they are destined for greatness, whether they actually achieve it or not. Athletes are those who always ran better on the playground, jumped higher than others in P.E. class, and could perform tasks on the first try. For those who don't have the natural talent, their spirit, hunger and dedication can in many cases close the gap. This is the beauty of sport. That said, all competitors have certain things that make them special. It's their passion, pursuit of greatness and obsession that provide what all spectators come to see.

During my time as an elite weightlifter, I must have experienced every emotional and physical stress possible. As a developing athlete, my stress levels were constantly changing from whether my technique was correct or how well I would do at a particular competition to how I looked or sounded during the competition in comparison to the older athletes. By the end of my career, having been a 3-time Jr. World Team Member (1995-1997), the sources of my stress were significantly more focused on making the Olympic team, staying ahead of the up and coming developing athletes, and maintaining high U.S. rankings. During this time, I developed some specific tricks to help me focus and stay at ease prior to and during competition. I teach these rituals to my athletes now and they have seen huge success, just as I did. Though not all of them have continued to practice my secrets, it certainly has allowed them to discover their own rituals to set them at ease in preparation for competition.

Pre-Competition

It is important as a coach to account for the smallest detail and prepare your athlete for anything. This begins with ensuring that he or she has their gear no matter what. It sounds so simple, so obvious, but the truth is that I have witnessed many competitions destroyed by an athlete's gear being lost by an airline. As a U.S. National Team member, I was always forced to travel with my gear close by. I could check a bag during flights, but the equipment that was needed to compete such as singlet, lifting shoes, belt and tape had to travel on the plane with me. This always brought comfort to me, since I knew that even if my luggage was lost in transit, I would still have my "stuff" to compete. You can have my toiletries, my extra clothing and my extra sneakers, but you're not taking my gear. I continue this practice with my athletes. It is mandatory that my athletes ensure they do not check in their necessary equipment but rather carry it on when traveling to competitions.

After arriving, gear in hand, preparation continues in the days prior to competition. Most importantly, the day before competing has always been a sensitive time for my athletes as it was for me. Training is a critical component the day before competition but it must be light, aimed at loosening the athlete up rather than being load intensive. Generally, I do not surpass 60%-70% in any given exercise. In fact, I recommend any coach who trains their athlete the day or evening before competition to do so by keeping in mind that the purpose is only to stimulate the nerves and keep an athlete's muscles firing sequentially. Not that they'll forget how to do so, but because this training session serves as a good stimulant prior to competition.

Following the training session, the waiting period begins. The evening leading to competition is even more important as this is often when anxiety builds. As a coach, helping an athlete to manage this anxiety is critical to achieving success the next day. Some best practices are as follows:

- Watch TV sitting up with all lights on as oppose to in dim lighting, lying down on the bed. Lying in bed with lights low tells your body it's time to sleep. When you don't follow through on this direction to rest, you will find yourself unable to sleep once the television is off and lights are out. By then, it is too late. The body accepted watching TV with lights low as a time to be awake. Unfortunately, you will spend significant time trying to reprogram your mind, but sleep will not come easy. Sitting up with lights on offers the athlete the opportunity to shut it all down and "wind down" for sleep later. Ever heard how the mind can play tricks on you? Well. guess what? You too can play tricks on it.
- Grooming is a ritual best done the night before competition. For me, shaving my face, getting a haircut, or attending to nails etc always gave me a fresh, new feeling. This serves to revitalize an athlete and allow them to feel prepared to give a huge

effort the next day. Yes, even in the sport of Weightlifting men may shave their legs. Of course, they're going to tell you that it was to minimize friction between the barbell and the shins on the first pull as well as the quadriceps during the transition and second pull (I began my career in a time when singlets were high cut, not the knee-length they are today) but, truth is they like the way it makes their legs look.

- Do not try sleeping early in an effort to "get a full night's rest." This is a big mistake. I have found with my own career and my athletes' careers that the best thing to do is to follow the points above and only lay for bed when one feels drowsy and sleepy, even if that results in the athlete only getting 6 hours of sleep. I realize this may contradict what many specialists have to say, but I speak from experience of not only myself but also of the athletes I've coached, which range from the 12-year-old developing athlete to the 20- year-old elite U.S. Jr. World Team to the 45-year old competing locally for the love of the sport. Attempting to go to bed early, especially if it is much earlier than normal bedtime, places the athlete at risk of a sleepless night. Their mind may wander and they are likely to stress out about the time of night and how they aren't in deep sleep, leading their body into restlessness. Now they find that they can't sleep and as a result sleep far less than the above example of 6 hours….or at least think they do. Perception is reality. If the athlete tosses and turns all night, most likely they do sleep some but feel as if they were in and out of consciousness all night long, whether they were or not. That feeling is not one to have before being asked to compete at maximal effort. So, I recommend allowing the athlete to read, watch TV or socialize quietly in a room until the point where they begin to feel drowsy. You may find this will actually come sooner as the athlete doesn't stress about getting to bed early and has the freedom and empowerment to sleep when they feel ready. By encouraging them to stay up until they feel sleepy, you will both reduce some unneeded stress and ensure that whenever they do decide to sleep, they'll do so with ease, thus providing quality sleep. 6 hours of wonderful sleep surpasses 9 hours of tossing and turning.

Day of the meet

Athletes tend to be superstitious people. The day of the meet is key in controlling anxiety and properly preparing an athlete for a perfect day. After waking well-rested and ready to compete, the athlete should do as they normally do to shower or dress. Once you're in the day of competition, there's no turning back. It's time to hit the venue and perform. I teach my athletes the following:

- Never change a routine. Competitions are not the place to try something new, especially new 1RMs, which I'll touch on in a moment. If an athlete never uses certain rituals such as sitting in a hot tub for hours the night before, then don't allow them to do so once in competition mode. I encourage athletes to maintain the same practices they normally perform during training. Remaining consistent is important. For example, I've caught some of my younger athletes "overdosing" on energy drinks right before competition when they normally don't in training. Without wasting space on how I feel about consuming these counter-productive products, I'll only emphatically state to keep your athletes (especially the young ones) away from them. I would certainly have a different opinion if what I have experienced was more positive but unfortunately, or fortunately, depending on how you look at it, I've only seen them cause problems. Drinking energy drinks to get "pumped up" to compete overstimulates the body. I've seen plenty of athletes get the jitters during warm up or the competition. As a result, they don't think straight and lose that very important connection between the brain, nervous system and muscular system--not to mention that their heart rate speeds, blood pressure rises, and their body temperature is higher than it needs to be, or that they could be violating USADA doping guidelines for competition without even knowing it. Isn't natural adrenaline, excitement, and overall anticipation enough to heighten the athlete's awareness? Now, I am not in any way bashing energy drinks for the purpose they serve. I just don't believe they have a place in competition, especially if the athlete is not used to consuming them in training. Why have energy drinks caused problems for an athlete's performance? Not because of the product themselves but because the athlete will more times than not consume too much. I've actually seen a young weightlifter kill two cans of a popular energy drink only to become nauseous and irritable, leaving them unable to perform.
- This next part applies primarily to Olympic Weightlifting focusing on maximal attempts. I've had a long lasting practice that tournaments are not the place to attempt new personal records with the exception of close competition where it's worth the risk in order to win. Training is the place to try 1RMs. Why? Because you have all day to try. There are not any judges, time is not of the essence and the pressure on the athlete is significantly less. This is the circumstance where continuous efforts can be made. In Olympic Weightlifting, the athlete has 3 attempts at a particular event. That's it. Athletes should make the best use of those attempts and ensure they are successful. My philosophy has always been that it doesn't matter what you do in training; if you don't do it in a meet, it doesn't count. After all, we're competitors. We don't call ourselves athletes because we only exercise. We call ourselves athletes because we compete, we fight, we challenge. What good is it to have a 150kg (330lbs) Clean + Jerk in training but you only successfully lift 125kg (275lbs) when in front of referees? It is important that attempts, especially the first two, are weights that have been executed a number

of times during training, perhaps in the range of 85%-95% of their current bests. If they're strong, those weights will be enough to place high in the competition. If they're not, well, why not keep the athlete in their comfort zone and let them walk away content with a good performance because they were not at the top of the class this time around? Now, as I said, there is an exception to this rule--and that is in the case of close competition. If you or your athlete is in a situation where personal records are needed to place high, and nothing else will matter, well then you do what you went there to do, win! Put it on the bar and give it your best. Perhaps the rush will give you the little extra strength and timing you need. Just keep in mind; you'll only have that one chance. There are no repeats.

- During competition, there are always situations where athletes and coaches have to abort their game plan and quickly change strategies. For weightlifting, it comes when other coaches manipulate the score cards to optimize their athlete's chances at winning but may leave you with less time to prepare or, in some cases, way too much time. It can also come from schedule delays but the most crucial component is still time on the clock. A strategy that always works for me is to not include the athlete in the decision-making process. Of course, you must know your athlete and make choices that do not negatively affect them. There are times when you consult with them to see how they feel about a scenario, but attempting to alleviate as much stress as possible is paramount. The athlete has much to worry about as is so leave them be. It's the coach's responsibility to filter unforeseen problems and reassure the athlete that they have nothing additional to stress about. Too often coaches wear their emotions on their sleeves, which will ultimately be reflected in the athlete who feeds off of the coach. If the athlete sees you stress and lose composure, they'll be thinking about the wrong thing when they're called upon the main stage. Then whose fault is it when the athlete is distracted and does not perform?
- Visualization is a huge part of mental preparation and stability. If an athlete can see it happen enough times in their minds eye, they are more likely to make it happen on the platform. I once would sit in a corner between every warm up set, staring at the ground, visualizing that I was witnessing myself commit the perfect lift. I encourage all of my athletes to find their best viewpoint and experience the movement, the strength and the meet in their head over and over again. Don't worry. They will snap out of it when their name is called. You won't lose them for long. Then I ask them to see it again and again. My viewpoint was third person and sometimes in the first person. Once athletes get comfortable seeing or experiencing a great performance in their heads enough times, they'll be amazed at how it becomes reality.
- Athletes need companionship during their moments of athletic execution. Even those who prefer to seclude themselves with earphones in a corner must know that not far away from them is their companion, their coach. The person who is

their only connection to the logistics of the tournament and who gives him/her the necessary information to proceed, to stand up, to get ready. It is good practice to never let your athlete feel lonely. They are in total control of their performance. Coaches prepare and mold the athlete but in the end, during those last seconds of testing, it is the athlete who has to make it happen. Nonetheless, knowing they have someone they trust nearby is essential. I make good practice of walking my athlete to the chalk tray and as far as I can until the official tells me I've gone too far. It is at that location that I wait for them on their return, whether successful or not. Even the toughest athlete needs that comfort. Give it to them.

There are people among us who are either born with, or develop the attributes of, being not only athletes but also competitors. It is their physical and neurological capabilities built on an unshakeable foundation of their spirit, pursuit, ego, and passion. Competitors are continuously striving for more. During training, they sacrifice themselves to pain and exhaustion, attempting to maximize every second of their sessions. They dedicate themselves tirelessly to be just one hundredth of a second faster than their competitor or just 1kg stronger than the next lifter. Prior to competition, they are in their hotel rooms staring at themselves in the mirror, moving through their technique in slow motion, visualizing being on stage. Their rituals give them the little extra edge needed for competition. Encouraging each athlete to develop their own practices before and during competition can and will reduce a certain amount of stress and bring them comfort. After competition is over, what do they talk about? The next meet.

I can tell you that I have always experienced a deeper meaning of hard work and athleticism. I had always enjoyed being an athlete, and now, coaching them, watching them grow, and feeling victorious. Athletes take with them a specific mentality to continuously strive in life when they embark on the "real world" after they have retired. Years after their athletic career is over, athletes are still dedicating themselves to something, be it work, school or family. Once an athlete, always an athlete. It's in us all to some degree but for those who choose, for whatever reason, to make sport an importance in their lives it is a wonderful thing. I may be a coach now but I'm always an athlete. Because us athletes, never rest.

MENTAL GAME COACHING:
AN INTERVIEW WITH BILL COLE PART 2
YAEL GRAUER

Internation Mental Game Coaching Association founder Bill Cole has been coaching and consulting in sports psychology for 30 years. He has served as a sports psychology consultant for various elite level athletes, including 2006 Olympic Gold Medalist and two-time world curling champion Russ Howard and the Performance Menu's own Aimee Anaya. "I am a much calmer and more consistent lifter, thanks to him," she said.

Cole has also worked as an NCAA Division I head coach, a sport psychology coach for the Stanford University Baseball and the Israeli Davis Cup Tennis Team and was the mental game consultant for the Irish National Cricket Team. We began discussing the importance of psychological preparation for athletic performance with Bill Cole last issue. This month we discussed mental training for various sports, and steps athletes can take to push through their own mental obstacles and limitations. Read on…

How do you know if you need to work with a mental game coach or not?

People call me because they are experiencing frustration in their sport performance in one of more of these ways:

1. They have lost their desire and passion to work hard and be committed.
2. Their sport is no longer fun and exciting.
3. They don't know how to win anymore.
4. They are in a slump.
5. They turn in a great performance, in the zone, but can't get there on command, again.
6. They are in transition in life or their sport, and lose their way.
7. Someone in their life is pressuring them to perform.
8. They play well in practice, but not in competition.
9. They have communication issues with key people.

My approach is to assess where they are, what got them there, discover where they want to go and help them devise a plan to achieve excellence.

My overall approach is to help people in these ways:

1. Improve their self-confidence in their sport.
2. Learn new and better mental approaches.
3. Improve their sports performances under pressure.
4. Discover new levels of awareness about themselves as an athlete.
5. Counsel them in the "big-picture view" of their sports career.
6. Help them transfer the many mental lessons from sport to the rest of their life.

No matter how good one's mindset, there are often other factors at play. How do you assure success for all of your clients? Is it possible for someone to not hold themselves back mentally but still not succeed for other reasons?

Sometimes athletes don't succeed in their events for a number of different reasons, none specifically mental. And sometimes these reasons are partly mental. Examples would be not playing smart tactically or strategically, not preparing properly, inadequate sleep and rest, and other fairly obvious causes.

To make sure my clients succeed I enlarge the reasons they come to see me. They come because their sport performance is falling short. I tell them that we will work on that, but that perhaps their performance issues in sport have larger ramifications. I do that to strengthen their motivation to change and to improve the quality of their lives beyond sport. Here's what I tell them:

Mental game coaching is an educational learning experience. It's an opportunity to grow as an athlete and as a person. It's an enlightening growth process, and a very interesting one. You will learn more about yourself as an athlete, and as a person.

Even though the main focus is to help you improve your mental game as an athlete, you will also discover ways to more consistently learn, change and perform in these other pursuits:

- Academic studies and exams
- Speeches, presentations and interviews
- Sales, networking and influencing situations
- Music, writing, art and drama
- Stressful life situations

As you master your mental game there will be easily measured, objective signposts that confirm your improvement in your sport. These might be records, times, win-loss outcomes, etc. You also want to notice the subjective measures of your progress with your mental game. These are less obvious, but they are just as real, and just as important. Here are 66 subjective mental game goals you can strive toward.

1. Improve your mental toughness.
2. Improve your concentration.
3. More confidence.
4. Enjoy competition more.
5. Understand yourself more as a person.
6. Understand yourself more as an athlete.
7. More positive self-talk and mental images.
8. Handle pressure better.
9. Enjoy your sport more.
10. Progress accelerates.
11. Skills become more automatic.
12. More happiness and satisfaction.
13. Reduce and eliminate a self-critical attitude.
14. Reduce and eliminate self-defeating anger.
15. Better ball judgment.
16. Make better decisions.
17. More control over your thoughts.
18. More control over your shots.
19. Enter the zone more often, and when it counts.
20. People who know you volunteer that they see you improving.
21. People you don't know volunteer that they see you improving.
22. Improve your positive mindset.
23. Overcome the fear of failure.
24. More patience with yourself and others.
25. Playing to win" more than "playing not to lose".
26. Reduce and eliminate self-sabotage.
27. Stay calmer and more poised under pressure.
28. Play as well in an event as you do in practice.
29. Reduce and eliminate perfectionism.
30. Reduce and eliminate mental blocks.
31. Fewer stress symptoms.
32. Fewer worry and nerves.
33. Better sportsmanship.
34. Analyze situations better and solve problems faster.
35. Improve motivation.
36. Better energy levels.

37. Better mental stamina.
38. Reduce and eliminate procrastination.
39. Better media relations.
40. Play better against weaker opponents.
41. Play better against stronger opponents.
42. Close out leads better.
43. Improve your stress control.
44. Keep slumps away and minimize them when they appear.
45. Reduce and eliminate choking.
46. Overcome the fear of success.
47. Better life-balance skills.
48. Handle setbacks better.
49. Handle opponent's mind games better.
50. Improve communication skills.
51. Improve anticipation skills.
52. Improve mental readiness skills.
53. Skills take less effort.
54. Better learning strategies.
55. Transfer mental lessons from sport to the rest of your life.
56. Reduce and eliminate fears and doubts.
57. Improve emotional intelligence.
58. Recover mentally from mistakes more readily.
59. Improve self-coaching skills.
60. Control your muscle relaxation better.
61. Control your breathing better.
62. Improve your will to win.
63. Not embarrass yourself in a competition.
64. Feel comfortable enough to try new things.
65. Keep your mental game together more regularly.

In essence, mental game coaching is a valuable, specialized educational experience, one that will benefit you far beyond your sport experiences. It's a lifetime investment in yourself as a person. The insights you learn and the skills you build will carry over to many important varied applications for school, business and life itself. I want to help you maximize your sport experience. I want you to succeed and to help you grow as an athlete and as a person.

How do you modify mental training for different sports? I'm assuming getting prepared for an individual sport like weightlifting is different than a team sport like football and different yet from, say, wrestling or other sports where you will compete with one person individually.

Almost all of the methods and approaches I use are applicable across all sports, and also to the salespeople, public speakers, actors, musicians and executives I coach in my work. The major common threads across these venues are:

1. Awareness
2. Learning
3. Development
4. Change
5. Habit Formation
6. Performance

I help my clients with these 16 critical performance issues:

1. Anxiety
2. Choking
3. Focus
4. Goal-Setting and Achievement
5. Perfectionism
6. Procrastination
7. Mental Preparation
8. Mental Practice
9. Self-Discipline
10. Getting In The Zone
11. Slumps and Confidence
12. Hecklers And Psych-Outs
13. Performing Under Pressure
14. The Fear Of Success
15. The Fear Of Failure
16. The Imposter Syndrome

I utilize these five major mind-coaching tools, but have a toolkit of hundreds of techniques.

Positive Thinking

Perhaps the most common mind tool of all, positive thinking involves being aware of thoughts and speech and making it as positive as possible.

Mental Practice

Mental practice is drilling or rehearsing your mind for an upcoming performance or shaping your mind to enhance a particular mental or personal quality.

Visualization

This involves using the "movies of your mind" to mentally practice, rehearse contingency plans, plan for goals, relax, energize, prepare or change mental, emotional and physical states.

Self-Hypnosis and Hypnosis

Once learned from a book, audio tapes, mind practitioner or a hypnotherapist, this mind-body skill may be utilized for a wide variety of mental training purposes. Uses include relaxation, visualization, habit control, fear reduction and performance enhancement.

Cognitive Restructuring

A more sophisticated mind tool, this involves changing thoughts and patterns of thinking so attitudes and mind sets are re-formed into desirable and intentional mental structures.

28 specific techniques and approaches I use in almost every session with clients include:

1. Managing The Inner Critic
2. Concentration
3. Recovery from mistakes
4. Mental Toughness
5. Mental Readiness Procedures
6. Championship Thinking
7. Maintaining Perspective
8. Breath Control
9. Affirmations
10. The Paradox of Letting Go While Maintaining Control
11. Relaxed Concentration
12. Closing Out Leads
13. Self-Fulfilling Prophecy

14. Paralysis By Analysis
15. Trusting Skills
16. Managing Expectations
17. Emotional Intelligence
18. Life Balance
19. The Imposter Syndrome
20. The Zone / Flow State
21. Fear Of Failure
22. "Playing To Win" Versus "Playing Not To Lose"
23. "Hating To Lose" Versus "Wanting To Win"
24. Emotional Management
25. Intrinsic Motivation
26. Influencing Skills
27. Extrinsic Motivation
28. Personal Narrative and Vision

You've coached some Hollywood stars in tennis, and some very high-level athletes, and I'm assuming some athletes who are not at that level yet. What are the differences that you've noticed? Or are the same patterns just amplified at different levels?

The amazing thing about mental game coaching across skill levels is when my lower level athletes discover that the world champions I have coached have the exact same mental issues they are facing. That is always a shock to them. But it's true. The difference? The high level people are more determined to succeed, have more mental toughness, and persevere in removing these mental and emotional obstacles.

Another unusual fact—many high-level athletes got where they are WITHOUT much mental training at all. They did it on pure mojo, desire and hard work and along the way they picked up mental toughness and personal success system. Kind of like they are on some sort of mental momentum. They feel they can't be stopped.

But then I often get calls from these same athletes when they hit a wall, go through a tough transition, say high school to college, or college to pro, and they lose their way. They forget how to be great, and they doubt themselves. That's where I remind them of their greatness, that they still have it, and give them ways to re-create that greatness, but with a new intentionality and focus.

So overall, the mental issues cut across all sports, levels and gender.

THE CASE FOR HIGHER CARB PALEO DIETS
SCOTT HAGNAS

I'd like to lay out a case for the inclusion of more carbohydrates in a typical Paleo diet. I've also been playing with my own diet this year—after quite a few years of eating essentially the same way—so I'll also relate my own experiences.

One common pattern I often see is the guy or gal eating a low carb, strict Paleo diet at, say, around 50 grams of net carbs per day. This person is training hard, hitting regular metcons, and perhaps doing some intermittent fasting on top of it. While this regimen may feel great at first, after a while this person becomes tired but can't sleep well. They find they can't drop some pesky belly fat, often develop a caffeine addiction and are cold all of the time. Finally, they end up with low libido. Yay for healthy living! (I realize not everyone follows a protocol like this one, but I see it often enough that I feel it needs to be addressed.)

First of all, a true Paleo diet—that is, how most humans actually ate over 10,000 years ago—isn't really low carb unless you are comparing it to a standard Western diet. It seems that most modern Paleo authors or authorities advocate a version of the Paleo diet that, from a macronutrient standpoint, more closely resembles how the Intuit Eskimos may have eaten. However, the diet of the Intuit is an exception; not the norm when it comes to contemporary hunter-gatherer diets that have been observed. Published ethnographic research shows that the average range of macronutrient intake for most early humans was likely 22-40% carbohydrate, 19-35% protein, and 28-58% fat. If we take the lowest end of this, 22% carbs, and calculate this over the paltry 1800 calories that our example athlete from above is likely consuming per day, that's still 100+ grams of carbohydrates a day! If one is consuming a more reasonable 2500 calories per day and we take the high end of that, you'd get 250 grams of carbs daily.

Even the few early humans living in the tundra consumed 6-15% of average daily energy from plant-based foods. Most authors state that early humans ate roots and tubers and mention the above macronutrient ratios, but then go on to recommend a diet that falls outside of this range. I understand their reasoning, as most people today have weight to lose, and low carb diets are very effective. However, if you are a fire-breathing athlete or are already lean, your needs are very different. If you've lost your desired weight eating low carb Paleo, now is the time to adjust your diet.

Let's look at what is going on with our modern Paleo metcon warrior. At first, he feels great eating low carb and fasting. Energy levels stabilize and even increase, thanks to elevated levels of catecholamines (adrenal hormones) and cortisol. The problem begins after these hormones have been elevated for a long period of time. When this happens, he will end up with either fatigued adrenal glands, or down-regulated receptor sites for the adrenal hormones. This may still happen eventually even with good sleep and low lifestyle stressors. Adding in poor sleep and a stressful, too busy life is like throwing fuel on the fire.

Large protein meals without significant carbohydrates still raise insulin levels quite effectively. Cortisol is then released to drive gluconeogenesis in the liver. Adrenaline is also released. If one is performing high intensity exercise regularly, there will be a greater need for gluconeogenesis to refuel the muscles for the next bout of activity. I suspect that this greater demand in an athlete is quite a bit more taxing for the adrenals than in a sedentary person eating low carb.

Many studies have shown a decrease in athletic performance following a low carb diet. However, all of the studies that I am aware of are very short term. There are certainly some longer term adaptations to low carb diets where we can see improved performance. Glycogen sparing and more efficient gluconeogenesis may be some of the longer-term adaptations. It would be nice to see a long-term study done. However, here's the rub: while both short duration alactic activities and long slow duration work can be fueled primarily by fat, glycolytic pathway work can only be fueled by glucose. Lactate can be recycled back to glucose thru the Cori cycle, a process that likely becomes more efficient with regular high intensity conditioning work. However, when the Cori cycle is very active, serum cortisol is higher. Cortisol is also higher in proportion to the demand for gluconeogenesis. This means that an individual performing glycolytic work while on a low carb diet will have higher levels of cortisol and catecholamines than one consuming more carbohydrates. From time to time, this situation would be natural, but when it is a chronic situation is when you will see trouble.

Secretory IgA is an immunoglobulin found mainly in mucus secretions in the body. One of its functions is to inhibit bacterial colonization in the gut. It is also anti-viral. Excessive cortisol or catecholamine levels suppress SIgA. This is not good, as your immune system will be weaker. You'll also have a greater likelihood of poor gut flora, which can lead to a leaky gut and a greater range of food sensitivities over time. It's not uncommon for a Paleo low-carber to develop additional food sensitivities over time, and this might be what's behind it. At least one study has shown that carbs taken during exercise can prevent the drop in SIgA.

Another thing that happens with prolonged ketosis from limited carbohydrates is that one begins to become insulin resistant. Higher free fatty acids during ketosis promote insulin resistance to spare whatever little carbohydrates are available for the central nervous system. Toss in high cortisol from stress due to excessive exercise and quite possibly other lifestyle issues, and you end up with chronically elevated blood sugar—even in spite of a strict low carb diet. If this continues unchecked, then eventually the adrenals cannot regulate your blood sugar effectively anymore. Do you wake up around 3am and have trouble getting back to sleep? Your blood sugar is now dropping too low, and your adrenals are called upon to release cortisol to bring it back up. However, your adrenals are already overtaxed, so insufficient cortisol is released to do the job. Your blood sugar drops even lower, then your body goes to plan B—adrenaline is released to get the job done. At this point, you wake full of energy and can't get back to sleep.

Cortisol and testosterone are manufactured from the same raw materials, so excessive demand for cortisol doesn't leave a lot left for testosterone. As a consequence, T levels go down. I've seen young guys with T levels comparable to a 65-year-old man. There is an interesting study of individuals undergoing the 62-day US Army Ranger training course. The physical energy expenditure is very high and the intake of calories is low. By the second half of the course, the Rangers had T levels that approached the level found in castrated men. While this is an extreme case, I think we can learn from it. Though the rangers' calorie intake was low relative to their huge energy expenditure, this was not a low carb diet. If it were, the result would likely have been even worse. Though your training and stress may not be that extreme, low carbs or low total calories will produce a similar result.

Carbohydrate restriction also can affect the thyroid hormones. The biology of starvation and carbohydrate restriction are nearly identical. Conversion of T4 to the active T3 is impaired, with the T4 getting converted instead to the metabolically inactive reverse T3. Body temperature and the metabolic rate drops when this happens, and blood glucose begins to run higher. This is correlated also with higher cholesterol levels. A high LDL level is not uncommon in the low carb trainee. Some authorities maintain that a higher protein diet will aggravate hypothyroid symptoms. Furthermore, omega-6 fats have been shown to suppress the thyroid. On a very low-carb diet, a large portion of the total calories will necessarily need to come from fat. As a result, the intake of omega-6 fats from nuts and oils will likely be fairly high, and this may suppress metabolism over time.

But what about ketones? In response to a low carb intake, production and utilization of ketone bodies does increase. The formation of ketone bodies does allow for a lower level of gluconeogenesis. The problem comes when we have excessive stress or exercise demand on the system. Stress actually increases glucose utilization in relation to total energy expenditure. Glycogen stores are depleted faster, leading (once again) to higher levels of cortisol and the catecholamines.

Finally we get to insulin. The popular belief that frequent high carb meals spike insulin too high, leading to insulin resistance, is incorrect. It is a much more complex process than that. Excessive use of processed, nutrient depleted foods, fructose and sugar consumption, omega-6 fats, poor gut bacteria and gluten intolerance are likely more important factors.

What then, should we be eating? First of all, if you are a 180-lb. male and are eating 1800 calories, just eat more! A lot more. Outside of this, I think there are several viable strategies depending on your situation. The first step would be to evaluate the status of your adrenals. This can be done a few ways. You can get a doctor to run an adrenal stress index test. Or, a simple test that I really like is Dr. Bruce Rind's body temperature test. You measure your body temperature at 3, 6, and 9 hours after waking. Average the three values and record. Track this for at least a week. If the values are consistently low, it would indicate less than optimal thyroid function at some level. If the values are irregular, jumping around from day to day, it indicates low adrenal function. Low and irregular values would mean both glands are performing sub-optimally.

If you test low for adrenal function, then I'd suggest eating some carbs with most every meal for now. 20-30 grams per meal might be a good starting point, but you can experiment with more. (I'd also suggest placing the metcons on hold for a while.)

If you have relatively healthy adrenals, then you have a few more options. I really like cyclic carbohydrate intake to get the best of both worlds. Low carbohydrate for 2-3 days, then a big carbohydrate re-feed day. You could also just go with a more random approach to meal composition. High protein and fat sometimes, carbs and moderate protein at others. Just remember that you want to balance things that raise catecholamines (low carb, fasting, underfeeding, stress, sleep loss) with things that lower them (carbs, overfeeding, rest, sleep).

If you are regularly performing metabolic conditioning, even if you limit yourself to 3-5 minutes of very intense activity, then I'd ratchet your carbohydrate intake upward. Consume your carbs not only in the post workout window, but also throughout the day.

If you are already insulin resistant and have high fasting blood glucose, then eating lower carb most of the time will still be your first priority. I'd still suggest a periodic carb re-feed, just less frequently—maybe one carb re-feed meal every 5-6 days.

If you haven't eaten significant carbohydrate for quite a while, you'll likely feel the effects of high blood sugar the first few times you eat carbs. Oral glucose tolerance tests on individuals consuming low carb diets normally show a high blood glucose level after administration of carbohydrates. This makes sense, as the body is somewhat insulin resistant to spare whatever little glucose was being consumed. After a week of eating carbs, though, you normally find that the test will show low blood glucose levels.

One final note on carbohydrates: emphasize starchy tubers and squashes. If one wants to adhere to a Paleo type diet, then yams and sweet potatoes are great options. There are many more varieties of tubers, though. A couple of my favorites are taro and yucca. Peel your tubers, as most of the toxins reside in the skins.

Processed carbs, grains, sugars of all types, and fruit may still cause problems.

This article is not a case for their inclusion in the diet. Fructose has proven uniquely damaging to both metabolism and insulin sensitivity. I still only recommend eating fruit in season. Nor am I advocating a truly high carb diet. Stick to 22-40% of calories, just as the ethnographic data suggests.

I'll finish by relating my personal experiences with reintroducing carbs. First of all, I was that guy above. For about 7 years. I stopped doing any regular metcon work over a year ago. My training has since consisted of mostly gymnastic strength work and mobility, along with some O-lifting; almost exclusively alactic pathway work.

I first experimented by reducing my protein and fat a bit, and upping my carbs. Total calories were still the same, a pathetically low average of fewer than 2000 calories per day. (How do I know? Because I track all of this crap daily. Want to know what I had as my second snack on June 21st, 2003? I could tell you.) My first result was better body composition, particularly in the abdominal region. Daily energy was noticeably better, and my sleep improved. General vigor and libido was up. I then did the temperature tracking and found my temperature very low (less than 95 degrees sometimes) and very erratic. After talking to Dr. G. (Garrett Smith), I took a month off from training and ate a minimum of 3000 calories daily for the month. I quickly laid down some body fat, mostly in the abdominal region. At the same time, my triceps, pecs and legs leaned out. This would be consistent with higher testosterone and reduced estrogen. After two weeks, the fat gain stopped, and by the end of the month I was leaning back out - still not training and still "overeating". My energy is now better than it has been in years, I have no need for coffee (which has always been a problem for me), and let's just say that my wife is very happy. I am consuming between 200 and 250 grams of carbs daily.

Time to get out the potato peeler and get to cookin'! It may be just the tool for increased performance, energy, and vitality.

THE MENTAL ASPECTS OF THE HANDSTAND
JIM BATHURST

Exploring and developing the mental aspects of the handstand can help you develop more confidence and consistency. Call it "clutch," or whatever you want, but focus and mental control can mean the difference between accomplishing-or not accomplishing-what you want when you want to.

I'm taking the safe assumption that there are more weightlifters reading this article than acrobats, but I believe the things I've observed over the years in both my clients and myself can be applied to other areas of training. My own training involves more than just gymnastic work, so I'll explain the relevance of each topic to various types of training.

I like to break down the mental aspects of the handstand into five different areas. The first is performing in front of other people. The second is becoming fearless of the exercise itself. Third is performing in different environments. Fourth is adding in variations. Fifth is the value of teaching to increase understanding and confidence. Each of these areas can come about naturally in your training over the years, but a dedicated effort to work on them can improve your "clutch" in any situation.

Handstands In Front Of People

If one routinely practices handstands alone, one avenue to develop confidence in the skill is to look for opportunities to perform in front of other people.

In both weight training and acrobatics, we may have our training partners and coaches routinely watch us during our workouts. Over time we become accustomed to, and perhaps even dependent upon, this gaze. We become comfortable. To develop further confidence, though, we need to find ways to make ourselves uncomfortable again.

I had the lucky opportunity to be part of Gymkana, an exhibitional gymnastic group, while I was in college. We performed handstands on various surfaces and situations in front of large groups of strangers.

In another lifetime, I did a lot of breakdancing. If you've never been breaking before, the thought of jumping into the middle of a circle of strangers while performing athletically AND keeping a beat is absolutely terrifying.

Getting in front of your peers - other b-boys who actually know what they're looking at (as opposed to drunken backspins at your cousin's wedding) is even more frightening. Making it through these experiences made me more resilient to the discomfort of people watching. It also gave me greater confidence to perform the handstand in front of anyone.

Esteemed Bulgarian weightlifting coach Ivan Abadjiev stated in a lecture that his athletes would perform in front of an audience three times a week. Ivan continued with the belief that the near competitive atmosphere stimulates the release of adrenaline and makes the desired training mechanisms adapt. He acknowledges the importance of the emotional factor. You can read the whole translated lecture here.

One may wonder whether frequent weightlifting competitions would accomplish the same thing. I believe that competition is an excellent way to develop mental control, but competition every week is not feasible for many reasons. Abadjiev knew this, so he attempted to recreate the same uneasy feeling with his team on a more regular basis. You can try to recreate this in weightlifting with a larger group of training partners observing you, training at busier times with more gym-goers watching, or simply having an existing training partner sit in front of you, as a judge at a meet would do. Actively look for opportunities to perform in front of others and it will have less and less of a negative effect on you.

Handstands From Different Heights – Becoming Fearless

I thought about writing this article after seeing a segment on Eskil Ronningsbakken, an acrobat who performs death-defying balancing acts on cliff edges and mountaintops. (You can see some absolutely astonishing handstand pictures on his website)

On Stan Lee's "Superhumans" show, Eskil was hooked up to a bunch of instruments that measured his stress levels. It was found that he was as calm and collected doing a handstand in the middle of a roof as he was on the edge of the roof. He was able to control his emotions and perform a stable handstand anywhere. Of course, Eskil didn't start off on rooftops. He built up his superhuman control of fear by working on progressively harder and more dangerous feats.

Now, I don't recommend anyone emulate Eskil's feats. My girlfriend has definitely forbidden me from even thinking about it (the first picture of this article has a large rooftop underneath me), but what we can learn is that we should be practicing fearlessness with progressively more challenging exercises and weights. This is different than the fear of a crowd. This is the fear of total commitment to an exercise and the repercussions if one fails. If one never practices dealing with this fear, then one will never conquer it.

A take-home exercise to try today is to perform a handstand on a small platform. Even a small box can be daunting at first. Provided you can come down out of a regular handstand safely, the handstand on the small platform is not that much more dangerous, but will still provide you with an uncomfortable situation. You can then increase the height of the handstand based on your goals.

In my thoughts about handstands and different heights, I always think about the advice given to me when I was first learning a chair handstand up on high. "It's just like a regular chair handstand, except higher."

These words are eloquent in their simplicity, but there's a message there. We focus so much on the repercussions (what if I fall/fail?!?) that we lose focus on the task at hand and it then becomes a self-fulfilling prophecy.

In a casual interview (with some choice words), weightlifting Champion Donny Shankle talks about the need to be fearless - - to try, to get knocked down again and again, but to never be afraid to get under that bar. "A master is a person without fear," he says. *Practice being fearless. Fall down. Repeat.*

Handstands In Different Environments

When I first taught myself a handstand, it was either outside in the grass or inside my small bedroom. Outside provided the challenge of uneven ground and a softer surface which made balancing harder. Inside provided the challenge of not kicking my nightstand. I had to be aware of my surroundings and control any fall. When I moved to practicing on a flat, open space-like a basketball court-it felt like a vacation.

Do you always practice your handstand in one spot? Have you ever tried practicing elsewhere? Do you know what the feeling of a handstand on asphalt feels like? How about grass? How about a sloped or irregular surface? How about the other subtle differences in lighting, temperature, and ambient noise? This is probably the easiest handstand variation you can try: practicing your handstand in a different environment.

One arm handstand practice on my old driveway

A change in scenery can strengthen up your handstand by providing a stimulus that is "same, but different." Although it's the same exercise, the subtle or not-so-subtle differences of your environment will throw you off. But from this you can start to feel the commonalities among each handstand you do and internalize your technique. As this internalization gets stronger, the external environment and variations you encounter will affect you less and less.

This may not seem to matter to some, but I am amazed when something in my client's environment changes (like practicing in a non-regular spot in the gym) and it results in difficulty in their technique for the first several attempts.

In the weightlifting world, everything needs to be honed and perfected in the predictable environment of a bar, plates and a platform. We are looking to lift and develop consistent technique with that equipment. What we can then do to apply this aspect is practice lifting on other platforms; visiting other gyms and getting into other atmospheres. If you've never lifted on a platform other than your own, then the unfamiliarity of new surroundings during a competition can throw you for a loop.

Visiting other gyms is a simple yet excellent idea, anyway. We are all part of a community that should already be traveling-exchanging ideas and stories with each other. Get in some lifting at other spots and soon you'll be comfortable anywhere.

Again, while entering competitions can fulfill this exercise, visiting other gyms can be done on a more frequent basis in a more casual environment.

Different Types Of Handstands

On the same theory of "same, but different" and in order to understand your own handstand better, working variations of the handstand can allow you to see the similarities constant throughout. Is your weight balanced forward on your fingers? Is your body tight? Are your elbows straight?

A few of the infinite variations you can try include fingertip handstands, handstands for your fists, chair handstands or even walking in a handstand.

A quick disclaimer on handstand walking: Please make sure you are performing this variation with control. Staggering about in a handstand is not walking; it's just an uncontrolled handstand. Work on better control and the ability to stay in place.

An old-time muscle beach tradition was partner acrobatic balancing–performing handstands and other such acrobatic moves with one or more people. Doing a handstand on someone, or supporting someone in a handstand, is much more difficult than it first appears!

Handstand at Urban Evolution

Another challenging variation is to perform a blindfolded handstand. I'd like to bring to your attention to one Eddie Motter. He was a gymnast in the 50s that, despite being totally blind, was able to hold a handstand for over 3 minutes.

In weightlifting, it's true that we are not looking at how to proficiently clean or snatch anything other than a barbell. In powerlifting, it's still squatting, benching, and deadlifting with just a barbell. I propose though that strongman and odd object lifting- deadlifting a stone, cleaning a keg, or pressing a log-can be fun and challenging variations that will actually help one understand the fundamentals of the lifts while giving a psychological break from only lifting a barbell (though it goes without saying that the basic clean and jerk and snatch should still occupy a large percentage of one's Olympic weightlifting training).

Teach A Handstand

There's the saying "when one person teaches, two people learn." I've had the fantastic opportunity to make a living doing what I love–coaching full-time for the past 5 years. I have also been requested to give gymnastic seminars at numerous gyms, which allows me to see many problems and pitfalls that people have with their handstand. This gives me such a fantastic insight into the skill.

In order to be an effective coach, you have to be able to simplify the complex--to give just the key points that the athlete needs to hear at that moment: no more, no less.

By teaching others, we see the exercise from a different perspective. Technique problems that we never had, and probably never even considered, are somebody else's bane.

This doesn't mean that you need to coach athletes full-time yourself, but offering to watch and help someone's technique in the weight room (if they are open to it) can help you in return. This back and forth exchange should be a normal part of everyone's gym, but it's not. How many of us have been to a gym where everyone is plugged into their headphones and no one helps anyone else? What community does that foster?

If you are still hesitant to teach, you can also observe a respected coach teaching. Watching him train and coach a fellow teammate can give you better insight into your sport. This improved knowledge will help improve your own technique and build your confidence.

Time

It needs to be said that excellent results in any skill takes time. Hard, consistent practice over years and years will always give you more confidence in your technique. I hope that you can speed up the process and explore areas you hadn't considered with the techniques I've described.

The pictures used for this article were taken over a decade of practice. I've done more handstands in the past 10 years then I can even begin to count. I still have plenty of room for improvement, but I have enjoyed myself every step of the way.

So what is the ultimate culmination of all these variations? Of training your handstand so that the confidence in your ability is unwavering?

How about handstand walking in your underwear on asphalt in the winter in front of a crowd of people?

Never forget to have fun with your training.

THE MOTHER OF INVENTION
MATT FOREMAN

New inventions. They're great little things, aren't they? Where would our society be if it wasn't for some creative thinkers who decided to develop ideas for things like penicillin, beer, rock and roll, cell phones, weightlifting shoes, pencil sharpeners and canned vegetables? Every one of those things has made life easier, usually for a lot of people. So here's what I want you to do with me. Let's think about a great invention that has really contributed something to how we live our lives. I've got it…how about Google? Google is a doohickey thingy on your computer that you can use to find out about anything, and I mean absolutely freaking anything, in the world. I could go to Google right now and type in something like "soil conditions in lower Russia," and I would get enough information about it to write a ninety-page research paper…in 0.13 seconds. Now that's what I call an invention, jack.

Next, I want you to think about another type of invention. This little sucker will be something that makes you scratch your head and wonder how on earth anybody in their right mind would ever decide to pay money for it. I've got a perfect one…let's look at the Shake Weight. I just took a look at an instructional video for the Shake Weight (that I found on Google) and I thought I was watching White House security videos from the Bill Clinton era. If you don't know what I'm talking about, get on your computer and check it out as soon as possible. The fact that somebody is making money on this contraption really tells you something about the world we live in. Reminds me of that old quote from W.C. Fields, "It's morally wrong to allow a sucker to keep his money."

All of this witty banter leads us to the topic of this month's article. We're going to take a look at the concept of invention as it applies to weightlifting training. More specifically, we're going to examine different ways in which people try to come up with new training programs or routines that will supposedly revolutionize the lifting world. There's no shortage of this type of stuff either. Lots and lots of people have claimed to have found (or created) the hidden keys to the strength kingdom. There's always somebody running around out there in the iron world that holds the secret…that magical combination of sets, reps, and technique that will stack more kilos on your total and send your performance into the next galaxy. Now, I think it's important to acknowledge that there have been a few people over the years that have done a pretty legitimate job of pulling this off. I know I'm making it sound like I think everybody with a new angle on training is a snake oil salesman, but I will be the first to admit that there actually are some coaches who have blended a little innovation with a lot of experience and come up with training ideas that really can make you stronger. So instead of throwing the baby out with the beef tallow, let's check out an example of strength training innovation that generates a lot of discussion on the internet forums and other shrines of intellectual achievement. Then, of course, we'll add some warnings so we can try to find a way to caution our treasured readers from falling for an "Improve Your Clean and Jerk with the Shake Weight" type of program. Boy, that last part is just begging for jokes, ain't it?

Westside

One particular method that carries a lot of popularity in the lifting world is Louie Simmons' Westside Barbell program. The more research you do on serious lifting these days, the more references you'll hear about this discipline. Now, I'm going to assume that those of you who are reading this already know some of the basic principles of Westside. I might be making a mistake with that because this program is rooted in powerlifting, and many Performance Menu readers focus on Olympic lifting. I'll be the first to admit that most true Olympic Weightlifting purists probably don't know much (and don't care) about Westside. However, one of the major trends in the iron game these days is to blend different types of training methods, often including powerlifting and Olympic lifting, to form a more versatile strength athlete. I think many of you who are reading this article probably fit that category, at least to some degree.

Louie Simmons is a powerlifting coach in Columbus, Ohio who runs a famous gym called Westside Barbell. Simmons has been in powerlifting for several decades, and he has developed a program that many people refer to as "the Westside method" or some other similar terminology. This Westside method is considered by many strength coaches and powerlifters to be a highly effective system for getting stronger. Westside's powerlifting results certainly speak for themselves, as some of the strongest squatters, benchers and deadlifters in the world have their roots either in Louie's gym or his training approach. And this is probably the point where many of you think I'm going to say something negative about Westside because you know I'm an Olympic lifter and there seems to be an eternal pissing war between powerlifting and Olympic lifting. That's where you're wrong. I'm going to speak respectfully here, because I think we can find something valuable in this examination.

Westside's approach to training is very complex and I'm not going to devote much of this article to it, especially since I do not consider myself an expert in their field.

But I've been reading Louie's stuff for many years and I think I can probably look at one aspect of what they do and try to apply it to Olympic lifting. One of the fundamental elements of Westside training, according to what I've read, is the practice of using a variety of different exercises to improve performance in a competition lift. In other words, lifters will train to get stronger in the squat by doing an assortment of exercises other than just the squat itself. Westside lifters will use box squats on a regular basis, where the lifter literally squats to a sitting position on a box before standing up. These box squats will be performed at various box heights (which changes the depth of the squat), using different types of barbells, applying different levels of resistance through the use of high-tension rubber bands, switching foot position and squat stance, etc. To get stronger in the bench press, lifters will use exercises like floor presses, which are bench presses with the lifter lying on the floor, which only allows the elbows to bend until the upper arms touch the floor (making the lift a partial bench press). Benches will also be performed with a variety of different grip widths, etc. The overall idea is that the body will grow and develop through the use of different specialized lifts, instead of simply practicing the actual competition lift over and over.

The question here becomes, "Will this approach work with Olympic lifting?" To be more specific, "Can an athlete train to snatch more weight by using other lifts instead of the snatch?" This is a major can-of-worms question, and the answer ties in very closely with other topics I've covered in past Performance Menu articles. The full answer is more complicated than I can cover in a couple of paragraphs, but we can definitely get some useful ideas out here. First of all, let's ask the question again. "Can an athlete become a better snatcher by using different training lifts than the snatch?" The basic answer to this is NO. Because of the amazing complexity of the Olympic lifts, an athlete cannot expect to improve performance without practicing the full lifts themselves. The snatch and the clean and jerk have to be developed through thousands of perfect reps, and that process will not take place if the athlete devotes significant training time to creative exercises like the ones mentioned above from the Westside method. Interestingly, many top Olympic lifting coaches over the last thirty years have built their training philosophy around the Bulgarian approach, which is a training method that consists almost solely of the snatch, clean and jerk, and squat. No assistance exercises, at least not any that are used to any important degree. At first glance, this seems to be almost a polar opposite of the Westside method.

However, there is more analysis that needs to go into this. It is clear from the success of the Russian and Chinese systems that auxiliary exercises are often used by elite weightlifters. The old Soviet weightlifting system (which Louie Simmons originally based his ideas on) involved a wide range of lifts and exercises that were worked into the training program along with the snatch and clean and jerk. Much of the thinking that goes into the idea of GPP (General Physical Preparedness) has its foundations in the preparation phases that Soviet coaches would use at different times throughout the competition year to increase the fitness and overall work capacity of their athletes. Different lifting exercises, such as kettlebells and bench presses, were implemented during this time, along with plyometric training and, sometimes, actual participation in other sports. But as the Bulgarian program rose to world domination in the 1980s, the stripped-down approach gained popularity. Many top coaches came to believe that training the snatch, clean and jerk, and squat was all that was necessary for serious Olympic lifters. I heard this sentiment from a lot of top weightlifting names during the prime years of my career. Now, here we are in 2011. China has emerged as the new weightlifting leviathan of the planet, and we are routinely seeing Chinese training videos on the internet where the athletes are using unorthodox lifts in training like pseudo-RDL snatch-grip pulls standing on a twenty-five kilo plate. Weird stuff like that, and they're kicking the crap out of the rest of the world. It's funny how the sport seems to go in cycles over the years.

So, can the Westside method have useful application to Olympic lifting? I guess we can say that creative auxiliary strength exercises can definitely be worked into a weightlifter's training program, but I still believe athletes who want to improve in the Olympic lifts need to focus the vast majority of their training time on the snatch, clean and jerk, and squat. I've heard it said over the years that, "The Westside program can put 100 pounds on your squat. If our American Olympic lifters were all squatting 100 pounds more, they would be able to snatch more." The simplicity of that idea sounds good on paper, but there's much more to it than that. We've had American weightlifters that could squat more than Anatoli Pisarenko, but Pisarenko had a 584 lb. clean and jerk and the American record is 523. Squatting more weight just isn't the solution to everything, as many people would have you think. The Russian legends of weightlifting have said that themselves.

The REAL point to all of this…

Sometimes, the furious quest for innovation simply results in spinning your wheels. I'm not going to attack the methods of any particular coaches because I don't like the way that approach comes across. But I will say that if you, the athlete/coach, are in the early stages of your strength career and you want to find somebody to listen to, make sure you're going with somebody who has some legitimate credibility. I'll keep it in generalities. I've spoken with a lot of coaches in the last few years that basically seem to take the approach that trying as many new things as possible is the best way to train. They think you get better by a system of almost constant experimentation, that type of notion. Much of this approach might be based on the Westside method and there is some merit to it. But the problem I see is that we create a situation where the entire training philosophy is based on never settling on one method. A kind of training ADD sets in, and there is never any real focused consistency to anything. Before you know it, two years have passed and you've tried every new idea under the sun...but you're still lifting the same weights. I believe that it's important to settle on one method. Furthermore, I think it's especially important when you're in the early stages of your lifting career to find somebody else that already has a proven method and let them teach you. This isn't the way a lot of our society likes to go because everybody with a little experience these days thinks that they're qualified to develop their own methodology. We're in the age of the five-minute expert. Bravo to the spirit of independence and creative thinking, but it often doesn't translate into success.

To my way of thinking, the process of becoming a good coach is first being an athlete in a successful system, and then moving on and teaching others the system you've learned. Finally, after you've developed a mastery of the teaching element and learned some plain old "what works and what doesn't" ideas, then it's time to integrate some of your own ideas into the proven things that have already worked. After time and experience have accumulated, you start to find ways to adapt the system for individual athletes and your own personal circumstances. Then you're ready to strike out on your own. Many of you who are reading this are coaches and you're probably relatively new to the Olympic Weightlifting game. If you've been working the Olympic Lifts for less than five years as either an athlete or a coach, you're still new. I don't mean that to sound condescending, but if you talked to most of the seasoned veteran weightlifting athletes or coaches out there and asked them to compare themselves at the present to where they were at the five-year point, you'd see what I mean.

People want to be innovators, and that's a great thing. America would never be where it is right now without the people who storm ahead and try to break through the walls of the old ways. But the people who are best equipped to break through those walls are the ones who have a solid foundation of time and experience before they pick up the hammer, and that experience was forged through a mastery of the bread-and-butter fundamentals. If you want to get creative and crazy with your training, go right ahead. My advice, however, would be to also never lose sight of the most basic elements of success. I was watching a documentary about the movie Jaws once, and horror director Clive Barker said something about it that I always remembered. "Some ideas are so obvious that they're right in front of us all the time and we just don't see them. How could we not have known that there was the best, exciting, suspenseful movie to be made about a f----ing huge white shark that ate you up?"

TAKE WHAT WORKS:
THE LESSONS OF PHYSICAL CULTURE HISTORY
CHIP CONRAD

"That there is an almost total neglect of the physical education of our youth in the home and school, as seen in the imperfectly developed frames...crooked spines, round shoulders and protruding shoulder-blades... flabby muscles... lung-starved and blood-poisoned bodies of our boys and girls, our men and women."

Plus ça change, plus c'est la même chose. Although the above quote could describe the slouched teenagers and frail hipsters ubiquitous in my neighborhood, it was written a bit before our time as an observation on modernization and the human condition... in 1892.

So what's new? Well, strangely enough, the quest for exercise, according to statistics of gym memberships, surveys and product sales, is greater per capita than it was 113 years ago. And yet our health, our holistic state of physical being, is actually declining. We might be living longer, but that's modern medicine prolonging our decay. We're fatter with a higher incident of a host of diseases that have simply replaced a bunch of other diseases that we've gotten rid of over the last century.

What's changed? We're no longer striving for health. We're trying to look better, health be damned! Our culture supports a fitness industrial complex that is as geared toward actual health as the cosmetics industry or plastic surgery lobby is. The booty shaking, bright lights and fake vocabulary of modern marketing seems to have us convinced that 'science' has evolved fitness into little pills and, well, the Shake Weight.

To be fair, the snake oil and gizmos were around a century ago as well, but the refinement and volume of modern marketing hadn't yet proliferated the nonsense in grand public view with three easy payments.

Fitness in the new millennium is an industry driven by a media-fed aesthetic ideal: endless gadgets and gizmos eking out every "pump" and "burn," allowing users to (supposedly) "tone," tighten and target problem areas. Almost gone are the days of health and ability for health and ability's sake, now replaced with constant striving for ripped abs, pert bottoms and "defined" arms.

There was a time when muscles and bodies were built for use, not just for show; when training called for strength and ability of the entire body, used to conquer obstacles and prove might - not just to swell muscles full of blood.

These were the days of Physical Culture, a bygone era, a relic of the past that seems wholly unfamiliar and irrelevant to gym members of the twenty-first century, but was in fact the foundation for everything we know about fitness.

For the past 2+ years a handful of us have been collecting research and interviews for a documentary about the history of fitness, which, as far as we're concerned, is a history of strength. Is that a slightly biased premise to our documentary concept? You bet, but we think a fair one.

Physical Culture is something in and of itself - not merely a performance aid or assistant to improved body composition. It is not a just sport or a training method. It is a world comprised of movement, obstacle, burden, success and perseverance; a philosophy that stresses strength, empowerment, self-improvement and personal victory.

With roots in ancient Greek philosophy (along with elements borrowed from Eastern thought and movement), Physical Culture drew its influence from the developing arts of gymnastics, wrestling and dance. It has a much richer history, though, in the deepest roots of human motivation: the desire to push against the un-pushable, move the immoveable and become victorious over the unconquerable.

The development of tools throughout the ages, from Indian clubs to dumbbells, to bicycles, barbells, kettlebells and more, has added to the evolution of movement and training. Physical Culture has been the toolbox for survival, an expression of national pride and a means for developing the body (for strength, sports and otherwise).

It found its name in the late 1800s at the hands of such Physical Culture luminaries as Bernarr McFadden, Professor Attila and perhaps most famously, Eugene Sandow. But the path had been laid generations before in the ancient Greek Olympics, in the Turnverins and YMCA's of the early 19th century, and by health and fitness legends like Catherine Beecher, Edmund Desbonnet and Johan Guts Muths.
Our current wish is to revive and reanimate the study of Physical Culture, excavating its ancient history, breath life into its antiquated countenance and uncover the hidden history of fitness. Perhaps a look into the roots of modern fitness will bring the current physical culture underground a bit more into the popular forefront.

Although idealized in many ways, as history can often become, Physical Culture had a few lessons that we can learn from by not repeating them. For instance, our current dot in chronology has no monopoly on gurus and experts. Despite the desire of our research to unveil nothing but pure holistic consciousness from a century ago, there are many correlations to our practices in the industry today that might be more about stubborn dogma than actual health.

The western concept of fitness is either entirely vague (lift weights + hop on treadmill = 6 pack abs) or completely specialized (I do yoga, or I powerlift, or I CrossFit, or I do Pilates). We strive for identity through our workout choices, and therefore choosing a trend or group fits our personality needs.

Although there are many stories of the classic strongman also having a background in several other disciplines of training, sometimes history has curious stories that might have us asking "what if?"

One of these stories is man responsible for bringing the barbell to popularity in America.

"Men looking to reshape and strengthen their body in fin de siècle America (particularly after Eugen Sandow's 1893 appearances at the Chicago Worlds Fair) discovered two major problems: the limited exercise literature available in this era almost universally espoused the use of lightweight training methods which did not build the kind of muscles owned by Sandow, and those who wanted to lift heavier weights—ala Sandow and other professional strongmen—could not buy such implements from any sporting goods company in America. Enter Alan Calvert, who solved both problems for American men by opening the Milo Bar-bell Company in 1902. His promotion of progressive resistance exercise using the adjustable barbells and dumbbells he manufactured launched a new era of strength and muscularity for America."

A Quick Story of the Barbell

About 50 years before the barbell was introduced to America via Mr. Calvert, Austria's Karl Rappo was using a revolutionary big bar with globes on it in his strongman act. Before that the closest thing you might recognize as resembling a barbell were 4 foot long wands with small globes on the ends, often weighing less than the mini-barbells used in Body Pump classes today.

But there was unknown prophecy in Rappo's act, as the door began opening wider to the concept of heavier training implements being integral not just to strongman acts, but to health and what the idea of strength meant to the eventual lifting public.

Weightlifting clubs started blooming around Germany and Russia, but while Europe was embracing the barbell and its heavy kin, here in America heavy athletics received a fatal PR blow when a stroke ended the life of its most popular spokesperson, George Barker Windship. Public opinion blamed strength training, especially the heavy kind, for Windship's sudden demise at 42. Then, according to historian Jan Todd, "during the 1880s and 1890s, heavy dumbbells and barbells were nearly impossible to find in America."

But let's not remember Windship by the bad public opinion that might have been unfairly levied on him and strength training. Windship can probably be credited with the original concepts for shot-loaded and plate-loaded heavy training implements, since he started toying with these concepts as early as 1850 when building the heaviest dumbbell he could, which was adjustable with loadable shot up to 180 pounds. This was followed 6 years later by a patent for a fantastic adjustable plate-loaded dumbbell, which was to have a range of 8-101 pounds--in half pound increments! According to the H.J. Lutcher Stark Center for Physical Culture, there might have never actually existed a finished product, since there isn't much suggesting that one was ever produced. But heck… a boy can dream!

America, being behind in the strength training trend by the turn of the century, finally had a voice for the cause when Alan Calvert opened the Milo Bar-bell Company in 1902. Calvert sold globe barbells that were both shot AND plate loaded, all in one. With the globe opened, you'd find a section for shot and another section with changeable plates.

There were a variety of barbell options throughout the beginning of the century, but it was the 1928 Olympics that heralded the official life of the barbell we recognize today. The Berg Barbell, which was the first to revolve, made the competition lifts much easier (try cleaning a heavy, fixed barbell and you'll see what I mean), and it was quickly copied by everyone and became the gold standard of weightlifting. What you get your hands on in most gyms today has not changed much in the last 80+ years.

So the barbell became the tool of choice for most practicing strength addicts of the time, a common tool of the that end of the Physical Culture spectrum, and Alan Calvert's words and instructions were gospel to any true iron head. But the iron game guru became the follower of Edwin Checkley, another physical culturist guru (he called himself a 'physicultirst') from the other side of the spectrum, who advocated breathing and less-than-vigorous bodyweight movements as the path to health and wellbeing.

Soon after Edwin Checkley's death, Calvert made the complete switch, denouncing barbell and heavy weight training and embracing, teaching and writing about the Checkley Method for the rest of his life. Even his friends weren't entirely sure why his philosophy switched so abruptly, and his followers were less than thrilled with his new ideas.

The Modern Correlation

Bruce Lee once said to take what works and discard what doesn't. History can now offer us a palate of successful ideas, but through Calvert, it might also teach us that applying Bruce Lee's concept would let us incorporate multiple disciplines rather than hop philosophical ships from one extreme to the next. Calvert could have taken the best from both worlds and created an entirely unique and holistic experience. That's the real curiosity… why didn't he?

Are you?

The lessons from history often don't come from the words or direct actions of those who came before us. It's the patterns over time that develop. Many folks, including modern historians, regal in the excitement of our current period, watching records continue to fall and strong men and women push boundaries far beyond what was thought possible.

But might be of more interest about modern strength is the limits we put on our definition of it, not the individual feats that represent this definition. We've gone from an ideal of being strong, in a broad, holistic definition that might be interpreted as 'capable,' to being the Best, which now means dominating one aspect of strength possibility.

Strength had a use... You were a benefit to the tribe, to the family, to your clan or country. Whether through actual physical usefulness or simply as a gauge of possibility, a strong person represented someone who could DO, who was useful, healthy and capable. This is even evident 100 years ago simply by perusing the iron game and physical culture literature of the time. From Arthur Saxon defining strength as the ability to endure the stresses of life, not just the gravity of a heavy barbell, to Bernarr MacFadden screaming from the masthead of every copy of Physical Culture magazine "Weakness is a crime, don't be a criminal," the one-trick-pony strength and sport world of today made as little sense to many of the early physical culturists as not training or lifting at all.

"Mind and body should be viewed as the two well-fitting halves of a perfect whole, designed and planned in perfect harmony, mutually to sustain and support each other, and equally worthy of our unwearied care and attention in perfecting." 1

Or to paraphrase an even older text, "Man know thyself, thou art fearfully and wonderfully made."

THE SOVIET SYSTEM VS. THE BULGARIAN SYSTEM OF WEIGHTLIFTING
RYAN KYLE

The Soviet system versus the Bulgarian system has been the question in the minds of weightlifting coaches, athletes, and administrators in this country at least since the rise of Bulgarian Weightlifting in the early 1970's. Prior to 1970, Bulgaria was a virtual unknown in the weightlifting world. However, with the appointment of Ivan Abadjiev to the helm and the implementation of the world's most intensive training program, Bulgaria quickly became a contender. With their success at the 1972 Olympics, they stood head-to-head with the Soviet Union at the top of World Weightlifting. In 1975, Carl Miller, who had been recently appointed the U.S. National Coach, went to Bulgaria to attend the European coaches clinic and brought back with him a picture of what the Bulgarian system was really like. This further added to the mystique of Bulgarian weightlifting. Their success in the 1980's boosted them to mythological status. The great question in the United States since those times has been "how should we train?" Should we do as the Soviets did, as some of the leaders today do? Or should we go the road less traveled and train as the mighty Bulgarians? Let's compare the two systems and then coaches can make their own assessment.

First, a disclaimer regarding the Soviet "system". I put system in quotations because there really is no Soviet training system. The Soviet Union was a massive country both geographically and population-wise. Therefore, each club/region/republic trained in their own manner, depending on the coach. Even the members of the National Team would train in their hometown facilities until it was time to gather together for the World or European training camps. These camps were more or less a gathering of potential candidates for the teams, but each would train in their own manner. The main idea was to gather the talent together to increase their quality of preparation.

There is also an important point to remember when discussing the Bulgarian training system (noticed I wrote system without quotes. This truly was a system of training). For the most part, when coaches listen to Ivan Abadjiev speak, he is talking about the training of his elite team. Recently there was a discussion on an internet chat board where it was reported that Ivan Abadjiev stated the back squat was essentially useless in the training of weightlifters. This caused near panic on the board with people bashing Ivan, and some were even speaking words boarding blasphemy saying he had "lost his mind" and "did not know what he was talking about." I highly doubt that a man who coached 9 Olympic Champions, 57 World Champions, and 64 European Champions, suddenly forgot what he was doing. You have to remember that for the most part Ivan Abadjiev coached the elite Senior National Team. While the team usually consisted of a fair number of Junior lifters and even some lifters who would be Youth lifters, they were good enough to compete in the Senior World Championships, they had no use for other exercises. If you have ever read Naim Suleymanoglu: The Pocket Hercules written by Yazan Enver Turkileri and published by Sportivy Press, you will see in the training section that in Naim's early training he did many exercises. However, it is stated in the book that the exercises were chosen for his development in the snatch and clean and jerk and by the time he was 15 and on the Senior National Team he was training with THE Bulgarian system. No doubt a lifter of lesser ability would be on these education programs for far longer.

General Training Program

For the purpose of this discussion, we will use for examination the classic Soviet model of periodization which begins with periods of low intensity and high volume gradually progressing to high intensity and low volume as the next competition approaches. This system of training requires a great deal of planning. You begin the program doing many reps in the exercises, usually about 5 reps per set. Once you reach a certain percentage, the reps drop from 5 to 3 and then down to singles. By this time, approximately twelve weeks have passed and the next competition is approaching. You would then have a light week of training which involves almost no training at all, and then you would lift in the contest. After the contest you would have new maxes of which to base your training.

The Senior Club Coaching Manual from USAW has a generic plan listed in it using the classic model of periodization. The outline is as follows:

	CYCLE 1	CYCLE 2	CYCLE 3	PRE-COMP
WEEK	1 2 3 4	5 6 7 8	9 10 11 12	13
INTENSITY OF TOP SETS	70 75 65 80%	75 85 70 90%	85 95 75 100%	80%
REPS PER SSET	5	3	2/1	

This program is a simplistic outline of the total program. To list each individual week with reps and sets would take up too much space and also is outside of the scope of this compare/contrast article. However, it does allow an insight into what the Soviet style of training is like. While the exact percentages may have been added later to give the learner of the program a general picture of the weights that should be lifted, the general idea is start with more reps and work your way down to heavy singles, hopefully with 100%. There would also be cycles where twice daily training was common, but usually for a shorter amount of time, say one month here and there, as opposed to the Bulgarians who almost always train more than once a day.

The Bulgarian system has a much more intuitive approach to it. The lifter trains up to a max each day; this could be a true max or it could be the max weight that can be lifted on that day. The lifter then may back off and work back up or drop down for some doubles with sub-maximum weights. This basic workout would be done several times a day in small increments. First would be squats followed by a break, then snatches followed by a break and finally clean and jerks. The afternoon would start with snatches, break, clean and jerks, break, and more squats. A third session later in the evening could be added if more work is needed. When lifters begin the training year, they may only reach 85%-90% of their best, but gradually as the year progresses they begin to lift closer to their true max more often. Also, at the beginning of the year they may only train once a day and then twice a day and then finally during the heaviest periods of training three times a day. As the major competition draws near (i.e. the World Championships) they begin to reduce the amount of training, but continue to lift maximum weights. The total training time during the lighter periods would be approximately 3-4 hours a day and the training time during the heavy periods would be around 6-8 hours a day. This would include the breaks.

Exercise Selection

Exercise selection is a hotly debated topic among weightlifting coaches and the Soviet and Bulgarian systems could not be further apart in their opinions on the exercises necessary in the training of weightlifters. The Soviets prefer a plethora of exercises and the selection really depends on the lifter and their personal coach. The Bulgarians, on the other hand, stick primarily with the snatch, clean and jerk and squats.

Again we will use the USA Weightlifting Senior Coaching Manual as our reference to the generic Soviet approach to weightlifting. The Senior Manual lists 38 individual exercises that can be used in training and this does not include combination lifts such as one clean + one front squat + one jerk. The exercises are subdivided into the categories Competition Lifts, Semi-competition lifts; Lift related exercises; Exercises for power and strength; and Remedial exercises. The exercises included range from snatch/clean shrugs, jerk recoveries, jerk dips, pulls, squats, snatch/clean and jerk down to medicine ball throws and abdominal work.

They do not suggest that all 38 exercises should be used during every training cycle. Rather, these exercises are on the menu from which the coach can select in order to tailor the training program to address each individual athlete. When the lifter is far out from a major competition, their training would primarily focus on the power and strength exercises as well as the remedial exercises. During the middle cycle, the training would incorporate more lift related exercises and semi-competition lifts. Finally during the last phases of training, there would be further inclusion of the competition and semi-competition lifts in order to get prepared to lift in the contest.

In contrast to the Soviet à la carte of exercises, in Bulgaria there is only one meal choice - snatches, clean and jerks, and squats and plenty of them. During the lighter phases of training, and by light I mean only training once a day for approximately three hours, the workout would consist of snatches, clean and jerks and squats to max. Sometimes when the lifters are very tired or have a minor injury, they will do the power versions of the lifts. As the year moves on and the program progresses, the lifters move from training once a day and begins to train twice daily, again to max both sessions (although heavier lifts are usually achieved in the afternoon). No matter how many times the lifters train in a given day, the program always stays the same - snatches, clean and jerks, and squats.

Another word regarding the Bulgarian system; the system has been ever evolving. Yes, the Bulgarians at one time did pulls, jerk from the rack and power jerks. However, as Ivan Abadjiev constantly reviewed his system and looked for more ways to improve it, he eventually began to throw out certain exercises and focus on the ones he knew would improve results. If you think about it logically, there is no definitive proof that hang snatches improve the snatch, or that lifts from blocks improve the competition lifts. Some people are able to lift 90% or more of their competition lifts in the partial lifts, while others can barely do 80%. However, if I snatch a new PR then I can say, yes I got better. A new PR in the hang snatch is useless if I still snatch the same. Since you only have a limited recovery potential, the Bulgarians would rather spend all of their energy on lifts they know they will get a return on instead of hoping the other exercises will result in gains.

What should you do?

So how should U.S. lifters train? Some coaches advocate the Soviet system because it provides plenty of variety in terms of exercises and because the training is not constantly at max effort, so it should allow for an extended athletic career. The Bulgarian system, on the other hand, is rumored to be only for the best-of-the-best--in other words it takes a special kind of athlete to handle the monotony and intensity of the training. While the Bulgarian system is incredibly difficult and it does take a special athlete to handle the system, it takes a special athlete in general to become a World or Olympic Champion. If you need help deciding which system/style of training you should take up you should consider your personality first. Are you the type that cannot wait to "go heavy" in training, or do you prefer to have a specific plan for your training that you can follow like a road map? If you are the type of person who wants to know what you are lifting on a certain day, and you want a specific dates for when you should try to PR, then I would suggest using the Soviet system. However, if you do not mind lifting heavy day after day nor mind missing PR attempts on a regular basis, then try the Bulgarian system.

Warning: Do not read this next paragraph if you do not want my opinion.

That previous paragraph was intended for the everyday lifter (aka the hobbyist). Now I will give my personal opinion. When it comes to our elite lifters in this country, I think they should all be training in the Bulgarian style. Many people argue that we should train like the Soviets because we have a small talent pool of athletes and we need to make sure their careers are longer. Because we have a small pool of athletes we should be training them as hard as possible. We really need to have the cream rise to the top. If they run, they were not meant to be a champion. We do not have the luxury of being able to throw a bunch of stuff at the wall to see what sticks like the mainstream sports in the U.S. We literally need to build mountains out of molehills in some cases, so we must push our athletes harder than anyone else. In 1972, Bruce Jenner placed 10th at the Olympics in the decathlon. He took a few weeks off after the Olympics and began training for the next games: six to eight hours a day every day for the next four years. The result - A GOLD MEDAL! How do we expect our lifters to win the Senior World Championships or the Olympics when they are only training five days a week for two hours. It is almost comical that anyone considers this difficult training. There are people in local health clubs who work out more, but we expect to win in World Weightlifting with such little training. The Bulgarian system does not guarantee progress through formulas or various set and rep schemes. It only guarantees progress through incredibly hard work and dedication. I was talking to a former Bulgarian lifter once and I asked him how much he trained (he was a Junior lifter at the time). He said they trained at least twelve times a week. Then he asked me how much we train in the U.S. I said some of our lifters only train five times a week. He told me this is no good. My response was that if you looked at our lack of medals, it is obvious it is no good. Then in eight words he told me the secret to weightlifting: "Exercise more, and there will be more medals." All of U.S. lifting needs to step back and evaluate if they are exercising as much as they can.

Notes
Jones, L. (1991). USWF Coaching Accredidation Course Senior Coach Manual. Colorado Springs: U.S. Weightlifting Federatoin.
Turkileri, Y. E. (2004). Naim Suleymanoglu: The Pocket Hercules. Livonia: Sportivny Press.

OUT WITH THE NEW, IN WITH THE OLD
MATT FOREMAN

Yesterday, I was walking through a Dick's Sporting Goods store, looking for their prices on iron plates (they're pretty good, incidentally). As I was making my way to the corner of the store where they keep the weight training equipment, I happened to pass through the kids clothing section. I stopped for a couple of minutes as I strolled past the racks of t-shirts, shorts, sweaters, etc. because I noticed something that made me think. The store had several racks of t-shirts with all kinds of little tough-sounding motivational phrases on them. You've all seen the shirts I'm talking about somewhere before, nothing new. But the thing that caught my eye was the actual slogans and words that were on the shirts. I guess we've moved way past the days of shirts that say, "No Pain, No Gain" and other overused mottos like that. The shirts I saw yesterday said things like "I feel YOUR pain!" "Dare to take ME on?" and "If you see ME, get used to second place!" As I said, these were all in the kids section of the store, so the shirts were probably meant for ages 9-12, something like that.

After I left the store and started driving to the gym, I found myself thinking a lot about what I saw. All of the words on those shirts were designed to sound cocky, arrogant, self-absorbed and disrespectful towards other competitors. The store had several racks of them, so it's obvious that these are big sellers. That means that we're living in a culture where parents are putting their kids into sports programs and then buying them clothes that are specially constructed to demonstrate self-worship and insulting attitudes towards opponents. The more I thought about this, the more connection I began to see with much of the adult behavior we see in the sports world today. The NBA is a pretty good place to explain this connection because it's one of the biggest sports venues in the world. Here we find situations where the sport's top stars announce their decisions to switch teams by getting on television and saying things like, "I've decided to take my talents to South Beach." And then when these stars get to South Beach, they hold outrageous spectacles at Miami's American Airlines Arena where they get onstage with two of their teammates (ignoring the rest of their team), and declare themselves "arguably the best trio ever to play the game of basketball." It doesn't stop there, because they have to continue to run their mouths by predicting that they will win "not two, not three, not four" NBA championships. They label themselves as the newest sports dynasty before they've ever played a game together. Yes, I'm talking about LeBron James and the Miami Heat.

So, the process seems clear. Little kids are enrolled in youth basketball, football, soccer, etc. by their parents. Then, their parents buy them the shirts I saw at Dick's so they can try to intimidate the competition. From there, the kids go through their sports careers and the most talented ones make it to the professional level, where they are given the highest possible pedestal to hold glorious celebrations of ME. Their self-absorption and disdain towards others is not only appreciated, but encouraged. Yeah, this sounds about right. Make no mistake about it; professional sports have become a public display stage for the absolute highest levels of selfishness and poor sportsmanship. And since you're all wondering, let me tell you where I'm going with this.

Many of you are coaches, parents, gym owners, etc. In other words, you're in positions where there are people under your instruction. You are an authority figure on some level. This means that you are responsible for teaching and administrating the people you work with. What I want to do with this month's article is examine what kind of job you're doing in these functions. I'm not talking about how you're teaching technique or programming to your athletes or kids; I'm talking about how you're teaching attitude. Let me make it clear right from the beginning that I'm going to be pushing my own personal opinion pretty hard with this one, because this is one area where I'm positive that I'm right. When it comes to training, exercise selection, snatch technique, etc., I've always tried to make it clear that I'm not the only one with the right answers. In this area, however, I think there's a pretty strong distinction between what's right and what's wrong. I'll try to explain my ideas as clearly as possible, and you should be able to find something in here that will make your gym, your home, and your life better.

Old School vs. New School

Everything about our culture has changed over the last hundred years. When people started competing in organized sports around the late 1800s and early 1900s, the personalities of the athletes were reflective of the general attitudes of society. People, for the most part, were much less boisterous and demonstrative than they are now. If you've ever had a chance to watch some of the earliest football, basketball, or weightlifting that was captured on film, you've probably noticed how the athletes acted during competition. There wasn't much celebration or emotion involved. Sure, you would occasionally see athletes jump in the air or raise their hands to the crowd after a successful performance, but it was nothing like the environment today where the sport of football has actually had to invent rules to restrain the celebrations of athletes after they score touchdowns.

This is what we're going to call "old school attitude." An old school attitude was what you saw when athletes just shut their mouths and did their job. If they won, they would probably show a little excitement and appreciation to the spectators, but there was definitely a sense of restraint and modesty. If they lost, they shook the hands of their competitors and blamed only themselves for their failure. There was no end zone dancing, choreographed celebration that lasted two minutes, or whining about bad referees after a loss. These types of behaviors were simply not part of the picture because they were considered undignified and self-indulgent.

Smack talking was often part of the picture with old school athletes, but it was done between the competitors and away from the public. There's no doubt that many great athletes from the days of yore, like Babe Ruth, Jack Johnson, and Norb Schemansky, engaged in some trash talk with their competitors. However, it was different then than it is now. Even if modern technology would have been present beck in 1948, I seriously doubt if you would have ever seen Tommy Kono getting on television and bragging that he was going to win "not two, not three, not four" Olympic medals. The attitude was simply different in those days. You just didn't do stuff like that.

However, fast-forward to 2011 and we've got the disgraceful type of narcissistic circus we see in so many modern sports. We'll call it the "new school attitude," where athletes brag as loudly as possible to as many people as they can, ridicule and insult their competitors, value themselves more than their teams, and refuse to take personal responsibility when they fail. If you watch ESPN long enough, you'll get a pretty good idea of what I'm talking about. Now, let me make it clear that not every athlete in the modern era has been contaminated by the new school attitude. I was just watching a Grand Slam tennis tournament last month where Rafael Nadal beat Roger Federer for the championship. The behavior of both these men was a pretty classy demonstration of old school behavior, as Nadal complimented Federer after the match by saying, "I respect Roger because he acts the same whether he wins or loses." These guys are clear examples of positive athletic behavior, and they're not the only ones in contemporary sports that act right. But the fact still remains that you can't watch sports for very long these days without seeing something that just makes you want to vomit because of how immature and negative it is.

When did everything change? When did we go from old school to new school? It's not something that happed instantaneously or because of one person, but I do personally believe that Muhammad Ali had a lot to do with changing the sports culture in this country. Ali was one of the greatest athletes in history, and his accomplishments in boxing were equaled only by his incredible personality. Ali's trash talking, disrespect towards his opponents, and self-promotion were done at a level that had never been seen in sports before. His image was so larger-than-life that he heavily influenced generations of young athletes that have grown up in his wake. Kids have actually moved through their athletic careers wanting to embody the same showmanship and bravado that Ali had. He is the point of origin for much of the new school attitude. Please understand, though, that I'm not committing the sacrilege of dumping on Muhammad Ali here. As an athlete, I hold Ali on a pedestal as one of the supreme competitors I've ever seen. I never liked his behavior and I still don't, but I would never deny his greatness as an athlete.

Therefore, we have a stark contrast between two very different methods. Based on how I've described all of this, you can probably guess where I stand in the evaluation of old school vs. new school. I am very much an old school personality, I require my athletes to be the same way, and I reject new school attitude as being childish, irresponsible, and shameful. Got it? Hopefully I made that clear enough. But then that leaves us with you. What kind of personality are you, and what are you doing to make sure your athletes, children, etc. are developing in the right direction? Let's take a look at this, and I'll give you a few handy dandy tips to make sure you're not contributing to the ramming of modern sports into the toilet.

The basic blueprint for not becoming a jerkoff

How do you represent yourself in the strength world? Because one thing you better believe is that when you're a coach, your personality will filter down into your athletes. Even if you're not a coach, your personality still will filter down to the other lifters in your gym, your children, friends who admire you, etc. There's a sense of accountability that has to be there. If you're in any position of authority or responsibility, the people around you will often act the way you act.

I've used the word "selfishness" quite a few times in this article, and obviously there's been a negative connotation with it. However, I should mention that being selfish is very important to an elite athlete. If you're in a position where you're competing at the top of your sport, you have to have a certain element of self-centeredness to be successful. High-level athletes have to see their training and their performance as the most important things in the universe. These aren't always the most endearing people to be around because they basically expect the whole world to stop and revolve around their workouts. For better or worse, this just comes with the territory. Championship athletes usually aren't very giving personalities. Hopefully, that all changes after retirement or once age sets in and real life gets started. Most elite athletes go through a lot of attitude changes when they make the transition to civilian life, and that's a good thing.

The negative aspect of selfishness that I'm describing here is the point where selfishness makes the transition to blatant punk behavior. It's fine to be totally focused on your athletic priorities, but we need to make sure that we don't cross over into the bragging, impertinence, and whining. Hell, I'll make this easy for you. Here are four simple things you can do that will keep you from looking like a turd:

1. Show a lot of interest, enthusiasm, and support for others. Simplest thing in the

world, right? Just start caring and getting excited about the people around you. You will absolutely never go wrong if you cheer for others during their workouts, congratulate them after they're successful, and throw them a little encouragement when they're down. This is 100% guaranteed stuff and it takes very little energy.

2. Don't talk about your accomplishments unless somebody asks you about them. The quickest way to make a bad first impression is to start throwing your resume in somebody's face without any reason. If you're a stud, people will either already know it when they meet you or they'll figure it out pretty quickly. You don't need to wave your gold medals around your head. It looks insecure and arrogant.

3. Don't coach people in the gym unless they ask for it. Let's say you're in a gym training and you see somebody who's clearly doing something wrong. If the person has a coach who is working with them, you need to just stay out of it. It's none of your business, so don't turn into to Butty McButtinstein. Now, if the person doesn't have a coach and they're doing something wrong, just ask them, "Do you mind if I give you a suggestion?" You'll know pretty fast if they want to listen to you or not, and then you can proceed accordingly. If it's obvious that they want you to keep your comments to yourself, then do it. You asked politely, so you're in the clear.

4. Don't get on the internet and talk @%*!. Ooohhh, I think I'm probably ruffling some feathers with this one. Look, the internet is the greatest medium in the history of civilization for people who want to unleash their anger and disgust over how stupid everybody else in the world is. But even if you're right and your opponent is wrong, you'll both still come away from the argument looking stupid. Just don't do it, baby.

Quick confession- Just so nobody calls me a hypocrite or thinks I'm sitting on my high horse, I'll openly admit that I've violated every one of these suggestions at some point in my life. Nobody's perfect.

In Conclusion…

A lot of the mistakes that come with new school attitude are connected with youth. It's pretty easy to act like a dork when you're young. We've all done it. It's part of growing up. And you coaches need to remember this, because most kids literally don't know how they're supposed to act. We sometimes make the mistake of telling ourselves, "Dammit, they should know better than that!" Well, maybe they DON'T know better than that. Maybe nobody has ever told them the difference between acting right and acting wrong. Remember, some of these kids you work with have been practically raised by wolves. They need some guidance.

And as always, I know there's the possibility that some of you might think everything I've just said is all wrong. If you just got back from Dick's Sporting Goods and you're excited to give little ten year-old Tyler a shirt you just bought him that says, "I'm number one and everybody can lick my butthole" so he can wear it to youth wrestling practice tomorrow, then I guess we probably have a difference in opinion. But here's some food for thought. What if Tyler shows up to wrestling practice with his cocky new shirt, and then he gets pinned in sixteen seconds by some tough little Mormon kid? At that point, we can safely say that Tyler is NOT number one, and that shirt is gonna look pretty stupid. Don't humiliate your kids.

Look, I'm not telling you to be boring. I'm not telling you that you have to be an emotionless robot as an athlete, and I'm certainly not telling you that you can't have a colorful personality. We don't have to stay stuck in the Stone Age; we couldn't even if we wanted to. Times change, and you have to be able to keep up with the changes. But not all changes are good. The shift we've seen towards total self-absorption and egotism is not good. Whining is not good. Insulting your competitors is not good. So do society a favor and take a stand against those things. Make your athletes take a stand against them, too, and maybe we'll all have a better experience in our sports lives. Let's give it a try.

REPETITIVE MOTION/OVERUSE INJURIES IN ATHLETES
DR. STEPHEN FLIKKE

Repetitive motion/overuse injuries, otherwise known as cumulative trauma disorders, are described as tissue damage that results from repetitive demand over the course of time. The term refers to a vast array of diagnoses, but is most common in repetitive motion and high impact activities. As the name indicates, the types of activities that are most likely to cause these types of injuries are those that require the same movement over and over again. Examples of this would be long distance running or swimming, or any activity in which the athlete is required to do the exact same movement in a repetitive motion. In strength training, you are more likely to see these types of injuries in which the routine is not changed or the lifter fails to work the opposing muscles, creating a muscular imbalance.

What is an overuse injury?

Overuse injuries are caused by an accumulation of micro trauma, or a small amount of muscle injury (important for muscle growth and strength), which builds up to macro trauma, which is a large amount of muscle injury that is not important for muscle growth or strength and will actually stop your training due to pain. When a weightlifting injury occurs, this can cause a weakness. There are three sources for a weakness due to an injury—the muscle, the joint and the nerve. The muscle may be damaged, shortened or deconditioned. If the joint separates at all (such as the shoulder), the muscles that cross the joint are not as strong due to the fact that they will not fully function in an unstable joint. If there is any pressure on the nerve, such as a herniated disk, this can decrease the neurological flow to the muscle and cause a weakness. Also, some new research has shown that nerve tension can decrease the muscle strength as well. You need to assess the muscles, joints and nerve supply to the muscles to determine if any of the structures are dysfunctional. If any of the structures are not functioning properly, they need to be fixed, then rehabilitated.

How are tissue and joints specifically affected by an overuse injury?

Joints

Joint injuries are either a compression or shearing injury that can cause pain and multiple muscle weakness patterns.

In the compression type of injury, the trauma is directed mostly to the joint itself. This type of injury has little or no tearing of the tissues and swelling, if present, is limited to the joint capsule. The stress of the weight affects mechanoreceptors and nociceptors in the joint structure. This type of injury appears to affect the internal structures of the joint that can exhibit a common finding of multiple muscle weaknesses, especially muscles that cross that joint. Joints that can be affected by this include the ankle, knee, lumbar, thoracic and cervical joints. The exercises that can affect these joints are usually ones with heavy axial loading such as heavy squats, deadlifts, shoulder presses, etc. These heavy loads can compress the joints enough to create an abnormal firing of joint receptors and change the normal tone and strength of the muscles that surround that joint. Repeated traction of these joints can normalize the firing of the joint receptors and reestablish the normal tone and strength of the muscles.

The second type of joint injury can occur from a shearing or tearing action that can injure multiple structures. This the most common type of joint injury and occurs when joints and related structures are strained and twisted, causing injury to muscles, ligaments, skin and receptors of the joints. Any joint in the body can be affected by a shearing injury by virtually any exercise. The shearing type of joint injury will cause weakness of the muscles that cross the joint. The weaknened muscle pattern will cause a strain on ligaments, which will cause residual pain over the ligaments. Ligaments are the structures that cross and stabilize the joint and when stressed abnormally, will cause a weakness in the muscles that cross that joint. There are certain receptors in ligaments that when overloaded will cause a reflex muscle weakness. This is because the muscles will not function properly or with full strength in an unstable joint; this is a protective mechanism to prevent further damage to the joint. Depending on the severity of the injury and the length of time before initiation of treatment, the patient will adapt to their injury and require treatment for muscle incoordination and imbalances. This will cause a secondary reason for pain and weakness in the muscle when doing the exercise, long after the initial injury. Limitation of range of motion can indicate an imbalance of the prime movers and synergistics and antagonists. An example of this would be doing the squat improperly and inducing an injury to the knee. This will cause an abnormal stress on the knee ligaments and cause a weakness of the muscles that cross that joint such as the quadriceps and hamstrings. If the injury to the knee is not treated and rehabilitated immediately and properly, this can cause an imbalance between the quadriceps and hamstrings and create more pain and weakness. If the imbalance is severe enough or is allowed to exist for a long period of time, this can also cause stress in other joints and weakness in other muscles unrelated to the original injury.

Muscles and Ligaments

Strength training injuries in the soft tissue can come from a variety of sources. Examples of this may be poor lifting technique, lifting beyond your capabilities or training too often without proper rest or recuperation. All of these sources can lead to micro trauma, or small injury, that can get worse over time. Because you don't recognize that the injury is there, you reinjure yourself frequently. This repeated micro trauma can eventually have a profound effect on the specific action of the joint and the surrounding tissues. The effects of the micro trauma include the micro tearing of the muscle, the sheath around the muscle and the adjacent connective tissue, as well as stress to the tendon and its bony attachments. The micro tearing of the muscle tissue leads to microscopic bleeding, all of which affects the entire area around the injury, contributing to what is commonly know as inflammation.

Most people assume that inflammation can be easy to detect, like the swelling around a badly sprained ankle. This is not always the case, however. Micro trauma causes a corresponding low level of inflammation that cannot be seen or palpated.

The body responds to this myofascitis (inflammation of the muscle and fascia) by forming fibrous adhesions, or scar tissue, in the muscle between the sheaths of adjacent muscle groups and between the fascia and the muscle sheaths. These fibrous adhesions limit the ease and range of motion of muscles and joints and can decrease the muscles lengthening and shortening capabilities. Once the normal biomechanics of the joint are altered, this can lead to further inflammation and the pattern becomes a vicious cycle of long-term wear and tear.

This fibrous adhesion pattern can be seen in people who do certain exercises such as bench press and complain of the same pain in the exact same spot. This doesn't happen by chance. The fibrous adhesion formed in the shoulder muscle is preventing proper motion and pulling on the various soft tissue structures like muscle, fascia, tendon and bursa when trying to perform the bench press. An option would be to alternate the barbell bench press with the dumbbell bench press. You are still able to target the same muscles but at the same time you are allowing other muscle groups to fire and create stability.

Managing Overuse Injuries

Three general rules to remember for managing and strengthening overuse injuries:
1. Muscles work best when they can move through their full Range of Motion (ROM).

If you have a joint that is limited, it will impact how the muscles around it work. This may not be the case with your injury, but without a known cause, it's best to cover all of your bases. If you do not have full range of motion in a muscle, you may want to focus on the antagonist muscle and decrease the weight that you are using or seek help from a manual therapist or ART practitioner who specializes in restoration of ROM in the muscle.

2. Each muscle group has a beginning and an end, or origin and insertion. In overuse injuries, one end is usually symptomatic and the other is not. While working to loosen the symptomatic area, it is crucial to remember to work on both ends to alleviate built up tension throughout the entire muscle. The best way to do this is make sure you run through the full range of motion. When you are doing a squat, if you do not complete the squat, you are only working the superior portion if the muscle group. By bringing the squat down to the full range, you are also using the lower hamstring muscles, for example.

3. Muscle groups work in pairs that work against each other in opposite directions— as one group contracts, the other relaxes. If one group of muscles becomes tight or fatigued, it will stop contracting fully. This means that the opposing group of muscles will stop being stretched when that happens and stiffen up and restrict motion as a result. Therefore, you need to work on the antagonist muscle groups. If your quads become over developed, for example, your hamstrings will become weak and fatigued, causing muscular imbalance and leaving you prone to injury. Your training program should always include antagonist muscle groups. Balance quad-dominant exercises with posterior chain work and low back-dominant exercises with abdominal work. As far as volume goes, antagonists should be trained at the same level as the opposing group.

Be aware of minor injuries building up over time. For home care, make sure you ice and use a foam roller. For more serious injuries, make sure you go to someone who specializes in overuse injuries such as a sports chiropractor or a manual therapist.

If you like to run or bike, realize that you also need to do strength training and if you lift, realize that your core strengthening is key to preventing injury. When you are lifting or training, especially in the off-season, make sure you mix things up. Don't just do what you feel you are good at.

THE FOUR PHASES OF WEIGHTLIFTING
MATT FOREMAN

Have you ever stopped and thought about how so many things in life happen in different stages? Almost anything you can think of in your life probably followed some kind of progression; it happened in a phase one, phase two, phase three kind of order. Let's look at a really easy example to make this more understandable. Many of you are in long-term relationships, right? Some of you are married, and others have had a boyfriend or girlfriend for an extended period of time. I know this has to be true because people who read Performance Menu are generally smarter and more attractive than non-readers, so we usually don't stay single for very long.

Your relationship with your significant other has developed in stages. Think back about the time period when you originally met this person and started going out on your first dates. Think about how you acted, how you talked, how you dressed, etc. Most likely, you were on your best behavior and trying to look extra hot because you wanted something to happen with this person. You cleverly concealed any personal glitches of yours that other people might find gross because you were on a mission to look as tantalizing as possible. That was stage one. Then, there was a time when you two decided that you were an actual couple, and the newness of the relationship started to wear off. You got used to each other, and you got to discover some wonderfully special personal habits your partner has. Some of these were charming and funny, while many others were probably disgusting and irritating. That was stage two, and many couples never make it through this one. Lots of casualties in this area.

If you decided that this person's lifestyle was something you could live with, then you might have even progressed to stage three. This is where you're serious, and you start talking and planning serious future type of stuff. You think about getting married and buying houses. Once you're in this stage, it's intense business. You're considering spending the rest of your life with this person, and that's pretty heavy stuff to think about. Nervousness and second thoughts are common here. Some couples stick it out, and some don't.

So… that brings us to weightlifting and strength training. You might not even know it, but your experience as a weightlifter has also happened in stages. This also true for all the people you coach, if you're a coach. What I want to do this month is take a look at the stages of a lifter's career, and all the different variables that accompany these stages. If you coach lifters, you need to have an understanding of what's going through their minds when they come into your gym. Because if you're oblivious to the thoughts and concerns of your athletes, there's a strong chance that misunderstandings and conflicts will pop up. These can make gym life pretty sticky, and they could even lead to a break-up. Just like your life with your special little love interest, it's pretty damn important to be able to see things not just from your own perspective, but from theirs, too. Mutual understanding will almost always make things easier, whether you're talking about snatching a personal record or shopping for an engagement ring. So, let's take a look at the stages that you, your athletes, and every other person who calls themselves a weightlifter will go through during your relationship with the barbell.

Stage One: Clueless Rookie

Even though the term "clueless rookie" carries a negative tone, this first stage of your weightlifting life is one of the most exciting times you'll ever get to feel. This is when you are brand spanking new to the iron world. You may or may not have had some athletic experience at this point and you might have even done some form of weight training, but the focused discipline of serious weightlifting training is a whole new ball game. You don't really know anything about weightlifting at this point, but you do know for sure that you're interested in it. You're full of energy and curiosity. This is when you're first learning the snatch, clean and jerk, or maybe the squat or deadlift if you're a powerlifter instead of an Olympic lifter. Every day that you come to the gym is a new experiment of teaching your body to do something that it has never done. Frustration is guaranteed at this point, no questions asked. The complexity of the Olympic lifts are challenging for even the most talented natural athletes. You probably get to wipe out in some creative way in this stage, either through nailing your chin with the bar in the jerk, falling on your butt when jumping under a snatch, or some other wacky accident. Veterans, do you remember those days? You got embarrassed because there were probably other people in the gym who were experienced lifters and you felt like genetic sludge when you biffed it in front of them. Hey, this is like the awkward stage children have to go through. You're like the little boy who came to school and found out the hard way that the cool kids don't pull their pants all the way down around their ankles when they pee at the urinal.

But the great thing about this phase is that you also get to have those moments when everything clicks. You hit your first snatch correctly, and you FEEL the proper movement for the first time in your life. If I could offer a word of advice to coaches at this point…make sure you celebrate and compliment your newbies when they have little technique breakthroughs. Even though they might still have five or six technical glitches that need to get fixed and they're a long way from perfect, you have to remember that it's very important for new lifters to feel like they're making some kind of progress. Even if it's the smallest of baby steps, make your people feel like they're moving forward. That's what will keep them coming back for more. I've seen aspiring new lifters quit the sport because their coaches were such perfectionists that they basically wouldn't give ANY positive feedback in this phase.

If you're the lifter, please try to remember that this phase will be rough. You're going to have little aches and pains in places that you never have before. You're going to have moments when you feel like you've mastered the technique of a lift and then, three days later, you lose that mastery and feel like you forgot how to lift correctly. The aggravation is going to be a part of this stage, but that aggravation is a good thing. If you get angry when you do something wrong, that means it's important to you. You have a hungry spirit, and you get pissed when you fail because you really, really want to be good at this. That's the right attitude, believe me. The people who don't care if they make progress are the ones who will never amount to jack squat because their performance doesn't mean anything to them. Just hang in there, baby.

Stage Two: Turbo Teenager

Whoa daddy! At this point, you've passed the rookie phase and now you're moving up in the world. Stage two is when you're no longer a newbie and you've actually started to perfect the lifts and make progress. In fact, you've probably made enormous progress in a short period of time. The Olympic lifts are very difficult to learn, but the athlete will make remarkable gains during the time when the technique has clicked and strength improvements have begun.

This is when you've been lifting for maybe a year, or possibly even two or three years. Now, you actually do know some stuff about weightlifting. You understand the technique of the lifts and the training process. You've lifted some solid weights, too. You can probably even beat many of the other lifters around you. This is when many of you have begun competing, and you now have some meets under your belt. You might have even competed at the national level. This is a great time because you're good at weightlifting and you know it. Most likely, you've even started to teach others. Full-time coaching probably hasn't become your thing yet because you're climbing the ladder as an athlete. But you've helped some people with their technique in the gym, or even taught some beginners who are in stage one, just like you were not too long ago. The stage one people look at you as an expert because you can lift a lot more than they can, which boosts your pride and self-image. Basically, things are awesome at this point.

However, there is one thing about this stage that can be funky. What am I talking about? I'm talking about the fact that you probably think you know every freaking thing there is to know about weightlifting at this point. Trust me, stage two is when you start to get pretty big for your britches. Because you're now a qualified weightlifter, you start to think that your expertise is a lot bigger than most of the people out there. This is when you get on the internet and argue with people about weightlifting because you're right and they're wrong, dammit. That's why this stage is called the "turbo teenager" stage. You're like a seventeen year-old kid who thinks they know everything about life. You don't want to listen to your parents because you think they're old, out of touch with reality, and they don't have a clue about what your life is like. You've got enough hormones pumping through your body to fuel an oil tanker, and you won't back down from a fight.

At this point, you think the best weightlifters are the biggest experts on weightlifting. That's how you see it. And let me say a word to the coaches at this point. This stage two will be a blessing and a curse, just like being a parent and raising teenagers. The blessing of this stage is that your athletes will do a lot of incredible things that make you very proud. They're developing quickly, and it's a lot of fun to guide them while they blast away new personal records and rise up into the higher ranks of the sport. However, the curse is that they'll be hard to handle, just like the teenagers. They're going to say stupid things that piss you off. They're going to disobey you and violate the rules you've asked them to live by. They're going to require some tough love if you want them to remember that you're the authority figure and you're still in charge of this operation. Don't be afraid to lay down the law here. You're going to have to do it anyway, and most athletes respond well when they know they're following an alpha.

Stage Three: Holy crap, you mean I'm human?

Now, things are tough. Stage three occurs when you've had some years of experience under your belt. You've risen to a high level and you have some legitimate accomplishments on your record. You can look back on what you've done so far and feel a sense of reward, but now there's a problem.

Stage three is when something has happened to knock you down. You've had your balloon popped and now it's painfully clear that you're not superhuman. This could be a variety of different things. It could be an injury. That's a pretty common one. Or it could be that you haven't made any progress in two years. That's a REALLY common one. You've continued training your butt off and giving it everything you have, but your results haven't improved. Whatever the actual cause is, something has happened to burst your bubble when you're in stage three. You've learned that you actually didn't know everything like you thought in stage two, and you're not at the highest level of knowledge and experience in the sport. To put it very simply, you've been humbled. If we're comparing this to real-life experience, this might be like a time when you're now an adult and you've been burned by something. Maybe it was a divorce, an arrest for DUI, or maybe you got fired from a job. You've been knocked for a loop, and you have to ask yourself, "Where do I go from here?"

Coaches and athletes, please pay close attention to what I'm going to say next.

Stage three is the end of the road for many lifters. The defeat they experienced, whatever it was, proved to be too much for them and they decided to hang it up. They let it beat them. If you've made it to stage three in your career either as a lifter or a coach, I can guarantee that you've at least thought about quitting. It crosses your mind, and you can't believe that it might actually be coming to an end. I think anybody who has been in this sport for an extended period of time has had moments when they thought about walking away. Brothers and sisters, this is when you really start to learn about being a weightlifter. All those little motivational slogans you've seen on gym wall posters over the years, the ones that say things like "It's not how many times you fall, but how many times you get up," you know the ones I'm talking about? Stage three is when those words become reality. You've fallen, and you have to find a way to get up. Nobody can help you, either. The only thing you have to rely on is the strength of your own character. Olympic champion Yuri Zacharevich once said, "There is simply a time in your life when you must clench your teeth and hang on." All of you experienced lifters and coaches who are reading this, do you know what I mean? I know you do. All of you newbies and greenhorns, do you know what I mean? Probably not, but you will someday.

Stage Four: Rebirth

This is the stage you hit when you've survived stage three. You took your lumps, got back to work, and found a way to become successful again. This is where you're finally mature. You've come back from your defeat and now you know that you don't know everything, and you never did in the first place. In fact, you know now that you'll never know everything because the world of weightlifting is a big complex place, and you've also learned that some of the old fogies who you dismissed in stage two probably knew more about weightlifting than you thought they did because they've been through stage three, maybe even more than once. Mark Twain described this time with his famous quote, "When I was a boy of fourteen, my father was so ignorant I could barely stand to have the old man around. But when I got to be twenty-one, I was astonished at how much the old man had learned in seven years."

You might not lift the biggest weights of your life when you're in stage four. You probably hit those when you were in stage two. But there's a difference between lifting the biggest lifts of your life and doing the best lifting of your life. I hit the biggest weights of my life when I was twenty-six, but I think I did some of the best lifting of my career ten years later as a master. My lifts as a master were much lighter than my lifetime bests, but being able to still snatch over 300 pounds and qualify for the Senior Nationals when I was thirty-six years old was, in my mind, some of the finest lifting I've done in my career. Believe me, I had to survive a lot of stage threes along the way. But those stage three moments are the things that have made this whole journey so much more rewarding. If you're a coach, you'll probably never have a greater experience than when you help an athlete make it through stage three, because this is where you learn that this whole road we're traveling is about much more than just lifting weights.

I guess stage four is when you're not a kid anymore. You've been around the block a few times, so to speak. You've had your share of defeats. Nothing is clearer to you at this stage than the knowledge that you're human, just like everybody else. That's a great thing to know in life. What is equally clear to you is the understanding that you should really enjoy and treasure the bright moments of your weightlifting life, because it won't always be sunshine, lemonade and baskets full of puppies. Sometimes, it will be outhouses and spoiled milk. Still, the persistent ones who have fought through stage three and made it to stage four are the ones who reap the biggest rewards. Lemonade tastes a lot sweeter when you've been dying of thirst for a long time.

COACHES AREN'T THAT IMPORTANT... RIGHT?
MATT FOREMAN

One of the best pizzas I've ever had in my life was from a little Greek place in Seattle called Santorini's. Tiny hole-in-the-wall restaurant, Greek owned and operated, and I've been saying for years that they put out one of the best pies I've ever chomped on. Anyway, I remember sitting in this joint several years ago, feasting and having beers with a friend of mine. This friend was an elite American lifter from the 80s...World Team member, American record-holder, the whole bit. He and I were in the middle of a conversation about former Olympic gold medalists in weightlifting who had gone into coaching after their athletic careers were over, and how many of them had been successful. It was a fun few minutes of weightlifting trivial pursuit while we tried to recall how many top lifters had gone on to become top coaches. Names like Alexeev, Suleymanoglu, Rigert, Kono, and other superstars come to mind, and we diagnosed how effective their coaching had been based on their country's world championship performance. In the middle of this conversation, I asked my buddy if he thought world champion lifters made good coaches. His answer was, "I don't know. Coaching is overrated anyway."

"Coaching is overrated." I've been thinking about that statement for fifteen years. The point he was making was that athletes either have the natural ability to become champions or they don't, plain and simple. The ones that have world championship ability will probably become world champions regardless of who their coach is because they simply have more talent than anybody in the world. And the ones that don't have world championship ability? You could give them the best coaching in the planet throughout their entire careers, and they'll never make it to the top. That was the general idea of the dinner banter.

I'm a coach, as many of you are. One of the beliefs that I think is common among all coaches is that we control how successful our athletes are. If they win championships, it's because we guided them to those championships. If they fail, it's because we didn't prepare them properly. The statement "coaching is overrated" punches a few holes in our basic belief system, because it basically says that we're just not as important as we think we are. I think this is damn fine material for an article. And as with most of the subjects we analyze here at Performance Menu, it's not a simple black-and-white issue. Like a good pizza, there are many different components involved.

Big Al and his Magic Towel…

Does everybody here know who Al Oerter was? Probably not, which is a shame. Al Oerter was one of the greatest athletes who ever lived, no question about it. An American discus thrower, Al won four Olympic gold medals. That's right, four of them. Even more impressive is the fact that Al set new Olympic records in all four of these performances, and he won a couple of them with torn cartilage in his ribs, neck injuries, etc. Al's greatness is beyond comparison, and one of the freaky things about him is that he was never really coached in his career. He basically taught himself. I heard an interview with him once where he was asked who his coach was throughout his prime years. Al said, "My coach was a towel."

What the heck does that mean? Al went on to explain that he didn't have a coach. All he did was set a towel out in the throwing sector at the distance he wanted to hit with the discus. If he wanted to throw 190 feet, for example, he would just take a white gym towel and lay it on the ground 190 feet from the disc ring. Then, he would just go through his workout and make sure he threw past the towel. No coaching, no input from others, no video, etc. He just put a towel out there and made sure he threw the discus past it. Using this method, he won Olympic gold four times. Seriously guys, I'm not making this up. The guy was from another galaxy.

Now, there are some things that we have to openly acknowledge about this example. Clearly, Al Oerter had a level of natural talent that was beyond human comprehension. The "towel method" worked for him because he simply didn't need much help from anybody. He was born with an unnatural sense of knowing how to make his body move in the most effective pattern, and he also happened to have the strength, power, balance, and coordination to perfect that pattern. These things are obvious. Equally obvious is the fact that athletes like Al Oerter are extraordinarily rare. People just aren't born with tools like this on a regular basis.

However, Al isn't the only example in history. Olympic weightlifting legend Vasily Alexeev was very similar. Alexeev won two Olympic gold medals and broke eighty world records during his ten-year reign of invincibility in the 70s. Like Al, Vasily trained alone and formed his own methodology. He was able to dominate the world for a very long time without any coaching, just by doing his own thing. In addition to these two men, there have been a few other cases throughout sports history where athletes reach world record greatness without being coached. However, do these examples prove to us that coaching is overrated or, perhaps, unnecessary? Well… here's another angle we have to look at.

Ivan Abadjiev

Okay, most of you probably didn't know who Al Oerter was. How about Ivan Abadjiev, do any of you know who he is? Anyone? Anyone? Dang it, I hope you're not zero for two. If you are, let me bring you up to speed. Ivan Abadjiev was the head national coach of the Bulgarian weightlifting team during the 70s, 80s, and early 90s. Bulgaria, in case you don't know, is a relatively small European country with very little weightlifting success prior to the early 70s when Abadjiev was hired. This man built Bulgaria into one of the most feared powerhouses in the history of the sport. The 80s were an insane rampage of world champions and world records from this tiny nation, as they toppled the massive Soviet Union to become the best weightlifting team on the planet. Abadjiev is widely considered the greatest coach in the history of the sport, and there is no question that he was an iron-fisted control freak who ran his program with a dictator mentality. Abadjiev's belief was that his program would produce world champions, plain and simple. He understood that most athletes would not be able to handle the inhuman workload of his training program. But the ones that could handle it would become the best in the world. And it worked.

This is an interesting contrast to the examples of Oerter and Alexeev. With those two men, you had a situation where coaching was irrelevant. They had their success with nobody telling them what to do. With Abadjiev and the Bulgarians, however, the level of success was almost entirely attributed to the coach. Through his vision and his direction, the national program was developed into a weightlifting machine. Year after year, the Bulgarians simply pumped new bodies into the machine the way meat is pumped into a sausage grinder. With Abadjiev cranking the handle, the Bulgarian program spit out world champions as reliably as the grinder churned out sausages.

We have examples where championships are won without any coaching at all. And then we have other examples where coaching is almost the sole reason for the championships. So, getting back to our original question, is coaching overrated?

It's All About Levels...

The answer to this question has to be a little long-winded, so let's break it down in a way that makes it easy to understand. Let's take a look at different levels of athletes:

Al and Alexeev Level

With these athletes, coaching isn't even necessary. They have so many God-given gifts that they can simply operate on their own and they will still rise to the top of their sport.

Okay, we understand. And we also understand that athletes at this level are one-in-a-trillion. They're the Haley's Comets of sports.

Not quite Al and Alexeev but still way ahead of everybody else Level

Here, we're looking at athletes who are extremely talented, but they still need coaching and direction. These are freaky studs, but they don't quite have the athletic genius to be able to operate on their own. The interesting thing about these athletes is that they will usually be successful no matter who their coach is. As long as they're being coached by somebody who knows the basics of training and knows how to manage personalities, these athletes will win championships. Their success doesn't come from their coach, not really. Their success comes from their natural gifts, and their coach is more of a "talent manager" than anything else. If you happen to work with athletes like this in your coaching career, the best advice I can give you is "don't over-coach them." These athletes will need much less input and instruction than most other athletes. With these cats, the coach basically just needs to make sure they train consistently and show up for the competition on time. These are the ones that make life easy.

The Massive Majority Level

Now we're talking about the area that almost all of your athletes will fall into. This is the level where the athlete has solid athletic talent and good work ethic, but they will not rise to the top without very well-planned training and preparation. These athletes don't have the same physical gifts as the athletes in the two higher levels that we just examined. And to be totally realistic about it, these athletes should not be able to beat the athletes in the two higher levels. However, this is where life can get interesting. Because if you have Massive Majority Level athletes who have astonishing work ethic and amazing commitment, and they're competing against Al and Alexeev Level athletes who have unparalleled physical gifts but also happen to be lazy and stupid, then you might just have a shot. Massive Majority athletes are not supposed to beat Al and Alexeev athletes, make no mistake about it. Donkeys don't usually outrun thoroughbred race horses in the Kentucky Derby. But if the coach, the program, and the mental qualities of the Massive Majority athletes are exceptional enough, then there could be exceptional results.

Genetic Cesspool Level

Groan… These are the athletes who, God bless them, just don't have it. They can barely stand up straight and cough at the same time. You could coach these poor critters until judgment day and they'll never win championships. You'll know these athletes when you see them. And you want to know the hardest part of it all? These athletes often have the highest work-ethic, commitment, and love for what they're doing. They suck and they know it, but they freaking love the sport and they'll bust their butts harder than anybody. Some coaches turn these athletes away, and I say shame on them for doing that. Because one thing I can tell you for sure is that these athletes can very easily become your best volunteers, most loyal supporters, and most faithful contributors. I always tell people that if they work hard, contribute something to the program, and don't cause trouble, then they're welcome members of the team. You should do the same.

Are we ever gonna get an answer?

"Coaching is overrated." True or false? We can say that this statement has some truth to it. At the end of the day, an athlete's talent level will be the deciding factor in his/her career. Average is not supposed to beat exceptional. Superior shouldn't lose to normal. These things are true, and coaching doesn't have much to do with it. I've seen some really phenomenal athletes who are coached by borderline incompetents. The athletes still win championships because they're just better than everybody else. Nothing complicated about it.

However, the best coaches are the ones who build great programs. A great program is one that produces high-level results year after year, even if there aren't any Al Oerters or Vasily Alexeevs running around. Abadjiev built Bulgaria into this type of program. Now, it's obvious that there were a lot of exceptional athletes in the Bulgarian program throughout the 70s and 80s. You can't be a world champion without being an exceptional athlete. But the point is that the Bulgarians achieved the highest levels of success for many years, and that success was driven by the coach who set the whole operation up.

One thing I would say about great coaches is that they can design effective training programs, but even more important than the program is the environment they create. Great coaches create great training environments. The "environment" is the atmosphere of discipline, enthusiasm, intensity, and respect for the team that you see when you walk in a gym. This is, in my opinion, the most important element of coaching. Athletes have to be able to actually feel a sense of responsibility and high expectation when the coach is present. They have to feel like everything is under control when the coach is there, because that is the feeling that will propel them forward to greater results. If a coach is panicky, disagreeable, or negative, then the athletes will develop those same qualities. Pretty soon, you've just got a gym full of losers.

Is coaching overrated? Well, I guess we can admit that nobody every turned horse manure into pancakes just by pouring syrup on it. None of the JV discus throwers on the track team I coach will probably ever break Al Oerter's record of four Olympic gold medals. But if I do my job as a coach, I might be able to get that JV thrower into the finals of the state championship in three years. At that point, we've seen exceptional results from an average kid. That, my friends, is where coaching is most definitely NOT overrated. We took something normal and we turned it into something special, just like a great pizza maker does. Anybody can spin dough and then toss some toppings on it. But think about the best pizza you've ever had in your life. Go ahead, think about it right now. That pizza was perfect because somebody took a bunch of ordinary ingredients and made something amazing from them. Not just any hick from the street could make that pizza taste as great as it did. It was great because it was made by a master. That's coaching, and it makes all the difference in the world.

ON LOSING: SEVEN WAYS TO PICK YOURSELF BACK UP
YAEL GRAUER

Pep talks and positive adages aside, losing sucks. There's no two ways about it. When all eyes are on you and you don't shine in that shining moment, aphorisms about "how you play the game" don't cut it.

Losing's also a part of competition and life. So how do you take as much as you can from an otherwise difficult situation and use it to become a better athlete or even a better person? And how do you help a friend, teammate or someone you're coaching bounce back?

After many losses of my own this year, and watching many people I care about go through the same experience, I was stumped on that one, so I consulted the professionals.

I spoke with sports psychologist Dr. Kate Hays of The Performing Edge in Toronto. She works with a wide range of clients, ranging from amateur athletes all the way through Olympians and professionals, in a wide variety of sports. I also spoke with Brady Greco of Above and Beyone Consulting. He works with elite athletes, primarily hockey players including high school freshmen all the way through the professional level. Greco played three years of D-1 hockey at Colorado College, and also played professionally for the Tampa Bay Lightning.

Whether you're struggling with your own mental frustration after a loss, trying to find perspective before or after the big game (or meet), or looking for ways to support friends, teammates or athletes you coach, here are some strategies to consider.

1. Before D-Day: Setting Multiple Goals

Dr. Kate Hays believes that setting several goals is important in going into a competition. "One goal might be winning/losing, but there are other types of goals that you can have for a particular competition. Another piece might be how well you stay with form, which might be very good even if you didn't win that particular competition. Another might be mental focus; how well you were able to stay focused and in the present rather than drifting off to some other thoughts," Hays explained.

The purpose of setting different goals before a competition allows you to review a variety of aspects of your performance after the fact, so that you can measure multiple performance indicators rather than just looking at things as black and white.

2. To Watch Or Not To Watch

Although it's useful to review your performance at a meet or game or competition, Dr. Hays points out that the timing of evaluating your performance is crucial.

"I find very often that people try to do that kind of evaluation right after the event, and that's probably the worst time of all because there's so much emotion from having done the event that you're not going to be in your right mind; you're not going to be able to be logical about it, so you're not going to learn anything from that review," Dr. Hays says. This is particularly true following a loss, where athletes may be beating themselves up for what they feel was a poor performance

If you want to learn from a loss as much as you do from an experience where you did well, gaining some distance can allow you to review what you did well and what you could do differently the next time with fresh eyes. The timing of this varies from person to person. "For some people, that's a couple of hours later, but for some people that's not until the next day. Each person needs to figure out what's best for them," she explained.

What about when you end up on the wrong side of someone else's highlight reel, or there's video footage that's particularly painful to replay? Dr. Hays offers a practical solution. "[I'd] encourage them to turn it off," she says. "You don't need to watch it over and over again. You don't need to open that wound again. It's 15 seconds that's going to pass as soon as somebody else does something else."

3. Supporting a Friend or Teammate

Trying to support someone you care about who just suffered a loss can be an awkward situation. "Very often if somebody's upset there isn't any right thing you can say," Dr. Hays said. "On the other hand its much more important to say something to somebody than not to say anything at all" because you are worried about possibly saying the wrong thing, she added.

One approach that works for her is a 1-2 approach of first providing empathy and really recognizing what they are feeling, and then following that up with a bit of perspective, reminding your friend or teammate that they have another competition the following week, or pointing out something which they did do well.

"If all you do is wallow with them, then they don't feel any better. But if all you do is provide this cheery 'whatever,' then they're going to say, 'No, no, you don't understand,' so that's why I like doing both pieces in that sequence," Hays said. Obviously coaches who do not get caught up in a one-size-fits-all approach would have a better sense over what individual athletes would respond best to.

Sometimes all someone needs is a sympathetic ear. "Sometimes its just a matter of being there for somebody and listening to what they have to say and letting them talk it through it to a friend or teammate," Dr. Hays said. "Just pay attention to what they're experiencing."

4. Finding Perspective

In her work at the Performing Edge in Toronto, Dr. Hays helps athletes break out of self-limiting patterns and gain some perspective, helping athletes recognize that "their performance in that particular moment is not the full definition of them; there are other aspects of them that are also really important and can be valued." It's easy to forgot in the heat of the moment, but there are a whole lot more elements and aspects of your life than just your sport.

5. Gaining An Edge

Brady Greco, who primarily works with hockey players, points out that losses can be useful in a team setting. Using hockey as an example, he points out that very few teams are undefeated in a season. "I think it's important from a team aspect that you lose, because that will help continue to motivate your team, whether it be in practice or the following game, to understand what they need to do in practice to improve both individually and from a team point of view as well."

Since good teams can get complacent, losing is a trip back to the drawing board which compels them to go back to the drawing board to practice and implement skills in the next game. This allows both individual players and teams to reach their full potential.

6. Gleaning Life Lessons

"I think your character really shines when you lose," Greco said. "It's not fun to lose, but you can take a lot from it depending on how you lose or what you actually when you do lose what specifically you take away from it. There could be life lessons learned, there could be character learning lessons, personally and as a team."

7. Games are Supposed to Be Fun

Greco believes losing in a team sport may be even more difficult than an individual loss because you may feel like you disappointed and let down a whole team and coaching staff.

"You always want to look to the positives in a loss," Greco said. "It's not the end of the world, obviously, even at the professional level. You play the game to have fun." An athlete no longer enjoying their sport will see a decline in their performance. "It's crucial for anyone to get over a mental barrier or get over a loss to go back to putting it in perspective and look at the big picture of things, of 'I started this game because I love the game and I want to have fun.' Once you stop having fun, that's when you see your sports performance decline, so it's important that if you do lose and you are mentally beating yourself up for that loss, that you take something positive from that loss and understand that this is a game and games are supposed to be fun."

So there you have it. Suck all the learning out of your losses that you can, and then get back on the field and have some fun.

DIFFERENT STROKES FOR DIFFERENT FOLKS: VARIATIONS IN PULLING TECHNIQUE
MATT FOREMAN

The Catalyst Athletics forums are turning into hot territory these days, that's for sure. I find myself on there a lot lately, reading up on the latest strength conversations instead of doing the little jobs around the house my wife wants me to take care of. That should make you, the Performance Menu readers, feel pretty special. I'm spending my free time reading your forum posts and pumping my brain full of your questions and dilemmas while my Christmas lights sit in a big pile in my backyard and my washing machine makes so much noise that it sounds like there's a severed head in there. That's my level of commitment to you, brothers and sisters. Hopefully you'll appreciate this if I come home from work one day and find all my clothes sitting in my driveway. I'm taking one for the team, baby.

Anyway, back to the forums. Technique, technique, TECHNIQUE! That's what people want help with, no doubt about it. The vast majority of the Olympic weightlifting stuff I see on the internet these days is focused on either technique or programming. Now, it just so happens that I've got one mother of a programming project going on right now that I absolutely freaking guarantee you'll be able to use to make yourself a better lifter or coach, regardless of what level you're at. But it has to wait a month or so, which means you'll have to keep reading the Menu. However, the technique area is one that we can get to right now.

Which area of technique are we going to look at in this article? Finishing the pull in the snatch and clean. That's it. More specifically, we're going to do an analysis of a topic that's probably causing one of the most interesting technique discussions in our sport these days. The topic is, "Should the lifter extend up on the toes or stay flat-footed at the top of the pull?" This is a seriously confusing question for new and intermediate lifters who are in the process of building their own technique. Most athletes are smart enough to study the technique of the world's best lifters as they're trying to develop their own personal lifting form. The internet has made this a thousand times easier for modern lifters than it was for the older generations because of the wonderful blessing of YouTube. Anybody can get online these days and watch hours of World Championship footage where you can do slow-motion breakdowns of the technique of the best lifters on the planet. But this is where things can get puzzling, because not all world record holders use the same technique. Some of them extend high up on their toes at the top of their snatch/clean pull, and then others basically keep their feet almost completely flat on the floor all the way into the turnover phase. If you're a newbie, you have to ask yourself, "Which way is the right one?"

Yeah, good question. It's a really good question, as a matter of fact. What do you say we find an answer to it, so you can start grooving in your own permanent lifting technique and get one step closer to the day when you might be at a World Championship meet yourself, with other rookies watching YOUR technique on YouTube and trying to figure out how the heck you can pop those insane weights.

Explanation of styles

Obviously, we can't start talking about which technique style is better until we get a clear understanding of each one. First of all, let's make sure we're all clear that this article is specifically analyzing the phase of the lift where the athlete is extended into the top position of the snatch or clean pull. This is the moment where the upward pulling movement is hitting its completion and the lifter is on the verge of jumping down into the turnover phase. When this stage is reached, we can start to see some variations in movement between different lifters.

We'll refer to the first type of technique we're going to examine as "toe-extension pulling," for lack of a better phrase. With this technique, the lifter drives and extends up onto the toes at the top of the pull. If you were to do a frame-by-frame video analysis of this technique and then pause the video when the lifter is at the absolute highest extension moment, the body position would closely resemble an athlete who is jumping off the ground. This is why some coaches actually use the verbal cue "JUMP" when coaching weightlifters. This cue can teach the athlete to reach full vertical extension with the feet, knees, hips and torso, which will lead to higher elevation of the barbell. When athletes use toe-extension pulling, there will usually be a loud slapping sound as their feet hit the floor when they jump down into the bottom position. If you're having trouble telling whether or not the athlete is using toe-extension pulling, this sound is often a dead giveaway. If you hear that slap, it's probably toe-extension. From a biomechanical standpoint, the basic idea behind toe-extension pulling is that the athlete will be able to lift the barbell to its highest possible point by extending the body to its highest possible point. Maximum force is generated through creating the longest extension line from the floor to the top of the athlete's body, and that extension line is lengthened by driving up onto the toes. That's pretty much how it works.

Now, there is another style of pull finishing that you'll also see if you study world record holders long enough. Again, we'll invent our own name for this style just so we can read this article more easily. Let's call this second technique "flat-foot pulling." Understanding what this technique looks like isn't too complicated. It basically looks the way it sounds. Here, the athlete is finishing the pull with the body extended, but has not risen up onto the toes prior to turnover. Most of the athlete's foot stays on the floor throughout the entire pull. With flat-foot pullers, you will likely still see a little rise from the heels at the moment of full extension. But it's nothing like toe-extension pullers, and you won't hear the loud stomping sound from the feet when they hit the bottom position either. Biomechanically, the reasoning behind flat-foot pulling is that the athlete will be able to continue generating force into the floor if they keep the surface area of their foot in contact with it. If you keep your feet on the floor, you can drive the body upwards harder. Without getting into scientific jargon, that's about as simply as we can describe it.

The absolute perfect place to see the contrast between these two styles is the men's 77 kilo bodyweight class at present day 2011. Two of the best lifters in the world in this weight class are Tigran Martirosyan from Armenia and Xiaojun Lu from China. These two have been taking turns winning the World Championship for the last three years. Their ability levels are extremely close, but their lifting styles are quite different. Tigran is a toe-extension puller, and Lu is a flat-foot puller. If YouTube is convenient for you, check out the World Weightlifting Championships from either 2010 or 2011 in the men's 77 kilo class. These two athletes have personal records that are within just a few kilos of each other. Tigran's best snatch is 381 (173kg) pounds, while Lu's is 383 (174kg). (I know, holy buckets of lizard spit...)They are two of the finest lifters in history in their weight class, and they're an amazing contrast between the types of pulling form we're examining here.

More examples...

Knowing that world record weights have been lifted using both toe-extension and flat-foot pulling, one of the obvious questions that pops up is, "Which technique is most common at the highest levels?" We want to know which style gets the greatest results the highest percentage of the time, right? It seems like the safest bet for which technique to model our own lifting after would be the one that has the widest track record of success.

If you study weightlifting long enough, I think you will probably see more toe-extension pullers at the top of the sport. Sometimes, you will see lifters who are extreme toe-pullers, like Zlatan Vanev from Bulgaria. Vanev is a lifter's lifter, a wild animal who has won multiple world championships with the intensity and aggression of a Norse Berserker. And if you want to see the ultimate example of what we're talking about when we discuss toe-extension pulling, watch this guy. His explosiveness when he jumps his feet into the bottom position is simply phenomenal. It's faster and more violent than almost any other lifter you'll ever see, with the exception of Iran's Behdad Salimi. Salimi, who recently snatched a new world record of 214 kilos (471 pounds), basically defies physical laws of movement with the power and acceleration he generates into the barbell. He's a textbook definition of toe-extension pulling. He and Vanev are what I would call hardcore toe-extension pullers, but there are many other examples of great lifters who use this technique with a more moderate level of foot movement. Soviet legend Alexander Kurlovich and women's world record-holder Svetlana Podobedova are pretty good models of this, along with being two of my favorite lifters of all time.

In a nutshell, you'll usually see more toe-extension pulling when you look at the best in the world. However, let's not make the mistake of thinking that there aren't some great flat-foot pullers in the sport. We mentioned Xiaojun Lu as a flat-foot puller, and it's worth pointing out that many other Chinese lifters also pull this way. I'm sure it's being taught over there, because you just see it too commonly from their top world-level lifters to be a coincidence. But if we're talking about flat-foot pullers, then we can talk about his royal majesty, the supreme imperial grand poobah of Olympic weightlifting, Pyrros Dimas of Greece. Dimas, for those of you who have been living under a rock, is a weightlifting titan who won three Olympic gold medals and was one jerk away from winning four, and he's a flat-foot puller. His heels come off the ground just a little at the top of his pull, but he absolutely keeps most of his foot on the ground throughout most of the lift.

That brings us to you. You're a lifter or coach, probably somewhere around the beginner or intermediate level, and you want to know which technique to use. You want to be good at this, so which way do you go?

Go Where the Spirit Leads You…

First, I'll share my own personal preference as a lifter and a coach. I'm a firm believer in toe-extension pulling, always have been and always will be. I've always felt like the only way I can really put some serious pepper on my pull is by leaving the floor, driving up to the tallest point I can get to in the pull before jumping into the receiving position with a good loud smack when my feet hit the platform. I've never tried to lift any other way. And when I teach the Olympic lifts to others, I have them do it the same way. Now, there's a delicate balance you have to hit when you're teaching other lifters to extend onto the toes and then jump their feet into the receiving position. You don't want them to get excessive with it. I've worked with a few lifters who bring their feet too far off the floor during the turnover, almost to the point that it looks like a jump-tuck when they're pulling themselves under the bar. You don't want those feet too far in the air because that will cause a little delay-separation moment in the turnover where the athlete is basically floating in space. That's not good. In my experience, I think athletes will find their own comfortable feel for the movement as they practice it. If you tell them to jump at the top of their pull, they'll eventually develop a motor pattern that works for them. Some of them will have that dramatic extension/stomp-the-feet technique we see from Vanev, and some will have a more restrained version of the movement. Once you've built a concrete knowledge base of what good technique looks like, and you've got some experience as a coach, you'll know when it looks right and when it looks wrong.

That's how I do it, and I personally think most lifters will learn the movements more effectively if they use toe-extension pulling. Flat-foot pulling? I've never taught it to anybody and I don't know if I would want to try. There's no denying that it can produce world-class results. I would never say otherwise because there's plenty of evidence to prove it. From a coaching perspective, I would let an athlete use flat-foot pulling if that's what they naturally grew into. Good athletes figure out how to use their bodies in the best way. Poor athletes won't be able to figure anything out. If you coach some of those, then just teach them the best you can and try to get them as far along as possible. If I taught a lifter to extend up on the toes but then, as we continued to practice the lifts, the lifter just started to pull with a flat-foot position, I would let them do it if it looked right. How do you know when it "looks right?" As I said, that's where experience, research, and a brain full of technical expertise will answer the question. If you're a competent coach, you'll know when it looks right, just like you'll know when it "feels right" as an athlete. But in either case, you have to put in the hours of study and learning. You have to have a model of good technique that's second nature to you, and you get this through analysis of the best. You have YouTube nowadays, so you have no excuse for not getting the job done in this area.

There's no one right way. Sometimes I get annoyed when I listen to philosophers, politicians, or religious leaders because it basically seems like most of them are saying, "Only I am right, and everybody else is wrong." That just doesn't work for me, because I believe that there is usually more than one solution to a problem. It's a complex world. All you have to do is watch one world championship and it should be clear to you that there's more than one way to lift big weights. Your job is to find your own way, the one that's right for you.

OPTIMAL STRENGTH TRAINING FOR ENDURANCE
STEVE BAMEL

Before we get into anything else, strength training wise, the first question that needs to be answered is WHY? Why is strength training for endurance athletes important? Frankly speaking, it is important for two main reasons: injury prevention and performance enhancement.

If you are an endurance athlete, whether competitive or non-competitive, than you live the endurance athlete lifestyle. Your days, nights, work, family functions, etc. revolve around you getting your training in. And if it's that important to get your training in, why would you let an injury, a preventable injury at that, get in the way of what you love to do? Ankle sprains, muscle, tendon, and ligament damage could be greatly reduced, even eliminated with a good, solid, strength program.

The second reason to strength train is simpler than the first: good, old fashioned, performance enhancement. Your times will be faster and the hardest parts of races and training sessions will feel easier.

When designing any training program, strength or otherwise, the first place to start is the annual plan. Since endurance training is your priority, that plan must be set up first. Once that plan is in place, then, and only then, can you move onto the strength training portion. It is of utmost importance that both your endurance training plan and your strength training plan match up in regards to volume and intensity. Periods or high volumes and/ or intensities in running, swimming and biking must match up with periods of high volumes in the weight room. The same goes for periods of low volumes and or intensities.

Over the course of the year, you will modulate your volumes and intensities based on your competition schedule. As you start to decrease your endurance intensity and/ or volume, you will also cut back on the intensity and/ or volume in the weight room. If it is a time during the year that calls for increased intensity and/or volume of your endurance work, then you will increase the intensity and/ or volume in the weight room as well.

As you approach a competition, the same rules apply. You will start to reduce the volume in the weight room in conjunction with your training volumes, as you reduce the training intensities, your weight room intensities will decrease, and then 2 weeks before competition you will cut out the weight room completely, and then pick it back up once you resume your post-competition training.

The volumes and intensities need to match up perfectly, as do the most important weeks, the rest/ recovery/ restoration weeks. Without these two plans matching up, inevitably, you will wear down your body too much. And we all know what happens once you start to feel rundown. You start cutting out the weight training and preserving your energy for your runs, or swims, or bike rides. Then, because there is no weight training, you start to feel better, more energized, assume the weight training was killing you, and never go back in the weight room. You must understand that this happened not because you were in the weight room, but because your training plan was flawed from the start.

Once your annual plan (which includes weight training) has been laid out, it's time to figure out what to do in the weight room. The most important thing to keep in mind when in the weight room is that you are not chasing weight room numbers. You are chasing performance. On bike, on road, on trail, in water, performance. Because of this, your goal in the weight room is simple: Do not do any more than what will help you the most. Do not do one more rep, one more set, one more exercise than the bare minimum it will take to improve your times. As an endurance athlete, you need to be ultra-conscious of any added volume to your body. And not just in the weight room. Walking around an amusement park for 6 hours with your kids will take its toll on your performance as well. That's why the strength training you include must be enough to enhance performance without becoming a liability to your body.

We need to keep it simple when it comes to exercise selection. Our primary exercises will consist of multi-joint movements, or movements that work more than one joint at a time. These are the best exercises for building strength. They will be squats, deadlifts, and the overhead and bench press. Our auxiliary exercises will include unilateral (one at a time) leg movements, posterior chain (backside) exercises, and upper body pulling exercises.

Depending on how many days a week you want to go to the gym, and how much time you have, will determine which layout you choose.

2X PER WEEK	
DAY 1	DAY 2
BENCH PRESS	OVERHEAD PRESS
SQUAT	DEADLIFT
PHYSIOBALL LEG CURL	STEP UP

3X PER WEEK		
DAY 1	DAY 2	DAY 3
SQUAT	OVERHEAD PRESS	BENCH PRESS
PHYSIOBALL LEG CURL	DEADLIFT	CHIN UPS
STEP UPS		

4X PER WEEK			
DAY 1	DAY 2	DAY 3	DAY 4
SQUAT	BENCH	OVERHEAD PRESS	DEADLIFT
PHYSIOBALL LEG CURL `	CHIN-UPS	LAT PULLDOWN	STEP UP
STEP UPS			

The best part about setting up your workouts like this is that week-to-week, you can choose whatever option works best for you. If one week you can find 20 minutes 4 days a week than choose that option. If the next week you can only find 2 days but have 45 minutes, then you can choose that option.

Now let's talk some sets and reps. For your major movements (Squat, Bench Press, Overhead Press, and Deadlift), every day you are going to warm up with 3 sets of 5 reps that get both your mind and body prepared for the working sets. Then once you've performed those warm up sets, you will perform either 3 sets of 5 reps (3x5), 3x4, 3x3, 3x2, or 3x1 of that movement, depending on what your training intensity for that week is. For the accessory movements (every exercise that is not Squat, Bench Press, Overhead Press, or Deadlift), you will perform either 5x10, 4x10, 3x10, 2x10, or 1x10, depending on what your training volume for that week is. You will change the sets as reps each week to correspond with your training volumes and intensities for that week. Progression will happen the next time that same set and rep scheme comes up. If 5 weeks ago you did 3x5 on the squat and today you have 3x5 again, look to see what you did last time and beat it by 5 lbs. The same goes for your accessory movements. If 3 weeks ago you did 3x10 on the lat pulldown, and again today you have 3x10, beat it by 5 lbs. I recommend starting off very light on every exercise and increasing by the smallest possible increments. For barbell work, that will typically mean increasing in 5 lb increments as 2.5 lb plates are usually the smallest you can find in a gym. For dumbbell movements, you will have to increase by either 2.5 or 5 lb increments, depending on what's available to you.

Now I know what your next question is going to be: "What do I do when I can't add any more weight?" First and foremost, this will not happen for a while--so stop looking for an out!! You will be starting light and increasing by the smallest possible increments. But, yes, at some point it will be hard to continue to add weight to the bar. And even though you are a good 2-5 years from that point, I will let you in on a secret. Once you hit that point, chances are you have achieved all the strength that you will need to reap the benefits of strength training for endurance. No other strength coach on the planet will tell you this, but I'm going to: There is an optimal level of strength for your given sport. What that level is depends on the individual and you will have to find that sweet spot for yourself. To get stronger would be to sacrifice one of the other elements that it takes to be successful in your given sport. Sure, you could keep getting stronger by adding body weight, but that extra weight is not going to feel too good when you're running or biking up a steep hill. At that point in your career, there are still going to be things you have to focus on to get better. Continue strength training with those weights that you are at and move onto the next aspect of your game that needs improving.

Consistency is the key to everything and where most endurance athletes fail when it comes to weight training. The problems arise from constantly adding and then removing weight training from your program. The fact the body never gets used to weight training is the killer. It would be like moving into an apartment on the 20 floor. For the first month you live there, you take the stairs every day. After a month it starts to become easier, and every subsequent month taking those stairs gets easier and easier to the point where you will actually go back upstairs to get whatever you forgot. Now let's just say after that initial first month of living there you decide to start taking the elevator. A month passes of you taking the elevator and then you decide to start taking the stairs again. When you go back to taking the stairs, it's going to be like you've never taken them before, even though when you first moved in you took them every day. Weight training is like those stairs. Stick with it, don't stop, let your body get used to the stress, and after a short time it'll start to feel normal. That's when you will start to reap those benefits.

Remember that strength is not only important, it is necessary component of any complete training program. Overlooking it could lead to injury and poor performance. Including it, in a simple to follow plan, will yield amazing results. Train hard, be consistent, and have fun.

GPP FOR THE COMPETITIVE ATHLETE: THE LOST TRAINING PHASE
STEVE BAMEL

If you have ever trained, worked with or been around competitive athletes, you know one thing about them. When it's game time, they bring it. Full speed ahead, non-stop, balls to the wall, go go go. Because of this mentality, when athletes and coaches set up training programs, they often do it the same way, full steam ahead starting at their first training session. However, it takes a carefully constructed plan to prepare their bodies for the upcoming off-season and in-season workouts, as well as practices and the competitive season. This time period is often referred to as the General Physical Preparedness Period or GPP.

Typically, following the competitive season of any sport an athlete will take a few weeks off, and depending on post-season play, maybe more than that. This post-competition period is commonly referred to as the Active Rest period. During this time, an athlete is encouraged to do anything active that is not related to their sport, or the weight room, in any way. We don't want them to sit on the couch for a month, but we also need to give their bodies a rest. You will commonly hear about athletes playing golf, scuba diving, surfing or going on trail hikes during this time. Nothing too strenuous, but enough to keep the blood pumping so they hold onto some level of fitness.

And that's why it's important to remember that athletes suffer short-term memory loss. Coming out of the Active Rest period, all they remember is what they used to be able to do. I could squat 500 lbs, I could snatch 100 kilos, my vertical jump is 40 inches, etc, etc. Yes that's what you could, but what you can do today, after a full competitive season and a few weeks of Active Rest, are none of those things. We need to build them back up. The purpose of the GPP period is to get the athletes body prepared to get back to competition level fitness. Because if it were up to them, they would start off right where they left off, balls to the wall training, and once their competitive season rolls around, all we would have is a broken down athlete. So following this Active Rest Period comes the GPP period. Make no mistake about it; this may be the most important training cycle of the year. If you want to be able to excel in off-season workouts and pre-season practices, as well as staying injury free, then including a GPP phase into your training is a must.

GPP will reacquaint the athletes with body weight movements, weight room exercises, as well as improve their work capacity and mental focus with a reality check of what their bodies really can do, not what they think it can do. The workouts will always begin with an extended dynamic warm up. Here's a typical warm up I use for our GPP sessions:

Dynamic Warm Up

2 minutes Jump Rope
Body Weight Squats x10
Body Weight Good Mornings x10
Forward Lunges x10 Lateral Lunges x10 (5 each way)
Walking High Knee Pulls x10 (5 each way)
Walking But kicks with a Grab x10 (5 each way)
Glute Bridges x 10
Supine Leg Kicks x 10 (5 each way)
Seated Side leg Swings x10 (5each way)
Iron Crosses x10 (5 each way)
Fire Hydrants x 10 (5 each way)
Push Ups x 10
Groiners x 10 (5 each way)
Chain Breakers x10
Shoulder Circles x 10 (5 forward, 5 backward)
Jog 20 yards
Backpedal 20 Yards
Lateral Shuffle x 20 yards
Light skip x 20 yards
Power Skip x 20 yards

As each session has a dynamic warm up, immediately following that, each session will also have time dedicated to improving, re-acquainting, and re-mastering all the important exercises that will make up the core of your off season workouts. In general, those exercises are the Olympic lifts as well as the back squat, deadlift, military press, and bench press. It is important to keep in mind that the exercise selections should mimic the exercises that you plan on incorporating in the off-season and in-season workouts. For me, these are entirely sport dependent.

After the technique work is finished, the daily workouts will begin. I typically will have my athletes do 3 GPP sessions per week. Each session will be a total body workout. For the first 2 weeks of GPP, our total body workouts will be limited to body weight exercises. No external loading. Full ranges of motion. We will perform these exercises circuit style in big or small groups. Here are 2 examples of these workouts:

Workout 1

Workout notes: For workout 1, you will perform one set of each exercise in each group and then repeat that group for the given number of sets. After all sets of the group are completed, you will then move onto the next group and perform the exercises in the same manner.

Circuit 1

> 1A Chin Ups 3x8
> 1B Step Ups 3x8
> 1C Mountain Climbers 3x15 each leg

Circuit 2

> 2A Push Ups 3x15
> 2B Lunges 3x 12 each leg
> 2C Burpees 3x12

Circuit 3

> 3A Dips 3x8
> 3B Hip Extensions 3x15
> 3C Double Unders 3x10

Workout 2

For workout 2, you will perform 1 set of each exercise and then immediately start back at the first exercise with no rest. You will continue in this manner for the given number of sets.

Big Circuit (3x through)

1. Bodyweight Squats x20
2. Diamond Push Ups x10

3. Pull Ups x 8
4. Crunches x20
5. Russian Twist x 20 each side
6. Step Ups x 20 (10 each leg)
7. Lunges x20 (10 each leg)
8. Moving Back Plank x20
9. Moving Side Plank x40 (20 each side)

After 2 weeks of bodyweight exercises, we will then begin to externally load the athletes as well as introduce low-level plyometrics. For weeks 3 and 4, each week will have 1 barbell, 1 dumbbell, and 1 bodyweight workout. The barbell and dumbbell workouts will be Javorek style complexes. (A complex is a group of exercises performed one right after another with no rest between exercises, but a set rest time between each giant set. The rest period we use is 60-120 seconds, depending on the athlete and sport.) There will be little to no weight on the bar, with the emphasis being placed on technique as well as speed through the complex. I know that sounds a bit like I want to have my cake and eat it too, but the reality is that you can move through the complexes fast, with good technique if your technique work during the sessions has been going well. Here is what a full week of workouts would look like during week 3 or week 4:

Workout 1- Barbell Complex x 5 sets, 6 reps each

> RDL
> Bent Over Row
> Hang Clean
> Front Squat
> Push Press

Workout 2- Dumbbell Complex (light) x 5 sets, 6 reps each

> Lunge
> Squat Push Press
> Lateral Lunge
> High Pull
> Upright Row

Workout 3- Bodyweight Complex x 5 sets, 6 reps each

    Pull Ups
    Dips
    Glute Ham
    Chin Ups
    Push Ups

Following week 4 it's now time for our final phase of GPP. During weeks 5 and 6 both the dynamic warm-up as well as the technique work will stay the same. However we will now move towards more traditional, I hate to use this term but I will, bodybuilding/ hypertrophy workouts. I know what you're thinking, bodybuilding workouts for an athlete? Relax; it's only 2 weeks and it's the best way to begin to introduce volume and load to the body. It's not enough time to see any change in mass of the athlete. These workouts will begin to introduce a lot of the accessory movements you will use in your off-season and in-season programs. Pull ups, chin ups, dips, unilateral lower body movements, glute ham raises, they will all be in there and they will follow the more traditional 3-4 sets of 8-12 reps scheme. Rest times will be 60-90 second between exercises and you will finish all the sets of the exercise before moving onto the next exercise. Here are 2 examples of workouts we will perform during weeks 5 and 6:

Workout 1

    DB Bench Press 3x10
    Bent Over Barbell Row 3x10
    DB Bulgarian Squat 3x10 each leg
    Glute Ham Raise 5x5
    DB Military Press 3x10
    Optional Gun Show Work

Workout 2

    Chin Ups 3x10 (or 30 total reps over the course of the
    Workout if the athlete cannot perform 10 in a row)
    DB Inc Bench Press 3x10
    Inverted Row 3x10 (or 30 total reps over the course of the workout if the athlete
    cannot perform 10 in a row)
    DB Walking Lunge 3x10 each leg

DB Shoulder Series (Front, Lateral, and Rear Delt Raise) 3x10 each exercise, circuit style
Optional Gun Show Work

The key to a successful GPP phase is remember that when you are training athletes you are training for specific goals and specific time periods as well as training to enhance specific qualities that will improve their performance in their given sport. That is why we move on from the GPP period with athletes, because it's GENERAL preparation. As we get closer to the competitive season, we need to specifically prepare the body for certain things that the athlete will do or encounter in their sport.

Just a quick note: If you are not training athletes, you can manipulate the sets and reps and the load and these GPP workouts can work for anyone looking to improve general fitness.

GET YOUR GUMP ON:
HAZARDS OF INTELLIGENCE IN ATHLETES
MATT FOREMAN

Okay, listen…the subject of this article has the potential to offend some people. And as I've gotten older, I've been working harder on not saying offensive things. When I was twenty, I thought it was funny to make belligerent comments and shock people. Unfortunately, that's probably part of being a young meathead guy with an underdeveloped brain. Now, being a wiser mature man with a really sensational personality, I try not to piss people off with unnecessary remarks that could be considered vulgar or cruel.

But for the subject I want to examine this month, there aren't many ways to dance around the issue. Let's get to the point and you'll understand my concern. This article is going to be about the difference between coaching intelligent athletes and unintelligent athletes. See what I mean? We're going to try to take a serious look at how coaching skills have to be applied to smart athletes versus dumb ones. Like I was saying, there are all kinds of possibilities for insults and inappropriate words. I mean seriously, how can we do a productive training analysis when we're basically labeling some of the people we work with as dumbasses? Well, the first thing we're going to do is avoid insulting names like the one I just used. I know many of us probably use words like "idiot" and "retard" on a regular basis. You say no, you don't do that? How about when you're alone in your car and bad drivers are all around you? Yeah, I rest my case. Most of us do it, but we probably don't make a habit of peppering our conversations with comments about how moronic and stupid other people are. It's a social turnoff, so we try to be polite and non-judgmental when we're talking about those special souls who don't exactly have brains leaking out of their ears.

Seriously, I think we can have a frank discussion of how intelligence plays into the training of an athlete. Let's quit tip-toeing around something that's pretty obvious and just take a blunt look at it. Many of you are coaches, apparently. If you've been doing this for a while, then you have to agree that you'll have a wide range of talents, both mental and physical, who join your program at different times. I've coached a few people in my career who were borderline geniuses, with the qualifications and stats to back up that title. And yes, I definitely have to also acknowledge that I've coached people who were on the far opposite end of the intelligence spectrum. Because we all know that coaching has an awful lot to do with how you merge your personality with others, it's fair to say that there are going to be differences in how you interact with these polar opposites. So, how can you pull this off? How can you successfully coach people with lower intellectual capability without making them think you're being condescending or mean? Likewise, how can you successfully coach people with higher intellectual capability who might be five steps ahead of you mentally, even though you're the coach and the authority figure?

Lots to think about, that's for sure. We should definitely start by not underestimating anybody, regardless of how light we think their brainpans are. As Alan from The Hangover reminded us, "Rain Man practically bankrupted a casino, and he was a......" See? I'm not going to say it. Aren't you impressed with how sweet I am?

A Quick Word About Stereotypes

I'm not sure where it started, but there's this old stereotype that jocks (power athletes in particular) are unintelligent. You've come across this, right? It seems like even back when I was a kid, the football players and weightlifters you saw in movies were always portrayed as Neanderthal dolts who weren't smart enough to do anything besides eat red meat, beat people up and make weird grunting noises that sounded like a rhino having sex. I think a lot of it might come from the old days when high school athletes didn't have to pass their classes to participate in sports. Or maybe it's just the common belief that athletes spend all their time working out and practicing instead of reading books or studying. Whatever the origin, a lot of people still think you have limited mental capacity if you look strong or muscular.

Back when I was in college, I can remember professors who openly tried to talk down to me and throw snippy little insults my way before they even knew anything about me. I looked like a weightlifter/football player, so they tried to hold this intellectual arrogance over me. There was one time when I had won the collegiate national championship and the campus newspaper ran a little story about it. One of my instructors approached me a few days afterwards and asked, "Hey, you're that weightlifter, right?" I said, "Yeah." He chuckled and asked, "What are you gonna do when you turn forty and all those muscles turn into fat?" This was a college professor asking me about something that's biologically impossible, and trying to have a little laugh at my expense. I knew he was responsible for my grade and I didn't want to make him mad, so I just said, "When that happens, I'm just gonna kill myself." He didn't talk to me the rest of the semester, which was what I wanted.

I've never thought I was a genius, but I also know I'm not an idiot. Many of you might fall into the same bracket I'm describing. You're sharp enough to qualify as a bright human being, even if you're not Aristotle. So let's look at some benefits and hazards to working with athletes who fall above the average mark on the intelligence scale.

Brainy Benefits

There are some pretty obvious benefits to working with intelligent athletes. One of the easiest ones to look at is memory. Smart people generally have pretty good memories. Maybe not photographic or anything, but they can definitely remember the important things you tell them. Here's a little training example of what I'm talking about. Let's say you're teaching somebody how to snatch a barbell for the first time. Before you can really start getting into the teaching of proper pulling mechanics, turnover, etc., there are a few little basic things the athlete has to remember on each rep. We're talking about how to set up, grip the bar, position the feet, and flatten the back. Every time the athletes go to perform a snatch, they need to have their feet set at a proper width that you've shown them, and they need to have their hands evenly gripped on the bar at a width that you've determined for them. You probably even gave them landmarks on the bar for where they're supposed to put their hands.

Have you ever worked with an athlete where you had to remind them every… single…time… to put their feet in the right place and grip the bar in the correct spot? Rep after rep after rep, they just don't catch on. You've patiently told them where to put their feet and hands, but they just keep forgetting. It gets to a point where you're having a really hard time teaching them anything about extending the body, jumping and shrugging, keeping the bar close, etc. because you have to constantly stop and remind them about their feet and their hands. I taught a young lady to do power cleans a few weeks ago where I literally had to repeat, "Point your toes straight, wrap your thumbs around the bar, straighten your elbows, and close your mouth" every single time she attempted a lift. The last command on that list was needed because she kept opening her mouth as wide as possible before each lift, and it was bugging the living crap out of me.

Some athletes are different (and much easier) to work with. After you've told them once or twice about getting their hands and feet set properly before each lift, they've got it. They remember what you taught them, and they do it right every time. This makes it a lot easier because then you can move on to teaching them more. To state it all very simply, intelligent athletes can memorize technique much easier. Because they have strong memory skills, they're able to process your instructions and execute them consistently. They also recognize little coaching cues better. If you say "tight" or "extend" to them, they'll understand what you're trying to get them to do. There's nothing worse than working with somebody who looks at you questioningly when they're in the middle of performing a lift. These are the ones that just cleaned a bar and they're getting ready to jerk it. You yell out, "Dip and drive!" to them and they look over at you (with a heavy bar sitting on their shoulders) and say, "Huh?" Ouch…

Now, there's an interesting point to mention here. Some of us have worked with people who are highly intelligent in some kind of intellectual field, but they've got absolutely no athletic intelligence at all. This is the PhD in biochemistry guy who decided he wanted to learn weightlifting, but you tried to coach him and he was as physically clueless as the ones we just mentioned. Conversely, there is no denying that there are some mental midgets running around out there with flawless technique and huge lifts. What the heck? How does this get explained? This is where we see that there are different types of intelligence. Gardner's theory of seven different types of intelligence tells us that human beings are usually more gifted in some areas than others. Some people have highly developed linguistic intelligence, and others are strong in mathematical intelligence. There are other types such as interpersonal, musical, and bodily-kinesthetic. People who have high levels of kinesthetic intelligence simply have a knack for knowing how to use their bodies. They can see somebody perform an athletic skill and then simply make themselves mimic that movement with very little coaching.

Whatever the particular composition of an athlete's brain might be, it's obvious that there are some big benefits if they're smart. Intelligent athletes will often know how to listen to their bodies a little better, which can lead to avoiding injuries. When they're sore or fatigued, they know it's just something they have to work through. When they're legitimately injured, they know they have to see a doctor and get it looked at. Lower-intelligence athletes can have a higher risk of handling this difference the wrong way. I once knew an athlete who injured his elbow on a second snatch attempt, lied to his coach and said he was okay, and then went out there to attempt a bigger weight on the third attempt. Result? Dislocated elbow; career-ending injury. Using some common sense would have kept this athlete safe, but it just didn't work out.

Big Brain, Potential Obstacle

Okay, let's just go ahead and admit it. There's also such a thing as being too smart for your own good, don't you think? There are some potential hazards that can go along with being an intelligent athlete, and overanalyzing is probably the biggest one. Aaahhh, I'll bet I'm hitting close to home for some of you. These are the people who practically paralyze themselves because they're just thinking way too hard. You give them some simple instructions, and then they dissect those instructions like a science lab frog. Please forgive me for sounding sexist here, but I think women battle this more than men do. Most of the gals I've known in my life have told me that females tend to over-think things, making their lives a lot harder than they need to be. Guys, on the other hand, don't seem to do this as much. I've said for years that men are a lot simpler than women think we are. We really only think about three or four things, and our women agonize over stuff that never even occurs to us. But I digress...

Intelligent athletes, both men and women, can suffer from the same mental overheating. Here's another way of looking at it. Let's say you've got a smart athlete who is getting ready to attempt a heavy snatch in competition. The lifter stands on the platform, staring at the barbell and trying to concentrate on technique, and thoughts keep popping into his head about how many times he missed this same weight in training leading up to this meet. His acute memory is working against him in this case, because he recalls multiple missed attempts with this weight and now he's starting to doubt himself. He walks up to the bar, and he's trying to ignore thoughts like "damn, I haven't made this weight in three weeks!" instead of focusing on his technique like he's supposed to.

Athletes with lower intelligence levels can actually have an easier time in this situation. They stand there on the platform looking at the bar, and the only thing that goes through their minds is, "I'm gonna snatch the hell out of this thing, and then I'm gonna go have a burrito." The fact that they missed this same weight nine times in training doesn't even enter into the picture. Many years ago, there was an elite American athlete who most people considered pretty low on the brain scale. I remember being at a meet once and watching this guy getting ready to attempt an American record. My coach leaned over to me and said, "The best thing about this guy is that he doesn't know he's not supposed to be able to do the things he's doing." Stop and think about that sentence for a minute. It made a lot of sense to me, then and now. This guy had a short memory, so he didn't remember prior failures. That kept him confident. He also had no fear of anything, which is one hell of a quality to have as a weightlifter. So…we've now got a situation where the qualities of lesser-intelligence athletes, like fearlessness and no comprehension of limits, are some of the best weapons you can have in your battle for maximum lifts. What's going on here? I thought this was going to be about how smart people are always at an advantage?

The Answer to the Riddle…

Listen, being smart is better than being stupid. I don't think I'm wrong about that. However, being smart doesn't always guarantee you an easier ride in weightlifting, or anything else for that matter. Your big intellect can get in your way sometimes. People with superior intelligence have ideas and thoughts hitting their brains so fast that they sometimes can't keep their minds clear and organized. We've all known at least one genius-type person in our lives who was socially inept, right? These are the people who can analyze calculus on a Good Will Hunting level, but they couldn't get a date if their lives depended on it. Remember those kids in high school who didn't fit in with the crowd at all, despite the fact that they had special mental gifts? Were you one of them yourself? These people usually hit their life peak a lot later than high school. And I'm pretty sure that's a good thing.

Which ones are easier to coach, smart athletes or dumb athletes? As with a lot of the things we examine in The Performance Menu, there isn't a clear-cut answer. Being intelligent doesn't mean that the individual is going to have the mental qualities to be a good weightlifter, and being unintelligent absolutely doesn't doom an athlete to failure. That kid who appears to have some serious cranial deficiencies? He might also have some amazing characteristics that will give him a big advantage in this sport. You can never really tell for sure. All you can do is give every interested newcomer the same treatment. You should always have the same positive attitude towards everybody, even if the person happens to be a freaking moron.

THE PULL FROM THE FLOOR: A BAD TIME TO SUCK
MATT FOREMAN

We've got pressing business this month, brothers and sisters. There are urgent matters at stake regarding your lifting technique, and this article is going to give you some important little thoughts that will keep your snatches and cleans from descending into a world of suckness. In the coming months, we'll get back to some juicy writing about motivation, coaching, and all the other tips-for-how-to-fix-your-whole-life stuff that we love so much. There's plenty of that on the horizon, but this month is focused on technique because we need to get some things straight NOW.

Some of you read the blog posts I put on the Catalyst Athletics website. A few weeks ago, I wrote some things about foot positioning in the bottom position of the snatch and clean because I had just attended a meet in California and I saw plenty of athletes who needed some help in this department. Well, this article is coming from that same direction. It's been a good month, because I've been fortunate enough to see a lot of weightlifting. I went to another local meet last night, and the webcast of the National Collegiate Championships has been playing all weekend. This is fun to watch because it's good to see the technique of lifters who aren't the best in the world. I know that sounds funny, but it's true. We all like to watch World Championship footage because we want to analyze perfect technique, but I think there are huge benefits to watching people who are still in the intermediate stages because you learn how to spot mistakes. Beginners and developing lifters do some things wrong, technically. This isn't insulting or disrespectful because we all know it's just part of the learning process. Every lifter has gone through a "still making mistakes" phase, including me. And these things have to get cleared up one way or another. Hopefully, the next few pages are going to serve that purpose for some of you.

The first pull from the floor, when the bar is lifted from the platform to the knees, is our focus area for this analysis. This short range of movement, when the bar travels up the length of the shins and arrives at the patella, is specifically what we're going to take a look at. This is when the lift begins, and it's tremendously important because there is very little chance of executing a lift correctly if the athlete makes a mistake in this first phase. There are some different schools of thought about how the lifter is supposed to combine speed and balance when the bar is being taken from the floor to the knees. Different coaches have varying beliefs about the proper way to do this. As I always say, I'm just going to share some ideas and thoughts about how I think it should be done. Is there going to be somebody out there in weightlifting land who does things differently than I say, and yet still manages to set records and hit huge lifts? Probably. Is there a right way and a wrong way to pull the bar from the floor, regardless of any minor technique differences you might see from various lifters? Certainly. The two areas we're going to concentrate on are A) bar speed and B) bodyweight distribution on the foot. I really want to drive home the point that this is crucial stuff. You can't fix a lift that starts out broken, just like you can't make a good pot of spaghetti if the first thing you do is screw up the sauce. Making errors in the first phase of a snatch or clean puts the athlete in a position where complete technical precision is basically impossible. And regardless of what you've been told by some guy at your gym who says that it's okay to do the Olympic lifts with crappy form, you have to make complete precision your goal if you're serious about getting good at this. Read on, and take from these words what you will.

Greasy Fast SPEED…

First of all, most of you probably understand the basic idea of speed in the Olympic lifts. The overall concept is that the first pull from the floor will be a slower movement, and then the athlete will accelerate after the bar passes the knees. This is something you can figure out just by watching weightlifting for a little while, at almost any level. Get on YouTube and type in Olympic Weightlifting, and you'll see it. The bar moves relatively slowly from the floor, and then it picks up speed as it starts to reach the level of the thighs. We all know this. But there's a tricky little fine line we need to take a look at when we're examining this part of the lifter's technique.

What I'm talking about is when lifters make the mistake of deliberately pulling the bar too slowly in this first phase. When I see lifters in local meets, and also some developing lifters at the national level, it sometimes looks like they're intentionally moving the bar really, really slowly from the floor to the knees, much slower than they should be. I think what's happening here is these lifters have been taught that the first pull is supposed to be slow and controlled, or maybe they've just learned this fact on their own if they don't have coaches. The mistake is that they're taking this notion too far. They're overdoing it, and the whole lift becomes inefficient as a result.

Here's the rule I learned as a lifter, and it's what I still believe now; the athlete should pull the bar from the floor as fast as possible while still maintaining proper position and balance. The only time a lifter should consciously think about slowing down the first part of the lift is if he/she is using speed to a degree that it causes a breakdown in form. In simpler terms, we can look at it like this. If the athlete is ripping the bar from the floor so fast that the back loses its tightness and starts to round over in a "turtleback" position, then there might be a reason to slow down the first phase. This happens with beginners sometimes. The athletes want to move quickly, but they can't maintain a good flat back posture because of a lack of strength. If this is a problem, then I think it's appropriate to have the lifters slow down at the beginning of the pull and focus completely on arching the back and staying tight. Regardless of anything, proper positioning of the back can't be compromised. The whole lift is a dead duck if this happens.

Another common problem that can occur when beginners pull too fast from the floor is falling forward. Because the lifters aren't strong enough to pull quickly, they start to shift forward onto the toes prematurely when they attempt to really rip the hell out of it. Basically, their butt is coming straight up while the shoulders are still low, which causes everything to tip over. The weight of the bar is winning the battle.

When a coach sees either of these problems, the athlete should be taught to correct them. I'm not a big fan of ever using the phrase "slow down" with a lifter. I would rather tell the lifter to focus more on staying tight, and let them continue to pull with good speed. In rare situations where the lifter is just trying so hard to haul ass that he/she can't maintain any kind of control, then saying "slow down off the floor" might be appropriate. Turtle-backing or falling forward are justifications for a slower first pull because the lifter is losing the fundamental positions that are required for a proficient lift.

Okay, we've got that concept nailed down. But we have to remember that what we're still trying to do is get the bar moving as fast as possible, as early as possible. As the athletes develop consistent motor patterns and gain strength, they'll be able to keep their posture tight. This is when speed needs to increase. If you want to study the point I'm making, the best place to look is the Bulgarian lifters of the 1980s. For those of you who don't know a lot of lifting history, the Bulgarians of the eighties lifted some of the biggest weights ever seen. Alexander Varbanov clean and jerked 215.5 in the 75 kilo class (that's 474 at 165 for you pound people). Asen Zlatev clean and jerked 225 at 82.5 (496 at 181). To this day, nobody has beaten those lifts. These guys were weightlifting machines like our galaxy has never seen.

But their technique is what I'm talking about. The Bulgarian lifters were famous for ripping the bar from the floor with speed that defied any accepted principles of gravity. It was freaky to watch them lift. Most of these guys would approach the bar, reach down and grab it with their hands, and then sit down on their haunches in a full squat for ten or fifteen seconds, getting ready to start the lift. Then, they would simply explode with pulling force as they tore the bar from the floor. Some of them would begin their pull so explosively that you could see the hair on their heads jump, and almost all of them screamed like banshees as those plates left the platform. They weren't starting with a slow pull and building up speed. They were mashing the gas pedal to the floor from a dead stop. However, because of the immense strength they possessed, their positions weren't compromised. Their backs stayed flat as boards and their balance never wavered.

This is what we're trying to do in weightlifting, my friends. It's the ultimate goal. Rookie lifters and coaches often make a very human, understandable mistake by teaching a first pull that's much slower than it needs to be. If the lifters are getting totally spasticated because the speed of their first pull is too much and they're not ready to go that fast, then explain to them that they need to modify what they're doing to keep their positions correct. But don't go crazy with this concept, because you could easily wind up with lifters who are just too freaking slow, plain and simple. I'm seeing a lot of this these days.

Heels? Toes? What the ****?

I'm going to be very direct and blunt in this section. First, let's just ask the question. "Should the lifters have their bodyweight on their heels or their toes as the bar is pulled from the floor?"

My personal answer is "neither." I think the lifter should try to feel their weight in the middle of their foot as the bar is pulled from the floor. Once again, you'll hear some conflicting views on this if you interview different coaches. I've read articles that say the lifter should immediately shift the weight to their heels as soon as the bar is pulled from the floor, and others who have argued for the toes. The heel argument is probably more common. One of the main reasons why there's disagreement on this point is that some world class lifters use different styles.

Going back to Bulgaria, they've had some world champions who used a pulling style that looks like a rocking chair if you watch their feet. As they pull the bar from the floor, the foot is flat on the platform. Then, as the bar is passing the knees, their toes rise slightly (obviously indicating that they've shifted their weight to the heels). Continuing, as the bar meets the hips and they extend into the top of their pull, their heels rise off the platform and they extend up on the toes in a jumping motion. So there's kind of a "flat foot-heels-toes" progression from the beginning to the end of the pull. They rock backwards, and then they rock forwards (albeit slightly). You don't see this from many lifters, but Ivan Chakarov did it this way.

On the other hand, some rare lifters appear to have their weight on the toes right from the beginning. I was in the warm-up room at a national championship several years ago when Oscar Chaplin was lifting. Oscar was a Junior World Champion and American record holder who snatched 166 kilos in the 85 kilo class, so he definitely qualifies as a world-class lifter. I was sitting in a chair directly behind the platform he was warming up on, probably three or four feet away from him, and I saw his heels separate slightly from the platform right at the beginning of his pull. This guy could snatch 365 pounds at 187 bodyweight, and his weight was obviously more towards the front of his foot when he started his pull from the floor. Different style than Chakarov, and he was still snatching amazing weights.

These are somewhat rare examples of different technique styles. You don't see tons of lifters who use either one. What you see most often are lifters who keep their feet flat on the floor until the bar reaches the level of the hips, and then they extend up on the toes. We covered this in an article I did a few months ago about the difference between flat-foot and toe-extension pulling. So, when the lifters have their feet flat on the floor, is their bodyweight shifted to the heels or the toes at the beginning of the pull? You basically need to ask the individual lifter, because you might get some different replies. As a guy who has snatched 341 pounds, I can tell you that I never thought about putting my weight on my heels. I tried to feel my weight on the middle of my foot when I pulled from the floor, and then I extended onto the toes and jumped at the finish. That's just one opinion from one lifter. I personally have no idea how anybody could do a snatch or clean effectively by shifting their weight to their heels and keeping it there throughout the pull. I can't jump forcefully without driving up onto my toes. Maybe you can, I don't know. If you can pull from your heels and snatch more than me, good for you. I'll buy you a can of Pringles.

At the end of the day...

Hopefully, you've learned enough to know that there's more than one way to lift big weights. Different lifters have individual nuances in their technique. This is pretty clear. But still, there are certain principles that hold true for everybody, and speed is one of the main ones. I don't know who said it, but I read somewhere at the beginning of my career that "a fast lifter with bad technique is better than a slow lifter with good technique." I believe this is true. Now, obviously a fast lifter with good technique is what we're all trying to grow into. That's easy enough to grasp. However, the quote I just gave you is an illustration of the fact that this is a speed sport, plain and simple. I hope all of you have the privilege of going to a national or world championship someday and watching the lifters in the warm-up room or training hall. I'm telling you guys...you just won't believe how freaking fast most of the top lifters are. You can see it on video, but it's a whole other world when you get to witness it in person.

You'll know what I mean when you see the best. It's not that their pull from the floor is slow and then their finish is fast. It's more like their pull from the floor is fast and then their finish is super turbo fast. Whether they have their bodyweight on their heels or whatever when they pull from the floor will be dependent on their anatomical structure, leg length, and personal feel for the movement. Will you be ready to use this kind of speed when you're a rookie? No, you won't. Speed is just like strength; it takes a long time to really develop. However, we always have to remember that we can't be good weightlifters by moving slowly. So let's just keep that thought in our minds as a cautionary note when we're working with newbies. We don't want them slow and properly positioned. We want them fast and properly positioned. At least, that's what I think.

OLYMPIC WEIGHTLIFTING: THE POWER POSITION
DANIEL CAMARGO

For those who have attended any of my seminars or who have trained with me, the term "power position" will be all too familiar. It is engrained in your mind and body by the end of the day's session through executing repetition after repetition. The power position is arguably the single most important aspect of the snatch or the c+j. Unfortunately, in the years I've spent training and now coaching the movements, it seems this portion of the movement is widely ignored by athletes and coaches, especially in the CrossFit arena. The astonishing difference experienced by the athlete once the power position has been either taught or reinforced is like the difference between night and day. It alone can fix many pre-existing errors such as an early arm-pull or the feeling of losing the weight forward. Though tough to describe in writing and illustrations, it is the goal of this article to define the power position, describe why it's important, what occurs if it is not practiced, and how to apply it to your technique.

Defined

The power position, once referred to as the "scoop" or "scooping," is the point during the snatch or clean where the lifter's torso is erect with knees slightly bent, flat footed, and the bar is in contact with the top of the thighs. Have you seen an elite lifter appear to "smack" the bar off their thighs and it appears to just catapult overhead or to the shoulders? Well, they are, except the contact isn't the primary goal of the movement, which is why beginners should never try to directly mimic this precise act as it could cause errors in other portions of the lift. The reason the "smacking" looks the way it does is because the lifter is practicing the use of the power position where the bar will make contact with the lifter. After learning the power position correctly, hopefully from day one, the lifter will develop the ability to hit the power position each time, maximizing his or her ability to generate the great explosion required to execute a maximal effort lift. The "smacking" is a secondary cause.

Why It's Important

The power position is so important because:

1. It allows the athlete to maintain the bar close to the body, which gives the athlete control of the center of gravity, thus optimizing the force applied to the bar.

2. It allows the lifter to be in the best position to jump or complete a triple joint extension, a term most are familiar with, for the second pull, and

3. It properly prepares the lifter to land in the best receiving position that follows, be it the overhead squat for the snatch or the front squat for the clean.

During the start position, you should have been taught to begin with the barbell against the shins. Failure to do so causes the bar to roll out in front of the lifter, and we all know how extremely difficult that makes it on the part of the athlete to successfully lift the weight. It is kind of like carrying your groceries out in front of you with locked arms rather than carrying them against your chest; a waste of energy and completely inefficient. Of course, the goal is not for the lifter to have bruises, scrapes or wounds on their shins from dragging the barbell against their leg as they lift off the ground, but while learning to control the barbell, you may find your shins a nice shade of black and blue! The closer the barbell is to the body the more control the athlete has maximizing the force applied during the lift.

Therefore, wouldn't it make sense for the barbell to travel just as close to the body the rest of the lift? The answer is an emphatic YES and hitting the power position accomplishes this goal. It's true that while picking up the barbell the center of gravity (if considering the lifter and barbell as a single unit) is towards whichever is heavier; the lifter or the barbell. Ensuring the athlete practices the power position will keep from letting that center of gravity shift further towards the bar, pulling the lifter forward, as it gets heavier.

As noted above, the power position places the lifter in the best possible position to conduct the second pull, also known as the triple joint extension. If the lifter doesn't use the power position, they will more than likely be "arm pulling" [PHOTO 4], or bending the arms too soon while still bent over. This puts the bar forward. Try jumping or conducting the second pull when the bar is forward.

Where will you and the bar end up? The answer is further in front of where you started and unable to receive it properly, snatch or clean, instead of vertical, which is where you need to land. Remember in the definition above, the power position is when "the lifter is erect with knees slightly bent, flat footed…." Lastly, with the lifter in the right position prior to the jump, the bar will then end exactly where the lifter needs the bar: directly overhead in the snatch or shelved right onto the shoulders in the clean. Perfect!

Consequences If Not Used

- Failure to utilize the power position technique will undoubtedly cause the following errors:
- forward placement of the bar, as a result having the bar win over the athlete
- slow the speed of the bar
- cause the athlete to bend arms too soon
- reduction in power output
- ruin the timing/ability to receive the bar in the correct position.

Remember, keeping the bar close to the body at all times is essential. The only way to ensure this is accomplished at the height of the thighs is with the institution of the power position. Not having it means the bar is left out in front of the lifter after the first pull (ground to the knees). Since our arms are not as strong as our hips, legs and buttocks (dominant muscles during power position), the arms alone will not be able to generate the speed and power needed to elevate that bar. The arms will try, which is why they bend too soon, but they will fail. This will in turn keep the athlete from truly producing enough velocity to make the bar weightless long enough to receive it. Thus, the landing or receiving portion of the snatch and clean will be rocky, unstable, and so awkward as to compromise the overall technique and likely cause a missed attempt.

Applying It To Your Technique

If you're not already using the power position, I have hopefully now convinced you to do so. The most efficient way to learn this great tool is to build into it with progressions. Start with an empty bar, not a PVC pipe or dowel rod, as the bar will have just a bit of resistance to let you feel the movement. It isn't necessary to belabor the proper progressions in this article, which is certainly the method used in my seminars, as I would need more space and illustrations. However, in a short and concise manner, I can recommend to start with the posture associated with the power position. From this position, with straight arms, jump the bar up from the thighs and into the receiving position. In the snatch, if you lock out overhead simultaneously as you land on your feet, you'll get a sense of the effectiveness of this technique. In the clean, rack the bar on the shoulders with elbows pointing as straight forward as possible at the same time you land, which will also result in the same feeling. Reset and repeat several more times until you feel consistent. Then try it from the hang position. Execute the same thing, but after you hit any hang position, making sure to return to the power position before actually jumping and receiving the bar. After several reps and sets of consistency, you can then try lifting from the ground.

Keep in mind that when you lift from the ground, you must hit all the positions including the power position prior to initiating the "jump" and "receive" steps. You'll know the very first time if you were successful. It is suggested that the athlete try several reps of slow motion execution to ensure all the positions are hit before jumping and receiving the bar. Practice your speed while hitting the positions, and then gradually increase the load on the bar.

It won't be long before the new power position implementation will be a normal part of the athletes' new technique. The challenge will be the first time a 1RM is attempted. The impatient will undoubtedly rush the form, bend the arms, miss the power position, and revert back to their old ways. So ensure the athlete has added speed and load while maintaining consistency for a good period of time before attempting serious loads with the new power position.

UPGRADE YOUR MEMORY, BREAK THROUGH PLATEAUS, AND IMPROVE YOUR COACHING (OR: WHY YOU SHOULD IMAGINE SHOVING YOUR ANKLES UP YOUR ASS)

YAEL GRAUER

If you've been coaching for any length of time, you may have noticed that it can be confusing to your clients when you delve into elaborate details about basic techniques. As fun as it is to geek out on the intricacies of fundamental movements, engage in heated debates on the internet (or productive discussions on the Catalyst Athletics forum), and dissect variations with other bright minds, you'll find that sharing theories on modifications and progressions with your clients doesn't always have the intended results.

Throw out terms like proprioception or rate of force development and you'll often see people's eyes glaze over. Only a small handful of your clients will understand what you're talking about, and your long-winded explanations are unlikely to help them grasp those few basic movements they're still struggling with in spite of your patient guidance.

This doesn't make your athletes dumb or unmotivated, or mean that they don't have the desire to squeeze the most out of their training sessions. It just means that these details can be overwhelming for them, however tempting it may be for you to offer nuanced explanations. Maybe some of them will want to explore these complex concepts in greater depth at some point in the future, once they're further along towards their goal (be it technical mastery, competitive numbers, or looking good naked--whatever their driving motivation may be). But first, they'll need to learn specific movements you're teaching them inside and out, and take that knowledge home with them, especially if they work out on their own in addition to working with you, or have any kind of competitive ambitions.

A widespread criticism of workshops and seminars, as reported by attendees, is that they can't remember all the cool things they learned. Even cutting the technical jargon out of your coaching, simplifying movements and providing helpful cues doesn't always do the trick. Something which worked so seamlessly when an instructor was there to offer guidance and coaching can often seem impossible for people to recall on their own. Your carefully chosen cues seem to go in one ear and out the other, and you wonder if your clients are actually learning anything at all.

And even with your knowledge and experience, and the systems you've developed to help your coaching run smoothly, there are probably a few things you have trouble remembering yourself. So let's take a step back and tap into some strategies to better use your memory. We'll address the skill of memorization itself, explore a couple of ancient techniques, take a brief look at the wild world of competitive memory sports and, with current and former U.S.A. memory champions as our guides, look at strategies you can incorporate into your own coaching and learning.

What Are We Doing, Again?

As someone who's watched videos on YouTube for exercise suggestions on new equipment, written a series of exercise names and cues on an index card, and summarily forgotten a good chunk of the details by the time I hit the gym, I'm all too familiar with being unable to recall basic information. I like to think I'm somewhat intelligent. I have a working knowledge of various topics ranging from Russian literature to MMA, and a repertory of everything from song lyrics to poems to Latin names of plants in the recesses of my mind. Yet I've often been frustrated at my own inability to remember the most basic of things. According to 2011 and 2012 U.S.A. memory champion Nelson Dellis, I'm not the only one. This is something many people struggle with.

"Everyone in some way or form has to memorize things every day, and sometimes people have difficulty with it--maybe not in every form, but I can probably go out there and everyone will tell me one thing they hate memorizing or have trouble memorizing," he said.

The world of memory sports, described in fascinating detail by science writer Joshua Foer in the bestselling memoir Moonwalking With Einstein: The Art and Science of Remembering Everything, is a bit of an eye-opener about what the human brain can do with practice. Foer himself did not set out to become a memory champion, but noticed his numbers rising to competitive levels through guided practice, and found himself winning the 2006 U.S.A. Memory Championship in what began as merely an experiment in participatory journalism. In the book, he weaves historical details, cutting edge scientific research, compelling personal anecdotes and intricate analysis into a fascinating narrative on this strange world where normal people regularly accomplish seemingly impossible feats.

Simply recalling information, described as the lowest form of learning in Bloom's taxonomy of educational objectives, sometimes gets a bum rap...at least at first. "People think memorization is dull, and if you tell them that you're the winner of memory championship, they think that's kind of nerdy and lame, but when I tell them what I'm capable of and how I do it, suddenly there's a tremendous amount of interest," Dellis says. In the 2012 U.S.A. Memory Championship, he memorized 303 random numbers in five minutes, 163 names and faces in 15 minutes, a previously unpublished poem in 15 minutes, and the order of a shuffled deck of playing cards in one minute and 3 seconds. He also memorized a series of random words in an elimination round, recalled details about strangers in a memorization game aptly titled "tea party," and memorized the order of additional playing cards in the final showdown, beating out all other finalists.

In addition to his memory prowess, Dellis, who trains at an I Am Crossfit affiliate in Miami, Fla., has also climbed Mt. Everest to raise money for Alzheimer's research. He managed to incorporate memory training into this climb, memorizing shuffled decks of cards without the aid of supplemental oxygen, and reshuffling the deck at each altitude change. (In a phone interview, Dellis was quick to promise that he wouldn't automatically memorize our entire conversation, though. "That's a common misconception," he explained. "I'm not a tape recorder.")

Mental Athletes; Physical Athletes

Joshua Foer points out that a surprising number of those who do well in the world of competitive memorization are physical athletes, and are often competitive runners. This includes 2005 and 2006 World Memory Champion Clemens Mayer, 2007 World Memory Champion Gunther Karsten, and 2008 U.S.A. Memory Championship finalist Paul Mellor, who has run a marathon in all 50 states.

Although many people who perform well in memory competitions are athletes, Dellis points out that this certainly isn't the case with all competitors. "For the most part, most memory competitors are not physically active," he said. "It would be your typical kind of nerdy guy who just sits at his desk all day, but maybe the people who do a little bit better have a little healthier lifestyle."

Foer, a recreational cyclist himself, believes the link is there because "these are people who like to push themselves. They like to push themselves mentally, they like to push themselves physically and see where their limits lie and see if they can go beyond those limits."

Smashing Barriers

The drive to overcome perceived limitations can be quite strong, and Foer is quick to point out that when any kind of world record is broken, it's usually not long until others hit the same record, no matter how impossible this feat previously seemed. "There is this kind of interesting phenomenon, basically, where there's no competitive endeavor where records don't regularly fall. So if there's limits to what we can do, we haven't figured them out in any competitive sport, which is rather remarkable. It does suggest that we haven't found our limits yet as a species in basically anything," Foer explained.

But not everybody gets past what Foer refers to as the OK Plateau, where you continue practicing a sport or activity for hours upon hours without any improvement. You're putting in the time, but your training is automatic, and you're not pushing yourself beyond your comfort zone... and therefore see no improvement for all of your practice. And yet Foer, who is quick to insist he wasn't born with a good memory, regularly found strategies to overcome plateaus in his training. Working with a coach to get immediate feedback on performance, and making a point to practice in areas in which you have difficulty instead of focusing solely on those you're already good at can help you break down these walls in both physical and mental endeavors.

Of course, we must offer the standard disclaimer that trying to overcome plateaus does not mean one should sacrifice perfect form and get themselves injured trying to get better numbers to throw on a gym's whiteboard. But we've all seen positive effects from friendly competition. When I went to an indoor climbing gym with a friend, I noticed he was sticking to the bottom of the wall and feeling incapable. Having a vague idea of his fitness level compared to mine, I knew he had the potential to step up his game, so I deliberately raced to the top of the same climbing route. It worked--he suddenly found the ability to navigate the foot and handholds with increased speed and make his way to the top on his second go-around. You've likely had similar occurrences, which showcase the importance of training with people who are better than you or will continue to push you, rather than being the top performer in the gym, or stepping out of your comfort zone to compete at a national level no matter the outcome, instead of easily winning states year after year.

Application in the Gym (Shove Your Ankles Where The Sun Don't Shine)
Speaking of competition, I asked Nelson Dellis if using memorization techniques can help in high-stress situations, where memory sometimes flies out the window. (Science writer Jonah Lehrer, interviewed in the May 2012 issue, recently wrote about the new nerurscience of choking in the New Yorker.) Boxers often forget to keep their arms up and elbows in during an actual match, basketball players miss what should be easily attainable shots, and athletes in every sport often see the fundamentals of their technique fly out the window.

"That kind of stuff is muscle memory," Dellis said, and not easily solved by the memorization strategies covered in this article. "You only can do that [kind of thing] naturally if you practice it so much that you don't think about it anymore. What the techniques I do, I think, is get information in our mind quicker. So if you're presented with something new, it takes awhile for you to really lock it in your brain, and then it takes a while before you really know it, whether it's a movement in sports or a language or whatever. [These strategies help with] that part of getting it into your head first, the steps of how to do a golf swing, but to actually do the golf swing like Tiger Woods... that takes practice until it becomes natural.

Dellis thinks the technique is especially effective for learning new movements, which brought up some confusion for me. Why come up with an unrelated visual to learn something you're seeing visually via a demonstration? He reminded me that the brain latches onto bizarre images best, and provided a particularly cogent example of how one might memorize proper form for an exercise. "Say you're learning how to do a squat, and one of the important things that you need to remember is you want to go all the way down; you want your ass to go low. So you can see that when somebody's demonstrating it to you, of course, but that doesn't mean that when you're doing it you'll necessarily see that picture. So what I would do is make that image of that step, that image of the squat into an image that is more out of the ordinary, something sort of bizarre. So I can imagine maybe driving my ankles up my ass, something like that, something really stupid and gross, but when I'm in the bottom of my squat, I'm thinking of that image, which is a little more disturbing. That'll make me think, 'Okay, I need to go a little bit lower; I'm not fully as far down as I need to go.' And that's the kind of idea and that's what I do when I'm memorizing numbers or cards or names; I'm turning all that information into these weird, kind of shockingly absurd pictures, because those are actually easier to latch onto for the brain," he said.

Depending on the culture of your gym, telling a client to visualize shoving their ankles up their ass might be a bad idea, but having them develop their own series of images in response to specific cues might be an alternative way to incorporate imagery into their training.

Other Applications

In addition to training for specific competitive memorization events, and memorizing the names and faces of those he meets, Dellis also has a practical gym application for his skill. He keeps his mind active while he's training by memorizing his running time, weights, sets and reps--in particular, his maxes.

These days, Foer makes regular use of the memory palace, or the method of loci, to give speeches without notes. This is an ancient technique which was used by Cicero and countless others to memorize speeches, and by medieval scholars to memorize entire books. It involves coming up with an image to represent each part of a talk, and placing it somewhere along a building you know well. Ever heard someone say, "in the first place" during a talk? Foer pointed out in a speaking event that this was originally used to literally refer to a physical location in the orator's memory, going back to the earliest Latin memory treatises. Even the word "topic" was derived from the Greek word topos, which means place--a vestige of spatial thinking used in delivering speeches.

For best results, your objects have to be a bit out of the ordinary, though--the more unusual, colorful or bizarre, the better. Engage all of your senses. Think comic books. Make things stink or make them explode. Make things gigantic or pornographic-

-or both. (It's an interesting footnote in history that the most pious of sermons were delivered using these, uh, non-pious memorization techniques.) As you walk through the building in your mind's eye and see the images along the way, you'll remember the topics they represent.

I tested this technique out myself while visiting Marcelo Garcia's Academy in New York. I wanted to write a gym review on my blog, but obviously couldn't take notes in the middle of back-to-back jiu-jitsu classes. Instead of trying to recall the details afterwards, I wanted to memorize specific things that stuck out to me during my visit. I actually used the building of the gym as my memory palace, because two things about it struck me as quite unusual and memorable. The first was that it was on the 6th floor of a building, and despite my awareness of real estate in NYC, I'd always imagined my BJJ mecca as its very own building rather than just a segment of one. Another surprising physical feature of the Academy was that the elevator opened right up to the gym--no walkway, nothing; one step off the elevator and your foot is on the mat.

The first image I created was of the building getting visibly taller...like an elevator to the sky. The second image I created in my mind's eye was hundreds of eyeballs of all sizes appearing on the walls. Third, I filled the entire building with smoke.

When I had a chance to sit down and compose my blog post, I was pleased to realize that I remembered the three images well. It took me a bit longer to figure out what they meant, though. I knew the eyeballs represented the watchful eyes of the many assistant instructors at the Academy. But what was the building becoming taller? Eventually I remembered that this was the image I'd created to remember the expansiveness of the techniques. (All Alliance affiliates utilize a series of choreographed techniques in their fundamental classes, to teach proper movement patterns. In this case, we worked on setting up a seated upright guard pass, then our opponent would take the underhook and we'd respond with a backstep, they'd pull half-guard, we'd post on their leg and post our hands on their opponents hands and slide off to the side, followed by a seamless transition to side control. That's a lot of steps. Some gyms just work on a single guard pass to side control.) And finally, the smoke. After about ten minutes, I remembered that the smoke was an image I created to try to symbolize the positive vibe in the gym, where everyone was helpful and friendly and there were no meatheads to be found. I didn't know how to create an image for 'vibe,' so I changed the word to atmosphere, and used smoke to symbolize that.

Although I clearly need some practice to be able to remember what the images I create represent, I can attest to the fact that this technique actually worked quite well on my very first attempt--in spite of my skepticism.

Memorizing Vs. Learning

Although both Dellis and Foer use these skills they've developed in their day-to-day lives, they are both quick to agree that memorization has its limitations. It's a step towards learning, but isn't learning itself.

"Memory is the basic building block of learning," Dellis said. "It gets information quickly in your head. That's not the actual information you want to learn, but once you have it in there, you can review it and make sense of it after that and that's where the actual learning comes."

Foer points out that although repeating something over and over again is mindless, memorization can actually be mindful by "forcing you to reckon with what it is that you're trying to learn." He views committing things to memory as a necessary first step for processing the world. "Understanding is essential, but sometimes you need a little extra help," he explained. "For example, say you memorize all the U.S. presidents, and what years they served. That's raw and kind of uninteresting information, and it's not that useful in and of itself, but it becomes useful when you are reading U.S. history and then all of a sudden this information that was kind of disconnected can provide context and structure to what you're reading and what you're learning." Remembering basic facts gives you a starting point to fasten other facts to. Awareness of this is embedded into the medieval mind. In fact, the Latin word inventio gave rise to the words invention and inventory, signaling, Foer believes, that one needs to stock their mind with knowledge to be able to project into the future with new creative insights.

Giving oneself permission to use memorization as a starting point for analyzing information in detail at a future time is actually quite relieving. Trying to understand and analyze everything can be overwhelming, but allowing oneself to indulge in a bit of rote memorization as a stepping-stone can make things easier in an age where it's easy to get oversaturated with details.

But although mnemonic devices are very effective for recalling structured information, the memorization techniques aren't ones you'll necessarily want to use for all kinds of learning. Embedding random images in your head instead of observing what's going on around you isn't always the solution. "I can imagine some situations where it would distract you by taking you away from something practically meaningful and relevant," Foer said. The memory palace, for example, "is a technique that's good for something that does not have inherent meaning to you; you're adding a layer of meaning where there is none." Yet the brain does prefer to take in information in the form of pictures, and as I mentioned previously, the more bizarre or disturbing these images, the better. Graphically sexual or violent images are surprisingly effective.

I asked Dellis whether associating a person with an image might change your behavior toward them. What if you come up with a disturbingly gruesome image of a nice old man, and suddenly see and treat him differently from then on, reacting to my image association rather than the individual?

Dellis put my mind at ease. "That never happens. You can always separate the two," he assured. "The thing with names is, you will meet people who might be constantly in your life and you meet people you might never see again. So sometimes you try to learn their names, but it's not important because you may not see them again. But another person may become your best friend or your boyfriend or girlfriend. What happens with the people that become more prominent in your life is that you end up just knowing their name. It's not that you always have to think of these images. These images and this technique help get the name in your mind faster. It's like a crutch; it goes away. Over time, if you develop a relationship with that person, eventually you just know them as that name and you don't have to think of that image. The image; that's just something to help you in the beginning because it is so difficult."

Additional Resources

Books: You Can Have Amazing Memory by Dominic O'Brien is a how-to guide, filled with tips and techniques from an 8-time World Memory Championship winner. The Road to Excellence: The Acquisition of Expert Performance in the Arts and Sciences, Sports, and Games by K. Anders Ericsson, and Expert Performance in Sports: Advances in Research on Sport Expertise (also by Ericsson) looks amazing, if you have $50+ to spend on a book. And, of course, we already mentioned Foer's Moonwalking With Einstein, which is more of a memoir.

Online Resources: Elliot Waite has a Remember Names Game, and Memrise can help you learn languages. Mnemotechnics has boatloads of information, an active forum, and they sometimes organize Google hangouts on Sundays to talk about memory. And, of course, you can always check out Nelson Dellis' blog (he plans to return to Mt. Everest in 2013) or pore through Joshua Foer's website. If you're looking for more on the method of loci, Foer seamlessly incorporates a memory place into his TED talk, and Dellis has a great video where he demonstrates memorizing ten random words for a magazine.

Remembering Names In Five Easy Steps

While you may not want to memorize the order of a deck of playing cards at each altitude while climbing the highest peak in the world, remembering the names of everyone at your gym is a useful, practical activity. Dellis, who's taught workshops to help Crossfit coaches memorize the names of hundreds of clients, shared his five-step method:

1. Pay attention and make sure you're actively trying to remember someone's name,

instead of just thinking about the next thing you want to say. Consciously telling yourself that you're going to learn someone's name, or learn as many names as you can, surprisingly makes a lot of difference.

2. Before asking for their name, find a distinguishing feature on their face--a large nose, bushy eyebrows, a dimple, a scar...something that will pop out at you the next time you see them. This serves as a kind of anchor which will help you in the process.

3. Ask them their name. This is where imagery comes in; you have to be a bit creative, and it does involve some practice. Come up with an image for their name, or the syllables that make up their name. As an example, Nelson pointed out that his own name sort of sounds like the words "nail" and "sun." One might imagine a big yellow sun with a nail being driven through it.

4. Take the image of their name and intertwine it with the anchor from their face. Envision the image happening along with the distinguishing feature. When Nelson asked me what his name reminded me of, I mentioned Nelson from the Simpsons. Pointing out that he has a larger nose, Dellis said I could imagine Nelson from the Simpsons, who's a bully on the show, punching him in the face--making his nose big because it's all swollen.

5. Whether you casually use the person's name in a sentence or not, try to picture that image in your mind throughout your interaction with them.

Make Your Training More Memorable

1. **Find ways to make ordinary things fun.** Dellis describes breaking up his many hours of memory training into smaller chunks to make it less tedious to get through. Foer, who is the cofounder of Atlas Obscura (a compendium of the worlds wonders, curiosity and esoterica), found ways to make otherwise tedious memorization fun by tapping into his creativity and finding enjoyment in the process. These concepts can also apply to your own training in the gym or on the field. Whatever you need to do to find joy out of your deliberate practice, make sure it's not so boring or repetitive that you stop doing it.

2. **Get constant, immediate feedback, however possible**. Foer referred me to Personal Best, an article in the New Yorker about the importance of coaching. If you can't work with a coach, or aren't getting the feedback you need, post your lift videos on a forum or show them to someone who can help. Sharing videos of failed lifts or tournament losses isn't much fun, but getting better is, so make sure to get tips on your areas of weakness in addition to celebrating your strengths.

3. **Eliminate distractions, when possible.** When competing in the U.S.A. and World Memory Championship, Foer copied a technique from the Germans. He wore industrial-grade earmuffs to block out distracting sounds, and special goggles

that reduced his vision down to pinpricks. Although this is highly impractical in most everyday situations, making a willful effort to cut out distractions isn't, so leave your phone in the locker room.

4. **Rise above perceived limitations.** Nelson Dellis rattles off memorized words and numbers with ease in memory competitions, but it probably wouldn't look so easy if he didn't practice 4-5 hours a day leading up to a competition or 2 hours in the off-season. And although Joshua Foer is clearly highly intelligent, he insists that memory isn't actually his forte--and yet he pulled off impressive scores with hard work and expert guidance. We are capable of so much more than we think we are.

5. **Break out of the rut.** No matter how dedicated you are to your training, falling into a mindless routine at the gym is always a bad idea. Stay interested in your sport or activity by finding new ways to anchor your memories, so one training session doesn't blend monotonously into the next. This might mean visiting a different gym, attending a seminar which piques your interest (even if you don't "need" it), finding a new trail to run or bike, or even just playing with a new tool--whatever it takes to keep things memorable and fresh rather than rote and prescriptive. What will help you be more present, make your training more relevant and meaningful to you?

OLYMPIC LIFTING FOR THE COLLEGE FOOTBALL PLAYER
CHAD PEARSON

Olympic weightlifting has long been used in numerous American football organizations to increase athletic performance. The University of Minnesota is no different. We utilize a wide variation of the Olympic movements to further enhance football performance.

First, let's take a look at how the two events are similar; the average football play lasts about five seconds and is performed at a very high speed with large amounts of strength necessary to overcome one's opponent. At the college level, there is a 40 second play clock before the next snap must occur, not accounting for timeouts.

Across the multiple positions, football is considered to be 90% Anaerobic and 10% glycolytic/intermediate energy system pathway. Weightlifting, in comparison, is performed at 100% of the anaerobic pathway. Not many sports other than certain field events in track and field (shot put, discus) are performed at intensity this high.

Along the same lines, both football and weightlifting are dependent on ground force application. If you refer to Newton's 3 law of motion, you'll know that every action has an equal and opposite reaction. With consideration to these two events, the harder you push into the ground, the more force you will be able to produce. A common phrase used among our staff is "the harder you push into the ground, the faster you run and higher you jump." The game of football is played with athletes' feet on the ground; therefore, it is vital to train with feet on the ground. The kinetic chain of power utilized to clean or snatch a heavy load is the very same chain utilized to propel one's body in a given direction.

In addition, the motor skill development of weightlifting carries over to myriad other skills. The greatest lifters in the world are not necessarily stronger than others, but rather, much more technically sound. The ability to contract and relax the muscles of elite Olympic weightlifters is second to none. Football, being a game of trying to outmaneuver one's opponent by multiple techniques, makes this contraction/relaxation ability a great asset to being able to utilize said different techniques to dominate one's opponent.

How Olympic Lifting Is Programmed at the University of Minnesota

Our objective as strength and conditioning coaches for football is to create the best football player we can. It's not to make elite Olympic weightlifters. If our goal was to create elite weightlifters, we would only use the full movements. With that being said, it is important to understand how we utilize the partial movements of the Clean & Jerk and the Snatch. A football player must be able to produce force at different body angles and also receive force at different angles.

Terminology

Clean: pulled from the floor, caught in a full front squat

Hang Clean: begins from hang position (standing position, bar at hips), caught in full front squat

Hang Power Clean: begins from the hang position, caught in "power position" (1/4 squat)

Power Clean: pulled from the floor, caught in "power position"

Block Power Clean: pulled from boxes with bar just below or just above knee, caught in "power position"

Block Clean: pulled from boxes with bar just below or above knee, caught in full front squat.

The Snatch variations are listed as the same, trading clean for snatch and bar is caught above the head in a full squat or "power position."

Teaching Progression

The snatch is the first full movement taught to our new players. We believe that the snatch is easier to learn once the fundamentals of the RDL/hip hinge, triple extension, and high pull have been established. With that being said, before either the snatch or clean, the athletes are taken through a progression that breaks down the movement into the above sequence.

Foot Placement – Feet should start in one's jumping stance, that is to say, feet underneath the hips.

Grip – We use the hook grip.

RDL – Knees are slightly bent, and athletes hinge at hips, pushing their butt back, loading their hamstrings and heels.

Triple Extension – Body weight transfers from heels to the balls of feet, and hips/knees/ankles simultaneously extend, bringing the athlete to tallest position possible.

High Pull – The explosive triple extension propels the bar upwards; the arms simply guide the bar up in close proximity to the body. Elbows remain above the wrists.

Catch – either snatch or clean catch.

The hook grip, RDL, Triple Extension, and High Pull are all taught as part of a complex during the first four to six weeks of a new athlete's training program. For example: 6x RDL, 6x Triple Extension/Shrug, 6x High Pull, 6x Front Squat. As you can see, the front squat is being taught in concert with the other movements, thus making a smooth transition to the clean catch once proper bar and body position has been established.

Simultaneously, on a different training day, the overhead press is taught in progression from a strict military press, to push press, to push jerk. This enforces proper bar placement overhead. We call it the "sweet spot;" the position overhead with the elbows locked dispersing the load of the bar throughout the entire body. Note that all presses are taught from the front rack position (front squat catch).

Positional Differences: The strength and conditioning program at the University of Minnesota is designed to progress the athlete for a full four years. As the athlete enters as a freshman in the summer or as a junior college transfer, they enter what we call Block Zero, similar to that of Coach Joe Kenn during his tenure at the University of Louisville. This is a phase of training where the teaching progressions take place. The importance is placed on quality of the movements rather than quantity. There is no interest in how heavily the athlete can lift a weight incorrectly. Further, the athletes will progress another 4 levels with the next level beginning in January. After the athlete finishes Block Zero and enters Level 1, they will be split into a Front-7 group (offensive line, tight ends, defensive line, linebackers, long snappers), or a Skill group (wide receivers, running backs, defensive backs, kickers, punters), or a Quarterback group.

The differences in these levels are subtle, as the main priority of each training day is the same. However, a basic understanding of the positional needs is met. A Front-7 player will begin each play from a static position and usually with a hand on the ground, especially the offensive and defensive linemen. Therefore, a majority of the Olympic movements performed will begin with the bar on the floor to emulate the static position to begin each play. A Skill player will commonly be in a more athletic position, often moving before the snap of the ball. Therefore, a majority of the movements are performed from a hang position. Rep/set schemes are very similar during individual phases of the year (in-season, winter, spring, summer), but commonly change between each one. The highest number of reps in a set is limited to six and often in the 3-5 rep range. In order to increase total volume, more sets are added to accomplish the desired training effect at the prescribed load.

It is understood that the security of a strength and conditioning coach is limited to the success of the football team. Therefore, it is vital that we are able to produce the best possible athlete in the safest possible way. Having a star player on the sidelines with an injury due to poor training (barring any freak injury) is a strength coach's worst nightmare. By utilizing the Olympic weightlifting movements to increase ground force production, motor skill development--and in conjunction with the athletes current speed training/conditioning phase--it is our desire that these athletic abilities will transfer to the football field, enabling the athlete to utilize their skills to become a great football player.

Notes
Arthur, Michael; Bailey, Bryan. Complete Conditioning for Football. Champaign, Ill: 1998. Human Kinetics
Siff, Mel C. Supertraining. Denver, Co: 2003. Supertraining Institute

GOLDEN GOPHER FOOTBALL

PEARSON

Monday

Warm Up		week 1			week 2			week 3		
Tumbling - A, Hurdle Mobility - A			x5 ea							
Goblet Squat			x6							
Hip Thrust			x12							
Frankenstein, A-Skip			2x15 yd ea							
Activation/Pre-Hab		%	rep	wt	%	rep	wt	%	rep	wt
Cossack Squat				x5 ea						
90/90 ABD w/ band				2x8 ea						
Monday		%	rep	wt	%	rep	wt	%	rep	wt
Hang Clean		60%	3	76	60%	2	76	60%	2	76
		60%	3	76	60%	2	76	60%	2	76
Hang Power Clean		85%	3	108	80%	2	102	80%	2	102
		85%	3	108	85%	2	108	85%	2	108
* 3x Tuck Jump		85%	3	108	90%	2*	114	92%	2*	117
		85%	3*	108	90%	2*	114	92%	2*	117
Squat		65%	4	245	50%	5	190	50%	5	190
		85%	4	320	65%	3	245	65%	3	245
		85%	4	320	80%	3	300	80%	2	300
		85%	4	320	90%	3	340	92%	2	345
DB Incline Press		85%	4	320	90%	3	340	92%	2	345
					90%	3	340	92%	2	345
		77.5%	6	78	82.5%	6	83	87.5%	6	88
		77.5%	6	78	82.5%	6	83	87.5%	6	88
		77.5%	6	78	82.5%	6	83	87.5%	6	88
Clean Pull			4			4			4	
			4			4			4	
			4			4			4	
			4			4			4	

Warm Up	Torso	Post Work
Tumbling - A, Hurdle Mobility - A	Single Limb Plank	0
	2x15 ea	0
		uni lb
	Pallof Press Hold	
Activation/Pre-Hab	2x15 ea	

Wednesday

Warm Up		week 1			week 2			week 3		
Court Warm Up										
Bear Crawl - Slow			2x10 yds			2x12 yds				
Activation/Pre-Hab										
Scap Push Up			x15			x15				
Band Pull Apart/Band Scap Row			x10 ea			x12 ea				
Wednesday		%	rep	wt	%	rep	wt	%	rep	wt
Push Jerk		65%	5	80	65%	3	80	65%	3	80
		75%	5	90	75%	4	90	75%	3	90
		85%	5	105	85%	4	105	85%	3	105
1-Arm DB Press		85%	5	105	85%	4	105	85%	3	105
		90%	4	105	90%	4	110	92%	3	115
Pendlay Row		80%	4	210	90%	4	110	92%	4	115
		80%	4	210	80%	6	210	80%	8	210
1-Arm Cable Row		80%	4	210	80%	6	210	80%	8	210
		20%	8 ea	70	20%	6 ea	70	20%	8 ea	70
		20%	4 ea	70	20%	6 ea	70	20%	8 ea	70
1-Arm DB Press		80%	4 ea	210	80%	6	210	80%	8	210
		80%	4	210	80%	6	210	80%	8	210
		20%	4 ea	70	20%	6 ea	70	20%	8 ea	70
Drop Push Up		20%	4		20%	4		20%	4	
12" box		20%	4		20%	4		20%	4	
		20%	8 ea		20%	8 ea		20%	8 ea	
KB Bent Press			5 ea			5 ea			5 ea	
			5 ea			5 ea			5 ea	
			5 ea			5 ea			5 ea	

Warm Up	Torso	Post Work
	Russian Twists	0
	2x12 ea	shldr
		rc
	Alt. Superman	
	1x12 ea	

Friday

Warm Up		week 1			week 2			week 3		
Tumbling - B, Hurdle Mobility - B			x 5ea			x 5ea				
Supine Band Squat			x6			x6				
S.L. Bridge			2x15 yd ea			2x15 yd ea				
LETH, Pwr Skip										
Activation/Pre-Hab										
Middle Toe Pull			2x5 ea			2x5 ea				
Outside Toe Pull			2x5 ea			2x5 ea				
Friday		%	rep	wt	%	rep	wt	%	rep	wt
Drop Snatch		30%	4	30	35%	4	35	40%	4	40
Hang Snatch		55%	4	55	60%	4	60	60%	4	60
		60%	4	60	62%	4	62	65%	4	65
Hang Power Snatch		80%	4*	80	85%	4	85	88%	4	88
		80%	4*	80	85%	4*	85	88%	4*	88
* 3x MB Scoop		80%	4*	80	85%	4*	85	88%	4*	88
		80%	4*	80	85%	4*	85	88%	4*	88
Front Squat		68%	5	95	73%	5	102	78%	5	109
		68%	5	95	73%	5	102	78%	5	109
GHR w/ weight		83%	4	83	85%	4	85	88%	4	88
w/ pause @ 45°		83%	4	83	85%	4	85	88%	4	88
		83%	4	83	85%	4	85	88%	4	88
TRX Y's & T's			6			6			6	
			4			4			4	
Snatch Pull			4			4			4	
Landmine Twists			10 ea	25		10 ea	25		10 ea	25
			10 ea	25		10 ea	25		10 ea	25
kilograms			10 ea	25		10 ea	25		10 ea	25

Warm Up	Torso	Post Work
Tumbling - B, Hurdle Mobility - B	Off-Bench Oblique	ankle
	2x12 ea	
	Stab. Rev. Crunch	
Activation/Pre-Hab	1x15	

Tumbling - A:
Fwd Roll
Fwd Roll w/ Jump
Bwd Roll w. Press

Hurdle Mobility - A:
#4 - front move from side
#5 - front move from center

Court Warm Up:
25 Jumping Jacks - full court run
20 Flings - full court run
15 Push Ups - full court run
10 BW Squats - full court run

Tumbling - B:
Judo Roll
Fwd/Bwd Roll
Leaping Fwd Roll

Hurdle Mobility - B:
#6 - duck under - low
#7 - duck under - pop up

LOCKED AND LOADED: A LOOK AT MEET WEEK PREPARATION
MATT FOREMAN

It's a great feeling when you've got a big opportunity coming up and you know you're 100% prepared for it. Know what I mean? Have you ever sat in a hallway, waiting to be called into an office for a job interview, and you basically know you've already got it in the bag before you even go in there? That's a nice little moment. All you have to do is walk in that room, sit down, turn on the charm, and they're going to offer you a gig that pays you enough money to get those credit card companies off your ass.

However, there's a flip side to this coin. Having experiences when you're totally unprepared for an important moment are miserable. Let me give you an example. I used to train with a buddy who had a chance to go on one of those TV court shows. You know the ones I mean, like The People's Court or Judge Judy or something. Anyway, for some reason he decided to go out and get insanely drunk the night before the show. So the next day, he was standing there in court with the cameras rolling, and he was hung over to the point that he was sweating booze out of every pore and trying as hard as he could not to crap his pants. That's what we call "lack of proper preparation."

These little examples lead us into this month's topic. Many of you are competitive weightlifters. Maybe you're a CrossFitter who decided to lift in a meet once, and now you've competed a couple of times and you're fired up to keep it rolling. Others might be long time veteran lifters with a lot of experience. There might even be some of you who have never competed in a meet before, but you're starting to get the itch and you've even looked around for some upcoming events in your area. And finally, some of you might be coaches who don't have any plans to compete yourself, but you've got people in your gyms who have expressed some interest in it.

This is why we're going to talk about meet week preparation in this article. Frankly, I'm surprised that I've been writing for Performance Menu for as long as I have without addressing this already, because it's one of the most important topics I can think of. I'm talking about the week of a competition, the Monday through Friday time period when your meet is on Saturday (or maybe Sunday). Let me tell you something people, this is an area where you don't want to make any mistakes. Think about it...you've been training for this meet for weeks, or maybe months. You've invested a ton of time and effort in it, your parents and friends are going to show up, your coach is excited for you, etc. The last thing you want to do is go out on that platform and look like some klutzbag who learned how to lift five minutes before the meet started. Well, that can happen if you don't do things right during meet week. I've seen lifters who trained really well for an entire cycle, and then they went out there and crapped the bed at the contest because they did something stupid in the gym during those last few days. You don't want this to happen to you, right? Okay, so let's figure out how to avoid it.

European Influences...

As with a lot of the topics we've analyzed in the past, there are different ways to do this successfully. One of the first things I want to do is look at what some of you have seen and heard about from top international lifters.

If you've spent some time learning about the sport, particularly if you've watched the World Championship training hall videos from IronMind, you've probably discovered that many of the best lifters in the world train with pretty high intensity and volume all the way up to a couple of days before they compete. It blows your mind when you first see it, because these suckers are in the gym hitting multiple singles with weights that are relatively close to what they're going to attempt in the competition, and they're doing it 48 or 72 hours before the meet. It's freaky because common sense tells us that those last few days before a competition should be mainly devoted to rest and recovery. If you want to be fresh and ready on the day of the meet, you need to drastically reduce the amount of activity you do in the last few days prior. Makes a lot of sense, doesn't it?

Sure it does. That's why it's confusing to see videos like the one of 2001 105+ World Champion Jaber Salem from Qatar snatching two singles with 200 kilos (440 lbs) just a few days before competing. Jaber snatched 210 kilos in the meet, so 200 was 95% for him. And he isn't the only lifter who we've seen this from. The majority of the top lifters in the world do it this way. Going up to 95% right before a contest sounds like suicide. There is no way you should be able to recover from a workout like that in time to be fresh for the meet, right? Well, wrong…in the case of the athletes we're talking about here.

The important thing to remember with world championship lifters is that they're completely adjusted to this type of work progression. In the months leading up to a major competition, going to 95-100% on a daily basis is normal for them. It doesn't sound humanly possible, but this is how lifters from China, Russia, and most of the other top European countries train. They often work out 12-15 times per week (or more), and they lift weights that are very close to their maximum in most of those sessions. This is why they don't fall apart at meets when they've had heavy workouts only two or three days prior. Their bodies are acclimated to the workload. The competition, where they're going to attempt their biggest lifts, is literally just another day at the office for them.

Now, it's essential to acknowledge that it takes a very structured training system to achieve these results. With these athletes, lifting is their job. It's their whole life, and they don't have any real responsibilities outside of the gym. Their training is funded, they don't have other occupations, and their coaches have put them on a highly developed plan that incorporates their training with advanced recovery measures such as massage therapy and, admittedly, performance enhancing drugs. I hate to be the one to have to tell you, but these lifters aren't doing this clean. One of the reasons they can recover from savage workouts so quickly is that their testosterone levels are high enough to repair tissues quicker than normal humans.

So the best lifters in the world train pretty heavy all the way up to contest time. They're able to do this because of highly developed workload adaptation and scientific recovery techniques. That brings us to you. You're not a Chinese weightlifter. You have a job, a family, and you're probably a little older than your late teens/early twenties, when your body can recover from almost anything at lightning speed. Considering all of this, how can we structure your meet week so you hit peak performances at the right time?

Calpian Method…

You've read a lot about how I trained with the Calpian weightlifting club during my serious competitive years. Well, our team had a meet week plan we followed pretty consistently, and it always seemed to work. Here is basically how we did it.

The last heavy full workout would be the Saturday prior to the competition. That was the last time we pushed for maximum weights in the competition lifts, along with heavy pulling and squatting. Then, during meet week, this was the procedure:

Monday

- Snatch- work up to five singles with approximately 90%
- Clean and Jerk- work up to three singles with approximately 90%

Wednesday

- Snatch- work up to five singles with approximately 80%
- Clean and Jerk- work up to three singles with approximately 80%

All other days- light stretching, foam rolling, possibly some light bar work

That's basically it. Our whole team trained the same way, so this is what we all did during our meet weeks. Now, there were times when our coach would make some small adjustments based on an individual lifter's situation. If somebody was considerably overtrained or trying to heal up a minor injury in time for the day of the competition, these percentages could be lowered or modified. There were also times when some of our lighter lifters who had much quicker recovery time would add some back squats during this week, using weights that were around the same as the athlete's projected clean and jerk at the meet. Little variations like that were possible, based on the judgment of our coach. But overall, this was what we did during meet week for many years.

Our method was based on a kind of informal principle we sometimes referred to as "supercompensation." This was the idea that the last few heavy training weeks prior to the competition should be extremely demanding. The athletes would be working at maximum levels in almost all lifts and exercises. Attempts at new personal records would often be daily, which would obviously place tremendous strain on the body. To put it more bluntly, we would be beat to hell by the time that last heavy training week rolled around.

Then, the meet week was designed to be a piece of cake compared to how hard we had been training in the previous weeks and months. During the five or six days before a contest, our bodies went through a huge "freshening up" process. Our joints got a break from all the hard pounding, the heavy pulls and squats were eliminated, and the result was that we showed up on the day of the meet feeling totally recovered and ready to rock. We hadn't lost any of the strength gains we worked so hard for, and we no longer felt like a train ran over us. I can positively say that this worked for me for many years, and for many other athletes as well. I can remember going to meets and starting my snatches in the warm-up room and thinking to myself, "Damn, these 50 kilos feels like an empty bar." That was what I remember most, how light the weights felt in the warm-up room compared to how they felt in those last heavy training weeks. And let me tell you something Jack, it's a huge psychological boost when you're warming up at a meet and everything feels light and snappy. That's when you know you're going to unleash hell.

Other Approaches...

Although the Calpian method was what I used for most of my biggest years, I've done some other things during meet week throughout my career. When I was twenty, I did a contest where I back squatted a new personal record on the Wednesday of meet week. This wasn't the normal procedure I was used to, but it was a small local meet and we were "training through it." I clean and jerked a new personal record at the meet, just three days after the back squat PR. I think a lot of it had to do with the fact that I was younger, and I had that speed-of-light recovery we talked about earlier. Interestingly, the only other time

I ever did heavy back squats during meet week was at another local competition about six years later. I squatted heavy on the Monday of meet week, and at the competition on Saturday I bombed out in the clean and jerk with a weight that was ten kilos below my personal record. My body felt slow and creaky, and I lifted like dog turds. As I said, I was 26 at this time and I was also about twenty kilos heavier in bodyweight than I had been in the other local meet six years earlier when I did the C&J PR.

That brings up another interesting reminder…superheavyweight lifters usually need more recovery time than lighter lifters. A lot of coaches have no idea how to train a superheavyweight. You have to approach it differently, plain and simple. If you try to train a SHW with the same methods you use for lightweights, it will probably fail. The big rhinos can't go heavy as often as smaller people, especially in the C&J and squats. I've noticed over the years that some countries always seem to have good superheavyweights, and others rarely do. It's pretty obvious that some of the national coaches in places like Germany, Russia, and Iran know how to prepare a superheavy. Other places…clearly not so much.

When I was in my early thirties, I actually lifted in several meets where I didn't touch a barbell or do any kind of activity for an entire week before the contest. Seriously, I did absolutely nothing. And my competition results were actually pretty good, believe it or not. I guess I wouldn't recommend this to anybody, but I also can't say it's a completely ridiculous idea because it worked for me more than once, and a couple of the meets I did it at were big national contests.

Here's the main idea to this whole discussion, and it's what you need to take away from this article. There isn't a perfect one-size-fits-all way to prepare during a meet week. I presented you with a few different ideas here. But if you talk to ten other coaches, you'll get ten different plans. Most likely, you'll find lifters who have had great success with all ten of them. The principle that really matters is that the meet week program has to be based on the athlete's previous training. In other words, you have to plan the seven days prior to the contest in connection with what the lifters have done in the gym over the weeks and months. For example, if you've used a training plan where the athlete always has a rest day prior to attempting maximum weights, then you better make sure the day before competition is a rest day too. See what I mean? You don't want to add things to a lifter's meet week that aren't part of the normal routine. You can subtract some things. That's fine. But adding new things is a risky idea.

The whole idea of competing is showing up on meet day with the body at maximum strength, but also rested enough to perform well. Some athletes require more rest than others, based on their age, experience, bodyweight, and the workload they're adapted to. Some coaches like to have their athletes work up to their competition opening attempts during meet week. Other coaches like to keep the weights a little lighter than this (myself included). I generally like to err on the side of caution during meet week, both with my own lifting and with the athletes I coach.

Finally, one thing we all know is that weightlifting is equal parts mental and physical. I think showing up for a competition with the mind prepared is just as important as having the body primed. If you do things during meet week that are going to make the athlete uncertain and under-confident, it's a problem. I would rather create a situation where the athlete trains like an animal for several weeks and then gets to see the meet week as a little break before the contest. The mental strain of nailing heavy weights gets eased back for a week, and everything is rejuvenated on the big day.

This might involve trial and error. But with common sense and an understanding of training, you should be able to get a good plan put together. Getting completely hammered the night before an important day like my buddy did before he went on TV doesn't demonstrate common sense. We all know this. So, as with many things in life, just don't be a moron and you'll be fine.

PRIORITIZING OLYMPIC WEIGHTLIFTING COMPETITION TRAINING
KYLE J. SMITH

CrossFit athletes around the world are hungry for quality programming that will give them the support they need to perform well in competition. Mainsite continues to only publish WODs for general CrossFit enthusiasts, so coaches far and wide are popping out of the woodwork with their own approaches to CrossFit competition training. Athletes searching for the next big thing and new secrets flood these coaches' blogs daily. But one thing is consistent from program to program: Olympic weightlifting is king.

In this article, we'll investigate why Olympic weightlifting has become so important in CrossFit, and I'll introduce you to a few coaches who are taking it to the next level with their programming. Then we'll end with a framework for how to add Olympic weightlifting to your personal programming. Strap on your weightlifting shoes, give Fran a call and let her know you're gonna be late to your date; let's rock and roll.

CrossFit Games Individual Events with Olympic Weightlifting Movements

2007
"Hopper"
Row 1000m then
5 RFT:
25 pull-ups
7 push jerks 135#/85#
2008
FT 30 clean & jerks 155#/100#

2009
3 RFT:
30 snatches 75#/45#
30 wall balls #20/14#
1 RM Snatch

"Chipper"

FT:

15 Cleans 155#/105#

30 Toe to Bars

30 Box Jump 24"/20"

15 Muscle-ups

30 Dumbbell Push Presses 40#/35#

30 Double Unders

15 Thrusters 135#/95#

30 Pull-ups

30 Burpees

Overhead Walking Lunge 45#/25#

2010

"Amanda"

9-7-5 RFT:

Muscle UpSnatch 135#/95#

7 RFT:

3 Clean 205#/135#

4 Ring HSPU

(Part 2 of 3 part workout)

3 RFT:

30 T2B

21 ground to overhead 95#/65#

2011

FT:

5 ascents 15' Rope climb

5 Clean and jerk 145#/115#

4 ascents 15' Rope climb

4 Clean and jerk 165#/125#

3 ascents 15' Rope climb

3 Clean and jerk 185#/135#

2 ascents 15' Rope climb

2 Clean and jerk 205#/145#

1 ascent 15' Rope climb

1 Clean and jerk 225#/155#

1 RM weighted Chest-to-bar pull-up for load in 2 mins

1 rep max Snatch for load in 2 mins

Jug carry for distance in 1 min

2012

3 RFT:
8 Split snatch, alternating legs 115# / 75#
7 Bar muscle-ups
Run 400 meters

1-rep Clean every 30 seconds with progressively heavier barbells
245#--->385#140#--->235#

For time:
10 Overhead squats 155#/105#
10 Box jump overs 24"/ 20"
10 Fat bar thrusters 135#/ 95#
10 Power cleans 205#/125#
10 T2B
10 Burpee muscle-ups
10 T2B
10 Power cleans 205#/125#
10 Fat bar thrusters 135#/ 95#
10 Box jump overs 24"/20"
10 Overhead squats 155#/105#

"Elizabeth"
21-15-9 RFT:
Clean 135#/ 95#
Ring dips

"Isabel"
FT:
30 Snatch 135#/95#

One need only look over that table for a moment to see that Olympic weightlifting movements are essential in competition. The day is long gone where being "okay" at the snatch is "okay." It's time to become technicians and artists in the lifts, ready to adapt your abilities to any setting, at any intensity, with a whole lot of weight.

Simply showing that CrossFit uses the lifts and their derivatives in competition isn't even the most compelling argument as to why you should prioritize them in your training. For that, we will look to the very heart of Olympic weightlifting.

How Olympic Weightlifting Translates into Everything

It is easy to see how training the snatch and clean and jerk also improves movements that are used in the lifts, namely the deadlift, squat and press. And it is not difficult to continue down this path and see how similar lifts can also be improved, for instance the thruster, box jump and handstand push ups. Let's dive even further by analyzing how the bare essentials of the Olympic lifts improve everything we do in CrossFit. As a foundation to understand the "bare essentials of the Olympic lifts" we will use the list from Greg Everett's seminal article, "Six truths of Olympic Weightlifting Technique."

Truth 1: The lifter and the barbell system must remain balanced over the feet.

Truth 2: The barbell and the lifter must remain in close proximity to each other.

Technique: No barbell movements are more highly technical than the snatch and the clean and jerk. Period. Athletes spend their entire lives perfecting just these two movements. CrossFit athletes have a huge library of movements they wish to be competent in, and it is impossible to practice every single one and ever see growth in all of them. By choosing to focus on primarily the Olympic lifts, however, we can see progress across the board. Use the Olympic lifts and basic strength lifts to get stronger and better, use everything else to be ready for the unknown and unknowable.

Truth 3: There must be no time wasted at the top of the pull.

Truth 4: The relocation under the bar is an active movement.

Power: The Olympic lifts are the most powerful lifts in the book. Nothing is going to teach you to move large loads long distance quickly (in relation to a barbell) better than these lifts. This "need for speed" teaches you how to move as a power athlete. Is there anything better than being strong and fast?

Truth 5: The receiving position must be strong and stable.

Confidence: When you are comfortable and confident in the snatch, a sumo deadlift high pull just ain't that frightening. When you have the clean and jerk in the bag, learning to do an atlas stone clean is fun. Coming into CrossFit, I had two years of experience in the snatch and clean and jerk. I watched myself progress much quicker than my peers because the barbell was my friend--nothing was scary, stupid or weird. Get to know the Olympic lifts; they're great friends, with benefits.

Truth 6: Consistency is more important than technical style.

Practice: If you want to be the best CrossFit athlete you can be, don't do it just like Annie Thorrisdottir, do it just like you. Learn from Rich, Coach and every fire breather in a 100-mile radius, then make it your own. No one can create a program for everyone; no one can devise a game day strategy for the masses. Best practices are awesome, helpful hints are cool, buy learning by trial and error is the key to unlocking your true potential.

Coaches Prioritizing Olympic Weightlifting:

If you want a specific Olympic weightlifting / CrossFit program, here are some coaches who are publishing workouts daily that you can follow. Note: follow one coach. One. These guys/gals are smart, they're big goal/picture kinda people who don't promise results from one day of ass kicking. They promise results by consistency, dedication, ass kicking/TLC and hard fucking work- so give it to them.

CJ Martin CJ Martin has a big brain in his bald head and his programming will not dissappoint. A big plus at his website is the Fitness/Performance/Competition breakdown for programming. Maybe you're a new box owner who wants to use some reliable programming while you perfect your game, or you're a novice athlete who needs a ramp up to elite level programming- here's everything you need on one website.

Aaron Landes "Lando," of CrossFit Southie, is new on my radar but his program has potential. I gotta give respect to any coach who publishes their workouts with the "why" and a request for feedback. Give it a shot for a few cycles, let me/him know if you get better at CrossFitting.

Greg Everett Greg is not a CrossFit coach, Greg does not program for CrossFit athletes. He is an Olympic weightlifting master level ninja warrior with the light sabers to prove it, so if you want to take a few months in your programming to truly focus on the lifts, there is no one better to turn to.

Basic Olympic Weightlifting Framework for CrossFit Competition Training

Instead of prescribing a specific program for Olympic weightlifting, let me suggest some foundational ideas from which you can build your own program. Of course, these are not ideas on which every program is/should be built:, this is simply a place to start. As you experiment as a coach/athlete, tailor these ideas to optimize your growth.

Note: I'm assuming you are able to perform a full snatch and clean and jerk. If you are not at this point, then this framework is not geared towards you. Check out this program instead. These ideas are for coaches or athletes writing their own programming.

Some of the ideas are for a strength cycle; when it's time to shift your focus to other areas of your fitness, take what's helpful and leave what's not.

1. Learn the lifts correctly.

This is obvious but worth saying out loud. Trying to mimic what you see the great or competent do can be very helpful, but you may miss out on delicate and essential actions like not shooting your hips up prematurely from the floor or the need to actively pull yourself under the bar during the third pull. Imagine training for a year and then taking a great seminar like the one offered at Catalyst Athletics and having to exclaim, "Shit! My feet are supposed to start where?!"

2. Perform heavy snatches and clean and jerks regularly.

As a beginner, there is a lot of ground to be gained by doing light technique work with the Olympic lifts. But eventually you will reach a point where you're not going to get any stronger in the lifts or hone your technique any further without getting under some serious weight. As an example, "pulling under the bar" is mostly hypothetical when the weight is light; you're strong enough to pull the thing over your head, there's really no reason to get underneath it. But when the weight is heavy, you actually have to pull yourself underneath the bar in order to finish the lift, and in order to have any idea how to do that for real, you have to have to do it for real.

3. Use derivatives of the lifts to fix holes in your game.

There are an infinite number of derivatives of the lifts that include adjectives like hang and pause, qualifiers like from-the-knee and while-drinking-beer. Later in your weightlifting career, you may use these lifts for strength and variety, but as you begin to prioritize the Olympic lifts in your CrossFit training, let's only use them to attack very specific problems. What do I mean? Use the snatch and clean and jerk to get better at the snatch and clean and jerk. When you notice that you could use more speed getting underneath the bar in the snatch, use a hang snatch. When time after time the bar is too far away from you at the knees during the clean, start with the bar on boxes at your knees. With a coach's watchful eye, you should be able to translate these techniques back into the full lifts. Because no derivative of the Olympic lifts perfectly recreates what's going on during the full lifts, let's use them with intention.

4. Use power versions of the lifts to emphasize speed and to recover.

I find taking a day off from the full lifts by doing the power versions to be rejuvenating, invigorating and fun (but I'm a nerd.) In order for the power versions to be helpful in developing the full lifts, they must be fast and precise. Sorry, 2012 CrossFit Games Regional competitors, your hang power cleans aren't going to make you better at the clean because your technique has gone to shit. When you catch your power snatch at a thigh position above parallel, can you ride it the rest of the way down into a proper overhead squat? Good for you, you're doing it right.

5. Squat. All the time.

This instruction does not read "Deadlift. All the time," and there's a reason for that. A traditional deadlift is not identical to its relative equivalent in the Olympic lifts. In a traditional deadlift, your hips are set too high from the start and the movement is often executed too slowly. A traditional squat (high bar back squat or front squat,) when performed correctly, builds very useful strength for the Olympic lifts. How much strength do you need? I'll let Greg tell you about that.

6. Start your training day with the Olympic lifts.

Much like Coach Rutherford's Max Effort Black Box template, putting Olympic weightlifting training at the beginning of your day allows for maximum focus, attention, effort and time. You don't want to be tuckered out, mentally or physically, before practicing the Olympic lifts as that will not allow you to perform at levels that will benefit you in the larger picture.

7. Don't use the Olympic lifts in your metcons until you are an artist and a technician.

This is probably the most controversial idea listed here and I also think it's one of the most important. Watch video of the early CrossFit Games and you'll see that lots of competitors lost all semblance of correct technique when intensity was layered on. Compare that to video of Rich Froning completing 12.2 from the 2012 Open.

12.2

Proceed through the sequence below completing as many reps as possible in 10 minutes of:

    75# Snatch, 30 reps
    135# Snatch, 30 reps
    165# Snatch, 30 reps
    210# Snatch, as many reps as possible

The Fittest Man in the World is arguably also the most efficient and technically proficient man in the world. So I have to wait until I'm Rich Froning until I can do the Olympic lifts in metcons? No, that's a dumb question. Just do yourself a favor and wait until you are so comfortable in your traditional Olympic lifting technique that learning how to handle the lifts in a metcon setting isn't going to waste all the time and effort you've spent learning them the right way. If there's a competition coming up and you think you'll need to use them in a metcon setting then practice them, but don't lose focus on the larger and more important goal: being the best Olympic weightlifter you can possibly be.

Chalk Up

Opinions aren't worth any more than the beers they're drank over and this is just one man's opinion on how to program for Olympic weightlifting and CrossFit. There are one million ways to do this and half of them are right, the other half would be right too if they would allow themselves to adapt and learn. As a coach, programmer and athlete, I hope to learn every day by discussing, arguing and reading. But at the end of the day, none of that matters if you don't pick up a barbell.

You know what to do.

WEIGHTING QUESTIONS YOU'RE AFRAID TO ASK
GREG EVERETT

It was suggested to me by our talented editor Yael that I write an article about "dumb" weightlifting questions. A better word would probably be basic. Here are a collection of questions you might be embarrassed to ask someone in person and my quick answers.

Do I need knee sleeves? Which ones should I buy and where do I get them from? Oh yeah, how do I get these things on? How often do I need to wear them?

Probably not. Start without them and focus on establishing proper mobility, warming-up adequately before training, and training with appropriate intensity, volume and frequency. If you're doing all of these things and still have achy knees, try neoprene sleeves. Wear them for squatting, cleaning and possibly jerking, and ideally only on your heavier sets. To get them on, make sure you have the right size. Then just slide them on up.

Do I need weightlifting shoes? Where do I get them?

If you want to do the lifts properly and safely, weightlifting shoes are a good idea. There are two primary points of lifting shoes: a hard, flat sole and an elevated heel. The former improves your stability and maximizes the transfer of generated power into the bar. The latter increases the range of motion of the ankles, allowing you to sit into better squat positions with a more upright posture to establish the structure needed to snatch and clean. You will need to order them online. Try ordering a half-size smaller than your street shoe. They should be snug enough that your foot doesn't move in them, and when they're new, err on the tight side because the leather will stretch out a bit with use. Invest in good shoes—they'll last a long time and their lifespan can be extended with repairs and resoling.

What are some basic weightlifting etiquette rules in the gym and in competition?

- Don't do anything that will distract a lifter. The big ones are not walking or standing in front of a lifter when he or she is lifting or preparing to lift and being quiet during those times; this goes for the gym and competition. Keep your phone on silent.
- In the gym, always ask to use equipment or space even if you think another lifter is done with it; they may be using it again momentarily.
- As much as possible, don't step over barbells. This is a nit-picky one, but it's considered by many to be a sign of disrespect for the bar. Similarly, try not to walk across the platforms when in transit in the gym if possible; try to walk in front or behind them if you can.
- Don't lift at the same time as another lifter, especially if they're nearby. It's distracting for the lifter, and a coach can only watch one lifter at a time.
- Be respectful of equipment and the facility. Use equipment properly and put it where it belongs when you're done. Clean it off when appropriate.
- Don't coach other lifters unsolicited, especially if they have coaches. And don't contradict that lifter's coach or be disrespectful if an athlete does ask you for advice. You may be wrong, and you may very well be missing an important part of the story.

How often should I train? Like how sore can you be and still show up?

How often you train depends on many things, such as what you're training for, how advanced you are, and how old you are. That said, you can train when you're sore. In fact, moving is the best thing you can do for soreness. If you're really sore, don't train as hard, but do something. Training frequently will improve your ability to recover.

I get to do lots of heavy-for-me doubles and triples, but the weight's still relatively light... how many weeks/months/etc. until this actually starts helping me with my sport?

The weight not being remarkably heavy doesn't necessarily mean it's not helping you improve your athleticism. Also, if the weight feels heavy for you, it's heavy. There's no magic numerical threshold where training suddenly becomes effective. It would be like saying the weights a 125 lb woman are lifting are not effective because they're less then the weights a 225 lb man are lifting.

What are light weights with many reps vs heavy weights with few reps doing to your muscles? Which is better for building strength?

Depending on how light and how many reps, they're developing muscular endurance and/or encouraging sarcoplasmic hypertrophy and strengthening connective tissue. Heavier weights are generally improving neurological function to increase strength and power and encouraging myofibrillar hypertrophy. The latter is better for increasing strength, but both have their places.

*Lifting Large ;) - so all the cues of "get back up top", "shoulders back up top", "keep the bar tight to the body" etc etc etc are all great, and I must be doing them wrong, but I feel like my lady friends are still in my way. Especially during pull exercises. *cringe* nothing more embarrassing then doing a pull right into your ta-ta's in a gym full of men....... Please help! I need to learn to keep my lady friends in check so I can continue to lift bigger weights! - of a different kind ;)*

Invest in smaller sports bras, which may be uncomfortable, but more comfortable than collisions with a barbell. You can also double up on sports bras. Basically, strap those things down as tightly as you can. In the snatch or clean, your mechanics need to improve. You need to move your body out of the way of the bar on the way under, and your lady friends are considered part of your body. Try some tall snatches and tall cleans to practice. If you're hitting them on pulls, add more weight so you can't high-pull it.

How do you determine whether an athlete should stick with their bodyweight/weight class, increase to a heavier weight class or decrease to a lighter weight class?

First you have to evaluate how competitive an athlete can be at the current weight class. The height of a lifter relative to the weight class will largely determine how effective he or she can be. You can see how you stack up with other lifters in your weight class casually, or you can actually find height ranges for each weight class put together by Soviet researchers.

Next you have to consider how easily a lifter can gain or lose weight. For some athletes, moving weight classes will be prohibitively difficult, in which case the issue is moot. Also consider how a lifter feels at a given weight. An athlete may seem to need to increase a class or decrease a class based on height, but when it's tried, the lifter feels terrible and doesn't move as well. This has to be considered along with the height indices to get the full picture.

Is it better to do two-a-days a couple days a week if you're training in another sport, to have extra rest days, or would you just stick to 3X Oly and 3X other sport?

Most athletes who have reasonably sound training, nutrition and rest regimens can handle training 5-6 days/week, so the two pursuits can be split into individual days. Double days would be appropriate if combining two relatively short workouts, or if scheduling outside the training itself requires compressing the training into fewer days per week.

Is it better to go through bulking/strength and cutting/maintenance phases or just to stay close to your weight class while training? Which will yield the greatest net strength/power gains?

I prefer lifters to say close to their weight class limit. You can still alternate strength-emphasis phases with more classic-lift-emphasis phases (as normally occurs in weightlifting macrocycles), but you don't want to treat it like bodybuilding and gain a huge amount of weight just to cut down. There is really no off-season in weightlifting, so the scheduling is much different, making such swings in bodyweight much tougher and less effective anyway.

How do you get the bar to the hip on cleans? The only way i can manage is a very minute break at the elbows. It feels like a much more solid position because i'm able to hit much higher but i know that will only go so far as my biceps will eventually not be able to pull.

Ideally you can keep the elbows straight and the arms relaxed and still have the bar contact closer to the hips. The three basic parts of this are having a wider grip, retracting and slightly elevating the shoulders near the top of the pull, and staying over the bar longer. These things will all allow the bar to come into contact higher on the thigh.

I can power clean way more than I can front squat. What's my problem?

You need to squat and clean more and power clean less. This is a much simpler problem than many people in your position believe it to be. More emphasis on squatting will increase your squat strength. More emphasis on power cleans will just increase the gap. Back off the power cleans for a while and do only cleans until you improve the ratio.

Can I still do 2 or 3 conditioning workouts a week?

You can do whatever you like, but understand that the greater the specificity of your training, the greater the rate of improvement will be, and the greater the ultimate degree of development will be. Aside from that, your body will be able to handle a certain total amount of training in a given period of time. Doing 2-3 conditioning workouts per week means the amount of weightlifting training will have to reduced to accommodate this, which means less progress in weightlifting.

How beneficial are overhead squats?

How beneficial or necessary they are depends largely on the athlete in question. For newer lifters, they're very helpful if not completely necessary. For more advanced athletes who are technically proficient, adequately mobile, and are strong in a manner specific to weightlifting, they may be completely unnecessary.

Will knee wraps make me stronger?

Technically, no. They will allow you to squat more by helping you rebound from the bottom position. Squatting more weight will help you get stronger generally speaking. The caveat is that the additional strength you develop in this manner will be incomplete in a sense because the wraps will reduce how much muscular force is needed to perform the movement in the lowest position of the squat. This is not necessarily a large amount or a problem, but you will notice a significant difference with and without them.

How often should you max?

It completely depends on the level of athlete, the goals for the training cycle, the date relative to competition, the size and age of the athlete, etc. During competition or pre-competition training mesocycles, a lifter may take max attempts multiple times per week. During preparation mesocycles, it's likely a lifter will not attempt max lifts for as many as 4-12 weeks. Obviously there are different programming styles, and some would have you taking max or near max attempts 3-6 days/week indefinitely. Each athlete needs to find what approach is most effective for him- or herself.

What is the best jerk method? Squat style or split style.

The split jerk is by far the most common choice of competitive weightlifters for very simple reasons. It allows a lifter to get fairly low under the bar while still being able to stand again, creates the broadest base of support possible in all directions, requires the least flexibility, and has the largest margin for error. The power or push jerk must be more precise in terms of barbell placement overhead and body position and the bar must be driven higher. The squat jerk requires the same kind of precision of bar placement but also a degree of flexibility that few lifters possess, along with requiring a huge amount of leg strength to be able to stand from potentially a dead stop at the bottom of a squat with a weight that you likely just struggled to clean.

Should you snatch or attempt to snatch if you have limited overhead mobility and a crappy squat?

You can do light snatches or power snatches to start working on the mechanics, but you should not be lifting heavy weights (even relatively so) if you don't have a structurally sound overhead and squat position.

In terms of developing/perfecting form...when/how do you differentiate between those who need to improve by just performing the full lifts more frequently, and those who need to supplement with auxiliary lifts/work to address weaknesses?

Case by case ultimately, but I don't believe any beginner who is in that much need of technical learning or improvement should be just doing the classic lifts. Even Ivan Abadjiev, the coach who created the "Bulgarian system" has said explicitly that it's not appropriate for kids and beginners. New lifters need to perform the lifts, of course, but accessory work like squatting, pulling and pressing variations will always have a place in their development. Generally, the newer the lifter, the smaller the volume of the competition lifts and the greater the volume of accessory work.

It seems I'm everything but explosive & am more slow twitch! How should I approach weightlifting to get the best results?

Basically the same way as everyone else, you just won't ever be as explosive as someone born with a higher ratio of fast-twitch muscle fibers. You can help yourself a bit by reducing or eliminating slow-twitch training (e.g. endurance and high-rep work), doing more explosive accessory work like jump variations, and training with lower reps, always focusing on maximal concentric speed.

Does weightlifting make girls look manly?

No, testosterone does. The majority of women will never have enough testosterone to have truly masculine physical development without exogenous supplementation. Additionally, "manly" is a rather subjective description. If by "manly" you mean having any kind of visible musculature, then yes, weightlifting will probably make you look manly over time. However, I would say that, while not unheard of, this is a severe opinion and women, from my perspective, look better and still completely feminine with some muscle. Women with no muscle don't look more femine, they just look prepubescent. This aside, it seems horribly depressing to me to think of foregoing an activity you may love because of an unfounded fear of a few uncultured men potentially not finding you attractive.

THE 10 MINUTE RULE: SIMPLISTIC GUIDLINES FOR EFFICIENTLY SCALING CROSSFIT WORKOUTS
RYAN ATKINS

If you're a CrossFit coach, you've likely heard this question over and over again. "How much weight do I use?" Or, if you've just shown your client the gamut of pull-up or handstand push-up modifications, they respond, "Yeah, but which version do I use?" Astute clients will realize that depending on how they approach the scaling of their workout, they might end up with light weights and exercises that are very easy to perform and don't require much rest at all for large number of repetitions or, alternatively, tasks that are extremely challenging and that need to be chopped up into mini-sets and rest breaks right from the beginning of the workout. Which is better, one might ask. Well, in the context that CrossFit is a program touting the benefits of general physical preparedness and the discussion is revolving around a single workout, "both" would be an appropriate answer. A workout scaled towards the easy side of things allows for quicker repetitions for the exercises and transitions between them, thereby emphasizing speed, stamina and endurance. Workouts that require extended breaks every couple of repetitions won't stress those same traits, but the work/rest ratio might start to resemble that of a strength based workout. Given CrossFit's goals, both of these workout's effects are important aspects to consider in overall training design. And ultimately we want a good portion of our workouts to fall somewhere between these two extremes.

The real mistake is made when a client consistently leans towards the same extreme, workout after workout after workout. Pretty much every gym owner will nod in knowing acknowledgment when a frustrated trainer discusses how Client A, despite always finishing first in the group class conditioning cycle, fights tooth and nail against adding 5 pounds to the barbell (you know, they don't want to get 'bulky') to start closing the gap (usually substantial) towards the Rx'd weights. Although not as common, another subset of clients insist on ALWAYS 'going Rx' (or even 'scaling up' via added weight or exercise difficulty). In this case, Client B slugs through the workout at a snail's pace but usually reminds onlookers (those that stuck around for the hour after class ended, anyway) just exactly how much weight they were moving.

At CrossFit Level One certifications, participants are instructed that workouts need to be scaled to ensure that the highest level of power output is achieved. Now we could start busting out the tape measure, calculating distances for barbells and bodies moved, but I'm guessing most clients won't be overly hyped about using class time to do this. Consider the possibility that many clients frequenting CrossFit gyms are professionals during the day and might just be coming to CrossFit to shut down that part of the brain for a while. CrossFit has traditionally used the stopwatch to measure the proficiency of and improvements in our athletes. It's arguable that this stopwatch has to have some guidelines in order to maximize the efficacy and feasibility for a good portion of our conditioning circuits, especially in the context of group workouts.

This is where the 10-Minute Rule comes into play and it provides a good number of benefits via the following:

- Giving a decent performance goal for a good number of classical CrossFit benchmarks and some easily adaptable workout variations discussed below.
- Giving trainers and clients alike an easy-to-follow game plan towards keeping a balanced approach towards steady progress to achieve those goals. The lightweight speed demons moving through workouts at a blazing pace are required to work towards heavier weights and/or more challenging exercises until they can proudly boast (hopefully to themselves and not others), "Yeah, did you notice I Rx'd that stuff? I'm so boss!" On the other side of things, slower moving monsters will realize that they might want to reasonably reel things back so they don't get a DNF next to their name as a result of a time cap.
- Reducing the chances of over-training. Unless we need to specialize for something longer, it's usually smart training to restrict the metcon to 10-15 minutes 90% of time.
- Reducing injuries, especially for people new to high intensity interval training. A shorter workout interval provides a better potential cut-off point, beyond which fatigue can lead to serious form degradation.
- Contributing towards more efficient group class planning and execution. This is especially the case when a coach may be working with a larger group whose capabilities may not be well known. One option is to have a 10-minute cap regardless of how far a person gets into the workout. This option works well for teams, military units or other large groups where having a huge span of finishing times might not always fit into the group's schedule. This benefit also makes sense in the light that most CrossFit gyms with effective programming usually incorporate some sort of strength/power work as part of their class. Given the time needed for general warm-ups, skill work and this strength/power work, a 10-minute metcon makes sense on most days for an hour-long class, in addition to the benefits listed above.

Here's how the 10-minute rule is applied:

- Clients work with the trainer to come up with a workout that is challenging but doable. In the beginning, this will largely be based off of a trainer's evaluation of movement and ability of the client (this makes sense if the client is new to this type of training – they won't have a reference point). Let's use the benchmark Fran as our example. A reasonable goal is for the trainer to set things up where the client can make it through about 15 repetitions of the thruster before they start questioning just exactly why they are doing this workout.
- The client works their way through the workout. Their performance will be used as a guideline for the structuring of future efforts with that particular benchmark.
- If they completed the circuit under the 10 minutes, then the next time they come across it, they work towards getting the Rx version of the workout, if they don't already have it. In the case of Fran, maybe they add five pounds to the bar, or choose a slightly thinner band for the pull-up assist.
- If they took over 10 minutes to finish, then they will stick with the same modifications and try to bring their time under that range the next time they perform that workout. Alternatively, coaches may opt for the 10-minute cut-off rule, in which case the client would attempt to complete, or at least progress further into the workout, than they did during the 10 minutes this time around.

Which Workouts Should I Use? Conquering the Storms

Fran, Elizabeth, Diane, Grace, Annie and Isabel are among the first of the classical CrossFit storms. They are also great examples of the type of minimal input, maximal return type of workout that we're looking to use for the 10-minute rule. Now I realize that when the client eventually obtains sub 10 minute scores doing the Rx versions of these workouts, they might not exactly be ready for Regionals, but they've likely obtained some pretty significant milestones in their fitness journey compared to where they started.

Some other classics that are a little more challenging to finish within the time frame when done as written include Helen, Jackie, and Christine. They differ from the other workouts in that, although it's possible for them to be completed in less than 10 minutes, you won't see further significant improvement (i.e. into the 3-5 minute range) like you can with the other workouts mentioned as athletes approach more of a top tier status.

Which Workouts Should I Use? Part 2: Adding a Piece of 'Heaven'

There's one thing that all of the workouts mentioned so far lack – burpees!!! We'll correct that oversight in this section. In about 2008, a trainer I was working with introduced me to a workout entitled 'Seventh Heaven.' It consists of seven rounds done for time of seven thrusters, seven pull-ups and seven burpees, and is one of those that look deceptively simple when written on the board, but is brutal in application. The addition of the third exercise and (slight) increase in the volume of the other two make this a great step-up once someone already has an Rx'd Fran under 10 minutes. I've also used variations of this workout modeled after Elizabeth (cleans/ring dips/burpees), Diane (deadlifts/handstand push-ups/burpees), Nancy (overhead squats/10' shuttle runs/burpees) and Helen-ish (heavy swings/pull-ups/burpees)

Which Workouts Should I Use? Part 3: 10 to 1s and Annie variations

Already did burpees this week? Need more options? Well, in that case you can take any of the couplet pairings (or make your own) and perform a 10 to 1 (first round, do 10 reps of each exercise, the next round, do 9 reps of each exercise, ending the workout with a single rep of each of the movements). This combo brings the total rep count to 55 reps, as opposed to 45 for some of the classics mentioned earlier, which increases the volume, but still falls within the rep range seen in for assistance exercises in some of the more well-known strength programs. If you want something even more challenging for this time range, incorporate a movement that has a higher cycle rate – burpees (or even, gasp, burpee pull-ups come to mind, as do hang cleans to press/jerk variations).

Need to get your double under game on? Annie, which involves a total of 150 reps of that exercise, is a good option, and once you have some decent skill with the jump rope, it should be fairly easy to finish under the 10-minute mark. As good as of a workout as it is, the spinal flexion (and implications for spinal health) involved in the same number of sit-ups will draw concern from some experts within the fitness community. Some will argue that heavy loading with a properly performed barbell movement will contribute more towards trunk stability/athleticism anyway. Pairing the 50-40-30-20-10 rep scheme for the double-unders with a 10-8-6-4-2 rep scheme for pretty much any of the barbell movements (no, Turkish get-ups don't qualify, sorry) gives a person to take the volume of a Grace or Isabel and adds another skill component to take things up a notch (once they've driven the scores of those two workouts into the sub-5 minute range or so). If they're not quite at that level athletically, this rep scheme set-up with a more basic movement, like front squats, deadlifts, or push-presses. Want to work bodyweight stuff? It's conceivable that pairing exercises besides sit-ups with the double-unders at the same rep range, like push-ups or air squats, would make workable options. Pull-ups probably aren't the best option, at least on a regular basis in this scheme, unless you are practicing for the CrossFit Games or are looking to obtain the same results with your clients' hands that Tony Robbins gets with his clients' feet (hint: hot coals + feet = no bueno).

Conclusion

It's arguable that one of the best things that CrossFit brought to the fitness table in the early 2000s was the popularization of high intensity interval circuit using elements of weightlifting, bodyweight calisthenics and/or short bursts of what was normally considered cardio (running, rowing, etc.). The addition of measuring the duration of the workouts became a great motivating tool, as was the concept of the shared group workout. Both helped to bring out the competitive nature of clients, which in turn helped drive results. I remember during the programming portion of some of the early CrossFit Level 1's that if you were forced to choose to work only one pathway, it would be best to go with the glycolytic as it lended itself towards improvements to both of the other pathways – phosphagen and oxidative. This held true to a large degree, especially for people new to some of the movements involved. As the years progressed, some coaches observed that those with a good foundation of strength would ultimately perform like monsters during metabolic workouts, once a tolerance was established. It's now more and more common to see affiliates using some sort of strength program as a prelude to the conditioning circuits that follow. The form that it takes varies (Westside, Starting Strength, CrossFit Football, Wendler, Olympic lifting, etc.), but it's often there in some way, shape or form. Given the additional time spent in class working on that modality compared to the earlier years, the 10 minute rule provides a format that will help to efficiently manage time, set goals, push results, and get the most of the glycogen pathway-based workouts while allowing for consistency of training.

IMMUNOLOGY AND EXERCISE
BRIAN TABOR

It's the time of year when goals are made and determination is renewed. We all hit the gym excited and overzealous to make 2013 the best fitness year ever. It's also wintertime, though; the time of year when people spread germs, get sick, run fevers, and lose progress or motivation to achieve their fitness goals. There are numerous factors that go into how likely you are to get sick, your fitness and exercise being a couple of them, and a bunch of super sciencey physiological things, too. In an effort to help you achieve your goals with fewer bumps along the way, it helps to have some understanding of how training affects your immune system and what you can do to avoid getting sick this winter.

The immune system is a very complicated matter and studying the effects of exercise with regards to infection has proven to be a difficult task. Many of the studies to date present contradictory results, and changes in particular measures don't always correlate with risk of infections as nicely as we might like. But we can start by looking at some of the markers of immune stress that are commonly measured and their roles in resisting infections and illness. There are several types of immunological agents or markers that are commonly investigated with regards to exercise, but we'll focus on leukocytes, cytokines, and immunoglobulins.

Leukocytes actually refer to white blood cells, which are then differentiated into a variety of subcategories based on the function of the cell in defending the body from outside pathogens and germs. Natural killer cells are one such subcategory of leukocytes, which act as one of the first lines of defense for the body. They destroy other infected cells without the need for specific antibodies; sort of like a rogue agent that gets to shoot first and ask questions later. Strenuous resistance training has been shown to result in an immediate increase in the number of white blood cells circulating in the blood stream (including NK cells), but during recovery, these white blood cell counts drop below baseline levels measured prior to training. [3,5,7]. This effect has been shown to last for hours after exercise. The resulting decrease in Dirty Harry-esque immune cells could potentially be an increased risk factor for infection after demanding training days.

Cytokines are a type of proteins that act as signaling molecules in the body. There are many types and these proteins play a big role in signaling both proinflammatory and anti-inflammatory responses. Recovery and adaptations from resistance training as well as general immune function both rely on these types of signaling molecules to mediate the response from various types of cells and organs within our body. Whether its a response to mediate a cleanup of muscle damage and activate protein synthesis pathways or a signal for your immune system to destroy cells infected by virus, cytokines work to flip the switch for these types of cell functions and pathways. After resistance training, though, circulation of cytokines signaling both types of responses are increased [4]. Whether or not this interferes or enhances the immune response following exercise remains to be seen, because it is unclear if the increased levels of cytokines due to exercise would enhance a response by the immune system or compete with it to enable certain signaling pathways and actions.

Finally, immunoglobulins are antibodies that label foreign particles and germs by binding with them. This allows for certain types of leukocytes to identify foreign and potentially infectious particles within the body and destroy them appropriately. Immunoglobulin A or IgA is an immunoglobulin found in saliva that is commonly measured to assess immune function and stress. It has been shown that salivary IgA levels are also reduced after prolonged bouts of resistance training lasting two hours. [4] This reduced level of salivary IgA potentially makes it more difficult for the body to label and identify foreign pathogens that enter the body, which could be yet another increased risk for infection.

In addition to studies investigating the effects of training on various components of the immune system, epidemiological studies have shown that runners engaging in high mileage training or races are at higher risk for upper respiratory infections. [2] A more recent study however, has shown that increased rates of illness could potentially be resultant of a lack of adequate recovery from prior illnesses before engaging in high intensity and duration running again, i.e. competing in a marathon. [1] No studies have looked at incidence of infection among predominantly strength-based athletes. However, studies examining the effects of aerobic exercise and the effects of resistance training have resulted in similar changes to leukocytes and immunoglobulins. It is reasonable to expect similar risks to infection so long as training is sufficiently strenuous in terms of volume and intensity.

Training status also plays a role in how exercise affects the immune system. As with DOMS or muscle damage, it seems that immune system factors are also subject to the repeated bout effect. When researchers have subjects repeat the same resistance training protocols and leukocytes are examined a second time, the effects of exercise on leukocyte concentrations are attenuated. [6] The body adapts so that the stress of exercise is reduced after repeated bouts. Seasoned lifters may not experience as much increase in risk of infection as noobs unless they are training to greater absolute volumes and intensities than they are accustom to.

All of this information ultimately leads to some very common sense interventions to be taken during this season of resolution chasing and germ swapping. If you are new to resistance training and exercise, by all means start easy and try to focus on learning based strength gains. Most initial adaptations will be neural in nature, so there is no need to risk illness by crushing the body. If you are an experienced lifter, be sure to take precautions after strenuous training days. Limit your exposure to the elements when you are still sweaty, and make sure to get plenty of sleep, food and recovery time in between training sessions. And remember, gyms are veritable petri dishes for the recent edition of the cold or flu. Wash your hands.

Notes
1. Ekblom, B, Ekblom O, Malm C. Infectious episodes before and after a marathon race. Scand Journ Med Sci in Sports. 2006;16(4): 287-293.
2. Heath GW, Ford ES, Craven TE, Macera CA, Jackson KL, Pate RR. Exercise and the incidence of upper respiratory tract infections. Med Sci Sports Exerc. 1991;23(2):152-157.
3. Kraemer WJ, Clemson A, Triplett NT, Bush JA, Newton RU, Lynch JM. The effects of plasma cortisol elevation on total and differential leukocyte counts in response to heavy-resistance exercise. Eur J Appl Physiol Occup Physiol. 1996;73(1-2):93-97.
4. Nieman DC, Davis JM, Brown VA, et al. Influence of carbohydrate ingestion on immune changes after 2 h of intensive resistance training. J Appl Physiol. 2004;96(4):1292-1298.
5. Nieman DC, Henson DA, Sampson CS, et al. The acute immune response to exhaustive resistance exercise. Int J Sports Med. 1995;16(5):322-328.
6. Pizza FX, Baylies H, Mitchell JB. Adaptation to eccentric exercise: neutrophils and E-selection during early recovery. Can J Appl Physiol. 2001;26(3):245-253.
7. Simonson SR, Jackson CG. Leukocytosis occurs in response to resistance exercise in men. J Strength Cond Res. 2004; 18(2):266-271.

CREATING AN ANNUAL PLAN
STEVE BAMEL

I've said this before, but you are going to hear it again. All exercise works, but unless you've been getting results, with the same people, for years, do not tell me that your haphazard, instinctual training program is the best thing since bacon. Only a properly structured plan will work and produce continued results over time. With that being said, I am now going to teach you how to get these results, not for the first day, not for the first week, not for the first year, but continual results for years to come. These results all start with the Annual Plan. The Annual Plan is THE MOST IMPORTANT STEP IN PRODUCING RESULTS. Have a goal, set up an Annual Plan and follow through. It is the overall game plan that takes you to the promised land of championships, greatness, jackedness, rippedness, and beastmodeness. Yes, those are all words.

What you are looking at is an Annual Plan that I set up for a Track and Field athlete that completed in throwing, sprinting and jumping events. Where did the template come from? It is a combination of, the best parts of, a few coaches' templates that I have come across during my career. These were all great coaches, all taught me a thing or two, and now I'm passing their knowledge, along with a bit of my own on to you.

I build out an annual plan from top to bottom, from the most basic details of the year, to more specific details, while keeping in mind that it's still just a plan to follow, it never gets too specific (sets/ reps/ weights/ exercises/ etc.), and that the actual workouts will be built off this, but that this is not the actual workout card.

The first category that I fill out is the number of training weeks the athlete has leading up to their most important competition. It could be the Superbowl, World Series, Olympic Final, etc., etc. In the plan I have above, we had 47 weeks, so I labeled them 1-47 in the category labeled Weeks. Complex, I know.

The next category I fill out is Dates. The dates correspond to the first day of each training week for the athlete. Usually I start training weeks on Mondays, but in some cases they may start on a different day, so I use that category as a guide.

After Dates, I fill out Stage. The Stage category refers to the stage of training that will be taking place during those weeks. Each stage will typically have a different number of weeks in it, so this helps me to lay out how each one will transition into the next. The stages I have above are pretty typical for one of my training programs. I begin all training programs with the General Physical Preparedness phase (GPP). It is during this phase that we prepare the athletes' bodies for the workouts, as well as practices, and the competitive season. I won't go any deeper into what happens during the GPP Phase, as I wrote an article for the PM a few months back titled , GPP for Athletes: The Lost Training Phase, so if you want more info on that, go read it.

Quick note: You will see a sub category called Program under the Stage category. This is just a quick reference I use for any notes that I will need when programming out the Stage. In this category, you will start to see where I program in the active rest and unload weeks. Remember, you are setting up an Annual Plan to give you a guide for your athlete and where to take their training. It's your guide. Make any changes you need to the template to make it work better for you. Put categories in, and take them out. I've seen way more and way less detailed annual plans. The important thing here is that you find the plan that works best for you.

After the GPP Phase, the athlete should be prepared for the heart of the Off-Season Training Program, which I call the Developmental Stage. This is the time where the athlete is going to make the most strides in raising their ceiling of potential. What I mean by ceiling of potential is they are going to raise the ceiling of their physical capabilities. Power, speed, strength, etc., all going to increase. So the potential for success in their sport is going to increase. However, it is only their potential ceiling because without specific sport preparation, it will mean nothing. Think of the strongest offensive lineman on a football team who doesn't start or even see the field because their blocking techniques are terrible. Because they are really strong, their potential is high, but because they are terrible at their sport, it means nothing.

During the Developmental Phase, we can do the most amount of work with the athlete, and have the least amount of distractions from travel, family, and competitions. You will see that my developmental period was 13 weeks, with an active rest week coming only five weeks into the stage. If you look up to the Dates category, you will see why I programmed active rest that week. That week corresponded with New Year's. In this case, the athlete decided to train through Christmas and to rest and see family the week of New Year's. I gave him the choice of what week he wanted to train and what week he wanted to rest, but I gave him that choice while sitting down and looking at the Annual Plan. I showed him that his previous active rest week was for Thanksgiving and that if he took off for Christmas, then he would have only gotten in 3 weeks of training before another rest week and how 4 weeks would be a more ideal situation for his training. By laying out the Annual Plan in front of him, it allowed him to make a better decision for his career. Without the visual aid to show him, I'm sure it would have been a way tougher argument for me to get him to train through Christmas.

After programming the Stage and Program phases, we come to the most important category: the Competition Stage. Barring any unforeseen last-minute changes, this schedule must be set in stone. In the case of a track and field athlete, you need to know which meets they will be training through and which meets to peak them for. For team sports, you will need to know when to start pulling the reigns in because conference tournaments, playoffs, etc. will be coming up.

The next Category is the Microcycle. This describes, more specifically, what will be happening during that week of training. A base week is a week that I am introducing something new. A load week is a week that we are getting after it. An active rest week is a week that the athlete will perform non-weight room workouts. An unload week is a light week in the weight room, and a maintenance week is a week that the athletes training percentages will be something that I know they can hit without a problem.

After the Microcyles, I then punch in the priority of training for that week, listed in order. Looking at the chart, for the first 5 weeks, we were in our GPP phase. That is our only focus. After the active rest week that followed the GPP Phase, we moved to a period where ME (Max Effort) training was the primary priority, RE (Repetitive Effort) work was the secondary priority, and DE (Dynamic Effort) was the tertiary priority. As the weeks progress, you will see the priorities of training switched, depending on what is most important during that time. DE will moved up, ME will moved down, and as we got into the most important part of the season, RE fell off to reduce the amount of volume on the athletes bodies.

I include Holidays as a separate section as we will train right through them, but we may need to adjust training schedules. As far as Uncontrollable Factors goes, these are things we can't plan for and 95% of the time it's something to do with the airlines. I include this only because if we get really twisted around and I have to make changes in the plan because of this, I will make a note of it in the plan so that after the season when I go back and look over the entire body of work, I can see why changes were made. The last three sections are all the actual working percentages that I will use for training during each Microcycle.

This is the exact plan that I will set up and review with the athletes and sport coaches prior to beginning training. During the offseason, everything is meticulously planned out as we cross our t's and dot our lower case j's (bonus if you know what movie that's from). As we get into season, I plan out the training percentages prior to the next week. I do this so that I can take into account any and all factors that may affect the workouts for that upcoming week. Travel days, fatigue, poor nutrition on the road, etc. Everything that is not recovery is something that is breaking the body down, which in turn is something that will affect training. It would be impossible to account for that, months in advance.

This article is solely about setting up training plans for athletes. However, the principles are the same no matter who you are, and what you are training for. Figure out your goals, set up your plan and then work that plan. Once you've completed your plan, look back at it, see where you could've gotten better results from, make the changes and work that plan again. By doing this, you will ensure continued results for as long as you are willing to put in the effort.

WEEK	DATE	STAGE	PROGRAM	COMPETITION	Microcycle	Priority of Training	HOLIDAYS	Uncontrollable Factors/ Notes
1	Oct. 22	GPP	GPP		Ana. Adapt	1=GPP		
2	Oct. 29				Ana. Adapt	1=GPP		
3	Nov. 5				Ana. Adapt	1=GPP		
4	Nov. 12				Ana. Adapt	1=GPP		
5	Nov. 19				Ana. Adapt	1=GPP		
6	Nov. 26				Active Rest		Thanksgiving 11/22	
7	Dec. 3	Developmental	Strength 1		Base	1=ME 2=RE 3=DE		
8	Dec. 10				Load	1=ME 2=RE 3=DE		
9	Dec. 17				Load	1=ME 2=RE 3=DE		
10	Dec. 24				Load	1=ME 2=RE 3=DE		
11	Dec. 31				Active Rest		Christmas 12/24,25	
12	Jan. 7		Strength 2		Base/ Unload	1=ME 2=RE 3=DE	New Years 12/31,1/1	
13	Jan. 14				Load	1=ME 2=RE 3=DE		
14	Jan 21				Load	1=ME 2=RE 3=DE		
15	Jan. 28				Load	1=ME 2=RE 3=DE	MLK Day 1/21	
16	Feb. 4		Strength 3		Base/ Unload	1=ME 2=RE 3=DE		
17	Feb. 11				Load	1=ME 2=RE 3=DE		
18	Feb. 18				Load	1=ME 2=RE 3=DE		
19	Feb. 25				Load	1=ME 2=RE 3=DE	Pres. Day 2/18	
20	Mar. 3	SSP			Unload			
21	Mar. 10		Strength/ Power	SDSU 3/14-3/15	Maint	1=ME 2=DE 3=RE		
22	Mar. 17				Load	1=ME 2=DE 3=RE		
23	Mar. 24			ASU 3/28-3/29	Maint	1-DE 2-ME		
24	Mar. 31			Pomona 4/5	Maint	1-DE 2-ME		
25	Apr. 7	Competitive	In-Season 1- Power	Sun Angel 4/11-4/12	Maint	1=DE 2=ME		
26	Apr 14			Mt. Sac Relays 4/17-4/20	Maint	1=DE 2=ME		
27	Apr. 21			UCSD 4/25-4/28	Maint	1=DE 2=ME		
28	Apr. 28			Steve Scott 5/3	Maint	1=DE 2=ME		
29	May. 4			OXY 5/10	Maint	1=DE 2=ME		
30	May. 11				Load	1=DE 2=ME		
31	May. 18			Home Depot 5/18	Maint	1=DE 2=ME		
32	May. 25				Unload	1=DE 2=ME	Mem. Day 5/25-26	
33	Jun. 2		In-Season 2	Endeavor 6/5	Unload	1=DE		
34	Jun. 9			US Olympic Trials 6/13	Unload	1=DE		
35	Jun. 16				Load	1=DE		
36	Jun. 23				Load	1=DE		
37	Jun. 30			Canadian 7/3	Maint	1=DE	July 4th	
38	Jul. 7		In-Season 3- Power		Load	1=DE 2=ME		
39	Jul. 14			USATF 7/16	Maint	1=DE 2=ME		
40	Jul. 21			USATF &/23	Maint	1=DE 2=ME		
41	Jul. 28			USATF 7/30	Maint	1=DE 2=ME		
42	Aug. 4		In-Season 4	Korea/ China Paralympic Team Training—Beijing (/6		1=DE		
43	Aug. 11					1=DE		
44	Aug. 18					1=DE		
45	Aug. 25					1=DE		
46	Sep. 1					1=DE		
47	Sep. 8					1=DE		

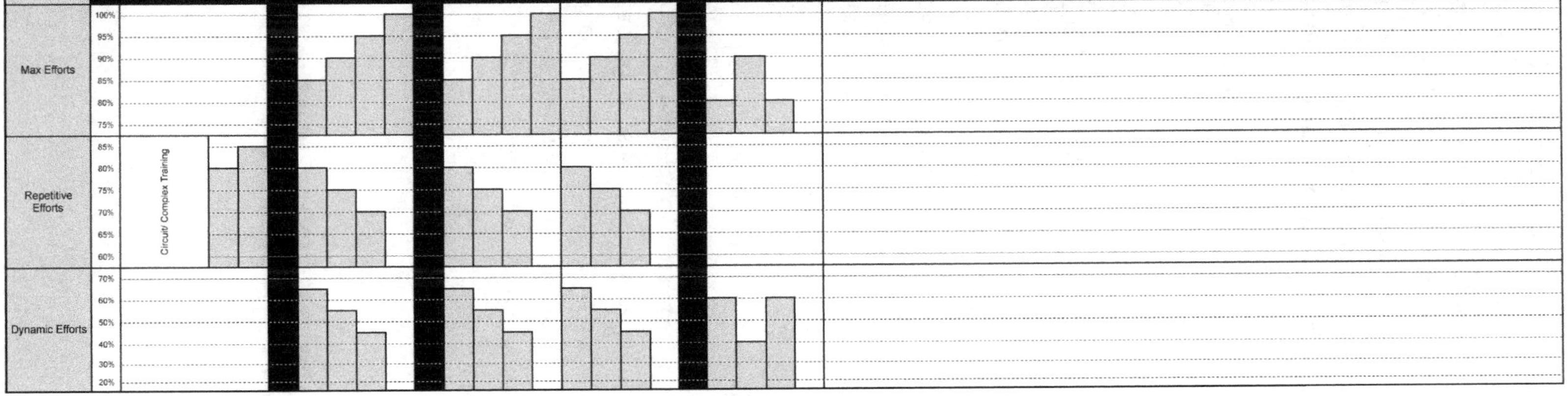

Max Efforts
100%
95%
90%
85%
80%
75%
Repetitive Efforts
85%
80%
75%
70%
65%
60%
Circuit/ Complex Training
Dynamic Efforts
70%
60%
50%
40%
30%
20%

DEVELOPING INDEPENDENCE IN A GROUP ATHLETIC SETTING
KYLE J SMITH

Imagine that you've been a student in a CrossFit or group training class for a while now. As these modes grow in popularity, you've noticed more and more strangers wandering into your gym. You're happy to see them, of course; they keep the place in business. But transitioning a new person into an established community can often be difficult. What can you do to help make their transition as easy as possible, while meeting your own needs? And if you're that new person, how do you make the situation as easy as possible for everyone? And if you're the coach, how do you make sure the regulars are happy and the newbies are engaged and hooked? Below is a list of ideas with the reasoning behind each one.

But before we get there, let's all agree on one thing: group training can never be perfect. There, I said it. I make my living off of group training classes, and I'm not ashamed to say the system is not perfect. Do I think it's one of the best possible solutions considering money, time, enjoyment and other variables? Hell yes. But do I think it's perfect? Nope. By realizing some of its imperfections, and then fighting the good fight towards peace and productivity, I think the everyday athlete can get a ton of value out of well-run group training classes.

Now let's get on to that list. (Each idea is shared with the athlete; some of them include notes for the coach at the end.)

Keep a workout journal, and then actually stick to it.

Wanna be stronger? Move more weight than last time. Wanna be faster? Do things quicker than last time. (Excuse my gross oversimplification.) Don't know what you did last time? Well there's your problem. Keep track of your weights, times and scores, and then do what your coach says. If you're hearing "Try to work up to a heavier weight than last time we were exposed to this movement," then actually try to do what's suggested.

Coaches: To keep an eye on your athletes' progress, consider having them log their scores into an online application. Make it easy for them to track, too. (At the end of each workout, I email my athletes a picture of the whiteboard so they can input it into their journals.) To keep them accountable, consider a pop quiz. "You guys should have these numbers written down somewhere. Can you show them to me now?" No? 15 burpees, please.

Come prepared.

On day one, it's okay to be wearing dress shoes. Everyone forgets their water bottle. It's funny the first time you whine because you didn't look at the blog to see what the workout was, and your coach won't mind if you stop him after his introduction to say, "Wait a minute, I have to pee." But come day two, all of the small flubs become pretty annoying. I don't say they're annoying because I hate n00bs. It's actually more annoying for the athlete because without the basic infrastructure in place and secured, you'll never have the productive, fun class you're paying for.

Make your needs known

Is your knee aching from a weekend ski trip? Back bothering you from pushing it too hard on "Diane" last week? Did you rip your hands practicing kipping yesterday? Your coach is happy to help you scale and modify, if they know that's what you need. Take a second to let them know while they refill their coffee cup before class, or as everyone is putting away their PVC pipes after the warm up.

Warm up what you need

A traditional warm-up starts generally, picks up the pace with some dynamic movement, and gets you ready for battle with specific focus. While the programming that follows is likely considering fine-tuned peaks and valleys that need to be respected, the warm-up is meant to do just that, warm up each individual athlete. A coach can write whatever he wants on the board, but he doesn't know exactly what your body needs. Change up the reps a little bit, add in some extra mobility (this is particularly important, as mobility differs so much from individual to individual), and unless they are purposefully adding extra volume into the warm-up, make sure you're not adhering to the advice of those terrible old t-shirts, "Our warm-up is your workout." (Hasn't everyone burned those by now?)

Ask questions

Is your coach Professor X? No? Then he probably can't read your mind. Do you have a question that you think is dumb? If you're following most of the advice shared here, it's probably not dumb. And even more importantly, it's likely that one of your newer classmates needs to know the answer even more than you do.

Coach: Make sure you're inviting questions regularly. As new students are familiarizing themselves with your style, they may be hesitant to "bother you" by asking questions, so make sure they know it's no bother at all; it's what you're getting paid to do!

Be a cheerleader

This advice came as a huge epiphany to me a couple of weeks ago. I was working out with a group, and thoroughly enjoying rooting on my fellow soldiers as we trudged through hell together. Why? Because I was in the moment of suck with them, and everything in my body was primed to "kick ass and take no prisoners." This is rarely a feeling you'll experience while coaching, and you probably shouldn't, as your attention needs to be spent elsewhere--dealing with priorities such as safety, range of motion, and intensity. If you encourage your students to be their own cheerleaders, the action will come from a more honest and excited place, freeing you up to focus on the important things.

Coaches: Consider designing workouts that allow your athletes to be cheerleaders while also getting a workout. Some examples include team workouts and intervals with staggered rest periods.

Trust your coach

Make them earn your trust, but once they have, give it happily. This trust goes for the big rocks like programming and recovery, and also the small rocks like "Please hold off on setting up your bars for the conditioning" and "Let's not do a toes to bar cash-out today." You're likely only focused on the day at hand due to all the other stressors in your life, whereas your coach is constantly considering the big picture, from next week to years down the road.

Give feedback, but don't whine.

Things never get better if there's not a constant flow of yays and nays, if many perspectives are not considered. Make certain your thoughts come in the form of "It's been my experience that... and I think the group would benefit from..." Then be open to hearing out your coaches on the reason behind their decision-making. Sometimes there's more to the picture than you're privy to.

Coaches: Be addicted to constructive criticism. One of the most important facets of your career is elite communication, so make sure you give and receive well.

Respect everyone's time

Don't live in a bubble. Every move you make in an hour-long class eats away at that hour for everyone, not just you. Make sure you're doing what you need to do in a timely manner, and be flexible in case things start to wander off the path.

Coaches: Tell your athletes what they need to know, and nothing more. Describing the journey of an entire class is going to leave folks confused and milling around at their heart's desire. Write instructions on the whiteboard as to exactly what time your athletes need to switch from one thing to another. That way there are no surprises and no one gets the rug pulled out from beneath them when you say, "It's time to move on."

Learn the curriculum

Coaches are happy to review technique for the snatch with a PVC pipe. They are less happy to remind half their class every time what a snatch is. Get the basics down so you can move on to the fun stuff sooner rather than later.

Coaches: We all know you've spent hours on the internet researching everything exercise since 1996. Share some of the more helpful resources with your students; coaching nerds with good questions is a challenging and rewarding experience.

Form meaningful relationships with the other athletes

Working out with friends who want to challenge and encourage you daily, and will hold you accountable, is a lot more fun than pumping iron with strangers. Get to know the other people you see regularly on a level that's a little deeper than, "What's your Fran time?"

Form a productive relationship with the coach

Your coach doesn't need to be your best friend, mom, pastor, counselor, alien overlord or dominatrix. Instead, he or she needs to be a classy conglomeration of all of these things. Give your coaches the respect they deserve, and the distance they desire, and let yourself learn from them everyday--I promise they're doing the same thing. Coach: Group training is strange in its ability to forge the most intense of relationships. The community and social aspect is vital. Just make sure you've drawn a clear line for yourself when it comes to these aspects. Do you see a relationship headed in the wrong direction? Consider pulling in your superior to douse the flame. And don't make any small decisions that leave your stomach even the tiniest bit queasy. That's your conscience talking to you.

Mind your manners

We get so caught up in other zone and hormonal surges that sometimes we forget not to be an asshole while working out. Don't be an asshole while working out. Were you an asshole to a fellow athlete or coach? Apologize.

Tailor the programming to your needs

"Needs" here ranges from duh to a bit controversial. When should you tailor the program to your needs?

1. Scaling: "Hang snatch 5x3" isn't super useful if you're not comfortable in an overhead squat. Should you do hang power snatch or overhead squat, though? Bring your coach in on the conversation.
2. Contraindication: If you tweaked your back last week, it may not be the best time to do heavy clean deadlifts. Let your coach know what's going on and have them help you assess your options.
3. Overexposure: Due to the way your schedule has fallen, have you done nothing but push presses over the past three weeks? Maybe your coach will deem it okay to perform horizontal rowing instead. Do make sure there's not a method behind their push press madness, though.

Learn how to be helpful

Logistically speaking, this is pretty easy to feel out--do what your coach says, when they say it, and help others out when you have a free hand (even if you're not their partner).

When it comes to coaching and cueing other athletes, it can be a little trickier. Some basic cues, derived from the objectives the coach laid forth at the beginning of class, are often great. More in-depth coaching may get you deep into territory that you're not ready for. Firstly, you aren't aware of the background of this athlete with the coach; perhaps they're working on specific things and won't be doing the same thing as everyone else for a while. And on the darker side of things, the coach is there to handle tricky and sticky situations involving athletes who have been struggling or underperforming for some time; you're just there to get your pump on with some buddies. If you see an athlete having a rough day or who clearly needs some extra guidance, grab a coach; they'll be happy to help.

Ask questions

Quick reminder here from a coach who is tired of trying to read minds. We, as coaches, want to be helpful. Your blank stares are rarely helpful. (I know it's early, 6:15 AM class, and I love you dearly.)

Listen to your body

Good programming will include balls to walls weeks, deload weeks, and a steady build. But no group program is perfect for an entire group. You must become master of your own domain, learn to perceive the signals your body is sending you so that you know intimately when you can push it, and when you need to rock and roll at 80 percent. Confused or worried about an ache or pain? Ask your coach first, then a doctor if necessary.

Always cool down

If any part of a class is going to get abbreviated for any reason, it's the cool down. Heading to the office with endorphins pumping and sweat dripping down your forehead is going to be uncomfortable and get your recovery off on the wrong foot. If your coach doesn't have a chance to lead the cool down, take a couple minutes on your own to stretch, roll or just walk. You'll feel much better all day because of it.

Coaches: Force yourself to constantly empathize with your students. Remember what it feels like to drudge through Karen or a run a 5k, then do your best to make your athletes comfortable when it's time to be comfortable. Remember to pull back as much as you push, to build up three times as much as you put down.

Learn outside of class

You may not have all day to read up and watch videos on exercise, but you can always take some of your free time to learn more about the goals you're pursuing. Take a few minutes to put your success in your own hands. You'll enjoy classes more when you understand more of the why behind the what.

Blame yourself

Is your group training not going as well as you'd like? Blame yourself first. Figure out what you can do to make the experience better for yourself and your peers. Then if it becomes clear, after a period of self reflection and non-gossipy conversations with some of your trusted classmates, that there are variables outside of yourselves that need addressing, find the most productive way to alleviate the issue.

Coaches: Blame yourself first. Are your athletes not doing what you would like them to do? Maybe your communication isn't up to snuff. Are you not seeing the results you'd like in your athletes? Perhaps there's something missing from your programming or extracurricular advice. Has coaching grown stagnant and boring? Push yourself to learn more, and start to add to your bag of tricks so that you can be the positive force you want to be for more people.

Bottom Line

The range of ideas shared here is pretty large, so how do you begin to implement them in your classes as a coach or athlete? Athletes, decide to make one change every week, and purposefully repeat it so that it becomes a habit. Coaches, don't be afraid to be didactic occasionally (especially if you tell good bad jokes.) Being independent in a group training session doesn't come naturally to everyone, and I'd bet a few people aren't going to read this article, so don't hesitate to share and do what you do best: coach.

HOW YOU ACT... AND WHY IT'S IMPORTANT
MATT FOREMAN

"Winning isn't everything. It's the only thing."

How's that for a cliché that's been beaten to death? We've all heard this quote more times than we can count. A lot of people think Vince Lombardi said it first, but I think it actually came from a college football coach at UCLA in 1950. Regardless of who said it, it's a load of crap. Winning isn't the only thing that matters in competitive sports, or life in general. Your actions, the way you behave, and your attitude are more important than winning. Much more important, if you want to know the truth.

Everybody who reads this can think of an athlete who wins a lot of contests, but also acts like a complete jackass. They're everywhere. When you watch these people, you don't really care that much about their championship titles or victories. The main thing you notice is their jackassness. You respect their ability, but not their character. It changes everything about how you see them. I'll even use myself as an example (and not in a good way). The only time my dad ever chewed me out after a weightlifting meet was when I was seventeen. It was the state championship, and I got pissed off after I attempted a new state record and failed. I took off my belt and threw it on the floor as I walked off the platform; everybody saw it. My dad ripped me a new one after it was over, telling me that I embarrassed myself and my family. He said I shouldn't even get on the platform to compete if I wasn't man enough to show some discipline and control when things don't go my way.

I won the meet, by the way. First place in my weight class and I also won the Best Lifter award. But all I remember about that day was disgracing myself and getting a verbal lashing from my dad. Everything he said was right, too. It didn't matter that I won the meet because I acted like an idiot in front of everybody. Like I said, winning isn't the only thing that matters.

Five or six years after that happened, I competed in a meet against a guy who had been a pretty big-name lifter. It was during a time period when I was still young and on the way up, and this other guy was starting to hit his downslide. I beat him, and you should have seen the tantrum he threw in the warm-up room afterwards. Kicking trash cans, throwing his shoes at the wall, screaming f--- so loud that the people in the audience could hear it. I remember looking at his wife while he was in the middle of it, seeing how embarrassed and ashamed she was. He wouldn't even come out and accept his second-place award. This was a grown man, by the way, not a seventeen year-old kid.

That stuff matters. When you lower your character to a point where other people lose their respect for you, it matters. It matters more than the color of your medal or seeing "1st" next to your name on the results sheet. What we're going to look at in this month's article is behavior.

When was the last time you got lectured about this area? Middle school, or maybe earlier? You're all adults and you're definitely past the point of needing little kiddie lessons about how to act. However, it doesn't hurt to hear a little reinforcement from time to time, especially if you're any kind of coach or administrator. The way you behave is either going to A) bring more clients to you or B) run them off. Trust me, your business can sink or swim based on the things you do and say. Knowing this, it's at least worth a few thoughts. And knowing that you found this magazine on the internet, why don't we start there?

Some ways to screw up your reputation online...

The internet. It's such an amazing thing, isn't it? It's one of the most important technological inventions in the history of civilization, no doubt about it. But it's one of those things you can love and hate at the same time, like reality TV or your spouse. One of the most fascinating aspects of the internet is that it gives you an opportunity to communicate with a whole new galaxy of douchebags you never knew existed. I can personally vouch for this. Some of the most incredible cornholes I've ever met in my life have popped up in my online travels. After arguing with them for a while, I have to assume their parents fed them a steady diet of paint chips when they were little.

Now, I learned a long time ago that a simple disagreement doesn't make anybody a moron. We all have our opinions, many of them are different, and most of us are pretty smart people. I'm cool with the idea that there's more than one way to look at something. When we're young, I think we tend to believe anybody who contradicts us is an idiot. That's not true. If you think that way, it's very possible you might be the idiot. However, as fair-minded as I like to think I've become, there's still one personality type I can't stomach. I'm talking about the schmucks who have basically zero experience in Olympic weightlifting, yet they write like they're experts who have the whole sport figured out. You could fit their weightlifting record on the back of a postage stamp but they'll still go on rants where they explain exactly what's wrong with OLifting in America...or offer some all-knowing analysis of how to become a world champion.

I hate to just come right out and say it, but your opinion on OLifting doesn't matter that much if you don't have any legitimate experience in it. Even if you've been highly successful in another strength field, you're not qualified to argue with people who have lived neck-deep in OL for years, produced high-level lifters, or had successful careers as athletes. Why the hell would you think you're a voice of authority in an area where you have almost zero accomplishment? Because you've read a lot of articles, watched a lot of videos, and even participated in it a little bit?

Listen; let's put this in a slightly different context. I like food a lot. I've been eating it for a long time, I know a few things about it, and I'm even a pretty decent cook. But you don't see me walking up to Rachel Ray and saying, "Hey you dumb skank, you don't know jack about cooking. Let me tell you how to do it right, because your food tastes like a bucket of goat balls."

I'm not gonna do that. Why? Because she's an expert in cooking and I'm not. I should be trying to learn from her, not argue with her.

And let's be fair. It's totally possible for somebody to have quality insight on something even if they don't have a big resumé in it. I'm not saying you have to lift in 30 meets or coach a national champion before you're allowed to open your mouth about weightlifting. That's not the point I'm making. You've got the right to get involved in any kind of weightlifting discussion that appeals to you, even if you're a total newbie, and you should be given basic human respect. Still, my personal opinion is that you should be trying to learn as much as possible when you're a beginner or intermediate lifter. It's probably not a good idea to argue with people who are much more qualified than you, and it's definitely not a good idea to posture yourself as an expert when you haven't really done anything important.

Also, let's wait a second before any of the paint-chip crowd jumps up and says, "Foreman's a jackass. He acts like he's a weightlifting expert, and it's not like he ever won a world championship or anything." Hold on, bubba. Put down the crack pipe. I'm not saying I'm the all-knowing voice of anything. I'm just a really attractive guy who's trying to give you some food for thought. That's all. Nobody is going to run to your gym to be coached by you if you're a reputed internet troll.

Back to non-internet behavior...

I watched a tennis match between Roger Federer and Rafael Nadal a few years ago. Federer lost…on TV…in front of millions of people. Afterwards, he shook Nadal's hand and congratulated him. In the post-match interview, he said, "I respect Nadal because he acts the same whether he wins or loses." That's good stuff right there.

If you're a coach, I believe it's your job to require honorable conduct from your athletes. You have to teach them to respect themselves, the sport, and their competitors.

You have to do this for two reasons. First, it's the right thing to do and everybody damn well knows it. Second, their shameful actions (if you allow them) reflect on you as the coach. Other people in the sport will see you the same way you see parents who let their brat kids run through a supermarket, screaming and knocking things over. You think these parents need to get smacked in the head with a brick, right? Correct, and the same goes for you if you let your athletes act like immature little morons.

Don't misunderstand this and think I'm saying that we should all act like boring zombies when we compete. I don't think that at all. I love it when athletes show emotion and go crazy after their successes. Screaming is cool. Jumping up and down is cool. It gets everybody fired up and adds excitement to the sport, both of which are good things. Go back and watch some old footage of Pyrros Dimas if you want to know what I'm talking about. And I also think it's good to get pissed off after you fail. I've said many times that I wouldn't give a plug nickel for somebody who screws up and isn't bothered by it. If you're gonna be a good athlete, you need to have zero tolerance for failure. Making mistakes has to bother you…a lot. But I don't think you should handle those mistakes by freaking out. Nothing good comes from that. Having an edge to your personality is good. Being a whack-job isn't.

Look, we're all competitive people and we all want to win. That's obvious. There's nothing better than fighting to the top of the mountain. It's also obvious that there are going to be people out there who have a different perspective on this whole issue. Some people think it's okay to act like a loose cannon, as long as you're still number one. They have the "you can say whatever you want if you're the best" mentality. I understand where they're coming from, and we can agree to disagree. This is just a little suggestion that maybe you should think about something more than just winning first-place medals. Maybe you should think about the example you set for others, and whether your actions make your example good or bad.

Does this sound like it's straight out of Sunday school? I don't know, maybe. Regardless of how preachy these ideas might be, you have to remember something if you're a business owner or a coach. People are either going to follow you, or they're not going to follow you. They'll follow you if you demonstrate the kind of qualities they respect and admire…the things they want to see in themselves. When you have this kind of personality and reputation, people will just start to show up more and more. Word of mouth will spread about you, and you'll start to get a lot of phone calls and emails from people who want to get in on what you're doing. These people will probably be the types you want to have around you, too.

I don't know many people who respect and admire immaturity, posturing, and mouthy foolishness. The people who follow these traits probably aren't the ones you're going to build a foundation for greatness on. If you're a tool, good people will see it and they won't follow you. You'll attract the bottom of the barrel, which is also where your gym will stay.

A final thought? I guess we leave with the simple idea that you should have a clear vision for what kind of identity you want people to associate with you. The whole "I don't give a f--- what anybody thinks about me, screw 'em all" thing? That's fine if you're pursuing a career in punk rock or professional wrestling. But if you plan to be a leader of others, it's probably smart to be a little more careful about how you behave. Just think about it. That's all I ask.

THE ELEMENTS OF A WEIGHTLIFTING TEACHING PROGRESSION
GREG EVERETT

The development of a teaching progression for the Olympic lifts is something that every coach who teaches the lifts will do one way or another—some will never move past the borrowing from others stage (which is fine, of course), others will gradually develop one over a long period of time (sometimes intentionally, sometimes just naturally), and others will set out right out of the gate to create an original progression (it may not be any good, but at least its original!).

This article will present some framework and foundational concepts that can be used to create your own teaching progression. This is based on the talk I gave at Ethan Reeve's annual clinic at Wake Forest University in January 2013.

Primary Elements

I consider there to be five primary elements of a teaching progression. That is, these are five things that must be addressed directly for the progression to be effective. These are positions, balance, posture, explosion mechanics, and relocation mechanics.

Positions

Squat

In the squat, the feet should be flat on the floor (this means fore and aft and side to side). This will be affected not only by general balance or imbalance, but also by the foot stance. For example, turning the toes out too much will often cause the feet to roll onto the inside edges, as will having too wide of a stance.

The spine should be in its neutral curvature or slightly hyperextended in the lumbar area and flattened in the thoracic area. The closer the trunk is to vertical, the closer the spine should be to neutral, as this is the position in which it best resists compressive force; the more forward the trunk is leaned, the more extended the spine should be (to its maximal degree of slight hyperextension) to both shorten the lever slightly, improve the ability of the spinal extensors to hold the spine in position, and create a hedge against injurious lumbar flexion.

The thighs should be approximately parallel to the feet—looking straight down at the thigh, it should be aligned with the foot and directly above it or very slightly inside of it. The hips should be open (thighs/feet turned out) to a degree that allows the athlete to sit into full depth with proper posture along with the proper alignment of the foot and thigh.

These positions will help ensure the optimal performance of the lifts, as well as help keep the lifter's joints safe.

Pull

In the pull of the snatch or clean, the lifter's spine should be extended slightly beyond the natural curve. The entire length of the spine is ideally set in a continuous arch by slightly hyperextending the lumbar spine and flattening the thoracic spine as much as possible.

The feet should be turned out slightly based on the athlete's comfort. Generally a stance that places the heels approximately under the hips is preferable, but this can be widened if the athlete feels it's more effective.

The arms should be internally rotated to orient the points of the elbows to the sides without the shoulders rounding forward. This will set the athlete up to relocate under the bar properly.

Overhead

In the overhead position of either the snatch or the jerk, the barbell should be located over the base of the neck with the head push forward slightly. The arms should be approximately vertical when viewed from the side. The shoulder blades should be retracted aggressively and upwardly rotated somewhat. This position can be achieved easily by attempting to squeeze the top inside edges of the shoulder blades together. The active and aggressive effort to maintain this scapular position creates a solid foundation for the arms to hold the bar.

The elbows must be extended completely and forcefully, with the bony points oriented approximately halfway between down and back. The exact orientation will change somewhat based on how the lifter is built. The bar should be resting across the palm of the hand, with the wrist extended and the hand relaxed to allow it to settle in securely.

In this position, the bar should be above the forearm (rather than behind it) very slightly behind its center point. The grip should be only tight enough to maintain control of this position—overgripping the bar will prevent the hand and wrist from settling into the proper position and will limit the speed and forcefulness of the elbow extension.

Clean Rack

The rack position of the clean will be an important factor in a lift's success. Most importantly, the barbell must be supported on the shoulders rather than in the arms. In order to position the bar properly, the shoulders must be protracted maximally and elevated somewhat while preventing the upper back from flexing. The protraction of the shoulder blades will create a space between the highest point of the deltoids and the throat in which the bar can settle securely—the bar must be in this groove, not on top of the shoulders, where it will not be secure from simply rolling down and forward. Elevating the shoulder blades will increase the depth of this groove for the bar, but will also keep it from contacting the clavicles, which can be painful, and will help prevent the carotid arteries from being occluded and causing dizziness. The shoulders should only be elevated enough to get the bar off the clavicles—there should not be significant space between the bar and the collarbones.

Generally the hands should be open with only the fingers under the bar and the elbows lifted as much as possible. In some cases, lifters will find it helpful to maintain a fuller grip on the bar. This should be used in such cases, but the lifter must still lift the elbows as much as possible to help secure the position and extend the upper back.

Jerk Rack

The rack position for the jerk is similar to that of the clean. The barbell should be supported on the shoulders instead of by the arms, the shoulder blades protracted and slightly elevated, and the bar sitting in the same groove between the tops of the shoulders and the throat.

However, the ideal position will move the palms of the hands under the bar rather than just the fingers, and the elbows should be move down (always at least slightly in front of the bar) and spread to the sides. This sets the lifter up for better pressing mechanics to relocate under the bar after the drive. The grip should be relaxed to ensure that the bar is settled in and connected tightly to the lifter's trunk to transfer maximal leg drive into it.

Balance

Squat

The weight should be balanced slightly behind mid-foot in the squat—I like to say at the front edge of the heel for an easy reference point. The balance and pressure over the foot will often shift forward somewhat in the very bottom of the squat, but this is acceptable as long as the athlete's posture remains intact and he or she moves the weight back to where it belongs immediately upon recovery from the bottom position.

Snatch & Clean

The balance over the foot should be slightly behind mid-foot like in the squat, although in the starting position, it will be balanced across the foot and immediately upon separation of the bar from the floor, it will be farther forward toward the balls of the foot. As part of the pull from the floor, the lifter must shift the balance back toward the heels immediately. The pressure on the foot will move from toward the balls of the feet as the bar first separates, back toward the heel during most of the pull, and then finish on the balls of the feet as the lifter extends in finish of the pull.

Jerk

The balance over the foot in the jerk should remain over the heel throughout the lift. This can be one of the most difficult things for many lifters to do. The pressure will shift from the heel during the dip and start of the drive onto the balls of the feet as the lifter finishes the drive and the ankles extend.

Posture

Snatch & Clean

In the starting position of the snatch and clean, the lifter's arms should be approximately vertical when viewed from the side, placing the shoulders directly above the bar (the leading edge of the shoulders will be very slightly in front of the bar). The trunk should be upright and the head and eyes directed forward.

Jerk

For the dip and drive of the jerk, the trunk must remain vertical. We imagine a vertical line passing through the lifter's ankle and hip and the center of the bar (when viewing the lifter from the side); these three points should never diverge from this line as the lifter dips and drives. In other words, the hips travel straight down and straight up through flexion of the knees only.

Explosion Mechanics

The mechanics of the final upward explosion of the lift should be taught properly to attain maximal performance of the snatch and clean. Athletes will naturally tend to perform this action less than optimally because the ideal position from which to initiate the explosion is not a comfortable or natural one.

The feet should be flat with the weight balanced toward the heel. The barbell should be in light contact with the mid- to upper-thigh, the shins vertical, and the shoulders slightly in front of the bar.

The movement of the final explosion from this position is a concerted violent extension of the knees and hips—the athlete will snap the hips open to slight hyperextension while punching the legs down against the floor. While this is occurring, the athlete must be actively pushing the bar back into the hips with the lats.

Relocation Mechanics

The relocation of the athlete under the barbell following the final explosion of the lift is an active and aggressive movement. The arms should still be internally rotated as they were set in the start of the lift so the athlete can pull the elbows up and out to the sides. This movement accelerates the athlete down while keeping the athlete and barbell in immediate proximity. Only after this aggressive pull of the elbows up and out is the bar turned over into the rack position (clean) or overhead position (snatch)—without the momentum generated from this movement, the turnover cannot occur properly.

The lifter must remain tightly connected to the bar throughout this entire movement—never should the two become separated, as this will prevent the lifter from completely controlling the position of the bar and body, and will result in the barbell crashing down onto the lifter in the receiving position, making its stabilization much more difficult, even if the position happens to be sound.

With these fundamentals in mind, competent coaches should be able to create drills that teach athletes to perform the lifts well. Don't be afraid to rely on existing teaching progressions until you feel comfortable branching out on your own; and don't be original for originality's sake if it compromises the effectiveness of your coaching and teaching.

SUPPLEMENTAL BODYWEIGHT TRAINING
MATTHEW MILLER

As the owner of Horespower Strength and Conditioning and creator of the Powerology training system, I work with athletes of all levels, ranging from complete beginners to professional athletes competing at the highest levels. No matter which client I am working with, my programs are focused on barbell training, jumping, sprinting and bodyweight training.

The foundation for strength and power training begins and ends with a barbell. The programs that I use are built around Olympic lifting, explosive barbell variations, squats, deads, and barbell lunges. With this programming, my athletes do a large amount of vertical pushing and pulling. Ninety percent of what we do is spent with the barbell over our area of balance (heel bone to balls of feet). This leaves a void that needs to be filled to make sure our athletes are well-rounded, working through a full range of motion, and keeping everything strong and flexible to maximize performance while making them less injury prone. I supplement in horizontal bodyweight pushing and pulling exercises at the end of every workout. I break our workouts down into push days and pull days. A typical push day would include the following exercises:

- Split Jerk
- Push Press
- Seated Box Jump
- Barbell Lunges
- Sprint Variation
- Bodyweight Push

A typical pull day would look like this:

- Cleans
- High Pull
- Box Jumps

- Squats
- Change of Direction
- Bodyweight Pull

Exercise Selection:

When I select each bodyweight exercise, I look to see if they meet the following criteria.

1. Does the exercise build strength?
2. Does it build speed?
3. Does it improve muscular endurance?
4. Are progressions measureable?

All of the exercises that I use in my programming hit at least one, if not more of the above criteria. In addition, I pick exercises to round out the workout with pushing and pulling from different angles than my athletes are getting from the barbell programming.

These are the exercise that I use for the bodyweight pushing and pulling. The sets and reps can be determined by each individual athlete's strength program.
Horizontal Pushes

Burn out Chain Pushups (4,3,2,1,BW) (suggestion 1- 4 sets)

✓ Start with four chains around the athletes neck hang freely to the ground (use chains weight appropriate with athletes strength level
✓ Do as many reps as possible with 4 chains, remove 1 chain
✓ Do as many reps as possible with 3 chains, remove 1 chain
✓ Do as many reps as possible with 2 chains, remove 1 chain
✓ Do as many reps as possible with 1 chain, remove chain
✓ Do as many Body weight reps as possible

Plyo Push Ups (Suggestion 5 sets of 5)

✓ Chest on floor, body laying flat on ground
✓ Hands off the floor
✓ Drive your hands down and push your body off the ground (Jump with your arms)
✓ Toes should stay on the ground the entire time (ultimate goal, push yourself to a standing position while keeping your back flat.
✓ Catch yourself with your arms, lower body back to start position

- ✓ Push Up Plank Sequence (Suggestion 5 Reps, 1-5 Sets)
- ✓ 5 Plyo Pushups, Plank walk 10 yards down, 10 Yard Back, Burn out Pushups

Horizontal Pulls

Rope Climbs (suggestion 5-10 Reps, 3-5 Sets)

- ✓ Start Laying flat on your back
- ✓ Keep back straight
- ✓ Heels on the ground
- ✓ Climb Rope hand over hand until in a standing position
- ✓ Once this becomes easy, the athlete can progress to rope climbs only using the upper body.

Single arm rope pulls (suggestion 5 reps, 3-5 sets)

- ✓ Start laying flat on your back
- ✓ Reach up as high as you can with one arm
- ✓ Explosive pull yourself to a standing position with one arm

Reverse Rows (suggestion 5-10 reps, 3-5 sets)

- ✓ Set a Barbell up at a height so the athletes back does not touch the ground when hanging
- ✓ Overhand or Underhand grip can be used
- ✓ Hands slightly wider that shoulder width
- ✓ Set a box for the athlete to put their feet on
- ✓ Explosively pull Chest to bar

Single Arm Reverse Rows (suggestion 5-10 reps, 3-5 sets)

- ✓ Every is the same as above, except we are doing the exercise with one hand
- ✓ Center your pulling hand on the bar

As I work through a training cycle with an athlete, strength improvements (increased reps), speed improvements, and height improvements are how I assess the gains with bodyweight movements. I progress athletes programming, moving to more difficult exercises as the athlete becomes stronger. I will add volume throughout the training cycle as the athlete's work capacity increases.

Example Push Day Programming

Push Day

Week 1
- 3xBO – 4chains/3chains/2chains/1chain/BW

Week 2
- 5x5 – Plyo Push Ups

Week 3
- 5x Push Up Plank Sequence

Week 4
- 3xBO – 2chains
- 3x5 – Plyo Push Ups

Week 5
- 3xBO – 4chains/3chains/2chains/1chain/BW

Week 6
- 5x5 – Plyo Push Ups

Week 7
- 5x Push Up Plank Sequence

Week 8
- 2xBO – 2chains
- 3x5 – Plyo Push Ups

Example Pull Day Programming

Pull Day

Week 1
- 5x5 Reverse Rows

Week 2
- 5x5 Rope Climbs (Ground to Standing)

Week 3
- 5x5 (each hand) Single Arm Reverse Rows

Week 4
- 5x5 (each hand) Single Arm Rope Climbs

Week 5
- 3x5 Reverse Rows
- 3x5 (each Hand) Single Arm Reverse Rows

Week 6
- 3x5 Rope Climbs
- 3x5 (each hand) Single Arm Rope Climbs

Week 7
- 5x 25' Rope Climbs

Week 8
- 5x25' Rope Climbs
- 3x5 Reverse Rows

Horizontal bodyweight pushing and pulling has been a great addition to the barbell programming that I do at Horsepower. This addition has helped to make sure that our athletes are working their strength at all angles, and builds the assistance muscles to keep progressing with their barbell training, which allows them to become stronger, better prepared athletes.

DEALING WITH BURNOUT
YAEL GRAUER

This isn't going to be another article on the importance of sleep. Chances are, if you're reading this, you've been inundated with information from Lights Out: Sleep, Sugar and Survival, already have f.lux installed on your laptop, and have at least contemplated buying blackout curtains.

This is about something slightly different: feeling exhausted and completely disinterested with work. This usually happens after months or years of doing just a little bit too much, of needing to take a break but ignoring those signals out of necessity (or obstinacy) or just due to circumstances outside of your control.

Whether you just opened a new box and have burned the midnight oil for one night too many, are juggling work and kids, volunteer work and school or your own unique combination of one thing too many, chances are that at some point in your life you've found that you've lost the drive for your work (or even play) and are simply going through the motions. You've done so much, for so long, that there's no way you can sustain that level of effort for a single day longer. And yet, it needs to get done, so there you are. What next?

Even the title of this article begs the question: how do you get the fire back? Obviously, that's going to be different for every person, but we know what doesn't work for everyone: ignoring those signals indefinitely and moving on forward, hoping that it doesn't catch up with you (and that nobody notices).

Typically, what's needed—and what's realistic—takes a completely different strategy-set than the one you've been using to burn the candle at both ends, but each situation is unique. So let's run down a list of options to contemplate, and you find something realistic that you haven't already tried, give it a shot, record the results, and repeat until you're back to your chipper self again.

Just realize that this is part of a process. It's like working out. Clearly, you'll need to recharge after a long period of excessive energy expenditure, and that's true for other aspects of your life as well. If you feel completely numb and disinterested in things that used to get you excited, take heart. You are not broken. You won't feel this way forever. But you do need to find a way to hit the reset button.

Take some time off.

A recent report by the Center for Economic and Policy Research shows that Americans are pretty stingy when it comes to vacation. And even when employees do dish out days off—far less than they do in other countries—Americans often don't take advantage of them. In fact, there are 175 million vacation days workers are entitled to but don't take each year.

There's really no substitute for going on a one or two-week vacation. Leaving your laptop and cell phone behind, going somewhere remote or beautiful (either alone or with family and friends), and finding activities to occupy your time that have nothing to do with putting out fires at work or dealing with office politics.

Unfortunately, truly taking time off can be difficult, depending on your specific job and circumstances. If taking a longer break is absolutely not an option, schedule something in the future when it will be.

A week or two off isn't in the cards for all of us, but almost everyone can take a single day, a weekend or even an evening off. Go on an extended hike and leave your phone behind and see if that helps you recharge. Had to pull an all-nighter? See if you can get someone to cover the next day. Take shorter breaks whenever possible if you can't take an extended one.

But remember: If you're truly burned out, a single day off or even a week off may lead you wanting more. You may not feel rested and replenished from a single evening away, and if taking months or weeks off isn't an option, make sure you don't just take a single day off and call it done. Just like you work rest days into your training schedule, plan days off into your schedule—an afternoon off every other week, for example. The trick is to address the issue before you're at the boiling point.

And this isn't just about days off. Even scheduling in time for sleep can be useful at this point.

Automate anything that's repetitive.

If you're a gym owner, think of all the things that leave you frazzled and scrambling every day and do as many of them as you can in advance. Here are some examples:

- Instead of jumping on Twitter between clients to try to come up with something clever to say day in and day out, use FutureTweets or TweetDeck or HootSuite to plan your tweets on in advance.
- Figure out exactly what's going on your blog ahead of time using an editorial calendar (perhaps with a regular, repeating theme for the days you post). Plan out your WODs far in advance so you're not scrambling every morning.

- Need to find a way to manage projects? Trello has saved me hours of time which I can spend taking naps and hot baths. (Wrike and BaseCamp are also nice.)
- Rather than writing a list of things to do on sticky notes around your office or little scraps of paper, use one of the thousands of list apps out there. (Do It Tomorrow, TeuxDeux and Remember the Milk are all options.)
- Write down all of your passwords that you keep forgetting somewhere (under lock and key, of course).
- Use Gmail's canned responses to answer questions from prospective members.

Figure out how to be proactive instead of responsive—or to leave time and energy for when you do need to be responsive. The more of this that you do, the more time you save, and if you're trying to save energy, eliminating even an hour of extraneous work each day is huge.

Outsource –or eliminate-- anything that's exhausting.

What drains your energy and takes tons of time away from what you're truly good at? For me, it's things like having to spend hours on the phone with service providers to tell them they messed up a bill or figure out what's broken. I spend $25/month to outsource that shit to FancyHands. Five tasks a month off my plate, freeing up energy for me to do what I do best.

This isn't about time; it's about energy levels. Got a class you're teaching that's leaving you drained and making it difficult to do what you need to before and after? Can you find someone else to teach or co-teach it? Over time, replace activities that aren't fun for you with ones that are. Think about what's win-win and what isn't. This may mean shifting things around, canceling certain events, or finding a way to get rid of that thing you really want to get rid of (and figuring out the details later).

It also means saying no.

Remember, we're talking about burnout. If you're feeling even on the verge of it, and can't get rid of the majority of you responsibilities, for God's sake, don't take on new ones! It can be hard to say no because it feels like we're letting people down or are too focused on just one aspect of our lives, but I've found people feel more let down if you say yes to something you don't really want to do and suffer through it when your heart's not really in it.

What can you say no to, today? Sometimes this is as simple as not calling to reschedule something with no-showed, or not rearranging your schedule to work with someone who came in late. It could be turning down that person who wants free sessions when you have clearly posted rates, or lowering the amount of workshops you host. Just stop yourself from trying to do everything when you don't even have the energy for what's on your plate.

It can be tempting to want to start something new, but don't think that the thrill and adrenaline rush of a new project is what you need to get you out of your funk. This is the time to focus on what you've already done—either celebrating your wins, or deepening the work you've already started.

This is also a very good time to allow other people to pitch in a bit more, if they're asking what you need help with.

Find activities that aren't work-related.

I know, I know. I just told you to cut back and take time off and say no to things and not start anything new, and now I'm telling you to find things to do that aren't work-related? But bear with me. Part of recovering from burnout is filling the well, and finding something to do that's not work-related doesn't have to be all-encompassing or time-consuming.

For me, it's reading fiction—something which I avoided for years, because I preferred to only read books that were directly work-related. It's watching movies or shows that I'm not planning to write about, or enjoying an evening of comedy, or spending time in my garden. What can you do that's enjoyable and not directly related to you job?

That also means you want to spend time with people who aren't asking you for things (or who you're not asking anything from). If you've been heavily networking and promoting your gym (or whatever), signing it from the rooftops, even, you may have forgotten what it feels like to just get coffee or drinks with friends. Likewise, if you're constantly doing what feels like unpaid consulting and letting people pick your brain on your 'off' time, you may be working even more hours than you think you are. Call up someone who really could care less about what you do and who you don't want to work with. It's energizing, especially if you're an extrovert. (If you're an introvert, let yourself have as much time holed away from the company of others as you need to reset, and cross some networking events off your calendar. You don't need to go to everything.)

Take care of yourself

Get enough sleep—and focus on sleep timing—even if you don't think it's helping. (Even a 10-minute walk outside and soaking in the sunlight can help reset your circadian rhythms if you find yourself up 'til 4AM each morning.) Get a massage or bodywork that's not ART or related to treating an injury. Pile up all of your gift cards and buy something frivolous.

What are your outlets, and how can you work them into your schedule? Many people throw themselves into work when dealing with (or not dealing with) personal problems, because it's easier to affect change…but ignoring the weight of those problems is a mistake. They'll pop back into your consciousness when you least want them to, unless you address them head-on somehow.

Another example of burnout is when dealing with medical issues. The added stress of bills (which means extra hours of work) combining with limited outlets to release that stress (due to whichever medical issues are causing the problem) means you've got more pressure and less of an outlet to release it. What can you do that makes you feel the same way (or similar) to the activities you can't do? Focusing on how you want to feel instead of all the things you want to do (and can't) can help you find surrogate activities until things are back to 'normal' again.

Bottom Line

If you're feeling so disinterested with your job and life that you're completely numb to things that would normally excite you, it's already been too long. Use some of the steps above to take a bit of pressure off, and use the time and energy you free up to take whatever steps you can (however large or small) to rise out of the ashes again.

STRENGTH TRAINING FOR FOOTBALL LINEMEN
MATT MILLER

Every high level lineman has brute strength, explosive hips, quick feet, hip mobility, mental toughness, and intelligence. The first five of these six elements can be built and improved upon in a properly planned strength and conditioning program.

There are very few sport-specific needs that carry over into the weight room as closely as those of a football lineman. The competition skills that are required of him are the definition of a power athlete: max force explosion, recover, max force explosion. In a football game, athletes give max effort for four to six seconds, followed by a rest period of 30 to 40 seconds. When an athlete is in the max effort explosion phase of their competition (the duration of a single play), he needs to drive quickly out of his stance, maximizing his ability to move his feet fast with a low center of gravity. This allows him to beat his opponent to the "spot," gaining a positional and leverage advantage to complete his assignment of blocking the defensive player/filling the gap.

Once the athletes are in position, they need to call on their hips (power) to move the opponent in the direction that they wish to take them. Once the lineman has delivered the "punch" to their opponent (hip driven punch with both hands to the chest of the opponent), he needs to rely on brute strength to handle and control the opponent until the end of the play. Throughout the duration of the game, the athlete needs to rely on mental toughness to continue to give max effort play after play in a brutal and emotional environment that has both positive and negative outcomes multiple times throughout the course of a single game.

Brute Strength

The job description of a lineman could be stated as simple as 'to push another person where you want them to go while they are trying to do the same thing to you.' This is why brute strength is so important to a lineman's success. Brute strength can make up for many deficiencies.

The foundation of brute strength training is squats, squat variations, deadlifts, deadlift variations, strongman training, and heavy upper body pushing. These elements need to be programmed in multiple times per week.

The most important lift that a lineman can do is back squat. This lift needs to be programmed every week, and should be the first lift done on your first lower body workout of the week. When squatting, it needs to be heavy and you need to have your hips below your knees. The depth is necessary for strength in all positions and hip mobility. The more time you spend driving out of the hole with heavy weight, the easier it is to play strong in a low position. Along with squats, you want to add in a variety of squat and deadlift variations. So we're looking at front squats, single-leg squats, deadlifts, Romanian deadlifts, and single-leg deadlifts.

In addition to your heavy lower body lifts, a key component to any lineman program is strongman training. The primary movement of a lineman is to push, so sled pushes and other pushing movements are the foundation of the strongman training that lineman should do. When you are having lineman push sleds, remember that you want to go max effort (speed, weight, or both) for a short period (four to six seconds) and rest for a longer period (30 to 40 seconds). This work to rest ratio will prepare them best for competition.

In addition to these pushing movements, I like to add in heavy pulling: sleds, cars, really any heavy object that you can have them pull. To round out the strongman training, use yoke walk, farmers walk, Atlas stones, tire flips, tire battles, and a favorite of mine to train the hips, the Hungarian core blaster. (Thanks, Sorinex).

To finish off the brute strength training for linemen, it is important that they have lifts with heavy pushing in their program as well. As I mentioned, they spend the majority of their time pushing, so is it is important that they have well trained and strong "push muscles." The pushes that are most important to lineman are push press, bench press, incline press, and floor press. It is also important to incorporate programming with a multi-grip bar that puts their pushing at a more sport specific angle.

All of these elements will raise the athlete's strength level and get them ready to have functional strength/power in every circumstance that a football game will present.

Explosive Hips

If you want to improve an athlete's hips, the very best way is through barbell power movements. The base lifts that will help a lineman's hips the most are cleans and snatches. Using a variety of cleans and snatches in programming will develop hips and make them explosive on the football field. The key snatch and clean movements that a lineman needs are the power snatch, power clean, hang clean, hang snatch, single-arm snatch, and single leg clean. When it is time for an athlete to work on explosiveness, it is good to have them do two pulling power movements back to back. When doing this, you want them to pull from different levels, pull to different spots, and incorporate single-leg and single-arm variations.

In addition to barbell power movements, jump training and sprint training are good ways to develop the athlete's hips. It is impossible to generate power in these activities without starting the movement with the hips. For lineman, max effort box jumps, long jumps, weighted jumps, and change of direction jumping are going to maximize the power development needed for football. When sprinting with a lineman, you want to make sure that everything is in the five to 25-yard range. All of the work linemen do is in short bursts, so train them accordingly.

Quick Feet

The best way to improve a lineman's feet is to make them stronger. This is taken care of in the brute strength and explosive hips area of the training. The stronger a lineman is, the quicker they can move their body. Once they have reached a solid level of strength, you want to incorporate supplemental training that focuses on speed. This can be done through sprinting, quick jumps (multiple jumps spending as little time with their feet on the ground as possible), and change of direction work. The more comfortable a big person gets moving fast, the better he will become at it.

Hip Mobility

The first and most important way to build hip mobility is to make sure that the athlete is working through a full range of motion in all of their lifts and exercises. In addition, you want to have them train mobility at the beginning of every workout. To play in a low athletic position, it is necessary to have ankle mobility and knee mobility along with hip mobility. Shoulder mobility is a key component to a lineman's success due to the amount of time spent pushing, and punching from multiple angles in a game. Thoracic spine mobility is also important due to the position that lineman play and have impact in. The more mobile a lineman is, the more comfortable they are playing in a low athletic position. In addition, their bodies become more resilient to injuries.

Mental Toughness

In order for a lineman to be successful, mental toughness is a must. To achieve at their highest level, lineman have to be able to give max effort confidently on every single play. Playing offensive line is demanding; it is squaring off against another person in a max effort war for territory. A lineman has to believe that he is the best player on the field and that he has the ability to physically dominate the person across the line from him.

Linemen have to have the ability to play every play with this confidence regardless of how they performed on the play before. When the ball is snapped, they need to go into attack mode, four to six seconds of ruthless aggression in order to dominate.

These are attributes that can translate from training to the football field. The bigger, stronger, quicker, and faster that a lineman becomes, the more confident they are in their ability to beat the person across the line. Improving builds confidence, period. When lifting, an athlete needs to train their mind to attack the barbell (or whatever equipment they are using) on every single rep. This helps athletes lock into what they are doing and commit to doing what it takes at max effort to succeed. Training puts athletes in a position where they are not comfortable; football is a game where things aren't comfortable. In training, you learn how to give 100 percent when you are not comfortable. This teaches athletes how to succeed when their body feels like it can't. It also shows them that the harder something is, the harder they have to push back in order to find success. Trying to move a 300-pound man is much easier when you have sat in the hole on a heavy squat and drove the weight up when it felt like there was no way it could happen. Training builds mental toughness by teaching athletes that they are capable of accomplishing more with their body than they believe in their mind. A proper training program for lineman will break mental barriers, build confidence, and teach them how to perform at a high level even when they are uncomfortable.

Programming

Take all of the information above and lay it into a proper program to maximize gains. The blueprint below is for an off-season training program. You would want to pull back volume and load when a lineman is in season. With power athletes, I will run them through a five-week cycle, the fifth week being a deload.

TAPERING FOR COMPETITION
JOHN GRACE

Athletes train to compete. More importantly, they train to win. Why else would they put in hours of training in a day just to come in second? Whether an athlete's season is three competitions or 20 competitions long, they should be at their peak performance levels for those few competitions that are the most important to have the best chance to come away with a victory. One way coaches can help ensure athletes are physically ready is a taper period.

A taper is a period of time in an athlete's periodized program when intensity, volume, and frequency are altered to elicit performance gains. Just as intensity, volume, and frequency can be altered to impose a training stimulus, these three variables can be controlled to encourage desired increases in performance. During a taper period and as you get closer to competition; the goal should be to keep adaptation rates high while minimizing fatigue.

The average improvement for a trained athlete given an appropriate taper is two to three percent, or zero to six percent, depending on the sport. Top athletes will most likely be at higher proportions to their "performance ceiling", so percentage improvements will generally be slightly less (half a percent to three percent). It is comparable to an overweight person with a goal of losing weight. The initial weight loss will come pretty easily with a moderate amount of work. As the person loses weight, it is much harder (and unrealistic) for that person to continue to lose the same amount of weight from month to month; just as it's hard for an elite athlete to see large gains when they get closer and closer to his or her "performance ceiling."

Tapering should start two to three weeks out from competition. Here are a few central fundamentals that should be taken into consideration when developing the competition taper:

- Volume
- Intensity
- Frequency

- Training Age
- Type of Athlete

Volume

Volume in this sense is the amount of work done (sets, reps, distance, time, etc.). Inigo Mujika, an expert on recovery and performance, suggests a 40 to 60 percent volume reduction over the course of two to three weeks. It is important to note that there should be an accumulation of volume over the course of a training plan, so there is something to reduce from when appropriate. The consequence of not accumulating volume can lead to a potential decrease in performance when tapering the suggested 40-60 percent. If you decrease too much from an already relatively low volume of work, you will short-change yourself on training stimulus.

Intensity

Intensity refers to the percentage you are working at relative to your rep max. Over the course of a training cycle, intensity should be gradually increasing until the taper period. At that point, intensity should remain relatively stable over the course of the taper. Maintaining intensity while dropping volume can assist in the ultimate goal: reducing fatigue while maintaining and improving strength and power.

Frequency

Frequency represents how many training sessions you or your athlete is performing in a given time frame. In a competition-tapering phase, frequency, like intensity, should remain unchanged if tolerated by the athlete (a maximum of 20 percent reduction in frequency if needed). For ease of example, imagine seven-day microcycles. Some elite athletes perform as many as 10+ training sessions in a given week, whereas other athletes may only train three sessions a week. There may be good reason to drop a couple of sessions from an athlete's program when they are training 10+ sessions a week, but if you're only training three sessions a week, there is no real logical reason to drop a training session from an already low training frequency.

Training Age

Training age can also be considered a component in this tapering equation. Training age refers to the accumulation of training time over the athlete's career. This doesn't mean that athletes with low training ages are necessarily young athletes. An athlete in their mid-twenties who has trained for a few months has a lower training age than a 16-year-old who has been training for three years, despite being chronologically younger. If an athlete has only trained for a few months, they are more than likely at a lower level relative to their genetic potential. When you or your athlete's performance levels are lower, you shouldn't need as much time to rebound from training because training is not placing as great of demand on your body.

Think of two identical Ferraris: One is consistently operating at 90 percent of its speed potential, while the other is operating at 50 percent of its speed potential. The Ferrari that is operating at 90 percent (the elite athlete) is stressing the components under the hood much more than the Ferrari that is operating at 50 percent. The Ferrari working consistently at 90 percent will need more maintenance checks and occasional recovery periods to make sure everything stays working properly. The same applies to elite athletes in comparison to novice or amateur athletes.

Knowing Yourself and Your Athlete

Certain types of athletes respond differently to these three training components (volume, intensity, and frequency). For the general athlete, these guidelines are best practice. However, there are always outliers to any guideline or rule-of-thumb. Over time, coaches can start understanding when to tweak certain components in a tapering period and what adjustments should be made.

When is an athlete in the most favorable position to be at their peak performance? Remember, this is where the real coaching comes in to play. Start the taper too late, and the athlete could potentially under-perform because they are still in a fatigued state. Start the taper too early, and you have an athlete that peaks early and is potentially on the downswing of the adaptation curve and subsequently under-performs.

Coaches and athletes alike can also start understanding what combination of volume, intensity, frequency brings out the best performances. Developing this coach-athlete relationship is beneficial to ultimately discover what combination works best.

This is a 6-week program for an athlete training three days per week. The program is geared to improve the full competition lifts with a max day at the end of six weeks.

The program starts at a relatively low intensities and moderate volumes. Over the course of the six weeks, volumes and intensities are trending upward. At the start of Week 5 (the start of tapering), volume is reduced while intensities are increasing minimally.

There are no changes in training frequency during the taper since this is only a three day per week program.

It should be noted that the sets and reps listed are working sets and there should be build-up sets proceeding.

WEEK 1

Tuesday	Sets/Reps	%
Snatch + Hang Snatch (AK)	6x1+2	75
Clean + Jerk	4x2+1	80
Back Squat	4x6	75+

Thursday	Sets/Reps	%
Power Snatch	5x2	77.5
Power Clean + Jerk	4x2+1	82.5
Front Squat	5x3	80+

Saturday	Sets/Reps	%
Snatch	4x2	80
Clean & Jerk	4x1	82.5
Back Squat	6x3	80+

WEEK 3

Tuesday	Sets/Reps	%
Snatch + Hang Snatch (BK)	5x1+1	80
Clean & Jerk	4x1	85
Push Press	4x3	85+
Front Squat	5x2	85+

Thursday	Sets/Reps	%
Power Snatch	5x1	82.5
Power Clean + Jerk	4x1+1	87.5
Clean Pulls	4x3	100
RDLs	3x10	-

Saturday	Sets/Reps	%
Snatch	5x1	85
Clean & Jerk	4x1	87.5
Back Squat	5x3	85+

WEEK 5

Tuesday	Sets/Reps	%
Snatch	4x1	90
Clean & Jerk	4x1	90
Front Squat	4x2	90

Thursday	Sets/Reps	%
Snatch	4x1	90
Clean & Jerk	4x1	90
Clean Pulls	4x3	105

Saturday	Sets/Reps	%
Snatch	3x1	92.5
Clean & Jerk	3x1	92.5
Back Squat	2x1	90

WEEK 2

Tuesday	Sets/Reps	%
Snatch + Hang Snatch (AK)	6x1+1	77.5
Clean + Jerk	4x2+1	82.5
Back Squat	4x6	+

Thursday	Sets/Reps	%
Power Snatch	5x2	80
Power Clean + Jerk	4x1+1	85
Front Squat	5x3	+

Saturday	Sets/Reps	%
Snatch	4x2	82.5
Clean & Jerk	4x1	85
Back Squat	6x3	+

WEEK 4

Tuesday	Sets/Reps	%
Snatch	5x1	85
Clean & Jerk	4x1	85
Push Press	4x3	87.5+
Front Squat	5x2	87.5+

Thursday	Sets/Reps	%
Power Snatch	5x1	85
Power Clean + Jerk	4x1+1	90
Clean Pulls	4x3	102.5
RDLs	3x10	-

Saturday	Sets/Reps	%
Snatch	4x1	85
Clean & Jerk	4x1	87.5
Back Squat	5x3	87.5+

WEEK 6

Tuesday	Sets/Reps	%
Snatch	2x1	92.5
Clean & Jerk	2x1	92.5
Clean Pulls	4x2	105

Thursday	Sets/Reps	%
Snatch	1x1	95
Clean & Jerk	1x1	95
Snatch Pulls	3x2	105

Saturday	Sets/Reps	%
Snatch	MAX	
Clean & Jerk	MAX	

Notes
David B. Pyne; Intildeigo Mujika; Thomas Reilly. Peaking for optimal performance: Research limitations and future directions. Journal of Sports Sciences. (2009). 27.3. pp 195-202
Hausswirth, C., Mujika, I. (2013). Recovery for Performance in Sport. Champagne, IL: Human Kinetics

TRAINING FOR THE TACTICAL ATHLETE
SAGE ADAMS

It's 3AM. The phone rings. Another call out. You had a lift and a high intensity interval session planned for the afternoon. So, what do you do? Do you try to squeeze it in somehow and just adapt and adjust? The unique demands of the tactical/combat athlete dictate the need for high levels of all-around fitness: strength, power, quickness, agility and extensive work capacity coupled with the ability to successfully navigate the stressful demands of the job and limited training time. While you can't control everything, there are ways to structure training and nutrition to mitigate the deleterious effects of high levels of stress and the divergent fitness demands of the tactical athlete.

Such unique all-around fitness often requires a significant amount of concurrent training, that is, training for strength/power and aerobic capacity simultaneously, rather than in separate periodized blocks of training. The idea of concurrent training and the interference effect is not a new concept. The debate as to whether high levels of strength and high levels of aerobic capacity can be developed at the same time without sacrifices in strength and power has long been discussed. Current research however, has elucidated some of the mechanistic factors that may help explain the potential for interference. These findings lend insight into how to structure training programs and individual training sessions to reduce potential confounding factors while still developing the necessary levels of fitness.

This interference concept is most important when seeking high-level strength and power gains. The development of maximal strength and power requires the recruitment of the high-end motor units within skeletal muscle. A motor unit consists of a motor neuron and all the muscle fibers that it innervates. This is most effectively illustrated within Henneman's size principle, as it explains the relationship between motor unit twitch force and recruitment threshold. This principle dictates that motor units are sequentially recruited based upon their recruitment thresholds and firing rates, with lower-end, larger, less fatigable motor units recruited first in most instances, followed by higher-end motor units as load and intensity increases.

With this in mind, we see that changes in skeletal muscle in response to exercise training are largely dictated by the stimulus provided. In order to elicit the desired changes, the muscle must receive a series of neural and biochemical signals that tell it how to adapt. Two important molecular signaling cascades that play a role in the changes in skeletal muscle in response to exercise are known as the mammalian target of rapamycin (mTOR) and its downstream effectors, as well as adenosine monophosphate activated protein kinase (AMPK) and its downstream effectors. These pathways are involved in mRNA translation initiation and thus have a significant impact on the end result of your training efforts.

Resistance exercise itself provides a mechanical stimulus for the activation of mTOR. This mTOR stimulation is an energy-requiring anabolic process that leads to protein synthesis. The subsequent accretion of myofibrillar proteins contributes to an increase in muscle size and strength. AMPK, on the other hand, is catabolic and because it acts as a cellular energy sensor, it can lead to adaptations such as mitochondrial biogenesis and the increased metabolic and work capacity of the muscle.

In essence, these signaling proteins represent opposite ends of the adaptation spectrum. Not only do these pathways elicit different effects on skeletal muscle, in many instances they interfere with one another because AMPK activation can block mTOR signaling. Taking these factors into account, it starts to become clear how endurance or interval-based activity can negatively affect strength and power gains. The catabolic cellular energy perturbations and metabolic by-product accumulation don't allow the anabolic signals to go through. You can't break down muscle and build it up at the same time.

So you may be thinking, this cellular stuff sounds well and good, but how does it apply to my ability to be strong and powerful? Well, in order to truly generate maximal force, those higher-end motor units we mentioned previously must be recruited and they must be recruited at a quick firing rate. When the ionic balance of the cellular environment is significantly disrupted (like after you perform very high intensity glycolytic intervals, for instance) the accumulation of metabolic by-products, low pH, disturbance in the Na^+-K^+ pump, etc., results in hyperpolarization. Hyperpolarization inhibits the neuron from firing and thus affects motor unit recruitment. As a result, it becomes difficult to recruit these high-end motor units and makes it difficult to achieve improvements in strength and power in this cellular environment.

Of course there are many athletes that are both very strong and have huge aerobic and anaerobic work capacity. And of course, it is not always necessary to separate these types of training sessions. Our focus here, however, is on the average athlete who may be experiencing a plateau in strength and power gains, or the tactical athlete who has limited training and recovery opportunities due to work, personal and other high-stress demands. Remember, the cumulative effect of your regular training program is what sets the stage for the phenotypic adaptation. Therefore, you want to construct a framework conducive to your desired long-term training goals. Fortunately, research in this area has pointed to a few strategies that can be effective.

One strategy involves leaving at least three hours between strength–focused and conditioning-focused training sessions. This three-hour window appears to be sufficient to mitigate the interference effect, provided the athlete does not remain in a negative energy balance. This can be achieved by performing two shorter training sessions per day separated by at least three hours, or by merely training the components on different days. If training must be performed in one session, performing the resistance-training portion of your training session first appears to be your best bet. This will allow you to embark on a lift prior to the resultant cellular energy depletion and accumulated metabolic by-products from interval or heavy aerobic training.

Nutrition

Nutritional intervention can also be an effective strategy to promote recovery and reduce the interference effect of concurrent training. In a study looking at the effect of an essential amino acid (EAA) and carbohydrate (CHO) drink and exercise on molecular signaling, the researchers found that the EAA-CHO mixture actually reduced AMPK signaling post-exercise and increased mTOR signaling, thus promoting an anabolic environment conducive to protein synthesis. This is likely due to the change in the energy state of the cell with the consumption of EAA-CHO beverage and/or the effects of leucine that has been found to act not only as a substrate but also potentially as an anabolic signal as well. Previous research has indicated that peri-workout nutrition also improved the hormonal environment by reducing cortisol and utilizing insulin and amino acids to provide an anabolic stimulus favoring protein synthesis. Coconut water and branched chain amino acids (BCAAs) would work well in this instance.

Stress

Stress is another important consideration with respect to overall health as well as training program design for the tactical athlete. Cortisol increases with acute stress. Chronic stress, including sleep deprivation, can also keep cortisol levels significantly elevated. If stress is not managed, this can eventually lead to compromised adrenal function, fatigue and adverse effects on health and performance. High cortisol has a two-fold negative effect on performance. Not only does elevated cortisol reduce testosterone, it also is a potent inhibitor of mTOR's downstream effectors. This inhibition blocks anabolic signaling and compromises protein synthesis. A reduction in testosterone and anabolic signaling means your ability to positively adapt to a resistance training stimulus is significantly compromised.

In this high-stress scenario, altering your training plan is important. Substituting a lift or a glycolytic interval session for rest, mobility training or a light active recovery workout consisting of lower intensity aerobic based activity will be more effective for overall fitness and health in the long run then gutting through a tough workout. As a guide for those of you who don't typically train in anything but fifth gear, keeping your heart rate below 130 beats per minutes is an easy way to quantify a "lighter" workout.

The following are a few simple templates to use in order to structure training in a way that can reduce the interference effect and manage recovery for the tactical athlete.

Once a day training session

MONDAY	TUESDAY	WEDNESDAY	THURDSAY	FRIDAY	SATURDAY	SUNDAY
LSD OR REST WORKOUT OPTIONS: -30-60 MIN-UTE RUN, BIKE, SWIM, ROW OR HEAVY BAG WORK OR LSD INTER-VALS: (WORK/ REST) -10MIN/1MIN -5MIN /1 MIN -2MIN /30S -1MIN/30S	LIFT WORKOUT OPTIONS: -SQUAT (4X5) -PRESS (3X5) -BSS (3X8EA) -PUSH-UPS (4X30) *BSS-BULGAR-IAN SPLIT SQUAT	INTERVALS WORKOUT OPTIONS: -15S/30S (X15-20) OR -5MIN/1MIN (X5) + 20S/40S (X10)	LIFT WORKOUT OPTIONS: -DL (4X5) -BOR (3X5) -LATERAL BB LUNGE (3X8EA) -INVERTED ROW (3X8) *BOR-BENT-OVER ROW	REST	SPRINTS WORKOUT OPTIONS: -6-8X100M (5MIN+ REST) OR -8-10X40YDS (2-5+ MIN REST)	MIXED MODAL + LSD OR LIFT WORKOUT OPTIONS: POWER CLEAN (5X3) FRONT SQUAT (4X3) PULL-UPS (4X8) BACK EXT/ GHD (3X10) OR 4 SETS OF: FRONT SQUAT (X8) 400M (OR 2MIN ON TREADMILL AT INCLINE)

Two-a-days

MONDAY	TUESDAY	WEDNESDAY	THURDSAY	FRIDAY	SATURDAY	SUNDAY
AM-LSD PM-MO-BILITY	AM-LIFT -SQUAT -PRESS -PUSH-UPS PM-INTER-VALS (1:2) (WORK: REST)	REST	AM-LIFT -DL -BOR -LATERAL BB LUNGE PM-INTER-VALS (2:1)(WORK: REST)	AM- LIFT -POWER CLEAN -FRONT SQUAT -PULL-UPS PM- MIXED MODAL OR LSD (30MIN)	REST	SPRINTS

*Based on a Monday-Friday work schedule. Adjust based upon work schedule, optimal training days and days needed for recovery. Additional rest or light long slow distance (LSD) days can be added to account for call outs and/or operation training, etc. Set and rep schemes will be dictated by phase of training and training goals. Additionally, decreasing strength training to 2 days a week and adding an additional conditioning session instead can be used for operators that need to focus on improved conditioning during a particular training phase.

Incorporating these concepts into a structured, linear or non-linear periodized training program can provide a solid quantifiable, progressive training program for a tactical athlete.

A GREAT OLYMPIC CHAMPION... AND YOU
MATT FOREMAN

I don't write about other people very often. It's not what I want to do, and I don't think it's what most of you are interested in reading. This magazine is called Performance Menu, which probably means most of the people who read it are looking for ways to improve their...performance. I don't think athlete biographies or weightlifting history articles are exactly what you're thirsting for, and I understand. As I said, it works out pretty well because that kind of stuff isn't what I want to focus on as a writer.

However, there are a few situations here and there where I think we can learn a hell of a lot by reading the stories of certain people. I love watching shows like A&E Biography and Inside the Actors Studio. When successful individuals sit down and talk about their lives, I almost always find something in their back story that connects really well with my own. Every single one of them has had defeats and obstacles, which is something we all like to hear because it makes us understand that we're not the only ones. Also, they've all usually had a point in their lives where they had to take some kind of huge risk. This gives us confidence about the chances we have to take in our own lives.

So, let me tell you some things about a guy most of you have never heard of (which is a damn shame). I'm going to write about Norbert Schemansky in this month's article. Norb was an American Olympic lifter during the 1940s, 50s, and 60s. You could make a pretty strong case that Norb is the best American weightlifter of all time. In fact, it's not a huge stretch to mention his name when you're talking about the greatest weightlifters in history...period.

STOP! Some of you might already be thinking about dismissing this article because you're not interested in spending a few minutes of your day reading about some weightlifter from the old dinosaur days. You want to read about training programs, technique, coaching, and all the other stuff we normally cover in this magazine. That's why I'm going to stop you dead in your tracks and tell you with 100 percent certainty that you can learn some of the most important lessons of your career by reading about Norb Schemansky. He's my weightlifting idol. And I'm not one of those guys who do a lot of "hero worship" with athletes, or anybody else for that matter. This guy is an exception to my rule, though. He's an exception to every rule you could ever think of.

Trust me, I'm not going to bore you with three or four pages of statistics and stuff like that. I'm going to connect this guy's life with your own. You're going to learn about Norb, but what you're really going to do is learn about yourself. By looking at what he did, you're going to get a clearer vision of what you want to do. By reading about what he went through, you'll see the things you're going through in a different way. And by learning about the kind of person he was, I honestly think you'll develop some new ideas about the kind of person you want to be.

I probably shouldn't use the word "was" in that last sentence, because Norb is still alive. At the time of this article, he's 89 years old. His career as an athlete is obviously in the distant past, but the accomplishments and legacy of this man will live forever because his spirit is in all of us. Yes, you read that right. His spirit is in you, me, and every weightlifter in the world. Let me prove it to you.

How's this for a resume?

Norb is from Michigan, the Detroit area (Dearborn, precisely). He was born in 1924 into a working-class Polish family. After growing up in a pretty normal way, he started playing around with barbells and weightlifting during high school. His training was interrupted for a few years by this pesky little inconvenience called World War II. No big deal. He joined the Army and served with an anti-aircraft unit in Europe, fought in the Battle of the Bulge, shot down German fighter planes…you know, the typical stuff we all did in our 20s. When the war was over, he did what most GIs did. He came home, got married, impregnated his wife a few times, and got a job. But he also decided to get back into the weightlifting thing because he was pretty good at it, and he was hooked. I'll give you the basics of Norb's career:

- Four-time Olympic Medalist (silver-1948, gold 1952, bronz- 1964)
- Three-time World Champion
- Nime-time US National Champion
- 26 WOrld Records (he set his last one when he was 38)
- 34 US National Records

Like I said, he's one of the greatest weightlifters of all time. That record stacks up against anybody, from any era. How much did he lift?

- Clean and Press - 402 lbs
- Snatch- 363 lbs
- Clean and Jerk- 445 lbs

Now, I need to give you a few bits of information about these numbers. First of all, weightlifting was a three-lift sport until 1972. Some of you might not know that. When you competed in a weightlifting meet, you did the clean and press (which is exactly what it sounds like, a clean followed by a standing overhead press), then the snatch, and then the clean and jerk. The press was eliminated in 1972. Ever since then, it's just been the way we know it now (SN, C&J). Stop and think about what it would be like to do a three-lift weightlifting meet like this. I'm telling you, the guys from the old pressing days were as hard as pig iron.

Second, Norb was a split-style lifter (as were most of the old timers from that era). That means he did split cleans and split snatches. If you don't know what these are, get on YouTube and type in "split snatch" or "split clean and jerk." Almost nobody does them anymore, but they used to be common practice.

Now, I listed above that Norb's best snatch was 363 lbs. That means he split snatched that weight. Stop and think for a second about split snatching 363 lbs. Once that image has kicked you in the brain, let me mention that Norb did this weight when he was 40 years old, after having a back surgery to repair a crippling injury that prompted doctors to tell him he might never walk again.

Yeah, he split snatched 363 lbs when he was 40 years old. He did it in a full three-lift meet. That means he had already clean and PRESSED 400 lbs, then he did the 363 split snatch, and then he split clean and jerked almost 450. When he was 40…after back surgery…while working a full-time job and supporting a family… We can reach a clear conclusion from these little details; this guy was the toughest son of a bitch in weightlifting history.

And by the way, he did all of this before the age of steroids. That means he was drug-free. Brothers and sisters, there has never been anybody like this guy. I know we've got some behemoth numbers in the sport these days. The top lifters in the world can snatch 450 lbs. and C&J 550. But when you look at all the pieces of the puzzle, and you take everything into consideration, this man's feats of strength are incomparable. Norb Schemansky is one of the giants of strength history, an iconic legend.

Work, diet, training, personality…

A guy named Richard Bak wrote a book about Norb a few years ago called Mr. Weightlifting. I hated the title, but loved the book. There was obviously a ton of information about his life and athletic career, but the best parts were the sections where Norb talked about the way he approached certain things. I'm going to break this down into a few short categories:

Nutrition

Obviously this is a topic that's hugely important to a lot of you. Eating for performance has become a field unto itself. Libraries of books and literature have been published about how to use nutrition to become a championship athlete. Well, let me give you the words of a guy who won more championships than almost anybody in history. When asked about his diet, Norb said, "Most of my diet is hamburgers, pizza, Polish sausage, and beer. If a guy needs a special diet to compete, I've already got him beat." Yeah, that's what he said. Based on that statement, you might think Norb had a sloppy physique. And you would be wrong. Norb was built like a Greek god. He actually competed in a few bodybuilding contests just for fun…and won.

Training

Programming is on everybody's mind. One of the main reasons you're probably reading this magazine is to pick up some tips about your own training regimen that will make you a better weightlifter. Here are some thoughts from Norb: "Don't attempt maximums in the gym. Some members of the U.S. lifting team couldn't believe how much more I could do in a contest, where it counted. I was never burned out. Attempts at limit weights should be restricted to once every three or four weeks. One should not work any more than 80 to 90 percent of his limit in training." That's straight from the horse's mouth. You might want to keep this concept in mind when you're planning your own training, since it comes from one of the greatest.

Work

Most of us have never trained at an Olympic level. I'm talking about the kind of training you have to do when you're the best in the world and you're trying to stay there. It doesn't take a rocket scientist to figure out that the intensity, stress, and all-consuming physical demands at this level are stupefying. Now, think about having to train like this when you're working a full-time job, worrying about paying your bills and supporting your family. Most of you are shaking your heads, and with good reason. It sounds like an impossible situation. Seriously, do any of us think the top lifters in Europe and Asia are working 40 hours a week at a brewery, struggling to afford their house payment, and then training to win the Olympic gold medal? Of course they're not. But Norb did. There's actually a famous story about how he once asked his boss at the manufacturing plant for some time off so he could train for the Olympics. The boss said, "Take all the time you want. You're fired." Then he had to go look for another job, while he trained to win an Olympic gold medal for his country.

Okay, okay…what does this have to do with ME?

After all of those neat little facts and quotes, how can we use the content of this article to make you better? I told you in the beginning that I was going to connect the story of this man to your life, right?

There are a couple of different ways we can do that. First of all, I want you to think about the concept of mental strength and determination. Now, look back at some of Norb's accomplishments. A 363 lb. split snatch at the age of 40, setting a world record at 38, winning four Olympic medals, making a comeback after a major back surgery, all that stuff. I want you to think about the phenomenal resilience and willpower it must have taken to do those things. Then I want you to think about your own lifting, your athletic career. Specifically, you need to think about the barriers and obstacles that are in front of you. Some of you probably have a mountain of crap standing in your way as you fight to reach your goals. Well folks, Norb's story is one of the greatest examples of overcoming obstacles in the chronicles of sports. Personally, I feel like his story gives me strength. This guy didn't believe in limits, and he never backed down. What kind of possibilities might be waiting for all of us if we simply apply those two principles to everything we do?

Second, some of the things Norb said about training and nutrition are obviously a lot different from what you read these days. Most current literature directly contradicts his ideas. Some might say we've progressed over the years, that our world has advanced beyond a lot of older methodology. We do things differently now because we're not in the caveman days anymore. Okay, I think that's true. But I also want to suggest the possibility that there are some old-school beliefs that we should reconsider, and maybe go back to. Everybody wants to think outside the box these days. Most people believe "thinking outside the box" involves moving past our old ways. Well, maybe one of the best ways to think outside the box is to GO BACK to some things that produced success in the past but got thrown in the toilet at some point because we were in such a hurry to reinvent the wheel. Am I telling you to quit eating Paleo and move to pizza, hamburgers, and beer? No. I'm just asking all of us to challenge the way we think and not reject certain ideas simply because they're from an older time.

Finally, I'm a big believer in the old transcendentalist concept of the Oversoul. This is the idea that the souls of all people are connected in some way, that we've all got the same spirit flowing through us and, on some level, we're all linked together. I think this is especially true in weightlifting. Why do you think weightlifters are so close-knit? Why do you think we stick together so tightly? Why do you think we're all so fanatical about what we're doing? It's because there's something intangible going on inside us when we become weightlifters. Nobody can put their finger on it exactly, but it's overpowering and it changes our lives. We're never the same after we've felt it. That's what connects all of you to Norb Schemansky. His career is one of the highest manifestations of the weightlifting spirit. He had something inside that propelled him forward, something that drove his engine beyond the limits of human ability. And you know what? You've got it too.

Look, I'm not a hippie. Some of you know me, and you know damn well I'm not a flower child, rolling around in a meadow and trying to communicate with nature. I'm an old-school guy, like Norb. But I definitely believe what I just wrote about the spirit of a weightlifter. We've all got it in our blood, just like he did. So, in some strange way, his life is a part of all our lives. That means his strength is part of our lives too. And that's a beautiful thing, brothers and sisters. A beautiful thing.

WALKING AWAY:
BREAK-UPS BETWEEN COACHES AND ATHLETES
MATT FOREMAN

I had a pretty good idea for an article recently. It was mainly a training-centered topic, about all the physical stuff you can do throughout a day to get prepared for lifting. I thought of it while I was on a plane, flying back to Chicago for my grandfather's funeral. Long flight, so I got a lot written down.

After the funeral weekend was over, I flew back home. I didn't have anything to read on the plane, so I bought a copy of Rolling Stone in the airport. Rock legend Lou Reed died a couple of weeks ago, and the issue I bought was mainly a tribute to him. While I was reading it, a different article idea occurred to me. It's another one of those things I can't believe I've never written about.

Probably because of the combination of my grandpa's funeral and the memorial articles about Lou, I started thinking about what it's like when things come to an end. These thoughts went in a weightlifting direction, and that's where the idea for this article started. We're going to talk about times when you have to end your lifting relationships. These are the situations where something isn't working right, and a big change is necessary. You have to leave your gym (or your team) and join a different one, or it could be when you have to make a coaching change...splitting from somebody you've been with for a long time. These are hard predicaments because something very big in your life is coming to an end. Even if you're doing it for the right reasons and the change is going to give positive results, the separation is still difficult. There's a lot of potential for ugliness and hard feelings.

These thoughts got pretty strong as I sat on the plane, because I've had to do this before and I'm pretty sure most of you will have experience with it at some point (or maybe you already have). You might be the athlete who has to break away, or maybe you'll be the coach who loses one of your lifters. During my flight, I borrowed a pen from my wife and wrote down this whole article in the margins of Rolling Stone issue 1196, with a big picture of Lou Reed on the cover. What you're reading now is just a typed transfer of the scribbled notes I made throughout the magazine. I have to admit, it was pretty cool the way it came together.

Break-ups suck, for the most part. Occasionally they feel really good because you hate the person you're splitting up with, and it's enjoyable when you kick them to the curb. But most of the time, these things are awkward and painful. We've all had to go through it in our romantic lives, and the next few pages are going to explore what it's like to go through it in your athletic life. Break-ups happen for different reasons. Sometimes, it's a "no harm, no foul" situation where everybody walks away without any bad blood. More often, it happens because somebody is unhappy or dissatisfied and there's fallout afterwards.

Almost every lifter I've ever known has had to switch teams or coaches at some point, and I'm pretty sure every coach in the world has felt what it's like when an athlete walks away. There are some definite good and bad ways to handle these moments, and that's what we're going to examine here. Thank god for boring plane rides, I guess.

Why it can happen…

We're talking about the situations where a relationship is over, between a coach and an athlete or maybe a whole gym. Because this whole area mainly deals with human interaction, there are literally countless factors and reasons that could be the cause. First of all, there are some times when the split has to happen because of simple life stuff. These are a little easier to manage because they don't involve any tension or resentment. If you live and train in Atlanta, and your employer is going to transfer you to Sacramento, there's not much you can do about that. It's disappointing and painful when you leave your gym, but everybody knows that it's not happening because of anything bad. Nobody is screwing anybody over and you all get to leave things on good terms. Great, lickety-split.

However, those aren't really the kind of predicaments I'm talking about here. We're looking at the break-ups that happen because there's some kind of problem. Common ones are:

- Betrayal. Some kind of major wrench got thrown into the works. Somebody lied to somebody, or there was some behind-the-back activity going on. Maybe the athlete was secretly working with another trainer behind the coach's back. Maybe the coach was talking crap about the athlete with other gym members. Maybe somebody screwed somebody else's boyfriend or girlfriend. You get the point. These are the really ugly ones, the big SNAFUs.
- Bad coaching. This happens a lot, unfortunately. When athletes stop making progress, they often blame their coaches. The thought process is, "I'm not getting any better, so my coach must not be training me correctly." At this point, the athletes usually notice other lifters who are having huge success, and they say to themselves, "Why are they all kicking ass, and I'm not?" If the athlete has the kind

of personality that leans towards finger-pointing, the coach can easily get blamed. These are the first seeds of a problem that could grow into a full-blown disaster.

- Toxic atmosphere. Here, the overall gym environment is the problem. It's usually not one specific thing you can put your finger on. More often, it's an assortment of dysfunction, adversarial personalities, weak leadership, etc. There might be one primary cause of the whole thing, like a prima donna athlete who contaminates the whole team dynamic. But it usually spills over into a lot of other areas, and you wind up with a place that's not much fun to train at.
- Uncoachable personality. This one is from the perspective of the coach. Here, the coach is thinking about dismissing an athlete, and it's probably because the athlete has become too difficult to deal with. For whatever reason, it's just not working out. You're a coach, but this is a person you simply don't want to have around.

What you should do...

Now, you're at a point where you're thinking about jumping ship. If you're the athlete, you're considering leaving your gym or switching to another coach. If you're the coach, you're thinking about cutting an athlete loose. Here are the factors that need consideration:

- Spend plenty of time making sure you have a good "plan B" before you pull the trigger. In other words, don't leave your coach or your gym until you've got someplace else to go. This might take a while, and it might create a situation where you have to stay with your current coach/gym longer than you want to while you're shopping around and putting your new arrangement together. Somebody once told me, "Monkeys don't let go of the branch they're on until they've got ahold of another one." Long story short, don't have your big bridge-burning moment until you've covered your ass and found a new coach/gym that's an improvement over the one you're leaving.
- When it's time to finally cut the cord, do it face-to-face. You need to show the other person some respect. When you break up with somebody through a text message or a phone call, it's cowardly. Arrange a sit-down, explain yourself, and give the other person a chance to respond. It's the right thing to do.

No way around it...

Once you've made the decision to do this, you have to accept the fact that feelings are going to get hurt. You can't avoid it. Somebody is going to feel like they're getting screwed over, and that's understandable.

This is where one of the prickliest concepts of the weightlifting life is revealed to us. I'm talking about the fact that the athlete's first loyalty has to be his/her own career. There has to be some selfishness involved. Don't get me wrong, I'm not saying it's okay to manipulate others and stomp all over people in your road to the top. Regardless of anything, there are basic principles of respect and decency that have to be honored in life if you don't want to be a complete scumbag. However, athletes shouldn't stay in bad situations simply because they don't want to hurt anybody's feelings. If you're a weightlifter and your career is going nowhere, or if you're in a crappy relationship with your coach that's making you unhappy, you have to think about yourself first. It's okay to be this way. At the end of the day, you're the one who has to live with the results you get on the platform. Those numbers are attached to your name, not anybody else's.

This creates a situation where you might have to be self-centered and walk away from somebody who you've previously built up a lot of loyalty with. Obviously, this sets the stage for all kinds of hard feelings. If you're a coach, you have to learn to be a professional about it. First of all, you enter into this profession knowing that situations like this are always a possibility. It's a risk you take when you decide to become a coach, because your lifters can take off at any moment. You'll get angry with them, and you'll probably think they're making a mistake. But you have to handle it like a grown-up. It'll still hurt, no doubt about it. Even if you have ice in your veins, you'll feel like somebody is sticking a dagger right in your chest because the coach-athlete relationship is incredibly powerful…and personal. When it ends, it's emotional. If it ends badly, it's painful and bitter.

But here's the bright side…

Your career as an athlete (or a coach) has a lot of chapters and phases. If you're going to be committing a large part of your life to this business, you'll have multiple seasons throughout the whole thing. Athletes are going to come and go. Coaches are going to come and go. Teams are going to come and go. It's all part of the game.

Here's a different way to explain it. I saw a movie once called "That Thing You Do." You might have seen it…Tom Hanks movie about a young rock band that makes it to the big time with a hit song. Anyway, there's a scene in it where a young drummer is in a bar and he meets one of his idols, an old jazz player who's basically a music legend. The old legend invites the drummer to sit down for some drinks, and they spend the night talking about the road you have to travel in your career. At one point, the young drummer tells the legend that he's worried because his band is about to break up and he thinks it'll be the end of his big chance. The old dude says to him, "Bands come and go. What you've got to do is just keep playing, with whoever."

The point he was making is basically the same one I'm giving you about your weightlifting life. It's a long journey you're on, and the faces will change from time to time. Most relationships don't last forever, and you shouldn't expect them to. If you curl up in a ball and contemplate retirement every time somebody lets you down or screws you over in this sport, you're not going to last long.

Having said that, make sure you also understand that a lot of thought and consideration has to go into a big decision like leaving a team/coach or firing an athlete. Most of the really successful people in the world don't live on impulsive, hasty moves. You can very easily throw away some great opportunities and situations if you have a habit of leaping before you look. I'm a pretty big believer that you should always give plenty of consideration to your options before you make a big switch.

Remember how I told you I got the idea for this article while I was reading about Lou Reed? Well, here's a final thought for you. Lou's career in music lasted from the mid-60s until his death in 2013. He played in a great band called The Velvet Underground, eventually went solo, collaborated with countless other artists, and took his music in several different directions over the course of thirty-something years. Decades passed and they brought a lot of changes, but he kept the focus on his music and the vision he had for what he wanted to accomplish. Your career in weightlifting will be the same way. It probably won't be permanently attached to any specific coach, team, gym, or program. Some of the phases you go through will end well, and some of them might involve some heartbreak. Ups and downs, you know? What you've got to do is just keep playing, with whoever.

PROGRAMMING AND PROGRESSIONS FOR YOUTH WEIGHTLIFTING: BUILDING WEIGHTLIFTING'S FUTURE
ERIK BLEKEBERG

PE programs are being cut, sports other than football or basketball get less money every year, and the injury rate of kids goes up as the movement quality goes down. I got into coaching the high school sector in strength and conditioning, but found it's about a lot more than just lifting weights. It is about building a program that develops kids that care about movement and how they do things, kids that have focus, goals and drive.

I have built an effective Strength & Conditioning program at Army and Navy Academy High School, but my focus has been on trying to make America a power in weightlifting again and that starts with the kids: they are the future lifters of the world, and if they are not going to be lifters, then they can at least be fans. I want to see more high school programs pop up because right now I am the only one in all of San Diego. What follows is a layout of what I have used to build an effective weightlifting program that in its first year sent three kids to Nationals to place in the top six. We have just gotten started and wish to see more schools follow suit!

First, you teach: How to teach a large group of kids to lift

To instruct a large group of kids in lifting, I use a concept I got from Coach Dan John, dumbbell yoga. This is a series of exercises, stretches and drills that's designed to help teach people the basic movements of lifting in a safe environment that allows for easy correction. The program is as follows:

Warmer (light jogging or jumping jacks)
hip flexor stretch
adductor stretch
T-Spine dynamic stretch
Yoga flow (eccentric pushup, cobra, child's pose, downward dog)- breath control emphasized

From downward dog – warrior one pose, both sides

Push-ups x10
Goblet squat x 10
Dumbbell deadlift x 10
Dumbbell snatch x 5
R Waiter walk - 20 yards
Dumbbell snatch x 5
L Waiter Walk - 20 yards
Repeat one more time

This sequence of exercises is done in a military large group format where reps are controlled and counted as a group. This allows for easy coaching and everyone can see everyone else to get feedback on how to properly perform the exercise while receiving coaching cues.

Then you must have a plan: A Periodized Year for High School Weightlifting Periodization seems to have mixed views nowadays. Some think it is the only way to do things and create success, others think it is devil's magic from a bygone Soviet era. Whichever way you look at it, you need to have a plan over the course of the year if you intend to take a kid from zero to a total. The layout of the year for me looks like this:

Late August/September – Learn/Teach Phase 1

Using dumbbell yoga as a warm-up, lifters then go through the main movements. Programmed lifts include trap bar deadlifts, push-ups, pull-ups, rows, kettlebell swings, back Squats, front squats and varying ab exercises.

October/Early November

Grow Phase Dumbbell yoga is no longer done; a joint movement warm-up is used instead. After that, we cover the technique of the snatch and clean with the bar/stick and use that as skillwork in 15-minute sessions before the main exercises. The main exercises included are the back squat, front squat, press, bench press, deadlift, RDL, good mornings, lunges, kettlebell swings, and varying ab exercises. The goal is hypertrophy and improved competency in more advanced lifts.

Late November/December (before winter break) Strength Test Phase

The exercises have not changed, but the focus is on lifting at a heavier percent of their one rep max. Max testing week is performed, but technique is carefully controlled. Most of these 1RMs could potentially be two to three rep maxes, but the body has reached technical failure so the lift is not pushed heavier. The Olympic lifts are still in their infancy but are progressing with technique plates. Still, the sn and c+j are done for reps of three, with a focus on position and consistency. We're now up to about 20 minutes of training time.

Early January - Review Phase

There is a two-week break following the Strength Test Phase, followed by a two-week get back in shape program that refocuses their mind and gets their bodies remembering the lifts.

Late January/February – Develop/Strength/Specialize

We now focus on the lifts, with more experienced lifters working in the 80 percent range on the snatch and the clean+jerk, while additional barbell work is kept in the 80-90 percent rep range and cycled through. The first developmental meet is in February. Only competent lifters may compete; others are required to attend to watch and learn.
March/April/May – Competition Phase

March marks our first major competition. Only top competent candidates are permitted in the first meet, but all must compete in the April meet. If technique is still in development, then the meet is treated as a technique meet for them. Volume is reduced overall and they are preparing for one meet a month. Those qualifying for Nationals will NOT compete in May but will enter an extended prep for that National meet. Otherwise, May will be the final meet.

June – Training for the future/Nationals Prep

Some will graduate and never see me again, while others are staying and training for Nationals. In the case of the former, I teach basic programming skills and explain how I structured their workouts and why, and make sure they can continue on at least for fitness if not for competition. The crew preparing for Nationals cycles week by week and the planned openers and lifts are decided at the start of the month and worked towards throughout the rest of the month. Youth Nationals typically takes place at the end of June.

Don't forget love: How to introduce lifting to kids

I don't just start teaching the kids the lifts. That makes them go through the motions. I first want wide-eyed fans. I show videos (the DVDs from Ironmind and YouTube) of different competitions and always dedicate at least the last 10 minutes of class to watching competitions and lifting, always World level lifters. The kids learn the names, they learn the format and they want to be like them, not only that they learn the technique.

I teach technique from the bottom up.

Snatch
Snatch Deadlift
Snatch High Pull
Muscle Snatch w/Squat
Power Snatch
Full Snatch

Clean
Clean Deadlift
Clean Pull
Power Clean w/Squat

Jerk
Dip and Extend
Power Jerk
Split (if necessary)
Clean + Jerk

I find this method has an easy sequential format for getting the kids to understand how the lift should feel, how to keep the pull long and how to be explosive. I always relate back to the videos to show the boys what they are learning and help them have better understanding.

And don't scare them away: Competitions done right

I am not someone who believes in holding a kid back for four years while he masters the technique and THEN letting him compete. By that same token, I don't think you should push the kid to max and shoot for PRs when he can't even do the lift right every time. All my boys compete in the spring, regardless of how long they have been in the program because I want them to learn format. If need be we will keep them on technique plates in the competition, and I give them notes and ratings on how they did. I don't care about their total. I care about how can we improve and most importantly, whether or not they had fun.

Competing should be fun for kids. Let them decide how serious they want to take it. The competitions that all the newer lifters do are ALWAYS on home turf so they feel comfortable. More experienced lifters go to a variety of locations, lift on different bars and get challenged. The key is building the confidence over time and making them see how much fun competitive weightlifting can be. It reminds them that they are spending all this time practicing for SOMETHING. You can't just keep a kid locked away for years on end; they won't be able to see the light.

Making it last: Build a team and culture

A team is a culture. It has a unified attitude, clothes, lifting styles, etc. You need to create a team because when someone is having a bad day, the coach doesn't need to help them out of it, the team can. They support each other, pitch in to do work or fundraise and make it a more enjoyable experience. There are plenty of articles and books out there on how to build great teams, but it's really just caring enough to make one. Get some shirts, have team breaks, have a record board and make everyone feel like they're a part of the club. It can go a long way and help make sure that all the technical work you put in to coach and develop the athletes does not go to waste.

Weightlifting is a precarious sport in the US and has some diehard followers. There have been many avenues to discover it but many people always wish they had discovered the sport earlier. Youth need the sport of weightlifting more than ever and they need it taught right. So get into the high school and youth sectors; teach, plan, build and grow, because weightlifting's future is learning to read and write right now.

PROGRAM DESIGN AND RECOVERY
TRAVIS COOPER

I have been competing in weightlifting for the past nine years. Over that time, my knowledge on weightlifting has expanded and evolved. I often get questions from people asking for my views on training and recovery. Here are the basic views and logic that I use when thinking about these two major components of training.

Programming

If someone told you today that if you did not add 15kg to your snatch in four weeks they would kill your family, what would you do? I have asked a variation of this question to both novice and veteran lifters and 99 percent of the time, a conversation similar to the following ensues:

> *Them: "I would snatch"*
> *Me: "How heavy would you snatch?"*
> *Them: "Heavy"*
> *Me: "How many times a week would you snatch heavy?"*
> *Them: "Probably every day"*
> *Me: "How many times a day would you snatch heavy?"*
> *Them: "Multiple times per day"*

After thinking of things this way, I cannot shake the notion that training the lifts heavy and often is the best way to make improvement. I believe that weightlifting is intuitive in nature, and the main thing that needs to be replicated to improve is not some secret training program, but the urgency to improve. In a situation where your family's wellbeing is at risk, it becomes necessary to get better. Instead of it being an option, you now have to get better. We have to somehow find a certain urgency to get better in the same way that we would have urgency to get to air if we were drowning. For this reason, my programming sticks close to the lifts taking the approach of going as heavy as I can, as often as I can, without getting hurt.

Glenn Pendlay, my current coach at MuscleDriver USA, has similar ideas. Over time Glenn has found that in the United States, for the drug free athlete, three max out sessions per week is a good balance between getting enough reps at high percentages to make continued progress, but keep lifters from getting injured. Let's face it; no one makes progress when they are injured. So Monday, Wednesday, Friday afternoons are heavy sessions in the snatch and clean and jerk. Those three sessions make up the backbone of our training. We also train in the mornings on Monday, Wednesday, and Friday, which are lighter technique sessions with no misses, working on crisp technique. On Monday and Wednesday after we do technique work in the mornings, we squat. Tuesday and Thursday are our recovery days where we do exercises that are easier to recover from. We may still go to max but we will do exercises such as power variations of the lifts or no hook grip work to limit the load we can use. Saturday is a strength day where we will squat heavy, push press, and do any other bodybuilding exercises that the individual athlete might do to stay healthy. We stick to singles in the lifts the majority of the year, but further out from a competition, we might do doubles or triples to max instead. In the strength exercises, we usually follow the Texas Method. A general template might look as follows:

	MON	TUE	WED	THUR	FRI	SAT
PM	SNATCH - MAX, 3X2@80%	POWER SNATCH - MAX	SNATCH –MAX, 3X2@80%	POWER SNATCH - MAX	SNATCH –MAX	SQUAT – HEAVY SET OF 5
	CLEAN AND JERK – MAX, 2X2@80%	POWER CLEAN AND JERK - MAX	CLEAN AND JERK – MAX, 2X2@80%	POWER CLEAN AND JERK - MAX	CLEAN AND JERK – MAX	PUSH PRESS – HEAVY SET OF 5
		PUSH PRESS – 3X5	PUSH PRESS – 3X5 (-10% FROM TUESDAY)			BODY-BUILDING
AM	SNATCH – TECH WORK		SNATCH – TECH WORK		SNATCH – TECH WORK	
	CLEAN AND JERK – TECH WORK		CLEAN AND JERK – TECH WORK		CLEAN AND JERK – TECH WORK	
	SQUAT – (3-5)X5 HEAVY		SQUAT – 3X5 (-10-20% FROM MONDAY)			

Recovery

In order to reach your potential as a weightlifter, recovery must be spot on so you can stay healthy and build higher work capacity to get those extra kilos! In my opinion, recovery is broken into two categories: the 95 percent category and the 5 percent category. Everyone always talks about the 5 percent category, which includes ice baths, chiropractic, massage, foam rolling, stretching, stem, etc. You can find tons of information on how these things will make or break your training. The truth is these are important tools for recovery; however, they will never make up for a lack of attention to the 95 percent category.

In the 95 percent category you will first find sleep. For the competitive weightlifter training five to 12 sessions per week, a minimum of eight hours of sleep is required. I personally sleep about eight to 10 hours per night. Oftentimes, the same people who are barely getting six hours of sleep are always looking for the secrets of recovery in the 5 percent category. Do not overlook sleep. You cannot overcome sleep deprivation through any other recovery method.

The second piece of the 95 percent category is diet. First and foremost, you have to get enough calories to recovery from the amount of training you are doing. That is not a problem for most weightlifters, so once you have that covered, the cleaner you can eat, the better.

The last piece of the 95 percent category is overall happiness. When I am training well, it is usually linked to happiness outside of training. This means that if you are fighting with your spouse, arguing with your kids, dealing with a lot of stress at work and so forth, training will suffer. In order to train well, you must minimize stress outside of the gym.

Sometimes the hardest things to change are in the 95 percent category. But trust me, if you organize your life to maximize your recovery, it will go much further than spending tons of money in the 5 percent category without changing the things you are lacking in the 95 percent category.

Conclusion

Keep in mind that these are my views and that no matter what, you must fully believe in what you are doing for it to work! The best program in the world will not work if you do not believe in it, and the worst program in the world will probably work if you are fully invested in it.

Train Hard, Sleep Well, and Eat Well.

COMPLEXES
GREG EVERETT

The excitement seems to be waning a little already, but at least momentarily, weightlifting complexes were the coolest thing on the internet. People had a cure for everything involving a lifting complex, and many blurred the line considerably between weightlifting and conditioning. Many articles included something about "getting shredded" in the titles, which to me is a sure sign that they're arbitrary combinations of exercises meant to just get you out of breath.

When you use a complex, make sure you have a reason to, and that it's a good one (i.e., not "complexes are cool"). It should serve a clear purpose and be the most effective and appropriate way to achieve that purpose for that lifter at that time. Sometimes a legitimate purpose is nothing more than variety to stave off mental staleness—but this is a short-term plan, and this isn't a reason to suddenly abandon all manner of training in favor of complexes only.

I use complexes occasionally in my lifters' programs when they serve a goal. This is usually a technique-related goal, which is why most of the complexes you'll see me use combine one exercise with either a snatch, clean or jerk afterward—they're allowing the lifter to practice something specific immediately prior to the lift in which I need them to correct that specific technical element.

The other reason I'll use them is strength-related (including mental strength). They may do a partial lift before a full classic lift to introduce a little fatigue before the classic lift and force them to fight harder for it.

Following are just a few complexes I use fairly regularly. The rep notation will be the first exercise + the second exercise. Numbers inside parenthesis are one series that gets repeated as many times as the number outside the parenthesis. For example:

- Halting Snatch Deadlift + Snatch – 1+1 means one halting deadlift followed by one snatch.
- Halting Snatch Deadlift + Snatch – 2(1+1) means one halting deadlift followed by one snatch, then one halting deadlift followed by one snatch for a total of four consecutive reps.

Halting Snatch/Clean Deadlift + Snatch/Clean

This is usually used to reinforce the posture and patience of the snatch or clean pull—that is, to help the lifter stay over the bar longer before initiating the second pull. In the snatch, I'll usually put the pause of the halting deadlift at the hip, and the upper thigh for the clean, and have them hold that position for three seconds. However, I also have them hold at a different position, such as the knee. I would use the knee in the case of a lifter who has a lot of trouble moving his/her weight back in the pull off the floor. This complex would allow them to focus on that initial lift from the ground that involves shifting back as well as moving up. If these complexes are done without straps in the snatch, they're also excellent grip training. The more technique work the lifter needs, the lighter the weights will need to be. You can take this complex very heavy, but don't exceed the weight at which the lifter is no longer able to maintain the proper posture, including a full back arch, and the full pause count, or you're defeating the purpose.

Snatch High Pull + Hang Snatch

This is a complex I use to train and reinforce the proper high-elbow, forceful pull under the bar that's needed for good snatches. The snatch high-pull allows the lifter to focus on both accelerating the bar upward maximally with the legs and hips, and then also the action of pulling the elbows high and to the sides, strengthening that movement at the same time. They then snatch from the hang (usually just above the knee) to perform that same arm action in the turnover. Doing the snatch from the hang instead of the floor means they will have to be aggressive in the pull under because of the limited time and space to get the bar moving upward, forcing the strong, high-elbow pull they're working on. It's also a good complex to help the lifter work on keeping the bar close in the turnover.

Clean + Front Squat

This is just a great strength complex, forcing the athlete to make a strong, accurate clean to have enough left over in the tank to make the front squat. The more technically sound the clean, the more energy the athlete will have for the squat. But even the best clean will make the following squat tough, so in any case, the lifter is forced to gut it out.

Snatch/Clean Pull + Snatch/Clean

This complex is great off the blocks as well. Performing a pull before the associated lift does a few things I like: It's an opportunity for the lifter to practice the proper movement from the floor to the point of explosion; it fatigues the lifter before the classic lift, forcing more focus and effort and making the body recruit more motor units; post-activation potentiation means the lifter should be capable of recruiting more motor units in the classic lift after the pull, and it helps lifters focus on a strong, upward leg drive at the top of the lift.

Snatch + Overhead Squat

This is a pretty obvious one—a lifter who is weak in the overhead position can easily get in more overhead/bottom position strength and mobility work by simply adding one or more overhead squats after his/her snatches.

Power Snatch/Clean + Snatch/Clean

I more often use the clean version than the snatch version. A power clean before the clean can be helpful in getting the lifter to be more aggressive in the finish and quicker in the turnover. The idea is to turn over and rack the clean at about the same height they did the power clean. Lifters who drop out from under their cleans and let the bar crash on their shoulders, or who cut their pulls short to rush under the bar in the clean, are the perfect candidates for this one.

Front Squat + Jerk

This is good for getting the legs a bit tired before the jerk to force the lifter to be more aggressive and follow through better, but also to simulate a jerk after a clean without having to do a clean first, which you may want to avoid for various reasons. Lifters who struggle to jerk from the rack (i.e. they tend to jerk better after a clean than when they take the bar from the rack) will often jerk better after a front squat because it helps them adjust into the jerk rack position better than they can straight from the rack.

Jerk Behind the Neck + Jerk

Lifters who tend to leave the bar a bit forward overhead in the jerk because they're not locking the shoulder blades into place well may find this helpful. Starting behind the neck allows them to set the shoulder blades tightly together where they should end up overhead, and the bar can move straight up into position instead of having to move back slightly. They can then aim to put the bar in the same place and get the same feeling of locking the position when they do the subsequent jerk from the front.

Pause Jerk + Jerk

Pause jerks are tough, and I think they can be effective in both helping improve the upward drive of the jerk and the balance in the dip and drive, but used alone, I've found they can interfere with a lifter's dip and drive rhythm. Because of this, I prefer to always have the lifter do a normal jerk after a pause jerk to maintain that rhythm. In the pause jerk, dip at a controlled speed and hold the bottom of the dip position for 3 seconds, then drive directly into the jerk from that bottom position (don't bounce or dip down at all before driving). Reset after recovering from that rep, and perform a normal jerk with no pause.

Push Press + Jerk

This is a good complex to use for a lifter who tends to drift forward in the dip or drive of the jerk, or who fails to finish the upward drive before splitting under. The goal is to drive the jerk exactly the way they drove the push press—all the way up, straight up—and then split the feet.

INTRODUCING PLYOMETRICS TO THE NOVICE OLYMPIC LIFTER
BRAD LESHINSKE

Olympic lifting is a sport in which explosive power and force production is key. In a sport where power production is so important, teaching new lifters to be powerful can be a tough thing to do, especially for the young Olympic lifter. A method in teaching power production, especially for the new lifter, is the introduction of plyometrics.

Plyometrics are movements or activities that enable a muscle to reach maximal force in the shortest time possible. There are three major components when looking at a plyometric movement:

1. **Eccentric phase** – the preloading phase in which the muscles store energy. The beginning position of this phase also resembles the landing position as well. This is also important because when the athlete gets into repeated jumps this phase needs to be done rapidly.
2. **Amortization phase** – the transition from the eccentric phase to the concentric phase. This phase is the most important as the quicker that we get through this phase the better force production and power we have.
3. **Concentric phase** – the actual jump. This is the body's response to the first two phases. The body will either use the energy provided and make the jump or dissipate that energy into heat.

With the sequences above in teaching plyometrics, we have to start with the ending first. The landing is probably the most important thing you can teach anyone new to jumping. This is because no one ever gets hurt jumping; they get hurt with improper landing. To learn how to absorb force, there are some coaching cues that need to be addressed. Teaching how to land:

· Hold the landing for two seconds. This allows the coach to see if the athlete can actually absorb the force and to check their ankle, knee and hip position.
· Good posture. Keeping the chest up and out is vital to a good landing and making sure that there are no big issues with the back alignment.

- Feet shoulder width apart. We do not want to see the athlete's feet inside shoulder width because of the force it puts on the knee joint.
- No hips sink when landing. Once you land, stick the landing, which is also called being stiff. Becoming a stiffer athlete is beneficial to force absorption and prevention of injury. But in reference to no hips sinking, in the two-second hold, you can definitely see if there is hip drop.
- Soft landing (don't put a hole in the box). We want to be able to control the force of the landing, especially in the beginning phase of jump training.

Once an athlete learns how to land, he or she can go on to work on force production. For Olympic lifters, teaching hip drive is crucial in throwing up big numbers in lifts. We can correlate the jump position to the power position in Olympic lifting. While the power position is important for the lifter, the pre-loading position is important to teach effective jumping. While Olympic lifting elicits more power production, novice or beginner lifters will benefit more from plyometric training because while learning the Olympic movements and really mastering the power position and certain pulls, plyometrics can help teach the athletes to generate power.

The same rule applies for jumping when talking power production. Here are some parallels from Olympic lifting to plyometric training.

PLYOMETRIC MOVEMENT	OLYMPIC MOVEMENT
1. LOAD POSITION	1. POWER POSITION
2. PUNCH AND DRIVE ARMS THROUGH, START TO GET EXTENSION IN THE HIPS	2. PULL THE BAR (DEPENDING ON LIFT) START DRIVING THE HIPS TO EXTENSION
3. GET FULL EXTENSION IN ANKLE, KNEES AND HIPS	3. GET HIPS THROUGH, START TO GET UNDER THE BAR OR INTO CATCH POSITION
4. SOFT BUT STIFF LANDING. CHEST TALL ARMS BACK	4. SOLID CATCHING MECHANICS

These parallels explain why plyometrics can be useful into teaching power production in an Olympic lifting program. Although there is way more to it than the cues above, this begins to show that there is a great comparison into certain cues and goals of both movements.

While those are the basic cues for simple jumps, you have to program correctly to elicit results over a longer period of time. For example, going right to max jumps on a box is setting the athlete up for injury or failure. Proper progression is needed in order to gain the results in the big picture. The progressions listed below are a way to progress correctly and safely to bigger and explosive jumps, while decreasing risk of injury. These movements are done in a two to three week block, progressing each week the new jumping mechanics listed below.

- Non-counter movement: No repeated hurdle jump or box jumping. Jump once, land and stick correctly then move on to the next jump.
- Jump with a mini bounce: An example of this is jumping over a hurdle, mini hop and jump over the next hurdle. This is a great transition from non-counter to the next phase of counter movement jumping. This ability to use the mini bounce helps teach the body to load and reload muscles and energy.
- Jump with counter movement: This is your repeated hurdle jump or what we call true plyometrics, the ability to jump and load that energy quickly and efficiently for the next jump.
- Advanced movements: Advanced movements like depth jumps are a key in taking your lifts to the next level when you're ready. Another advanced jump is a concentric jump where you sit on a box and jump to a higher box. This is pure power development because there is no loading on the body.

The next question is where do we put these movements in our training for novice athletes? Well, depending on your athlete's ability to lift, which at the beginning will be more technique based, I suggest putting them in at the beginning of the program for their power work and then teaching technique post jump training. This will allow the body to learn to produce power. As your athlete advances out on the platform, you decrease the volume of jumping and move on to other protocols for plyometrics.

Setting up the program for a novice lifter has to be constructed with landing mechanics in mind. As mentioned above, landing is crucial to moving into generating more power both on the platform and also with regard to jump training. When looking at new athletes and even older athletes, the incorporation of corrective movements or a stretch in between is important. For our correctives, I tend to lean toward the Functional Movement Screen Correctives. These are selected after we screen them for any mobility or stability issues. With our Olympic lifters, we can also include shoulder flexibility as well.

With regard to core movements, we want to introduce them to stabilizing movements such as planks, side planks, anti-rotation and other exercises that improve that strength. Because they are Olympic lifters, we do not have to worry so much on rotational strength as we would with a baseball or football player. Olympic athletes are very strong and explosive and we do not want to crush the central nervous system and compromise their lifting.

A typical program for a novice athlete will look like this in teaching the landing, generally taking about one to two weeks for most athletes depending on age. You will then move in the order mentioned above with regards to the non-counter movements, jumps with a mini bounce, jumps with counter movements and then finally more advanced movements. These phases can last anywhere between two and four weeks depending on the age of the athletes as well as their movement. You also would only want to include this one to two times a week if lifting four days a week for a novice lifter. If the athlete is on a two to three day lifting program, mix the plyometrics in on just one of those days. For our advanced athletes, we do a plyometric movement every lifting session, depending on sport and a needs analysis (what the athlete is weak in). For example, our baseball pitchers do not Olympic lift. Instead we provide them with a lot of plyometric movements and med ball rotational power movements.

Novice Athlete Landing Program

Weeks One and Two*

> A1 - Drop squats 3X5 (standing tall and dropping down to a squat)
> A2 – Flexibility work or corrective work (based off of FMS screen - example would be hip flexor stretch off the box)
> B1 – Box jumps 3X3 (start at an 18-24 inch box)
> B2 – Core exercise (front plank 3X15s)
> C1 – Single Leg Hops 3X3 (great for teaching stability and injury prevention)
> C2 – Core Exercise (side planks 2X10s)

Once learning has become efficient on landing mechanics, move on to the jumping. Generally see the athlete through two to four weeks and increase in box height if landing is sufficient.

Weeks Three and Four*

> A1 – Box jumps 3x4
> A2 – Corrective or flexibility (again FMS based, incorporate any weakness you see with mobility or start putting in Olympic lifting stretches, things for forearms or shoulder flexibility)
> B1 – Hurdle hops non-counter movement (start with 12 inch hurdles)
> B2 – Core exercise (front plank 3x20s)

Plyometrics with a mini bounce. This is done in weeks four to six and is the final stage before the advanced movements begin. Again, check for good landing mechanics and power output.

Weeks Five and Six*

A1 – Box jump with increased height

A2 – Corrective or core movement

B1 – Hurdle hop with mini bounce

B2 – Corrective or core

C1 – Single Leg hurdle hops with mini bounce 3X3 (teaches great control and eccentric strength)

Intermediate training is done when you feel the athlete establishes a great base of power. If the athlete is progressing fast on the platform, check the volume of the jumps and decrease them. The use of other exercises to compliment the power on the Olympic movements can be done with addition of depth jumps and broad jumps.

BONUS! Intermediate: Weeks Seven and Eight

A1 – Box jumps with weighted vest 3X3

A2 – Corrective exercise or core   (either a plank movement or shoulder corrective)

B1 – Depth jump to a squat jump 3X3

B2 – Corrective or core exercise (anti-rotation core movement)

C1 – SL hop, no stick or mini bounce

C2 – Core exercise (side plank)

Where do we put this program with regards to their lifting? As previously mentioned we want to do the plyometrics prior to the weightlifting portion of the workout. A sufficient warm up is needed then we can get to the jump training. For an athlete working out four days a week, make sure you have 48 hours of rest in between plyometric workouts. So if you want to hit the jump training on a Monday and Thursday, that would be fine. This allows for proper rest. If you're only lifting two to three times a week, add the jump training in on one of those training days. Again, making sure you have some rest is ideal.

The above are great guidelines in a novice program and will take four to six weeks to get through. Teaching proper explosive movement not only comes in the form of Olympic lifting, which we train every kid in, but can start with plyometrics and then be weaved into the Olympic setting. Most everyone will want to know what kind of results you will get when going through a jump training program. With a six-week program, you can expect to gain a couple inches in your vertical. With Olympic lifting and plyometrics combined, big lifting numbers are sure to follow.

*Athletes may stay in a phase longer or progress through one quicker if the coach sees that the objective is being met and the athlete can both jump and land correctly.

STRENGTH: EASY AS PI
JON DEMOSS

When my athletes ask me how to get faster, or get more powerful, or how to make plays worthy of SportsCenter's Top 10, I always answer the same: "Get stronger!" A quick trip around the interwebs reveals seemingly infinite methods and programs for increasing strength that often leads to more blank stares than a grade school geometry class. Don't make it harder than it has to be, though. At the core of each of these programs lies only a few principles to get stronger. Learning these simple principles of strength will help focus your efforts and drive your weights up. As Dan John famously quipped, "Simple does not mean easy," so be prepared to put in some work! I hope you brought a notepad and something to write with because the school bell is about to ring.

Basic Rule #1: Show Up to Class

For the weights to climb, you have to continually get your practice under the bar. To hone their skills, baseball players get in the cages, golfers hit the driving range, and swimmers take laps in the pool. Strength is also a skill and, just like any skill, requires consistent effort to gain proficiency.

Basic Rule #2: Listen to What I SAID

Spend any amount of time around seasoned strength addicts and/or read scientific research on resistance training and you will come across the SAID principle (Specific Adaptation to Imposed Demands). You cannot work your way to four wheels on the bar by doing things that got you to three wheels on the bar. The intensity of the challenge must be increased to break through plateaus and reach new levels of strength. (Note that the intensity must increase and understand that intensity can mean training load, volume, resistance, playing with leverage, altering base of support, and just about a thousand or so other ways to make your program more challenging. These topics will be addressed in the Master's course.)

Basic Rule #3: Avoid All-Night Cram Sessions

In their exuberance, many strength students tend to over-complicate and over-reach. "Why don't I just keep adding plates or do as many reps as possible?" Because neither option is unsustainable. Strength increases are only linear for the novice, or the weak, so a focused plan that manages load will serve you better than attempting to just pile on the plates. Plan to keep a couple of repetitions in reserve as trying to fit as many reps into one training session not only jeopardizes your quality control as fatigue sets in but could also interfere with your ability to bounce back for your next workout. If you cannot repeatedly put forth the same level of exertion to match the increasing intensity of each training session, expect to see your strength numbers burn brightly before quickly going up in smoke!

Course Requirements

1. **Do your prep work:** This program works under the assumption you know the fundamentals of each movement and have a high degree of proficiency. This is a strength program, and if you do not know how to properly execute the movements, then you showed up to Geometry class without first knowing how to add. Get with a coach and hammer your form until you can confidently, and competently, complete the exercises.

2. **Do the work:** Get in the gym and attack your training with purpose (you're here to get stronger, remember). Heavy weights with controlled exposures means that every rep counts, so be sure all repetitions are completed successfully! Technique becomes more and more important as the weight on the bar climbs, so keep your form dialed-in. Give it a fair shake and follow the program as outlined. Do not mix in other programs, ask how cardio fits into the routine (once again, you showed up looking for strength), or question the percentages/sets/reps, etc. Only when you have completed the program in its entirety can we have a proper discussion about adjustments and future direction.

3. **Do your homework:** Staples for any training program should include proper nutrition, adequate rest, and appropriate bodywork (mobility, stability, correctives, sports medicine, and so forth). Before you go scheduling an "arm blaster" day, be mindful that the goal of homework is to replenish and restore so you can come back again and again to put forth a consistent level of exertion for each training exposure.

4. **Check your work:** Make sure you are current with the program projections and successfully meeting the increasing intensity. Adjust prep work and/or homework accordingly to benefit your desired goal. Speaking frankly - if you

are eating garbage, staying up late to watch the Game of Thrones marathon, or running five miles a day then no, you should not expect full benefit of the outlined program.

The Curriculum:

Did someone say pi? No, not blueberry or pumpkin, but the mathematical ratio of a circle's circumference to its diameter. Let me guess, you fell asleep that day in math class too, huh? The Pi Program uses an undulating rep scheme within the workout that gradually increases to 3-1-4-1-5 (hence, Pi). This wave loading allows the athlete to increase the weight of their 1-rep max lift and gradually add repetitions with sub-maximal weight over time. The intent of increasing maximal strength through additional repetitions at sub-maximal efforts, a concept first posed by Marty Gallagher, adds a new dimension to the Pi Program. To avoid over-reaching with the increasing training load, the total volume of the program is controlled to allow consistency of effort. The Pi Program is meant to address true strength lifts that require a massive amount of motor unit recruitment (typically anything with a barbell - Deadlift, Press, Squat, Olympic Lifts - work best). I recommend finding the areas you need to add strength the most and focusing your efforts on those lifts.

The Pi Program is short in duration - only 10 workouts per cycle. You may string cycles together based on needs, but always incorporate alternating cycles of training to avoid stagnation (Power, Hypertrophy, Metabolic Conditioning, etc.). For the sake of explanation, I will detail a deadlift program one of our athletes recently completed.

WORKOUT	REPS (WT. USED)
1	1 @ 350 LBS. 1 @ 365 LBS. 1 @ 380 LBS. 1 @ 390 LBS. 1 @ 400 LBS.
2	2 @ 360 LBS. 1 @ 360 LBS. 1 @ 360 LBS. 1 @ 360 LBS. 1 @ 360 LBS.
3	3 @ 360 LBS. 1 @ 370 LBS. 1 @ 360 LBS. 1 @ 370 LBS. 1 @ 360 LBS.

WORKOUT	REPS (WT. USED)
4	3 @ 360 LBS. 1 @ 380 LBS. 2 @ 360 LBS. 1 @ 380 LBS. 1 @ 360 LBS.
5	3 @ 360 LBS. 1 @ 390 LBS. 3 @ 360 LBS. 1 @ 390 LBS. 1 @ 360 LBS.
6	3 @ 360 LBS. 1 @ 395 LBS. 4 @ 360 LBS. 1 @ 395 LBS. 1 @ 360 LBS.
7	3 @ 360 LBS. 1 @ 400 LBS. 4 @ 360 LBS. 1 @ 400 LBS. 2 @ 360 LBS.
8	3 @ 360 LBS. 1 @ 410 LBS. 4 @ 360 LBS. 1 @ 410 LBS. 3 @ 360 LBS.
9	3 @ 360 LBS. 1 @ 415 LBS. 4 @ 360 LBS. 1 @ 415 LBS. 4 @ 360 LBS.
10	3 @ 360 LBS. 1 @ 420 LBS. 4 @ 360 LBS. 1 @ 420 LBS. 5 @ 360 LBS.

Training Notes:

- Max Lift start: 400 lbs./ Max Lift end: 420 lbs.
- Sub-Maximal reps at 360 lbs. start: 6 (completed in workout 2) / Sub-Maximal reps at 360 lbs. end: 12
- This athlete completed a subsequent cycle of the Pi Program (with the new training max of 420 lbs.) and completed 440 lbs. at the end of that program! 40 lb. increase in 20 workouts
- Results have consistently averaged between 15% - 20% increase on tested lifts per cycle

The Workout:

5 days per week
30 to 45 minutes per day

Warm-Up:
Keep it basic! The point is to get your CNS primed and the gears of your body lubed-up for activity. If you have special concerns (tight hip flexors or a tricky shoulder from an old rugby injury) that require extra stretching or activations, they would be addressed here. Our athletes use the following kettlebell warm-up:

> Heavy Get-Ups: 1 set of 5 R / 5 L
> Heavy Goblet Squat: 1 set of 10 repetitions
> Heavy Carry (Double Rack or Farmer Walk): 1 set of 1 minute straight (Do NOT set the KB's down until the clock stops)

A Day: Monday/Wednesday/Friday

Completed in Circuit format - 5 rounds total

- Deadlift: Pi Programming
- Push-Ups: 8 repetitions first week, add 2 repetitions to each set every week
- Corrective/Mobility/Stability/Core

*Listed in this particular order based on priority. If you need Corrective work, then choose an appropriate drill. If you do not need a corrective drill but could use some Mobility/Stability work, then choose an appropriate stretch. If you are solid on the Corrective or Mobility/Stability front, then you are a unicorn and can proceed to extra core work. Please be mindful with your core work choices as you are lifting heavy and do not want to exhaust the muscles that will be protecting your spine, nor do you want to miss lifts because you went too aggressive on side planks.

B Day: Tuesday/Thursday

Completed in a Circuit format - 5 rounds total

- Heavy Swings: 10 repetitions

- Can substitute moderate (75%-80%) Cleans if more experienced with this lift opposed to KB Swings: 5 repetitions if selecting Cleans
- Pull-Ups: 5 repetitions first week, add 2 repetitions to each set every week
- Corrective/Mobility/Stability/Core *See A Day explanation for this portion of the workout

Pay attention more to the format of the program rather than the specific exercises listed. This example features the Deadlift. The Pi Program template has been used successfully for ALL major lifts including squats, presses, and Olympic lifts.

HANG CLEAN VS. POWER CLEAN:
WHICH SHOULD BE TAUGHT AT YOUR FACILITY
BRAD LESHINKE

Every college, university and high-level athlete uses Olympic lifting to increase power output, speed on the field, and agility. These movements are very specific, intense to learn, and take a long time to perfect. So much so that, as the name suggests, it is an Olympic Sport. Weightlifting is not something that is a recreational sport. It takes years to perfect these movements, even with great coaching. With hundreds, if not thousands, of kids getting taught in sports performance facilities the good old question arises: which type of lift is more applicable and which should be taught to athletes that are not Olympic lifting athletes?

Lets start off by agreeing that both the hang clean and power clean will get you big results no matter what your goal is: speed, power or agility. The complex movement and the speed it takes to move the bar work the body like no other movement. Any other movements cannot mock the power that is transferrable to sport. With that being said, great coaching and time is needed for both movements and which one is more practical is something that has to be taken into consideration.

The power clean is a staple in Olympic weightlifting and is a movement that is complex and straight up powerful. All sports can and would benefit from the teaching and use of the power clean in their programs. The power clean is a mainstay in many collegiate strength and conditioning programs throughout the United States, but is rarely taught in the private sector that caters to your HS athletes. This is because the athlete that generally hits the sports performance facility is only there on average two to three months and is sometimes in season during those months. The issue is not only the athletes making time to get better while in the off season, but for sports like soccer, baseball, basketball, softball and volleyball there is no off season anymore. The athletes play all year round with AAU and tournaments. This makes it very difficult to teach, progress and ensure that the Olympic lifting is taught properly. With that being accounted for, most athletes are taught the hang clean.

The hang clean is a great movement that was founded off of the power clean as a segment for getting better in the power clean. The hang clean puts the athlete in an athletic position past the first initial pull of the power clean. This position is where the transfer of power comes. The hip drive is the whole goal of the clean. The difference between the hang and power clean is the speed of the movement. The power clean generates more power through the movement because of that first pull. The hang clean has to be done with some downward movement first to generate some momentum for the hip drive to take place.

The question becomes this: if the power clean generates more power then why not put it into the private sector? There are three main factors I believe are the reason you do not see this more in the private sector.

1. Economy of training. I am not talking about money here, but time. The time it takes to teach the segments of the power clean is much longer and way more detailed. The hang clean is a more simple movement and takes less time to master. While it is still a technical lift, the teaching of the pull off the floor and body position of the PC is more time consuming. Having athletes for only a short amount of time we want to be as efficient as possible. With many sports performance facilities classes only lasting 60 to 90 minutes, time is crucial--and it's a business, so time is money.
2. Coaching. I believe that a great coach is needed to teach the power clean. Since it is a very technical lift, a qualified coach who is experienced should be teaching it.
3. Risk vs. Reward. I am a firm believer that with the amount of kids that you have for only 3 months, you get better results with the hang clean because you can load faster. This is because it is slightly easier to teach and you can progress quicker once mastered. The power clean, as mentioned, takes longer to teach and thus longer to progress with weight until perfected.

These three reasons are why the hang clean is more beneficial in the private setting. Within the college domain you have the time to teach, perfect and load the power clean properly. Private Olympic lifting gyms also have this luxury because this is what they do, perfect Olympic movements. Again good coaching plays a huge role in the ability to teach either lift. Both are phenomenal producers of power and you need one of them in your program to create the best athletes possible.

INCORPORATING OLYMPIC LIFTING IN YOUR PROGRAM TO INCREASE SPEED DEVELOPMENT
BRAD LESHINKE

For years, Olympic lifting has been worked into training programs of athletes looking to get stronger. What most people do not realize is that Olympic lifting is a huge component of speed development. While Olympic lifters do not have to add a speed development program to their regimen, athletes looking to get faster need to add Olympic lifting to theirs. This speaks highly to those athletes who compete in the Olympic lifting realm.

There are few concrete things we must look at when talking about speed development. First, speed is needed and is a game changer in all sports. It can make or break an athlete looking to get a scholarship. Second, plyometrics is a key ingredient that all athletes, including Olympic athletes, can use to benefit or complement power and become more elastic. Finally, science tells us that the output in sprinting directly correlates to the vertical jump. This is important when trying to show that Olympic lifting is vital to sprinting. We use the vertical jump as a test of power. We know that the vertical jump is a triple extension movement and shows the elastic ability of the athlete. With that being said, Olympic lifting is directly correlated to power output and increasing the vertical jump. These direct correlations from lifting to jumping to speed development speaks highly of why Olympic lifting is needed in your program.

In order to understand why Olympic lifts need to be added to an athlete's program, we first have to understand power and its job within sports performance. Power is the rate in which work is being done. What does this mean for athlete? The more efficient the work is being done, the faster the work will get done. When we look at sprinting, jumping, and lifting, we look at the ability to overcome gravity. In all movements previously mentioned the athlete starts from a static (non-moving) stance. This stance or potential energy needs to be activated as quickly as possible. Whether it's for a box jump, a power clean or a 40-yard dash start, the reaction needs to be fast and responsive. The mixture of these different movements is a cascading event. Speed is a very technical movement to learn because of all the moving parts and, unlike lifting or jumping, the movement takes place over a distance in a linear fashion. With Olympic lifting and jumping, most of the movement is measured in time of reaction or weight lifted as fast as possible. Olympic lifting is also a very technical. Whether teaching the snatch, clean, or jerk, it takes years to master theses movements. There is a reason why Olympic lifting is a sport unto itself. Having a qualified coach teaching these movements is essential to the success of the athletes.

The National Strength and Conditioning Association released a study on the effects of the hang clean relative to speed in March of 2008. The result of the test determined that the athletes who tested well in the hang clean were faster because of the gained power through the Olympic movement. The test also concluded as mentioned above that the athletes with better hang cleans had better vertical jumps. This correlation again speaks to the fact that explosiveness is a key component to increasing an athlete's speed. With this being said, every program designed to create faster athletes needs to incorporate Olympic weightlifting. So how do we program this into the sports performance realm?

When looking at a sports performance program, we must first recognize that athletes training for soccer and other various sports are not Olympic athletes. The base of the program will be geared to movement quality, injury prevention and increasing speed and agility. It is important to note that while they are not Olympic athletes, there needs to be time dedicated to teaching the Olympic movements correctly. This could take a few weeks in teaching new athletes proper positions. You must relay this message to the athletes in order for them to buy into the system. Letting them know it's a process in learning a highly technical movement. The proper order of gross movements would be the following:

Full Warm Up, including:

- Foam rolling
- Activation
- Mobility
- Dynamic warm up (including some ladder drills)

Plyometrics and Core

- Focus on the landing component first, then progress to more elastic movements when the athlete is ready
- Superset core with some jump work to allow legs proper rest

Speed Development

- Focus on technical movements, then apply the movements to actual speed work
- Focus on reaction last and skill movements specifically for the sport

Power Development

The first portion of lifting will be your explosive lifts

- Hang/power cleans
- Snatch
- Squat

Type of lift will depend on the day and the program in which they are involved. Remember, train based on the athlete and not just your program.

Core Lifts

- Various squat, bench and major muscle movements
- Again depends on the athlete and sport

Accessory Lifts

- Work on single leg training and smaller muscle groups

Having the proper order of movement and lifting is crucial to the correct outcome that one is seeking as an athlete. Setting up the program for the athlete to succeed is the goal of every strength and conditioning coach. Within the structure that the coach sets up for the athlete, teaching proper form in the Olympic movements and combining the above mentioned areas of sports performance results are sure to be gained.

As you can note from above, Olympic lifting is a key cog in a sports performance program. Understanding why these lifts are crucial to speed development and overall power development will encourage you to learn and add these movements into your program. Taking proper time in teaching the movements is needed because of how technical they are. Understanding that the mixture of plyometrics, Olympic lifting and speed development are all needed in creating the best and most dominant athletes. When a complete program is created, progressed and mastered the athlete will become more explosive, and therefore faster.

PUTTING THE CART BEFORE THE HORSE: LIFTING PREREQUISITES
TRAVIS MASH

Lately a lot has been done to revive the popularity of Weightlifting in America. The 2013 American Open was the biggest competition in the world that year with over 400 athletes. The 2014 Youth Nationals was the biggest weightlifting event ever with over 530 athletes. The sport is exploding, and I am loving it.

More people than ever are taking interest in a sport that I have loved my whole life. Less and less people are asking me what I bench when I tell them I compete in weightlifting. People of all ages are interested in learning the snatch and clean & jerk. Now as much as I love this, the new interest needs to be handled properly. The snatch and clean & jerk can be rough on the body and downright dangerous. A preparation phase along with proper technique should be the focus of any rookie lifter's program.

All too often, I see athletes performing the snatch or clean & jerk with terrible technique and/or bodies that are not ready for either. I am not just referring to CrossFit. I am talking about the garage warrior, the strength and conditioning athlete, and even people at globo gyms that happen to offer a weightlifting section. I am talking about any athlete trying to snatch and clean & jerk without a proper foundation.

Shane Hamman, arguably the greatest American Heavy Weight of all-time, spent a month with an empty bar practicing technique before one weighted snatch or clean & jerk. He spent time preparing his body with general exercises that world strengthen his body properly for heavy snatches and cleans. Shane's coach made sure that he had the proper mobility that would be required for the main lifts. When discrepancies were found, they were addressed first before moving forwards. This is the proper way to prepare someone for weightlifting.

Coaching an athlete that is new to weightlifting is a challenging but also rewarding endeavor. There is nothing like seeing an athlete complete his first full depth snatch with a perfectly vertical back. It's art! Without a solid foundation, instead of art you get the crap that we are all privileged to see on YouTube where you might see someone drop the bar on their head or worse. There are two exercises that I recommend having a new athlete attempt before beginning a program with them: the overhead squat and the front squat.

With the overhead squat, I am looking for proper depth, a vertical spine, and the bar directly above or slightly behind the ears. In the front squat, I am looking for solid protraction of the shoulder, the bars ability to sit on the shoulder, proper depth, a vertical spine, and the ability to keep their elbows up. If an athlete isn't able to perform these two movements properly, then mobility in these patterns is priority number one. There is no point in beginning to teach the snatch and clean & jerk if the athlete doesn't have the movement required. If you try to teach them at this point, their body will compensate with faulty movement patterns that could take a lifetime to correct. Spending a little extra time will pay off for the athlete in the long run.

Wes Barnett, two-time Olympian, was my first ever weightlifting coach. He was still an athlete when I met him, but he was a great coach. My athletes can thank him for a lot of the coaching methods that I use today. When I started with him, I spent months performing exercises that would strengthen my body for the upcoming training. For the snatch, I performed Sotts presses, overhead squats, snatch balances, snatch grip push presses, snatch pulls, and muscle snatches. For the clean, he had do front squats with as many of my fingers as possible on the bar, back squats, and clean pulls. For the jerk, we did presses from the split, jerks from the split, push presses, and standing presses. We also did some general strengthening with pull-ups, bench press, dips, and bent over rows.

Wes spent the rest of the time teaching me the proper technique of the snatch and clean & jerk. It wasn't glamorous, but it worked. I moved up quickly in the world of weightlifting after I took some precious time to learn the sport correctly. Coaches all too often rush into teaching weighted snatches and clean & jerks because they don't want to make the athletes mad. Today's athletes are impatient, and the coaches don't want to lose a client. I suggest girding up your loins, and remembering that you are the coach. These athletes have to trust that you have their best interests when you are coaching them. If they can't trust you, let them hit the road.

When you build a gym full of athletes that are snatching and clean & jerking like bosses, then people will be knocking the doors down to be coached by you. Nothing is more of a sign of good coaching than walking into a gym full of people lifting with beautiful technique. Nothing says "this coach is a joke" more than a bunch of people attempting snatches, cleans, and even squats with technique that looks more like a seizure or fit than real lifting. Weightlifting should look like art. If it doesn't in your gym, then change your program.

A beginner's program could look something like this:

Monday
Clean Grip Sotts Press
Snatch Bar Technique
Clean Bar Technique
Front Squats paused in bottom
Clean Pulls
Push Press

Wednesday
Snatch Grip Sotts Press
Snatch Technique
Clean Technique
Overhead Squats
Snatch Pulls
Snatch Grip BH Neck Press

Friday
Muscle Snatch
Split Jerk Position Presses BH Neck
Back Squats
RDLs
Dips
Bent over Rows

There are other ways to group the exercises, but you get the drift. The goal in the foundation stage is to prepare the body by strengthening the shoulder girdle, hips, and entire posterior chain. It is also to program perfect movement patterns that will be used by the athlete forever. Take your time in this phase, and the payoff will be huge!

DOES YOUR ATHLETIC EXPERIENCE DETERMINE YOUR COACHING ABILITY?
MATT FOREMAN

Weightlifting coaches are like fruits and vegetables. They come in all shapes and sizes. If you've been in the game for any length of time, you've probably seen a lot of coaches at meets, in gyms you've trained at, etc.

Coaches are different from lifters, because lifters all basically look the same. They're muscular, and they look like...well, like weightlifters. Different hair and faces, and some variations in body structure, but you know you're looking at a lifter when you see one walk in the room. Coaches aren't like that.

Some of them still look kinda physical and strong. You can tell they used to be athletes when you look at them. Others look like they they've never lifted a weight in their lives. Some coaches are fat and frumpy. Some are skinny and rangy. The young ones usually have some physical presence to them, but many of the old ones just look like the geezers you see walking around a mall. Some look good, and some don't. The coaches that represent Catalyst Athletics are attractive and sensually arousing, while many others are ugly and displeasing.

Does it matter what coaches look like? If they're good at their jobs and they help you make progress, does anybody give a crap if they've got an impressive appearance? Everybody will have their own opinion about it. Right now, you're probably rolling your eyes and asking, "Is this whole damn article going to be about what coaches look like? Is this all we're gonna talk about?" The answer, fortunately, is no. This article is going to be about the question of whether it's important for coaches to have personal athletic experience in the sport they're teaching.

Aaahhh, now it's a little more interesting. You see, I led off this article with the subject of physical appearance because that's something that people judge pretty harshly in our society. You know how it works. The way you look determines a lot about how people treat you, whether any of us like it that way or not. But when it comes to weightlifting, sometimes there's a different kind of judgment that takes place. I'm talking about the way lifters judge their coaches. Some athletes think it's a pretty big deal for their coaches to have successful backgrounds as lifters. They feel more comfortable taking orders if they know the coach accomplished some big things on the platform back in the day.

Others don't give a damn about that. As long as the coach does a good job and makes them successful, they could care less if he/she was ever a high-level competitor. So…obviously this discussion is directed towards you. Some of you are athletes. Some of you are coaches. Many of you are both. I want to take a look at how lifters view their leaders, because it's a topic that has some importance. Additionally, we need to confront the question of whether athletic experience in a sport is required to become an effective teacher of it. In other words, we're really asking two separate questions. "Do you need to have a strong competitive background in weightlifting to be a good coach?" and "Is the coach/athlete relationship impacted by the competitive experience of the coach?"

Quite the little pickle we have here. Having been both an athlete and coach myself, I've got multiple ideas about this. Since we all understand that the connection between coaches and their lifters is one of the most crucial components of this whole business, it's probably a good idea to have a clear perspective on it.

Examples? Examples?

Some of you might know who Naim Suleymanoglu is. If you don't, he's generally considered the greatest weightlifter of all time. Three-time Olympic Champion from Turkey, known as the Pocket Hercules…any of that ring a bell? He snatched 152.5 kg (336 lbs.) and clean and jerked 190 kg (418 lbs.) at 60 kilo bodyweight (132 lbs.) at the 1988 Olympics. Pound-for-pound, that's the best weightlifting performance in history.

The reason I'm mentioning him is because of this coaching thing we're talking about. After he won his first Olympic title in 1988, he announced his retirement. Turkey made him their head national weightlifting coach, figuring he was the perfect choice since he was the best lifter of all time. According to what I've heard and read, it didn't work out very well. Suleymanoglu wasn't a coach. I read an article in Sports Illustrated back in 1992 (I think) that described how it went. First of all, he wasn't ready to be finished as an athlete. He retired after the '88 Games because he had been lifting all his life and I'm sure the gold medal probably seemed like it was the top of the mountain. But then he started coaching and he watched other athletes win the World Championship in his weight class. The SI article described how he openly expressed some bitterness towards the athlete who won the 60 kg class at the 1989 Worlds. I've never met Naim and I obviously can't speak on his behalf, but I think he probably felt like they were taking HIS World Championship. Even though he had transitioned to coaching, he couldn't let go of the competitive instinct he felt as an athlete. The new job clearly wasn't working out, so he went back to training and eventually fulfilled his legacy by winning two more Olympic crowns.

Being a great athlete doesn't guarantee that you're going to be a great coach.

That's a fact that we need to establish right from the get-go. People sometimes think it works this way when they look at the game from the outside. If somebody's the best on the platform, they should be the best at teaching others, right? No way, Jack. That's not how it works.

You don't necessarily have to be a champion athlete to become a successful coach. I'll go ahead and use myself as an example for this one. I'm a high school track and field coach. Specifically, I coach the throwing events (shot put and discus). At the time of this article, I'm getting ready to start my 18th year on the job. I've qualified over 100 throwers to the state championship throughout my career, along with producing multiple state, region, district and city champions. I've probably got a stronger record than the vast majority of throws coaches at the high school level. And do you want to know how much throwing experience I had as an athlete prior to this? One year of high school track, and I wasn't even very good. Seriously, that's my whole personal throwing resume. Sure, I threw in some masters meets when I was in my early 30s just for fun, and I've also thrown in the Scottish Highland Games. But in terms of real shot put and discus experience, I have very little.

I started educating myself when I got my first job, I've worked with some of the best coaches and throwers in the world, and I made it my mission in life to develop a successful coaching system in the throws. My weightlifting background also factors into the equation because my throwers are usually pretty solid in the strength department, and I know how to teach them to compete. In addition, I'm good at working with athletes from the standpoint of motivation, personality stuff, and all the little nuances. Combining all of this with years and years of honing my skills, I've done well as a coach.

The point I'm trying to make is that prior athletic experience isn't necessarily a requirement or a guarantee when it comes to coaching success. Naim Suleymanoglu and I are on opposite ends of the spectrum in many ways, but the lessons are the same. I could list plenty of other coaching situations that further these examples, in both directions. Dan Gable was the greatest wrestler in the world, and he went on to be the greatest coach in the world. On the other hand, two of the top weightlifting coaches in the United States, Dennis Snethen and Gayle Hatch, don't have championship records as athletes in the sport. There's no one-size-fits-all formula for this issue. Every scenario, and every coach, is unique.

So, how do the athletes look at it?

Despite all the examples in the world, we also need to examine how lifters see the whole issue. As we know, most athletes are pretty stubborn. When they get a thought in their heads, sometimes you can't change it regardless of all the practical examples and common sense thinking you can muster.

That means athletes are going to have their own perspective on coaches. Sometimes this perspective might be sensible and intelligent, and other times it might be completely devoid of any rational thought. Some athletes think it's pretty important for their coaches to have strong backgrounds as athletes. I was definitely this way when I was young. It really mattered to me that my coaches had actually been weightlifters. I wanted to be guided by somebody who had walked the walk. Fortunately, that mentality led me to John Thrush. John had competed in two Olympic Trials back in the 70s and he also held the national collegiate record in the C&J for several years, so he had street cred. The fortunate part for me, however, is that he was also a great coach. I got lucky with him. Back in those days, it would have been pretty easy for me to migrate towards a lousy coach, just because he had been a world champion in the past. The prestige would have been enough to suck me in, just like it sucks in a lot of young athletes who don't know any better. The fact that I went to a great lifter/great coach was just luck of the draw, plain and simple.

Here's another story, and I won't mention any names. I used to train with a female lifter who was getting ready to compete in a national championship. During the months of preparation for the meet, she had exchanged several e-mails with a coach from a different part of the country who she had never met (or seen). He was basically just contacting her to give encouragement and support. He was a fan of hers, and he wanted to pump her up for a big performance. She was really excited to meet him at the nationals. I remember going with her (I was competing too) and listening to her talk on the plane about how she was looking forward to finally being introduced to the dude. When we got there and she bumped into him in the warmup room, the two of them had a short conversation. After it was over, we all went our separate ways. She told me later that it was a total disappointment when she met the coach. I asked her why, and she said she had it built up in her mind that he was going to be some big, strong, impressive guy. This particular coach was older and, quite frankly, not physically remarkable. He was one of those older coaches I spoke about earlier who look like an average Joe. Interestingly enough, this guy actually was a highly successful coach. Many of you would probably recognize his name (and the name of the gal). But this was an example where an athlete was underwhelmed by the "look" of a coach, and it changed her perspective on him. She thought he was going to look like a former lifter with some leftover beef, but she lost interest when he didn't fit the profile.

Is this shallow? Yeah, it is. It's pretty crappy, if you want my opinion. But as I said earlier, athletes have funny ways of thinking. I don't have any solutions, really. I guess these stories were simply supposed to offer you a chance for more understanding about how some of those meathead weightlifters think.

The bottom line…

Listen, it doesn't matter if a coach is (or was) a good snatcher. What matters is that the coach can teach others how to snatch well. This is why I definitely think a coach needs some level of athletic experience in the sport they're working with. There are things about weightlifting that you can't learn from a book, or video, or conversations, or clinics, etc. The only place you can learn about them is by living the life. So yes, I absolutely 100 percent believe weightlifting coaches need to have been weightlifters themselves. You can never truly understand this sport unless you've done it.

However, that doesn't mean the coach needs to have been a champion. That part is much less important, in my opinion. Championships are determined by talent, remember? Athletes who have more ability than everybody else will be the winners. You can have a legitimate weightlifting career without becoming a world champion. You might not have the talent to win a gold medal, but that doesn't stop you from developing a heightened understanding of the sport. At that point, you've got the knowledge. If you also know how to teach and you're good at working with people, you're likely in a position to do some damage as a coach--and I mean "damage" in a good way.

Most lifters are young, remember. When you're young, you're not always smart. Judging the ability of a coach based on physical appearance is foolish. Judging a coach based on how many medals he/she won as an athlete can be very misleading. You have to know this sport as a weightlifter before you're really ready to be a coach, but that doesn't mean you need to have an Olympic medal hanging over your fireplace. The sport has a lot of funny little relationship quirks in it, but the only thing that really matters is results. If your coaches lead you to excellent results, do you really give a rat's ass whether they used to be national champions? You might, but you shouldn't. Judge them on their coaching ability, not on their snatch PR or their biceps.

HEY COACH, IT'S NOT ALL ABOUT YOU
MATT FOREMAN

Greg Everett once told me that a large percentage of the people who read this magazine are coaches. I always try to keep this in mind when I write articles. Some of you might not be coaches presently, and your focus is entirely on your own lifting. That's cool. But as I've said before, it's almost impossible to spend an extended amount of time in this sport without somebody asking you to coach at some point. This means you'll probably do some coaching someday, even if you're not doing it right now.

Your technical expertise and programming skill are tremendously important when you're a coach. Those things are the nuts and bolts of the business. However, I personally think the most important aspect of coaching is how you act. It's the ultimate deal-breaker. You can be the most technically skilled coach in the solar system, and you'll still have an empty gym if you act like a jagoff. Nobody will want to be around you, whether you design great training programs or not.

I'm going to give you some miscellaneous tips about how you should act when you're a coach. Is this information going to be one-sided? Absolutely. My personal opinion is going to be a big part of it. So you're completely within your rights if you want to read this stuff and then toss it in the dumpster because you don't agree with me.

At the risk of making this article too scattered, I'm going to concentrate on one specific area. I'm talking about the degree of self-absorption, ego, and me-me-me behavior that's appropriate when you're a coach. Most coaches have big egos. It's part of the business, and there's nothing wrong with it. If you really want to know the truth, it's actually pretty important for a coach to have a big ego. However, the way that egotism is communicated through words and behavior...that's a different topic. This is where athletes (and just people in general) can get totally turned off if you don't give off the right vibe.

What I'm trying to say is that we're going to take a look at this idea: When you're a coach, you can't make everything about YOU. You have to make everything about YOUR ATHLETES. It's a slippery slope because we all have a basic element of selfishness in our personality. It's human nature. We want good things for ourselves. Coaches want good things for themselves, too. However, there's a specific way to handle this selfish impulse so you'll come across like a good coach instead of a self-centered toolbag.

It's easy to spot coaches who think it's all about them. To tell you the truth, it's also an easy trap to fall into when you're a coach. If you're good at what you do, you probably get a lot of praise and compliments. It's the most natural thing in the world for this praise to go straight to your head. Before you know it, you're a good coach and a good person who acts like a jackass because you've started to believe your own headlines. Everybody tells you how wonderful you are, and it just creeps into your bones.

I've been guilty of this from time to time. Maybe you have too? So let's read about this subject, shall we? Hopefully, we'll finish with something that will help us all keep our heads and actions straight.

First, an example of how to act right…

Let me tell you about one of the most impressive things I've seen in my weightlifting years. I think I can just about guarantee it'll make you a better person.

The 2000 Olympic Trials was held in New Orleans, Louisiana. I was there. Every Trials is special, but this one was historically significant because it was the first ever Olympic Trials for the women's division. For those of you who don't know, women's weightlifting had been up and running since the 80s, but it wasn't admitted into the Olympics until the conclusion of the 1996 Atlanta Games. The ladies had been competing at national and world meets for years, but the 2000 Olympics in Sydney was their first time at the big dance. The buzz was working overtime about who was going to be on America's first women's Olympic Team.

Our top men and women showed up to New Orleans and battled it out. When the smoke cleared, the Olympic Team was Oscar Chaplin and Shane Hamman for the men. And our first US Olympic Team in women's weightlifting was Tara Nott, Robin Goad, Cara Heads-Lane, and Cheryl Haworth.

After the competition was over, a banquet was held for the athletes, coaches, and officials to celebrate our newly crowned Olympians. It was a pretty special gathering for everybody in US Weightlifting. I went to it mainly because I heard they were serving prime rib, but I also wanted to see the festivities. One of the coolest moments of the banquet was when the organizers presented a special tribute to Robin Goad. You see, Robin was the only member of the Olympic Team who came from the early days of women's weightlifting. She had been on the scene almost right from the beginning and she actually won the World Championship in 1994. Most of the women from her generation had retired before 2000 rolled around, so they never got their shot at the Games. But Robin had continued fighting and she was basically the last of the nationally-ranked Mohicans from the first generation of female lifters. Needless to say, it was a big damn deal when she made the Team.

So at the banquet, they called her up to the podium and gave her a tribute. If I remember correctly, Jim Schmitz actually presented her with the first team trophy our US women ever won at the World Championship. Lots of tears in the room when that happened, I can tell you. In the middle of all the emotion and celebration, Robin got to step up to the microphone and say a few words.

That moment was supposed to be about her. If she would have wanted to, she could have talked about her career, all the glory she was experiencing, all the obstacles she had conquered, how good it felt to make the Team after all those years…that kind of stuff. It would have been totally appropriate for her to be a little selfish and maybe pat herself on the back, because everybody knew how hard she had worked to get to the top.

But she didn't take it in that direction. Instead, she dedicated her whole Olympic experience to all the women from the old days who started the sport with her and never got the chance to reach the pinnacle. She didn't make the moment about herself. She used those few minutes to honor other people, all the ladies who had trained and competed with her over the years and built up the women's movement in our sport. Her speech was completely devoid of any self-indulgence or me-me-me talk. She took the tribute that was supposed to be about her…and used it to pay homage to her former teammates and competitors.

It was probably one of most respectable things I've ever heard because it was just so humble and unselfish. It didn't surprise me at all, either. Robin was a good friend of mine. She had actually married one of my teammates and training partners, Dean Goad, and we had all spent some great years lifting together back in the 90s. The speech she gave at the Trials was completely consistent with her character. She was just a very classy gal, plain and simple.

People respond to this kind of behavior, know what I mean? They admire it, and it makes them feel good. They respect you more when you do things like this. Hell, I still remember it after almost 15 years. To me, this is a prime example of the way you're supposed to act. If you disagree, that's fine. But I'm right, and you're wrong.

So, are we not allowed to have ANY pride or ego?

In other words, I'm saying you can only be a coach if you're 100 percent altruistic, right? You literally can't have any self-interest. Every single thing you do and say has to be modest, humble, and completely devoid of any personal desire for recognition. Correct?

No, that's not the way it is. There's a connection between having a big ego and acting modestly. All of the best coaches and athletes have big egos. It's actually an important part of being successful. A big ego gives you belief in yourself. When you get in jams, you expect to be successful simply because you have a lot of faith in your ability and you know you'll be able to handle the problem. You see yourself as being strong enough to succeed, so that's what you do.

But that's different from acting like a jackass. That's the balance of the two. You want to have a big ego but ACT humble and unassuming. You've met champions who were very modest, right? These are the people like Robin and other great legends who don't wave their pride around like a big sausage. They've got a list of accomplishments longer than your large intestine, but they don't shove it in your face. Trust me, they've got big egos. But they don't act like buttholes, which is the perfect combination. There's a difference between what's going on INSIDE you and what you project OUTWARDLY to others. Seeing yourself as a champion is a great thing. Behaving like a d-bag isn't.

Obviously, we have to acknowledge the great ones who also act like arrogant d-bags. They're out there. Professional sports, particularly mainstream American sports, are great places to find them. Some of you might like that attitude. You might prefer "swag" to modesty. I understand that. I don't agree with it, but I understand it. But make sure you understand that these types usually don't inspire people in the same way as the champions with humility. It's a lousy experience when you meet a champion and they disappoint you by acting like idiots. It spoils the respect you have for them. But when you meet a champion and they're friendly and encouraging, it's the best feeling in the world. That's what we should all aspire to.

When you're a coach, you have goals. These goals are the things you personally want to accomplish. This is a good thing. However, that's where the caution comes in. Remember, your goals are going to be accomplished by other people. You're the coach, but the athletes are the ones who walk out onto the platform and hit the big lifts that make your goals happen. Knowing this, it creates a situation where your self-interest is dependent on the performances of others. This means one of your top priorities has to be preparing your athletes in the best way, and that includes managing your relationships with them. Your relationship will suffer if the athlete doesn't like you, and most athletes don't like coaches who wear their selfishness around like a bright red jacket. To make a long story short, the coach gets what he wants if the athletes get what they want. And athletes want to feel like they're valued. If the coach makes it clear that his number one priority is himself, it's going to put a dent in this whole thing.

Are you a "me" coach or a "we" coach?

You're asking yourself, "How can I make sure I handle this the right way? What are some tangible things I can do to give off the right impression to athletes?"

I'll give you a really easy one. Just use the word "we" as much as possible. Every time you use it, it creates the idea that this whole thing is a group effort. Giving strength to the group is how teams are built. Great teams make great programs, and they usually produce great results.

As I mentioned earlier, it's easy to slip into the me-me-me quicksand. All it takes is a long stream of praise and compliments without anything to humble you down. Before you know it, you've started to believe you're above everything…and everybody. All coaches, if they're good at their jobs, will suffer the occasional bout of this. The hardest thing is that it happens invisibly and usually without your knowledge. The only thing that solves it, unfortunately, is some kind of comeuppance. Something has to happen to neuter you back a little bit, and it'll probably be something that's a little embarrassing and painful. Those things are good for you though, know what I mean? They remind you that you're not a golden god. As Tom Hanks once said, "You never really learn anything unless you get your ass kicked first."

So there you have it, brothers and sisters. A bunch of Matt Foreman's personal opinions about how you should act when you're a coach. The bottom line is that it's hard to go wrong when you treat other people well. I know that's not rocket science, but it's easy to overlook sometimes. We all need occasional reminders of the basics.

BOMBING OUT
MATT FOREMAN

I'm surprised that I've never written about bombing out before. It's a juicy topic for competitive weightlifters, but I think it's also something you can apply to any area of your life. I just recently realized that I've never explored it in an article, so here goes.

First, I need to explain what we're talking about. In Olympic weightlifting and powerlifting, a "bombout" is the common description of missing all three competition attempts in a meet. In competitive lifting, each athlete is given three official attempts in each lift. In OLifting, you get three snatches and then three clean and jerks. In powerlifting, you get three squats, three bench presses, and three deadlifts. I'm talking about the attempts that happen on the competition platform. There's a warmup room backstage at every meet, which is where the lifters prepare themselves, but the only lifts that actually count are the three official attempts.

You have to successfully complete at least one attempt in each lift to finish the competition and be eligible for overall awards. And you have to be pretty precise about the weights you pick on these attempts, because you can't lower the weight if you fail. So let's say you attempt 200 lbs. on your first snatch in a competition and you're unsuccessful. You can't go down and attempt a lighter weight. You have to make the 200 lbs. on either your second or third attempt, or you can go up and add more. But you can't ever move down.

If you miss all three of your competition attempts in any of the lifts, it's referred to as a bombout. You won't finish the competition with a total, which basically means you have no shot at placing in the overall standings. In other words, it's the worst possible result you can end with. Bombing out, simply stated, is every weightlifter's worst nightmare.

Fortuntely, bombouts are relatively rare. Most lifters avoid them because they (and their coaches) select the right competition attempts based on sensible training and preparation. They aren't frequent, but they do happen occasionally.

A bombout really screws with your head. It's the ultimate badge of shame, and there's nothing worse than having to explain it when you go home after the meet and your friends start asking you, "So, how did you do?" Bombing out basically means you completely failed. You trained your ass off and prepared for this competition, and you walk away with nothing to show for it.

Because of this, bombouts usually produce a feeling of extreme disappointment in both athletes and coaches. They're very tough to swallow, and it's not uncommon to start asking yourself some really terrible questions if it ever happens to you. That's why I want to write about them. If you're not a competitive weightlifter, you should still be able to get something out of this article because we're essentially talking about how to handle a moment of complete failure. Hell, this kind of moment can happen in any sport. It can happen in your professional life. It can happen when you're raising your family. Like it or not, most of us are going to have big defeats at some point, the kinds of things that can make you consider quitting.

I don't want you to quit. You don't want to quit, either. So let's examine the best strategies for handling a bombout, whether it happens in weightlifting or life.

Examples usually help…

Here's my personal experience in this department. At the time of this article, I've competed in 109 meets, and I've bombed out five times. All of them were in the early years of my career.

I've had a very successful run as a competitive lifter, I'm fortunate to say. My record stacks up pretty well against the most athletes. However, I've tasted failure more than once. All of those five bombouts were crushing defeats. Two of them were at the American Open, which is the 2nd most prestigious competition in the United States. I bombed out of the Open twice in a row (1994 and 1995). Yup, you read that right. I also bombed out of the Olympic Festival, which used to be one of the main spotlight competitions in the country. Without a shadow of a doubt, I can tell you these things sting much worse when they happen on the big stage.

As I said, this all happened when I was young, very much in the intermediate stages of my development as a lifter. Each of these bombouts was my own fault. My coach wasn't to blame, there wasn't any kind of freak situation that knocked me for a loop… nothing like that. I just didn't get the job done, plain and simple. I tried my best, but I blew it. What caused the crappy performance? Mainly it was just a combination of nerves and immaturity. Looking back at it now, I understand that. It took me a while to figure out the right way to compete mentally. During that "figuring it out" process, I screwed the pooch a few times. I was a head case for a while, but I grew out of it.

You probably don't know this, but almost every high-level weightlifter in the world has bombed out at some point. You can mention the names of the greatest studs in the history of the sport, and I can probably point out a bomb somewhere in their careers.

Ever heard of David Rigert? He was a Soviet lifter from the 1970s, and he was the weightlifting idol for most of my generation. He's generally regarded as one of the best ever, a true icon in the sport. 1976 Olympic Gold Medalist, six-time World Champion, 68 world records in his career. Rigert was an animal with a body and physical presence that made your jaw drop. And do you want to know something interesting about him? He bombed out of the Olympics twice. That's right, folks. He bombed in 1972, won gold in 1976, and then bombed again in 1980.

Naim Suleymanoglu of Turkey is probably THE greatest weightlifter of all time. Three Olympic Gold Medals, seven World Championships, six European titles, and 46 world records. 152.5 kg snatch (336 lbs.) and 190 kg C&J (418 lbs.) at 60 kg (132 lbs.) bodyweight, which is pound-for-pound the greatest performance ever. And do you want to know something interesting about him? He bombed out of the Olympics in 2000.

Vasily Alexeev, the Soviet legend who did the first 500 lb. C&J in history back in 1970…remember him? Two-time Olympic Champion, 80 world records, bombout at the 1980 Olympics.

I could go on. Seriously, I could. I was amazed when I progressed throughout my weightlifting career and learned about all the champions of the sport. These athletes seem like they're inhuman. Their performances and victories are the stuff of legend. They stand at the top of the mountain, while the rest of us struggle to rise to their level. And almost every single one of them has bombed, at some point. Some of you have read my book Bones of Iron, where I told a story about the time I bombed out of the 1994 Olympic Festival. After I missed all three of my snatches, I was ready to throw myself on a spike. I walked back into the warmup room and saw Mario Martinez standing there, who was a three-time Olympian and one of the greatest American lifters of all time. Despondently, I walked over to him and asked, "Hey Mario, have you ever bombed out of a big meet?" He just smiled and said, "Yeah, sometimes. It happens."

After 20 years, I've still never forgotten that he said that to me. Mario is an iconic figure in US lifting, and he basically explained one of the most painful truths of the sport (and life) to me in one sentence. Failure and defeat are part of the game, brothers and sisters. Nobody, regardless of how incredible they are, is exempt from that rule. There are examples all over the place to prove it. So if you ever experience a bombout, try to remember that you're in good company. In my opinion, that's one of the best ways to deal with it. When you understand that the great champions have all had to go through the same thing, it gets a little easier. None of us are perfect, even if we've got Olympic medals in our closet.

Why it happens, and how to deal with it…

You want me to explain to you why bombouts happen? No problem. Trust me folks, it ain't the Riddle of the Sphinx.

When you're a weightlifter, you push the absolute limits of your physical capabilities. When you're a competitive weightlifter, you push these limits under the most stressful, complicated, unpredictable circumstances imaginable. If you push these limits frequently, there will be times when you come up short. I once read an interview with a great home run hitter in baseball who also had tons of strikeouts on his record. His explanation for the strikeouts was, "I swing really hard. Sometimes, I miss." I love that quote.

Bad days are just a part of being an athlete, and there's nothing any of us can do to change that. It's not rocket science, for god's sake. Look at the examples you see in other sports. In American football, Denver Broncos quarterback John Elway led his team to the Super Bowl AND LOST three times before they finally won it in 1997 and 1998. How about track and field? Ask the average track fan who the best pole-vaulter in history is, and the name you're going to hear most often is Sergei Bubka. Bubka, like David Rigert, bombed out of two Olympics (it's called a "no-height" in vaulting), but he also won it in 1992 and elevated the world record to over 20 feet in his hall of fame career. The two no-heights didn't diminish his greatness.

When you bomb out, your job as an athlete is to figure out why it happened. This is usually a tricky process because, most of the time, there isn't a clear-cut cause that you can point your finger at. It's typically just a short mental lapse, a break in your concentration, excessive nervousness, or something like that. Figuring out why these things happen requires you to figure out your brain, which isn't a simple task. But you have to try your best, because the only way you can keep a problem from happening again is to locate it and solve it.

Personally, competition got a lot easier for me as I grew up and matured. As a young lifter, I had a lot of mental obstacles that were mainly caused by my obsessive need for success and complete lack of tolerance for failure. You have to be a perfectionist if you want to be a great weightlifter, but perfectionists sometimes have problems because they simply get wrapped up too tight in their struggle to control everything. That mental "tightness" can cause some freaky performances, because most people do their best work when they feel relaxed and comfortable.

You can overanalyze a bombout, but it usually won't lead you to any reliable answers. In my experience, it's best to learn what you can from a bad day and then forget about it. The longer you analyze a bombout, the longer you're keeping it in your mind. The best thing you can do as an athlete is leave it behind and start moving forward. Hopefully, you'll be able to move forward with some understanding of how to prevent future screw-ups. The most important thing is that you move forward with determination that it'll never happen again.

And stay off the s**t pile...

Aaahhh yes, self-loathing and judgment. These are such wonderful feelings to live with, aren't they? Listen, a bombout will make you feel terrible. It's the pinnacle of failure, and it doesn't help when your coach gets a crappy attitude towards you and tosses you on the dung heap. Coaches, do you hear what I'm saying? The worst thing you can do to athletes is kick them when they're down. Coaches obviously feel just as badly as athletes when a bombout happens because it's a reflection on both of them. I know some coaches who treat athletes like dirt if they perform poorly.

First of all, the athletes are going to remember that you weren't there for them when they needed it. They tried their best and came up short, and you handled it by being selfish and pissing on them. It's not like they wanted to bomb, know what I mean? But coaches sometimes get an attitude with them anyway. This can be one of the first steps towards the athletes looking around for a different coach. Second, being a coach means you're a leadership figure. If you're a leader, you're expected to handle difficulties in the right way. You have to be the positive one, the voice of reassurance, and the reminder that bad days are just temporary. When your people look at you and they see that you can't maintain a strong attitude in the face of obstacles, they start to think you're not tough enough to cope with harsh times. Then they start to lose faith in you. At that point, it'll never be the same.

The bottom line is that you should be pissed as hell if you fail, either in weightlifting or in life. Regardless of the sport or life field we're talking about, it should make you angry when you experience defeat. However, that anger is something you have to control and eventually dismiss. Nobody makes any improvement by continually dwelling on failure, know what I mean? If you hang on to it, how can you expect to move forward? You're not the first weightlifter to bomb out. The best athletes have done it too. Learn whatever you can from your bad days, even if it's not that much. After you've learned, turn your thoughts towards your upcoming goals. That's what all the great ones have done, and it's one of the main reasons why they're great.

CALM LIKE A BOMB: PROPERLY APPLYING AGGRESSION
GREG EVERETT

Weightlifting is a very mental sport. A lot of coaches have been heard to say things along the lines of, "Weightlifting is 90 percent mental." I get the point and agree in principle, but it should be obvious to anyone that this is hyperbole. I don't care how focused and mentally strong you are—if you don't have the physical capability to deadlift 200 lbs., you're certainly not going to will yourself into snatching 300 lbs. I prefer my joking version of this saying: Weightlifting is 100 percent mental if you have 100 percent of the physical ability.

Aggression and psychological arousal are critical elements of successful weightlifting. Performing maximal snatches and clean & jerks isn't possible without a high degree of aggressiveness channeled into the task. This is true for many sports, but weightlifting differs in the sense that the nature and duration of the aggressiveness is very specific. In sports like football, aggression needs to be expressed for a longer period of time—for example as a lineman, for the duration of a play to allow him to continue battling with the opposition to either protect their own players to allow them to make a play or attempt to access the other team's players to stop a play. The duration of a play in football may strike you as brief, but relative to a single snatch or clean & jerk, it can be fairly protracted.

Because the degree of aggression in weightlifting must be so great, there is a limit to its possible duration. Few athletes have the energy reserves to maintain a high level of arousal for a long period of time and have any leftover to put into lifts. Antics in the gym or in competition, in my opinion, are simply drains on the athlete's finite energy reserves and a distraction of focus. That's all energy that could be put to better use in the performance of the lifts.

There are exceptions, but most high level weightlifters are fairly calm at all times outside of performing the actual lifts, whether in training or in competition. They remain still and focused on the upcoming lift until it's time to do it. I call this state being calm like a bomb (credit goes to Rage Against the Machine—this is one of their song's titles). Imagine an armed bomb—nothing about it betrays the explosive potential of the device. It's still and quite and unassuming. But when it's detonated, the power is beyond comprehension.

This is the way I believe weightlifters should behave. Every last drop of energy and aggression should be channeled into the task of lifting the weight. None should be wasted on shows for attention. Nothing will impress weightlifting fans more than successful big lifts.

This doesn't mean that the gym atmosphere should be funereal. Too sedate of an environment can drain energy from any lifter. The atmosphere should be upbeat while remaining focused—you can't sacrifice the ability of lifters to perform for the sake of having fun between lifts. Talking and joking and having fun is all well and good, but not if it's disruptive of athletes trying to lift. Athletes need to know when to cool it and allow a lifter to focus.

Learn to channel your energy into your lifts rather than allowing it to leak elsewhere, and you'll find yourself more consistently able to hit big lifts.

MINDFULNESS AND MUSCLE:
HOW THINKING ABOUT TRAINING CAN BE TRAINING
CAMERON CONAWAY

"As you think, so shall you become."
—Bruce Lee

The mindfulness movement is gaining popularity, and it's finding application in just about every sector. Google is bringing in Zen masters to help their employees cultivate mindfulness practices that spark insight and create happier work places. Educators in the USA, England, Canada, New Zealand and Thailand are achieving remarkable results by incorporating science-driven mindfulness lessons into their curriculum. But when it comes to the world of fitness, these practices have mostly only found homes in yoga studios. Those who take strength & conditioning seriously should be taking the science of mindfulness seriously, too.

I speak as a former MMA fighter and current NSCA-Certified Personal Trainer when I say that there are only so many physical ways to get faster, stronger and more conditioned. I speak as one who has studied with Zen Master Thích Nh t H nh when I say that we trainers and athletes have yet to explore the profound depth that practices such as a deep visualization can have on physical performance. Sure, we speak of performance being "90 percent mental," but we seem only to explore this in the realm of inner toughness and poise. In the past decade, science has proven that it's time to leverage the untapped dimensions behind our words. Here are insights culled from four of those studies:

2004

The results of an NIH-funded study titled "From mental power to muscle power—gaining strength by using the mind" were published in Neuropsychologia, an international, interdisciplinary and peer-reviewed journal based in Oxford and Boston that focuses on cognitive neuroscience. The purpose of the study was to determine if and to what extent mental training alone could induce physical strength gains. Thirty adults were taken